S0-ARN-301

Fundamentals of
Sports Injury Management

Fundamentals of Sports Injury Management

Marcia K. Anderson, PhD, LATC

Professor

Director, Athletic Training Program

Department of Movement Arts, Health Promotion, and Leisure Studies

Bridgewater State College

Bridgewater, Massachusetts

Susan J. Hall, PhD

Professor of Biomechanics

Department of Kinesiology

California State University, Northridge

Northridge, California

Contributing Author:

Cheryl Hitchings, MAT, MHP, LATC, PA-C

Assistant Professor

Department of Movement Arts, Health Promotion, and Leisure Studies

Bridgewater State College

Bridgewater, Massachusetts

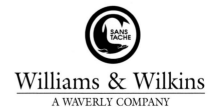

Williams & Wilkins
A WAVERLY COMPANY

BALTIMORE • PHILADELPHIA • LONDON • PARIS • BANGKOK
HONG KONG • MUNICH • SYDNEY • TOKYO • WROCLAW

Editor: Donna Balado
Managing Editor: Victoria Rybicki Vaughn
Marketing Manager: Christine Kushner
Production Coordinator: Marette D. Magargle-Smith
Senior Project Editor: Jennifer D. Weir
Typesetter: Bi-Comp, Inc.
Printer & Binder: RR Donnelley & Sons Company

Copyright © 1997 Williams & Wilkins

351 West Camden Street
Baltimore, Maryland 21201-2436 USA

Rose Tree Corporate Center
1400 North Providence Road
Building II, Suite 5025
Media, Pennsylvania 19063-2043 USA

All rights reserved. This book is protected by copyright. No part of this book may be reproduced in any form or by any means, including photocopying, or utilized by any information storage and retrieval system without written permission from the copyright owner.

Accurate indications, adverse reactions, and dosage schedules for drugs are provided in this book, but it is possible that they may change. The reader is urged to review the package information data of the manufacturers of the medications mentioned.

Printed in the United States of America

Library of Congress Cataloging-in-Publication Data

The publishers have made every effort to trace the copyright holders for borrowed material. If they have inadvertently overlooked any, they will be pleased to make the necessary arrangements at the first opportunity.

To purchase additional copies of this book, call our customer service department at **(800) 638-0672** or fax orders to **(800) 447-8438.** For other book services, including chapter reprints and large quantity sales, ask for the Special Sales department.

Canadian customers should call **(800) 665-1148** or fax **(800) 665-0103.** For all other calls originating outside of the United States, please call **(410) 528-4223** or fax us at **(410) 528-8550.**

Visit Williams & Wilkins on the Internet: http://www.wwilkins.com or contact our customer service department at **custserv@wwilkins.com.** Williams & Wilkins customer service representatives are available from 8:30 am to 6:00 pm, EST, Monday through Friday, for telephone access.

97 98 99 00 01
1 2 3 4 5 6 7 8 9 10

Preface

The primary goal for *Fundamentals of Sports Injury Management* is to integrate basic medical concepts and related scientific information to provide a foundation in the prevention, recognition, assessment, management, disposition, and rehabilitation of sport-related injuries and illnesses. Any individual responsible for providing on-site health care to sport participants should be able to recognize life-threatening injuries, determine a possible fracture or major ligament damage, manage the immediate injury, and determine whether referral to a physician is necessary.

Whereas *Sports Injury Management* was prepared with the professional athletic training student in mind, *Fundamentals in Sports Injury Management* is designed as an introductory text for students in coaching, exercise science, health education, health fitness, physical therapy, recreation, physical education, and youth sports. Both texts use a unique format whereby the student is introduced to new topics through a problem-solving approach using pertinent case studies. The text is easy to read and is supplemented with detailed line art, photos, and tables to further promote understanding and retention of the material.

CONTENT AND ORGANIZATION

The text is divided into six parts. Each part opens with a special feature highlighting a noted professional in the athletic training field. Those featured are:

Earlene Durrant, PhD, ATC
Director, Athletic Training Curriculum
Brigham Young University
Provo, Utah

Kathy Fox, MA, ATC, PT, SCS
Director of the Sports Medicine Program
Braintree Hospital Rehabilitation Network
Braintree, Massachusetts

Ron O'Neil, LATC
Head Athletic Trainer
New England Patriots Professional Football Team
Foxboro, Massachusetts

Yoshitaka Ando, BS, LATC
Head Athletic Trainer
Lincoln-Sudbury Regional High School
Sudbury, Massachusetts

Maria Hutsick, MS, LATC
Head Athletic Trainer
Boston University
Boston, Massachusetts

Marsha Grant, MEd, ATC
Head Athletic Trainer
Sterling High School
Somerdale, New Jersey

These interviews introduce individuals who work in both traditional and nontraditional athletic training settings. The athletic trainers provide a unique look at the field of athletic training and discuss how they got interested in athletic training as a career. Each individual speaks frankly about the ups and downs of their job and many share personal stories about why athletic training is so important to the overall health care of sport participants.

Part I: Foundations of Sports Injury Management (Chapters 1 and 2). Chapter 1 opens with an introduction to sports injury management and outlines the key role athletic trainers play as part of the primary sports medicine team. In addition, standards of professional practice, legal liability, record keeping, and career opportunities in athletic training are discussed. Chapter 2 provides the student with information on the mechanics of injury to soft tissues, bones, and nerves. The healing process for specific tissues, the basis of pain, and factors that mediate pain are also explained.

Part II: Sports Injury Management (Chapters 3 to 7). Chapter 3 introduces the HOPS format (**H**istory, **O**bservation and inspection, **P**alpation, and **S**pecial tests) used in basic injury assessment and relates this process to emergency procedures. In Chapter 4 this process is further expanded as it relates specifically to sport injury assessment. Chapter 5 discusses therapeutic exercise and therapeutic modalities used to facilitate healing. Chapter 6 discusses protective equipment used to prevent injury to specific body regions. Chapter 7 demonstrates specific taping and wrapping techniques for the upper and lower extremity.

Part III: Injuries to the Lower Extremity (Chapters 8 to 10). Part IV: Injuries to the Upper Extremity (Chapters 11 to 13). Part V: Injuries to the Axial Region (Chapters 14 to 16). Each chapter begins with a general review of anatomy of the joint or body region. Next, prevention of injury is discussed, followed by information on specific sports injuries and their management. Finally, a step-by-step injury assessment of the region is presented using the HOPS format and examples of rehabilitation exercises are provided for the treatment plan.

Part VI: Special Conditions Related to Sports (Chapters 17 and 18). Chapter 17 discusses injuries and conditions related to the reproductive system, including injuries to the genitalia, bloodborne viral diseases, and menstrual irregularities. Chapter 18 concludes with other health conditions that may affect sport performance, such as respiratory tract infections, gastrointestinal problems, diabetes, anemia, epilepsy, hypertension, substance abuse, and disordered eating patterns.

PEDAGOGICAL FEATURES

As educators, we have highlighted information in the text by incorporating several pedagogical features to enhance the text's usefulness as a teaching tool. This is designed to increase readability and retention of pertinent and necessary information. These in-text features include:

Learning Objectives

Each chapter opens with a list of learning objectives. These objectives highlight the most important concepts in the chapter that the student should focus on during reading.

Key Terms

Key terms used in the chapter are highlighted at the beginning of each chapter. These words are then defined in the margins and listed again in the glossary.

Thought Questions

Thought questions, identified by a question mark logo, are found at the beginning of each major section within each chapter. These questions encourage the student to critically analyze information and solve problems in the scenario presented. The answer to each thought question is provided at the end of that written section, identified with a light bulb logo.

Marginal Definitions and Tips

The key terms that are listed at the beginning of the chapter are also in bold print within the text and their definitions are provided in the margin. This allows the student easy access and better retention of new vocabulary terms. Important statements to assist in the learning process are also summarized in the margin.

Tables

Several chapters have numerous tables that expand upon pertinent information discussed in the text. This allows a large amount of didactic knowledge to be organized in an easy-to-read informational summary.

Field Strategies

A unique feature in this book is the use of Field Strategies to clinically apply cognitive knowledge. In Parts III, IV, and V, for example, the charts move step by step through the signs and symptoms of a specific injury, list immediate management, and provide several rehabilitation exercises for the condition. This careful integration of cognitive knowledge and the practical application of that knowledge is designed to give the student an overall picture of total injury management.

Art and Photo Program

Art plays a major role in facilitating the learning process. The editor and authors have worked hard to incorporate appropriate illustrations and photos to supplement material presented in the text. Two graphic artists with extensive experience as medical illustrators have provided realistic and accurate figures to depict anatomical structures and have devised innovative approaches to illustrate injury mechanisms. Each illustration was carefully reviewed to assess detail and accuracy.

Summary

Each chapter has a summary of key concepts discussed in the text. Several chapter summaries also contain a list of injuries or conditions that necessitate immediate referral to a physician for further care.

References

Any valuable teaching tool must include a listing of cited references used to gather information for the text. This provides the instructor and student with an accurate bibliographic reference that can be referred to if additional information on a specific topic is needed.

Glossary and Indexes

At the end of the book, the student will find an extensive glossary of terms, many of which appeared as marginal definitions. Furthermore, the comprehensive index contains cross-referencing information to locate specific information within the text.

SUPPLEMENTS

To facilitate the classroom experience, we have developed several teaching tools to assist the instructor in presenting information and in assessing student retention. In addition, material is also available for the student to add further reinforcement of the material presented in the text. These features include:

Instructor's Manual

Written by Dr. Melissa Martin, Director of the CAAHEP accredited undergraduate athletic training curriculum program at the University of South Carolina, the Instructor's Manual provides suggestions and exercises to supplement material presented in each chapter. Modules include chapter objectives, vocabulary terms, and laboratory exercises using injury scenarios to facilitate the learning process. These scenarios parallel those presented in the Student Manual. At the end of the Instructor's Manual are over 400 sample test questions from the text.

Computerized Testbank

For your convenience, this computerized test bank offers a flexible, time-saving method to create original, challenging tests utilizing over 1000 test questions in the testbank. With this program, you will be able to create, format, edit, and print exams that fit your specific needs. This Testbank is available to adopters of the text for Macintosh- and IBM-compatible computers.

Student Manual

Developed by Dr. Melissa Martin, Director of the CAAHEP accredited undergraduate athletic training curriculum program at the University of South Carolina, the Student Manual utilizes a problem-solving approach to challenge the student in the clinical application of cognitive knowledge presented in the text. The injury scenarios parallel those presented in the Instructors Manual and are designed to move the student step by step through the HOPS format, emphasizing proper vocabulary, skills, and techniques to thoroughly assess and manage each injury. In addition, short answers/questions are provided for students to review the basic concepts presented in each chapter.

Acknowledgments

The authors would like to express sincere appreciation to our many friends and colleagues who reviewed the text and made critical suggestions for improvement. These colleagues include Linda Barker, MS, ATC, EMT—University of Tennessee at Martin; Julie Felix, ATC—Virginia Tech; Mic McCrory, MEd, LATC—University of Mary; Dan Miller, MS, ATC—Chabot College; and Tim O'Brien, MEd, LATC—Mayville State University.

In addition to the reviewers, special thanks are extended to Cheryl Hitchings, LATC, PA-C, for preparing Chapter 7, and Theresa Joseph, LATC, RPT, who assisted in the development of the rehabilitation exercises listed in the individual joint chapters. Frank Forney of BioGraphics and Lydia V. Kibiuk of Illustrations Unlimited did a superb job on the illustrations and Denise Passaretti of Passaretti Photography and Susan Symonds of Main Frame Photographics did an outstanding job on many of the set shots used in the text. A special thanks to my devoted companion, Demeter, who had to forego her daily walks in the park to sit quietly while I worked on the computer to complete the text.

We would like to acknowledge all the help, direction, and guidance provided by our good friends at Williams & Wilkins, especially Donna Balado, Vicki Vaughn, Jennifer Schmidt, and Mary Finch, who took on the ominous task of polishing the manuscript and marketing the text. Thank you!

Marcia K. Anderson
Susan J. Hall

Contents

Preface   v
Acknowledgments   xi
Field Strategies   xxvii

Section I Foundations of Sports Injury Management

1 **Sports Injury Management and
   the Athletic Trainer**   5
   Sports Medicine   6
   Responsibilities of the Primary Sports Medicine
      Team   7
      Team Physician   8
      Primary Care Physician   8
      Athletic Trainer   8
      Coach or Sport Supervisor   9
      Sport Participants   11
      Student Athletic Trainer   11
      Physical Therapist   11
   Standards of Professional Practice   12
      NATA Certification for the Athletic Trainer   13
      Continuing Education Requirements   14
      Registration and Licensure   14
   Legal Liability   15
      Negligence   16
      Failure to Warn   16
      Informed Consent   17
      Foreseeability of Harm   17
      Product Liability   18
      Confidentiality   18
      Preventing Litigation   20
   Medical Records and Record Keeping   20
      Preparticipation Exams   20
      Medical Data Information Cards   21
      Accident Reports   21
      *Injury Management, Rehabilitation, and Progress
         Charts*   24
   Career Opportunities in Athletic Training   27
      High School and Collegiate Settings   27
      Sports Medicine Clinics   28
      Dual High School/Clinic Athletic Trainer   28
      Industrial Health Care Programs   29
      Professional Sport Teams   29
   Summary   29

2 The Mechanics of Tissue Injury and Healing   **31**

Injury Mechanisms   32
  Force and Its Effects   32
  Torque and Its Effects   36
Soft Tissue Injuries   38
  Anatomical Properties of Soft Tissue   38
  Skin Injury Classifications   41
  Other Soft Tissue Injury Classifications   42
  Soft Tissue Healing   44
Bone Injuries   46
  Anatomical Properties of Bone   46
  Bone Injury Classifications   49
  Epiphyseal Injury Classifications   52
  Bony Tissue Healing   52
Nerve Injuries   53
  Anatomical Properties of Nerves   54
  Nerve Injury Classifications   54
  Nerve Healing   55
Pain   55
  Neurological Basis of Pain   55
  Factors That Mediate Pain   56
  Referred Pain and Radiating Pain   56
Nutrition   57
Summary   58

Section II Sports Injury Management

3 Emergency Procedures   **63**

Emergency Situations   64
Obstructed Airway   65
  Partial Airway Obstruction   65
  Total Airway Obstruction   66
Cardiopulmonary Emergencies   66
Unconscious Athlete   66
Hemorrhage   68
  External Bleeding   68
  Internal Hemorrhage   70
Fractures   70
Shock   73
Hyperthermia   74
  Internal Heat Regulation   75
  Measuring the Heat Stress Index   78
  Preventing Heat Emergencies   78
  Heat Cramps   79
  Heat Exhaustion   80
  Heat Stroke   80
  Emergency Care for Heat Stress   81

Hypothermia	81
Preventing Cold-related Injuries	82
Frostbite Injuries	83
Systemic Body Cooling	84
Emergency Plan	85
Primary Injury Assessment	87
Assess Unresponsiveness	88
Open the Airway	88
Establish Breathing	91
Establish Circulation	93
Secondary Injury Assessment	96
History of the Injury	97
Observation	99
Palpation	102
Special Tests	105
Determination of Findings	106
Moving the Injured Participant	107
Summary	109
4 Sports Injury Assessment	**113**
Anatomical Foundations	114
Body Segments and Anatomical Position	115
Directional Terms	116
Regional Terms	119
Joint Movement Terms	119
Assessing an Injury	120
On-the-field vs. Off-the-field Assessment	120
History of the Injury	121
Primary Complaint	123
Mechanism of Injury	123
Characteristics of the Symptoms	123
Disability Resulting From the Injury	124
Related Medical History	125
Observation and Inspection	125
Observation	127
Inspection of the Injury Site	129
Palpation	129
Special Tests	132
Joint Range of Motion	132
Resisted Manual Muscle Testing	133
Neurologic Testing	135
Stress Tests	136
Functional Testing	138
Injury Recognition	138
SOAP Notes	140
Subjective Evaluation	140
Objective Evaluation	140
Assessment	141
Plan	141
Summary	142

5 Therapeutic Exercise and Therapeutic Modalities   145

Psychology and the Injured Participant   146
Developing a Therapeutic Exercise Program   147
Phase One: Controlling Inflammation   148
   Control of Inflammation   *150*
   Protect and Restrict Activity   *150*
Phase Two: Restoration of Motion   151
   Joint Range of Motion   *153*
   Flexibility   *153*
Phase Three: Developing Muscular Strength,
   Endurance, and Power   156
   Muscular Strength   *157*
   Muscular Endurance   *160*
   Muscular Power   *160*
   Open- vs. Closed-chain Exercises   *161*
Phase Four: Return to Sport Activity   163
   Coordination   *163*
   Sport-specific Skill Conditioning   *164*
   Cardiovascular Endurance   *165*
Therapeutic Modalities and Medications   165
   Cryotherapy   *167*
   Thermotherapy   *171*
   Neuromuscular Electrical Stimulation   *175*
   Intermittent Compression Units   *177*
   Continuous Passive Motion (CPM)   *177*
   Massage   *177*
   Medications   *178*
Summary   179

6 Protective Equipment   181

Principles of Protective Equipment   182
Protective Equipment for the Head and Face   184
   Football Helmets   *184*
   Ice Hockey Helmets   *186*
   Batting Helmets   *186*
   Other Helmets   *186*
   Face Guards   *187*
   Mouth Guards   *188*
   Eye Wear   *189*
   Ear Wear   *190*
   Throat and Neck Protectors   *190*
Protective Equipment for the Upper Body   192
   Shoulder Protection   *192*
   Elbow, Forearm, Wrist, and Hand Protection   *192*
   Thorax, Rib, and Abdominal Protection   *193*
   Sport Bras   *194*
   Lumbar/Sacral Protection   *195*
Protective Equipment for the Lower Body   198
   Hip and Buttock Protection   *198*
   Thigh Protection   *198*

Knee and Patella Protection	*198*
Lower Leg Protection	*201*
Ankle and Foot Protection	*202*
Summary	206

7 Protective Taping and Wraps **209**

Principles of Taping and Wrapping	209
Uses of Tape and Wraps	*211*
Types of Tape and Wraps	*211*
Application of Tape	*213*
Application of Wraps	*216*
Common Taping and Wrapping Techniques	217
Taping and Wrapping Techniques for the Lower Extremity	*218*
Taping and Wrapping Techniques for the Upper Extremity	*236*
Summary	243

Section III Injuries to the Lower Extremity

8 Foot, Ankle, and Lower Leg **249**

Anatomy Review of the Foot, Ankle, and Lower Leg	250
Bones of the Foot	*250*
Ligaments of the Foot and Ankle	*250*
Plantar Arches	*252*
Muscles of the Lower Leg and Foot	*255*
Nerves and Blood Supply of the Foot, Ankle, and Lower Leg	*255*
Major Muscle Actions of the Foot, Ankle, and Lower Leg	257
Toe Flexion and Extension	*259*
Dorsiflexion and Plantar Flexion	*260*
Inversion and Eversion	*261*
Pronation and Supination	*261*
Prevention of Injuries	262
Toe and Foot Conditions	266
Turf Toe	*266*
Hammer and Claw Toes	*267*
Ingrown Toenail	*267*
Blisters and Calluses	*267*
Morton's Neuroma	*270*
Bunions (Hallux Valgus)	*270*
Bursitis (Pump Bump, Runner's Bump)	*270*
Athlete's Foot	*272*
Contusions	272
Foot Contusions	*273*
Lower Leg Contusions	*273*
Acute Compartment Syndrome	*273*

Foot and Ankle Sprains   274
   Toe and Foot Sprains/Dislocations   274
   Lateral Ankle Sprains   274
   Medial Ankle Sprains   275
Acute Strains of the Foot and Lower Leg   276
   Muscle Cramps   277
   Lower Leg Tendon Strains   277
   Achilles Tendon Rupture   277
Overuse Conditions   278
   Plantar Fasciitis   278
   Achilles Tendinitis   279
   Medial Tibial Stress Syndrome (MTSS)   280
   Exercise-induced Compartment Syndrome   280
Fractures   281
Assessment of the Foot, Ankle, and Lower Leg   284
History   284
Observation and Inspection   285
Palpations   286
   Bony Palpations   287
   Soft Tissue Palpations   287
Special Tests   288
   Joint Range of Motion   288
   Resisted Manual Muscle Testing   288
   Neurologic Assessment   288
   Stress and Functional Tests   290
Rehabilitation   292
Summary   294

9 The Knee   **297**
Anatomy Review of the Knee   298
   Tibiofemoral Joint   298
   Menisci   300
   Joint Capsule and Bursae   300
   Ligaments of the Knee   300
   Patellofemoral Joint   301
   Muscles Crossing the Knee   301
   Nerves and Blood Supply of the Knee   301
Major Muscle Actions of the Knee   304
   Flexion and Extension   304
   Rotation and Passive Abduction and Adduction 304
   Patellofemoral Joint Motion   305
Prevention of Injuries   306
Contusions and Bursitis   306
Ligamentous Injuries   311
   Unidirectional Instabilities   311
   Management of Ligament Injuries   314
Meniscal Injuries   316
Patella and Related Injuries   317
   Patellofemoral Stress Syndrome   317
   Chondromalacia Patellae   318

	Acute Patellar Subluxation and Dislocation	*319*
	Patellar Tendinitis (Jumper's Knee)	*319*
	Osgood-Schlatter Disease	*320*
	Extensor Tendon Rupture	*321*
	Iliotibial Band Friction Syndrome	321
	Fractures	322
	Assessment of the Knee	325
	History	325
	Observation and Inspection	325
	Palpations	327
	Bony Palpations	*327*
	Soft Tissue Palpations	*327*
	Palpation for Swelling	*327*
	Special Tests	328
	Joint Range of Motion	*328*
	Resisted Manual Muscle Testing	*328*
	Neurologic Assessment	*330*
	Stress and Functional Tests	*330*
	Rehabilitation	334
	Summary	337
10	**Thigh, Hip, and Pelvis Injuries**	**339**
	Anatomy of the Thigh, Hip, and Pelvis	340
	Bony Structure of the Thigh, Hip, and Pelvis	*340*
	Hip Joint	*341*
	Nerves and Blood Vessels of the Thigh, Hip, and Pelvis	*342*
	Major Muscle Actions of the Hip	344
	Flexion	*344*
	Extension	*345*
	Abduction	*345*
	Adduction	*346*
	Medial and Lateral Rotation of the Femur	*346*
	Prevention of Injuries	347
	Contusions	351
	Quadriceps Contusion	*351*
	Myositis Ossificans	*351*
	Hip Pointers	*353*
	Bursitis	354
	Sprains and Dislocations	355
	Strains	356
	Vascular Disorders	359
	Hip Fractures	360
	Assessment of the Thigh, Hip, and Pelvis	364
	History	364
	Observation and Inspection	364
	Palpations	366
	Bony Palpations	*367*
	Soft Tissue Palpations	*367*

Special Tests   367
   Joint Range of Motion   368
   Resisted Manual Muscle Testing   368
   Neurologic Assessment   369
   Stress and Functional Tests   370
Rehabilitation   374
Summary   375

Section IV Injuries to the Upper Extremity

11 Shoulder Injuries   **381**
Anatomy Review of the Shoulder   382
   Sternoclavicular Joint   382
   Acromioclavicular Joint   383
   Coracoclavicular Joint   383
   Glenohumeral Joint   383
   Scapulothoracic Joint   384
   Muscles of the Shoulder   386
   Bursae   386
   Nerves and Blood Vessels of the Shoulder 388
Major Muscle Actions of the Shoulder Complex   389
   Throwing   389
   Coordination of Shoulder Movements   391
   Glenohumeral Flexion   392
   Glenohumeral Extension   393
   Glenohumeral Abduction   393
   Glenohumeral Adduction   393
   Lateral and Medial Rotation of the Humerus 393
Prevention of Injuries   394
Sprains to the Shoulder Complex   398
   Sternoclavicular Joint Sprain   398
   Acromioclavicular Joint Sprain   398
   Glenohumeral Joint Sprain   401
   Glenohumeral Dislocations   402
   Recurrent Subluxations and Dislocations 404
Overuse Injuries   404
   Rotator Cuff/Impingement Injuries   404
   Bursitis   406
   Bicipital Tendon Injuries   406
Fractures   407
Assessment of the Shoulder   410
History   410
Observation and Inspection   410
Palpations   411
   Bony Palpations   413
   Soft Tissue Palpations   413
Special Tests   413
   Joint Range of Motion   413
   Resisted Manual Muscle Testing   414

	Neurologic Assessment	*415*
	Stress and Functional Tests	*415*
	Rehabilitation	421
	Summary	426
12	**Upper Arm, Elbow, and Forearm Injuries**	**429**
	Anatomy Review of the Elbow	430
	Bony Structure of the Elbow	*430*
	Ligaments of the Elbow	*430*
	Muscles of the Elbow	*431*
	Nerves and Blood Vessels of the Elbow	*431*
	Major Muscle Actions of the Elbow	433
	Flexion and Extension	*434*
	Pronation and Supination	*435*
	Prevention of Injuries	436
	Contusions	436
	Olecranon Bursitis	440
	Sprains and Dislocations	441
	Strains	443
	Overuse Conditions	444
	Medial Epicondylitis	*444*
	Lateral Epicondylitis	*445*
	Impingement of the Ulnar Nerve	*448*
	Fractures	448
	Assessment of the Elbow	449
	History	449
	Observation and Inspection	450
	Palpations	451
	Bony Palpations	*451*
	Soft Tissue Palpations	*453*
	Special Tests	453
	Joint Range of Motion	*454*
	Resisted Manual Muscle Testing	*454*
	Neurologic Testing	*454*
	Stress and Functional Tests	*454*
	Rehabilitation	458
	Summary	459
13	**Wrist and Hand Injuries**	**463**
	Anatomy Review of the Wrist and Hand	464
	Bones and Articulations of the Wrist and Hand	*464*
	Muscles of the Wrist and Hand	*465*
	Nerves and Blood Vessels of the Wrist and Hand	*465*
	Retinacula of the Wrist	*467*
	Major Muscle Actions of the Wrist and Hand	470
	Flexion	*470*
	Extension and Hyperextension	*470*
	Radial and Ulnar Deviation	*471*
	Carpometacarpal Joint Motion	*471*
	Metacarpophalangeal Joint Motion	*471*
	Interphalangeal Joint Motion	*472*

Prevention of Injuries   472
Contusions and Abrasions   473
Sprains   473
    Wrist Sprains   473
    Gamekeeper's Thumb   474
    Interphalangeal Collateral Ligament Sprains   474
    Dislocations   475
Strains   477
    Jersey Finger (Profundus Tendon Rupture)   477
    Mallet Finger   477
    Boutonniere Deformity   478
    Tendinitis and Stenosing Tenosynovitis   478
    Ganglion Cysts   479
Fingertip Injuries   480
Nerve Entrapment Syndromes   480
    Carpal Tunnel Syndrome   481
    Ulnar Neuropathy   482
Fractures   483
    Distal Radial and Ulnar Fractures   483
    Carpal Fractures   483
    Metacarpal Fractures   485
    Phalangeal Fractures   486
Assessment of the Wrist and Hand   486
History   487
Observation and Inspection   488
Palpations   488
    Bony Palpations   489
    Soft Tissue Palpations   489
Special Tests   491
    Joint Range of Motion   491
    Resisted Manual Muscle Testing   491
    Neurologic Testing   491
    Stress and Functional Tests   492
Rehabilitation   494
Summary   495

Section V Injuries to the Axial Region

14 Head and Facial Injuries   **501**
Anatomy Review of the Head and Facial Region   502
    Bones of the Skull   502
    The Scalp   503
    The Brain   503
    The Eyes   504
    Nerves and Blood Vessels of the Head and Face   505
Prevention of Injuries   506
Cranial Injury Mechanisms   507
Skull Fractures   508

Cerebral Hematomas 510
Epidural Hematoma 511
Subdural Hematoma 511
Concussions 513
Grade I Concussion 514
Grade II Concussion 515
Grade III Concussion 515
Grade IV Concussion 515
Grade V Concussion 515
Grade VI Concussion 516
Second Impact Syndrome 516
Scalp Injuries 516
Assessment of Cranial Injuries 517
Vital Signs 518
History 519
Observation and inspection 520
Palpation 520
Special Tests 520
Determination of Findings 521
Facial Injuries 524
Facial Soft Tissue Injuries 524
Facial Fractures 524
Nasal Injuries 525
Epistaxis 526
Nasal Fractures 526
Oral and Dental Injuries 527
Lacerations of the Mouth 527
Dental Injuries 528
Ear Injuries 529
External Ear Injury 529
Internal Ear Injury 530
Eye Injuries 531
Periorbital Ecchymosis (Black eye) 531
Foreign Bodies 532
Conjunctivitis (Pinkeye) 533
Corneal Abrasion 533
Subconjunctival Hemorrhage 533
Hemorrhage into the Anterior Chamber 533
Detached Retina 533
Orbital "Blowout" Fracture 534
Displaced Contact Lens 534
Summary 535

15 Injuries to the Spine 539
Anatomy Review of the Spine 540
Vertebrae and Intervertebral Discs 540
Ligaments of the Spine 542
Muscles of the Spine and Trunk 542
Spinal Cord and Spinal Nerves 542

Major Muscle Actions of the Spine 545
  Flexion, Extension, and Hyperextension 546
  Lateral Flexion and Rotation 546
Anatomical Variations Predisposing Individuals to
  Spine Injuries 547
  Spinal Curvatures 547
  Pars Interarticularis Fractures 548
Prevention of Injuries 549
Cervical Spine Injuries 555
  Cervical Strains and Sprains 556
  Cervical Fractures and Dislocations 557
Brachial Plexus Injuries 558
Thoracic Spine Injuries 560
  Thoracic Contusions, Strains, and Sprains 560
  Thoracic Spinal Fractures and Apophysitis 560
Lumbar Spine Injuries 561
  Low Back Pain 562
  Lumbar Contusions, Strains, and Sprains 563
  Sciatica 564
  Lumbar Disc Injuries 565
  Lumbar Fractures and Dislocations 565
Sacrum and Coccyx Injuries 566
Assessment of the Spine 566
History 567
Observation and Inspection 568
  Posture 568
  Scan Exam 569
  Inspection of the Injury Site 569
  Gross Neuromuscular Assessment 570
Palpations 570
  Anterior Aspect 571
  Posterior Aspect 571
Special Tests 572
  Joint Range of Motion 572
  Resisted Manual Muscle Testing 572
  Neurologic Assessment 573
  Stress and Functional Tests 573
Rehabilitation 577
Summary 578

16 Throat, Thorax, and Visceral Injuries 581
Anatomy Review of the Throat 582
Anatomy Review of the Thorax 583
Anatomy Review of the Visceral Region 585
Prevention of Injuries 591
Throat Injuries 592
Thoracic Injuries 593
  Stitch in the Side 593
  Breast Injuries 594

Strain of the Pectoralis Major Muscle   594
Costochondral Injury   594
Sternal and Rib Fractures   595
Internal Complications   596
Hyperventilation   597
Pulmonary Contusion   597
Pneumothorax   597
Tension Pneumothorax   598
Traumatic Asphyxia   598
Hemothorax   598
Heart Injuries   599
Sudden Death in Athletes   599
Abdominal Wall Injuries   600
Skin Wounds and Contusions   600
Muscle Strains   600
Solar Plexus Contusion ("Wind Knocked Out")   601
Hernias   601
Intra-abdominal Injuries   602
Splenic Rupture   603
Liver Contusion and Rupture   603
Appendicitis   604
Kidney and Bladder Injuries   604
Assessment of the Throat, Thorax, and Viscera   605
History   605
Observation and Inspection   607
Palpations   607
Special Tests   609
Summary   611

Section VI Special Conditions Related to Sports

17 Conditions Related to the Reproductive System   **617**
Anatomy of the Genitalia   618
Female Reproductive System   619
Male Reproductive System   620
Injuries and Conditions of the Genitalia   620
Male Genital Injuries   621
Female Genital Injuries   622
Dermatologic Conditions   623
Bloodborne Viral Diseases   624
Hepatitis B   624
AIDS   626
Menstrual Irregularities   627
Dysmenorrhea   627
Exercise-associated Amenorrhea   628
Birth Control and Sport Participation   629
Pregnancy and Sport Participation   629
Summary   631

18 Other Health Conditions Related to Sports   **633**

Respiratory Tract Conditions   634
  Common Cold   634
  Sinusitis   634
  Pharyngitis (Sore Throat)   635
  Influenza   636
  Allergic Rhinitis (Hay Fever)   636
  Acute Bronchitis   637
  Infectious Mononucleosis   637
  Bronchial Asthma   637
  Exercise-induced Asthma   638
The Gastrointestinal Tract   640
  Gastroenteritis   640
  Diarrhea   640
  Constipation   641
The Diabetic Athlete   641
  Diabetic Coma   643
  Insulin Shock   644
  Exercise and Diabetes   644
Epilepsy   645
Hypertension   646
Anemia   648
  Iron-deficiency Anemia   648
  Sickle Cell Anemia   648
Substance Abuse   649
  Therapeutic Drugs   649
  Performance-enhancing Drugs   650
  Recreational Drugs   650
  Signs of Substance Abuse   650
  Drug Testing   650
Disordered Eating   653
  Disordered Eating Not Otherwise Specified (NOS)   654
  Bulimia Nervosa   654
  Anorexia Nervosa   655
  Exercise and Weight Management   656
Summary   658

Credits   **661**
Glossary   **663**
Index   **677**

Field Strategies

1.1	Physical Examination Record	22
1.2	The Two-minute Orthopedic Scan Exam	23
1.3	Mass Station Screening Exam	24
3.1	Management of External Hemorrhage	71
3.2	Management of Internal Bleeding	72
3.3	Principles of Emergency Splinting for Suspected Fractures	74
3.4	Management of Shock	76
3.5	Management of Heat-related Conditions	82
3.6	Reducing the Risk for Cold Injuries	83
3.7	Management of Frostbite	84
3.8	Developing an Emergency Care Plan	86
3.9	Management of an Obstructed Airway	92
3.10	Primary Survey	95
3.11	Determining the History of Injury and Level of Consciousness	100
3.12	Protocol for Head-to-toe Palpations	103
3.13	Transporting an Injured Individual on a Stretcher	108
4.1	Injury Assessment Protocol	121
4.2	Developing a History of the Injury	126
4.3	Assessment of General Appearance and Symmetry	128
5.1	Acute Care of Soft Tissue Injuries	151
5.2	Fitting and Using Crutches and Canes	152
5.3	Range-of-motion Exercises for the Lower and Upper Extremity	155
5.4	Using Static Stretching to Improve Flexibility	156
5.5	Power and Strength Exercises	161
5.6	Lower Extremity Exercises to Improve Balance and Proprioception	164
5.7	Cardiovascular Conditioning Exercises	166
5.8	Techniques for Using a Whirlpool Bath	173
6.1	Proper Fitting of a Padded Football Helmet	185
6.2	Fitting Mouth-formed Mouth Guards	189
6.3	Fitting Football Shoulder Pads	193
6.4	Factors in the Selection and Fit of Athletic Shoes	205
7.1	Application Techniques for Taping a Body Part	217
7.2	Application Techniques for Wrapping a Body Part	218

8.1	Exercises to Prevent Injury to the Lower Leg	263
8.2	Prevention and Management of an Ingrown Toenail	268
8.3	Prevention and Management of Blisters	269
8.4	Prevention and Management of Athlete's Foot	272
8.5	Management of a Lateral Ankle Sprain	276
8.6	Management of Plantar Fasciitis	279
8.7	Management of Medial Tibial Stress Syndrome	281
8.8	Developing a History of the Injury	285
8.9	Postural Assessment of the Lower Extremity	286
8.10	Determining a Possible Fracture in the Foot and Lower Leg	287
8.11	Rehabilitation Exercises for the Lower Leg	293
8.12	Foot, Ankle, and Lower Leg Evaluation	294
9.1	Exercises to Prevent Injury at the Knee	307
9.2	Management of a Ligamentous Injury	315
9.3	Management of Patellar Tendinitis	320
9.4	Management of Illotibial Band Friction Syndrome	322
9.5	Developing a History of the Injury	326
9.6	Knee Evaluation	337
10.1	Exercises to Prevent Injury at the Thigh, Hip, and Pelvis	348
10.2	Management of a Quadriceps Contusion	352
10.3	Developing a History of the Injury	365
10.4	Hip Evaluation	376
11.1	Flexibility Exercises for the Shoulder Region	395
11.2	Strengthening Exercises for the Shoulder Complex	396
11.3	Management of a Sternoclavicular Sprain	400
11.4	Management of an Acromioclavicular Sprain	401
11.5	Developing a History of the Injury	411
11.6	Postural Assessment of the Upper Extremity	412
11.7	Range-of-motion Exercises for the Glenohumeral Joint	422
11.8	Rehabilitation Exercises for the Shoulder Complex	423
11.9	Shoulder Evaluation	426
12.1	Exercises to Prevent Injury to the Elbow Region	437
12.2	Management of a Posterior Elbow Dislocation	442
12.3	Management of Muscular Strains	443
12.4	Management of Epicondylitis	446
12.5	Developing a History of the Injury	450
12.6	Determining a Possible Fracture in the Upper Arm and Forearm	452
12.7	Elbow Evaluation	460
13.1	Management of a Subungual Hematoma	481
13.2	Developing a History of the Injury	487
13.3	Observation and Inspection of the Wrist and Hand	489

13.4 Determining a Possible Fracture to a Metacarpal   490
13.5 Wrist and Hand Evaluation   496

14.1 Management of a Suspected Skull Fracture   510
14.2 Cranial Injury Evaluation   523
14.3 Wound Care Using Steri-Strips or Butterfly
      Bandages   525
14.4 Management of a Nasal Injury   527
14.5 Removing a Foreign Body from the Eye   532
14.6 Eye Evaluation   535

15.1 Prevention of Spinal Injuries   551
15.2 Preventing Low Back Injuries in Activities of Daily
      Living   563
15.3 Reducing Low Back Pain in Runners   564
15.4 Developing a History for a Spinal Injury   568
15.5 Scan Exam for a Spinal Injury   570
15.6 Assessment for a Spinal Injury   579

16.1 Management of Tracheal and Laryngeal Injuries   593
16.2 Management of Rib Fractures   596
16.3 Management of Suspected Intra-abdominal Injuries   603
16.4 Developing a History of the Injury   606
16.5 Observation and Inspection of the Thorax and
      Viscera   608
16.6 Assessment of the Thorax and Visceral Region   610

17.1 Management of Tinea Cruris   623
17.2 Preventing the Spread of Infectious Diseases in the
      Athletic Training Room   625

18.1 Steps to Prevent a Cold   635
18.2 Exercise Strategies for Exercise-induced Asthma   639
18.3 Management of Diabetic Emergencies   645
18.4 Management of an Epileptic Seizure   647
18.5 Guidelines for Safe Weight Loss and Weight Gain   657

Fundamentals of
Sports Injury Management

Foundations of Sports Injury Management

Chapter 1: **Sports Injury Management and the Athletic Trainer**

Chapter 2: **The Mechanics of Tissue Injury and Healing**

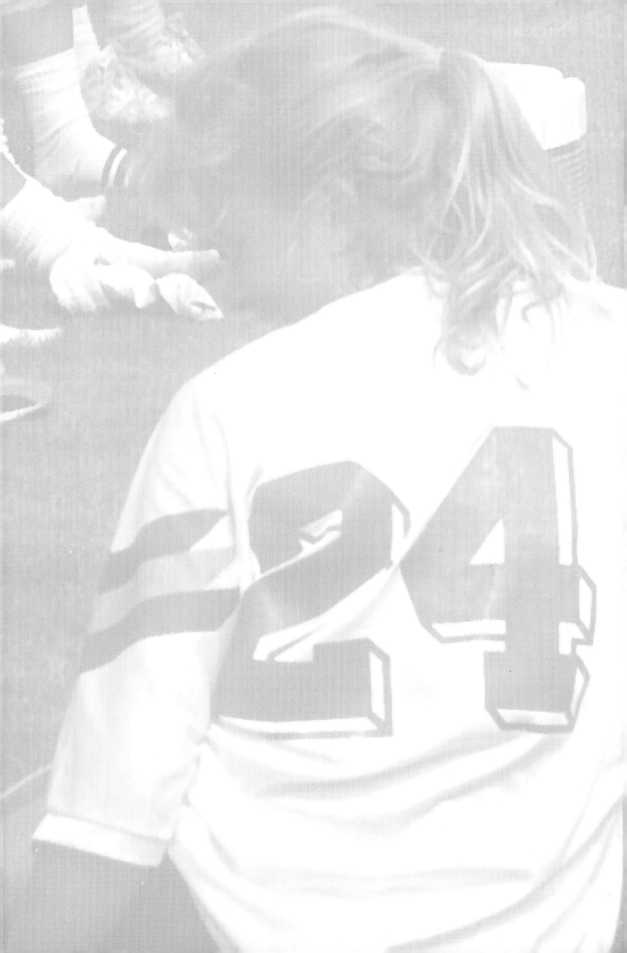

Earlene Durrant, PhD, ATC

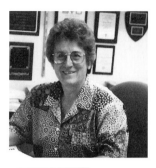

I came to BYU in 1973 to complete my Ph.D. in Physical Education. Title IX had just been passed and the university realized they needed a women's athletic trainer. Because I was the only female on the staff who had ever taped an ankle, I was elected. My clinical hours were completed under the direction of the certified staff trainers at BYU and I became certified in 1975, when there were fewer than a dozen certified women in the United States.

I started out as the Women's Athletic Trainer for 10 Division I teams and 6 extramural teams. In 1980, when the athletic training curriculum was approved by the NATA, my workload tripled when I became the primary educator and administrator of the curriculum program. Despite this, I love the job and would not trade it for the world.

As a curriculum coordinator, I am responsible for the day-to-day functional running of the academic program, including recruiting students, interviewing and testing students for admissions into the program, academic advising, scheduling, working with the clinical instructors, doing annual reports for the NATA and NATA Board of Certification, and developing the curriculum to keep our students abreast of the information and research they need to compete in this profession.

The best thing about teaching in a curriculum program is working with dynamic students who are not afraid of a challenge. Teaching athletic training gives me the opportunity to inspire these students to grow both professionally and personally. It is personally gratifying to know that I had a major role in making them better professionals, who may someday shape the direction of our profession. It's exhilarating to see the excitement in their eyes when they finally grasp the concepts in the classroom and translate them into the practical application of providing quality health care to their patients. To see them take personal interest in the welfare of their athletes and to unselfishly give of themselves is inspiring to me as a teacher. Many of my students continue to write to me or call just to say hello and thank me for introducing them into this challenging profession.

That is not to say that my assignment does not have its downside. Being a professor at a large university carries with it an obligation to do active research and publish. In addition, I raise funds to supplement the clinical program. I recruit donations from area physicians, physical therapists, schools, and clinics to provide stipends for the students to complete clinical hours at off-site locations. All of this takes time away from the personal interaction with my students.

For students considering a career in athletic training, I would recommend broadening your academic background with another program, such as teaching or health promotion, to make you more marketable. Realize that competition in the field is keen, and today you have to be better at your job than your clinical instructor is. Commitment is the key. Athletic training is a people-oriented service profession and you have to be willing to give of yourself 12 to 15 hours a day, 7 days a week. Get involved in the profession as a student by attending your state, district, and national conferences. Get to know those in the field and begin to develop your own networking system. Always remember that you are a professional. You have to act like a professional, and dress like one. That is how you succeed. Welcome to the athletic training profession.

Dr. Earlene Durrant is a Professor and Director of the Athletic Training Curriculum Program at Brigham Young University in Provo, Utah. As one of the first athletic trainers ever to receive a Ph.D., she was the first woman elected President of the Utah Athletic Trainer's Association and the first woman ever appointed to chair a national NATA committee.

Chapter 1

Sports Injury Management and the Athletic Trainer

After completing this chapter, you should be able to:

- Define sports medicine

- Identify members of the primary sports medicine team and their responsibilities in sports injury management

- Explain basic parameters of ethical conduct and standards of professional practice for athletic trainers

- Specify academic and clinical requirements necessary to become a National Athletic Trainer's Association (NATA) certified athletic trainer, and continuing education requirements needed to maintain certification

- Explain standard of care and describe preventative measures to reduce the risk of litigation

- Identify record keeping used in sports injury management

- Discuss potential job opportunities for an individual interested in athletic training as a career option

Key Terms:

Expressed warranty	**Negligence**
Foreseeability of harm	**Sports medicine**
Implied warranty	**Standard of care**
Informed consent	**Tort**

Sport, with the inherent risks involved, leads to injury at one time or another for nearly all participants. Physicians and athletic trainers responsible for the health and safety of sport participants are called sports medicine specialists. These individuals are essential in the prevention and care of sport injuries. Furthermore, these individuals serve as a valuable resource to educate and counsel sport participants to prevent chronic degenerative injuries and diseases through life-long activity-related fitness and health education.

This chapter examines the role of the physician and athletic trainer within the primary sports medicine team. In the absence of an athletic trainer, the coach or designated supervisor of the sport-related activity must assume the role of the immediate health care provider. Standards of professional practice and criteria for national certification as an athletic trainer are presented in detail. Legal liability surrounding sports injury care will be presented relative to reducing the risk of litigation. Finally, potential job opportunities for individuals interested in athletic training as a career are discussed.

SPORTS MEDICINE

? *Many medical and health care professionals refer to themselves as sports medicine specialists. Think for a minute about what this term implies. Where do sport supervisors, coaches, and athletic trainers fit into the scheme of health care for sport participants?*

Sports medicine is a broad and complex branch of health care encompassing several disciplines. Essentially, it applies medical and scientific knowledge to prevent and care for injuries or illnesses related to sport, exercise, or recreational activity, and, in doing so, enhances the health fitness and performance of the participant (1). Sport performance is enhanced through several mediums:

1. Provision of a clean, safe, and accessible participation environment
2. Prevention of injury through preparticipation screening, development and supervision of physical conditioning and exercise programs, the design, use, and fitting of protective equipment, and proper skill instruction
3. Assessment and recognition of a sport injury or illness
4. Management and disposition of an injury or illness
5. Injury rehabilitation through therapeutic exercise, reconditioning, and analysis of skill technique
6. Continued education and counseling to maintain life-long fitness and good health

The primary sports medicine team provides on-site supervision to prevent injury and deliver immediate health care. This team includes the primary care physician, athletic trainer, coach or sport supervisor in the absence of an athletic trainer, and the sport participant (2). Others readily accessible to the primary sports medicine team, but not necessarily on-site, include many of those professionals listed in **Table 1.1**.

Providing a safe, healthy, and accessible environment that is properly supervised will prevent many injuries. Due to the inherent risks in some sports and the forces involved in contact and collision activities, injuries will still occur. The National Athletic Trainers' Association (NATA) has projected that nearly 25% of

Sports medicine
Area of health and special services that applies medical and scientific knowledge to prevent, recognize, manage, and rehabilitate injuries related to sport, exercise, or recreational activity

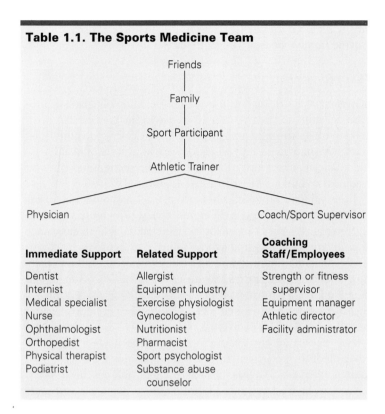

Table 1.1. The Sports Medicine Team

Friends

|

Family

|

Sport Participant

|

Athletic Trainer

Physician   Coach/Sport Supervisor

Immediate Support	Related Support	Coaching Staff/Employees
Dentist	Allergist	Strength or fitness
Internist	Equipment industry	supervisor
Medical specialist	Exercise physiologist	Equipment manager
Nurse	Gynecologist	Athletic director
Ophthalmologist	Nutritionist	Facility administrator
Orthopedist	Pharmacist	
Physical therapist	Sport psychologist	
Podiatrist	Substance abuse	
	counselor	

all interscholastic athletes are injured each year. For this reason, it is imperative that the primary sports medicine team work together to provide quality, comprehensive health care to all sport participants.

Sports medicine is the health care area that applies medical and scientific knowledge to prevent and care for injuries or illnesses related to sport, exercise, or recreational activity, and in doing so, enhances health fitness and performance of the participant. The athletic trainer, coach, and sport supervisors are responsible for daily on-site health care.

NATA projects that nearly 25% of interscholastic athletes are injured each year

RESPONSIBILITIES OF THE PRIMARY SPORTS MEDICINE TEAM

Think for a minute or two about the individuals who make up the primary sports medicine team. What duties should each individual be responsible for?

Total health care encompasses the prevention and care of sport injuries and illnesses. No single profession can provide the expertise to carry out this enormous responsibility. As such, the team approach has proven to be the most successful method of addressing health care for sport participants. The primary sports medicine team is the pivotal group of individuals with the neces-

The team approach has proven to be the most successful method to provide health care to sport participants

sary specialized training and expertise in their chosen field to provide immediate on-site health care.

Team Physician

A team physician directs the primary sports medicine team and is the final authority to determine the mental and physical fitness of athletes in school programs

In organized sport, such as interscholastic, intercollegiate, or professional athletic programs, a team physician may be hired, or may volunteer their services, to direct the primary sports medicine team. This individual supervises the various aspects of health care and is the final authority to determine the mental and physical readiness of athletes in organized programs (1,2).

In an athletic program, the team physician should administer and review preseason physical exams; review preseason conditioning programs; assess the quality, effectiveness, and maintenance of protective equipment; diagnose injuries; dispense medications; direct rehabilitation programs; educate the athletic staff on emergency policies, procedures, health care insurance coverage, and legal liability; and review all medical forms, policies, and procedures to ensure compliance with school and athletic association guidelines (1,2). This individual may also serve as a valuable resource on current therapeutic techniques; facilitate referrals to other medical specialists; and provide educational counseling to sport participants, parents, athletic trainers, and coaches.

In many high school and collegiate settings, financial constraints may prevent hiring a full-time team physician. Instead, several physicians rotate the responsibility of being present at competitions and are paid a per-game stipend. Primary care physicians, orthopedists, and other specialists with an interest in sports medicine may serve as team physicians. The team physician should be present at competitions, particularly with high risk sports, such as football, hockey, or lacrosse, to conduct emergency injury assessment and to manage and treat any immediate injury or illness.

Primary Care Physician

In the absence of a team physician, the primary care physician or family physician assumes a more pivotal role in providing health care to the sport participant. This individual can provide: information on the growth and development of an adolescent, immunization records, and medical history. In addition, they may administer preparticipation exams, provide initial clearance for sport participation, diagnose sport injuries, prescribe medication, and clear an individual for sport participation after an injury (2).

Athletic Trainer

Athletic trainers are the critical link between the sport program and medical community, and are certified by the NATA

Athletic trainers are the critical link between the sport program and medical community and are certified by the NATA Board of Certification (BOC). Although athletic trainers work under the direction of a physician, they provide a much broader range of direct services to the sport participant on a daily basis (**Fig. 1.1**).

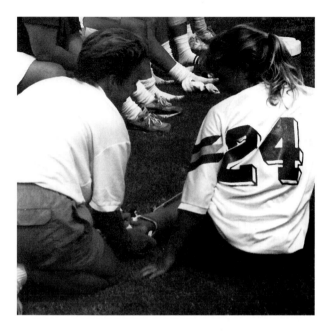

Figure 1.1. After evaluating an injury, the athletic trainer can determine what action is appropriate to manage the situation. This may include sideline treatment to control inflammation or immediate referral to a physician.

Athletic trainers have a strong background in human anatomy and physiology, kinesiology or biomechanics, psychology, health and nutrition, exercise physiology, first aid and emergency care, injury prevention, assessment, therapeutic rehabilitation, use of modalities, and health care administration. Because of this broad background, the athletic trainer serves as the facilitator and liaison between the physician and athlete, and the physician and coach. Their primary duties and responsibilities are summarized in **Table 1.2** and include (3):

1. Prevention of athletic injuries
2. Recognition, evaluation, and immediate care of athletic injuries
3. Rehabilitation and reconditioning of athletic injuries
4. Health care administration
5. Professional development and responsibility

Coach or Sport Supervisor

A coach is responsible for teaching skills and strategies of a sport. A sport supervisor may not be a coach, but instead may be responsible for supervising recreational sports or activity areas within health club facilities. In the absence of an athletic trainer, the coach and sport supervisor are expected to evaluate the physical condition of all sport participants prior to any activity, properly fit and use quality safety equipment, teach proper skill development and technique, and reinforce the importance of safety and injury prevention on a regular basis. All coaches and sport supervisors should maintain current certification in cardiopulmonary re-

Table 1.2. Duties of the Athletic Trainer

Injury Prevention

Identify physical conditions predisposing the individual to increased risk of injury through appropriate preparticipation screening

Design, fabricate, and fit custom protective devices

Apply appropriate taping, wrapping, or prophylactic devices to prevent injury

Evaluate the use and maintenance of protective devices and athletic equipment

Educate parents, staff, coaches, and athletes about the risks associated with participation, and unsafe practices, to enable an informed decision concerning sport participation

Recognition, Evaluation, and Immediate Care of Athletic Injuries

Obtain a medical history from the individual to determine the pathology and extent of injury/illness

Inspect, palpate, and perform special tests to the injured area using bilateral comparison to determine the extent of the injury/illness

Determine the appropriate course of action by interpreting the signs and symptoms of the injury/illness in order to provide the necessary immediate care

Administer appropriate first aid to facilitate efficient transportation and referral to appropriate medical personnel

Rehabilitation and Reconditioning

Evaluate the injury/illness status to determine appropriate rehabilitation programs

Restore normal function utilizing appropriate therapeutic exercise and modalities

Assess functional status in order to ensure safe return to activity

Educate parents, staff, coaches, and athletes about the rehabilitation process to ensure success

Health Care Administration

Create a plan that includes emergency, management, and referral systems specific to the setting

Establish written guidelines for injury/illness management

Comply with safety and sanitation standards by following universal safety precautions

Manage daily operations of the facility

Maintain all health records

Professional Development and Responsibility

Maintain knowledge of contemporary sports medicine issues through continuing education activities

Develop interpersonal communication skills by interacting with others in a professional manner

Adhere to ethical and legal parameters that define the proper role of the certified athletic trainer

Assimilate appropriate sports medicine research by using available resources to enhance professional growth

Educate the public about the roles and responsibilities of the certified athletic trainer

suscitation (CPR) and emergency first aid care. In addition, they should meet regularly with their respective staff and community Emergency Medical Services (EMS) to develop and practice emergency procedures, skills, and techniques. At least one staff person should have advanced training in emergency care. For brevity's sake, coaches and sport supervisors will henceforth be jointly referred to as sport supervisors.

Sport Participants

Sport participants can maximize injury prevention by maintaining a high level of fitness, eating nutritional foods, wearing protective equipment, playing within the rules of the sport, and seeking immediate first aid should an injury occur. Sport participants should also refrain from ingesting alcohol and other chemical substances, such as anabolic steroids, human growth hormones, and amphetamines, to enhance performance. Each can impair judgment, alter coordination, and place the individual at risk for injury. If sport participants understand and practice preventative measures, the number of injuries associated with sport participation can be reduced.

Student Athletic Trainer

Student athletic trainers provide the work force in organized sport programs to implement the policies and procedures of daily health care at team practices and games (Fig. 1.2). Many students gain practical experience on the high school level and enroll in a college or university to pursue a degree program in athletic training, human performance, physical education, or a health-related area. On the college level, NATA-certified athletic trainers supervise and guide the student athletic trainer through the clinical application of sports injury care. Initially the student athletic trainer may only observe the staff athletic trainers in action and assist when needed. As the student's skills and knowledge improve, the athletic trainers will help the student learn NATA competencies in athletic training and prepare the student to meet the NATA Board of Certification Standards. Student athletic trainers can view first-hand the contributions athletic trainers provide in the total health care of sport participants.

Physical Therapist

Physical therapists are not a part of the on-site primary sports medicine team, yet they provide a unique and valuable resource in the overall rehabilitation of a sport participant. Although the athletic trainer typically works with healthy athletes, the physical therapist has a broader background in treating patients of all ages, with a wider variety of physical problems. Physical therapists often supervise the rehabilitation of an injured sport participant in an industrial medical clinic, hospital, or sports medicine clinic. In

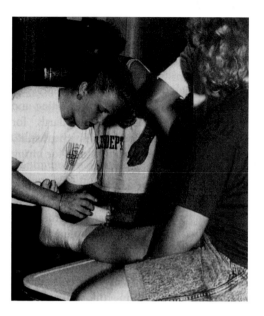

Figure 1.2. Student athletic trainers provide the work force to implement the policies and procedures of daily health care to sport participants.

many cases, athletic trainers are also registered physical therapists. Likewise, many physical therapists are also working toward certification as athletic trainers. Dual certification is a strong asset in the job market.

💡 *Within the primary sports medicine team, did you determine that the athlete trainer is the critical link between the sport program and medical community and provides a broad range of direct services daily to the sport participant?*

STANDARDS OF PROFESSIONAL PRACTICE

❓ *If injured, what standards of care and professional conduct should an athlete expect to receive from the immediate health care provider?*

Standards of professional practice are ethical responsibilities that guide one's actions and promote high standards of conduct and integrity to assure high-quality health care (4). These standards reflect what appropriate actions fall within the realm of the profession and, based on sound medical judgment, defines what actions are right and wrong. Individuals should be informed of the risks for injury, be protected from injury whenever possible, and receive expedient health care and rehabilitation if an injury occurs. Participants also have a right to confidentiality about their health status. Athletic trainers, sport supervisors, and physicians should be sensitive about dissemination of health information and should honor the wishes of an individual not to make the information public. Individuals who choose athletic training as a career option have

Standards of professional practice are ethical ideals that guide your actions and promote high standards of conduct and integrity

Sport participants have a right to confidentiality about their health status

a professional responsibility to meet entry-level competencies and to stay current on new techniques and protocols for treatment.

NATA Certification for the Athletic Trainer

Individuals seeking to become NATA-certified athletic trainers must complete the following core requirements:

1. Clinical athletic training hours (these may not begin to accumulate until after the high school degree has been completed)
2. Proof of graduation at the baccalaureate level at an accredited college or university
3. Proof of current Basic CPR (American Red Cross or American Heart Association) or EMT equivalent
4. At least 25% of all clinical athletic training experience hours must be attained in actual (on location) practice and/or game coverage with one or more of the following sports: football, soccer, hockey, wrestling, basketball, gymnastics, lacrosse, volleyball, and rugby.
5. Endorsement of certification application by a NATA-certified athletic trainer

An individual may qualify for application through two options: (1) by graduating from an undergraduate or graduate institution that has an educational program accredited through the Commission on Accreditation of Allied Health Educational Programs (CAAHEP) and passing the national certification examination, or (2) by completing an internship route to certification and passing the national certification examination. Students in CAAHEP-accredited entry-level programs must complete formal instruction in the following core curriculum subject matter:

Human anatomy
Human physiology
Psychology
Kinesiology/biomechanics
Exercise physiology
Prevention of athletic injuries/illnesses
Evaluation of athletic injuries/illnesses
First aid and emergency care
Therapeutic modalities
Therapeutic exercise
Personal/community health
Nutrition
Administration of athletic training programs

In addition to core subject matter, additional course work is highly recommended in chemistry, physics, pharmacology, statistics, and research design. Students are also required to complete 800 clinical hours under the supervision of a NATA-certified athletic trainer at the college or affiliated site (i.e., area high school or local college).

Students who do not attend a college or university with a CAAHEP-accredited entry-level program may complete requirements for certification through an internship. Requirements for this option are established by the NATA Board of Certification (NATABOC) and include the following subject areas:

Health (i.e., nutrition, drugs/substance abuse, and health education)
Human anatomy
Human physiology
Kinesiology/biomechanics
Physiology of exercise
Basic athletic training
Advanced athletic training (one course in therapeutic modalities and rehabilitative exercise are acceptable alternatives to satisfy the advanced athletic training requirement).

If seeking certification via the internship route, the NATABOC requires 1500 hours of athletic training experience under the supervision of a NATA-certified athletic trainer. Of these, at least 1000 hours must be in an athletic training facility at the interscholastic, intercollegiate, or professional sports level. The remaining 500 hours may be completed at a sports medicine clinic, campus health center, industrial health facility, other health-care facility, and/or sport camp setting under the supervision of a NATA-certified athletic trainer. These hours must be accumulated in no less than 2, nor more than 5 years.

Continuing Education Requirements

Continuing education programs provide athletic trainers with an opportunity to acquire new, innovative skills and techniques and learn about current research within the profession. Once certified as a NATA athletic trainer, the NATABOC requires eight continuing education units over a 3-year period. These may be accumulated by attending workshops, seminars, conferences, conventions, speaking at a clinical symposium, publishing professional articles, enrolling in related correspondence or postgraduate education courses, or becoming involved in the NATA certification exam testing program. In addition, current proof of CPR certification is required at least once during the CEU requirement period. For current standards of certification and continuing education requirements write to: NATA, 2952 Stemmons Freeway, Dallas, Texas 75247, or to NATABOC, 3725 National Drive, Suite 213, Raleigh, NC 27612.

Registration and Licensure

In addition to NATA certification, over 30 states now require athletic trainers to meet specific standards to practice within the individual state. This is referred to as state licensure, certification, or registration. These laws establish the legal parameters under which the athletic trainer can operate within that state and may define the specific clientele and services that may be rendered by the athletic trainer in the various work settings. Although standards vary, nearly all states accept the successful completion of the NATA examination as a basis for obtaining licensure (5). In nontraditional settings or in states that do not have licensure laws, athletic trainers may be restricted in the services they provide. Being properly licensed and practicing within established standards of practice are two of the strongest safeguards against litigation.

Did you determine what standard of care and professional conduct you should expect to receive if injured during an organized sport activity? If you determined the individual should be an NATA certified athletic trainer, you are correct.

> State licensure laws define the role of the athletic trainer and set legal parameters under which the athletic trainer can operate within that state

LEGAL LIABILITY

A sprinter on the high school track team injured her right hamstring during a race and was seen the next day by the family physician. The physician determined the runner should not participate in any activity except mild rehabilitation exercises and treatment until the next week, when she would be re-evaluated by the physician. The athletic trainer learned that over the weekend at an away meet, the coach entered the athlete in a relay, and, as a result, the runner injured the leg more severely. What implications exist concerning the athletic trainer's legal responsibility to this athlete? What action(s) should be taken relative to the coach who disregarded the physician's instructions?

Preventing injuries and reducing further injury or harm is a major responsibility for all athletic trainers. Legal action involving the practice of athletic training is typically tried under tort law. A **tort** is a civil wrong done to an individual whereby the injured party seeks a remedy for damages suffered. In lawsuits, actions are measured against a standard of care provided to those individuals for whom you have a duty to provide direct care. **Standard of care**, or liability, is defined as what another minimally competent individual educated and practicing in that profession would have done in the same or similar circumstance to protect an individual from harm or further harm (6). For example, an individual responsible for providing athletic training services would be held to a standard of care expected of a NATA-certified athletic trainer. Therefore, in states with specific registration, certification, or licensure laws, valid NATA certification and registration or licensure would be minimal protection against litigation for individuals providing athletic training services.

Duty of care is measured by what is learned, or should have been learned, in the professional preparation of an individual charged with providing health care. For example, coaches or sport supervisors should be able to assess and recognize potentially severe injuries, provide emergency first aid, and initiate appropriate referral for advanced medical care if necessary. Completing

> **Tort**
> A wrong done to an individual whereby the injured party seeks a remedy for damages suffered

> **Standard of Care**
> What another minimally competent professional educated and practicing in the same profession would have done in the same or similar circumstance to protect an individual from harm

The team physician is the final authority in measuring an individual's status for participation, regardless of the age of the participant

Negligence
Breach of one's duty of care that causes harm to another individual

To find an individual liable, the injured must prove that:
- there was a legal duty of care
- there was a breach of that duty
- there was harm caused by that breach
- the harm was a direct cause of the breach of duty

a basic athletic training class and having current certification in basic first aid and CPR would be minimal protection against litigation.

The team physician is the final authority in measuring an individual's status for participation regardless of the age of the participant. In the absence of a team physician, the final authority rests with the family physician. Parents of minors cannot assume the risk involved in sport for their child (1).

Negligence

Athletic trainers are expected to teach, supervise, inspect and provide quality safety equipment, ensure a safe environment, and provide a duty of care to all sport participants (7). Failure to provide this care can result in liability, or **negligence**.

To find an individual negligent, the injured person must prove that (1) there was a duty of care, (2) there was a breach of that duty, (3) there was harm (e.g., pain and suffering, permanent disability, or loss of wages), and (4) that the resulting harm was a direct cause from that breach of duty (7). If a spectator notices a large hole in the field prior to a game, and a player steps into the hole and breaks an ankle, the spectator is not liable because that individual has no duty of care for the player. An athletic trainer, however, does have a duty of care to the participants to check the field for hazards prior to competition. As such, the athletic trainer could be held liable for injury sustained by the participant. Although a sport participant does assume some risk inherent in any sport, the individual does not assume the risk that the professional will breach their duty of care. Negligence may occur as a result of an action or lack of an action. Situations that may lead to litigation are listed in **Table 1.3**.

Failure to Warn

Athletic trainers and coaches should inform potential athletes of the risks for injury during sport participation. Participants and parents of minor children must be informed that risk for injury exists, and understand the nature of that risk so informed judgments can be made about participation. Understanding and comprehending the nature of the risk is determined by the participant's age, experience, and knowledge of pertinent information about the risk. An advanced gymnast, for example, would know of, and appreciate, the risk of injury much more than a novice gymnast. Therefore, it is crucial to warn the novice of all inherent dangers in the activity and continually reinforce that information throughout the entire sport season. Warnings may be communicated at a preseason meeting with parents and participants, posting visible warning signs around equipment, requiring protective equipment, and discouraging dangerous techniques. Other methods that may be used are listed in **Table 1.4**.

Table 1.3. Actions That May Result in Litigation

Failure to warn an individual about the risks involved in sport participation

Treating an injured party without their consent

Failure to provide safe facilities, fields, and equipment

Being aware of a potentially dangerous situation and failing to do anything about it

Failure to provide an adequate injury prevention program

Allowing an injured or unfit player to participate, resulting in further injury or harm

Failure to provide quality training, instruction, and supervision

Using unsafe equipment

Negligently moving an injured athlete before properly immobilizing the injured area

Failure to employ qualified medical personnel

Failure to have a written emergency care procedures plan

Failure to properly recognize an injury or illness

Failure to immediately refer an injured party to the proper physician

Failure to keep adequate records

Treating an injury that did not occur in the school athletic environment

Informed Consent

Informed consent implies that an injured party has been reasonably informed of needed treatment, possible alternative treatments, and advantages and disadvantages of each course of action. To be valid, consent can only be obtained from one who is competent to grant it, that is, an adult who is physically and mentally competent, or, in the case of children under 18, only the parent can grant consent on behalf of the minor. For minors, exceptions exist in emergency situations when parents are unavailable. Authorization to treat in the absence of the parent, or in the event the individual is physically unable to consent to treatment, should be obtained in writing prior to beginning sport participation. This consent may be obtained during preparticipation meetings as part of the documentation depicting consent to participate in that activity.

Foreseeability of Harm

To recognize the potential for injury, then to remove that danger before an injury occurs, is another duty of care for athletic trainers. **Foreseeability of harm** exists when danger is apparent, or should have been apparent, resulting in an unreasonably unsafe condition **(Fig. 1.3)**. This potential for injury can be identified during regular inspections of safety equipment, athletic training facilities, and athletic areas. For example, unpadded walls under the basketball hoops, glass or potholes on playing fields, slippery floors near a whirlpool, exposed wiring, and failure to follow universal safety precautions against the spread of infectious diseases all pose a threat to safety. Unsafe conditions should be identified, reported

Informed consent
Condition whereby an injured adult, or parents of minor children are reasonably informed of needed treatment, possible alternative treatments, and advantages and disadvantages of each course of action, and give written consent to receive the treatment

Consent can only be obtained from one who is competent to grant it, that is, an adult who is physically and mentally competent, or, in the case of children under 18, the parent

Foreseeability of harm
Condition whereby danger is apparent, or should have be apparent, resulting in an unreasonably unsafe condition

in writing to appropriate personnel, restricted from use, and repaired or replaced as soon as possible.

Product Liability

Athletes, parents, coaches, and athletic trainers place a high degree of faith in the quality and safety of equipment used in sport participation. Manufacturers have a duty of care to design, manufacture, and package equipment that will not cause injury to an individual when used as intended. This is called an **implied warranty**. An **expressed warranty** is a written guarantee that the product is safe for use. Strict liability makes the manufacturer liable for all defective or hazardous equipment that unduly threatens an individual's personal safety (7,8).

Athletic trainers, coaches, fitness specialists, and sport supervisors should know the dangers involved in using sport equipment and know how to properly fit it. Furthermore, they should continually warn participants of the inherent dangers if the equipment is used in a manner for which it was not intended.

Confidentiality

A major concern affecting all individuals involved in providing health care to a sport participant is the athlete's right to privacy. If the individual is over 18 years of age, release of any medical information must be acknowledged in writing by the sport participant. This permission should identify what, if any, information should be shared with an individual other than the patient's physi-

> Manufacturers have a duty of care to design, produce, and package safe equipment that will not cause injury when used as intended

Implied warranty
Unwritten guarantee that the product is reasonably safe when used for its intended purpose

Expressed warranty
Written guarantee that states the product is safe for consumer use

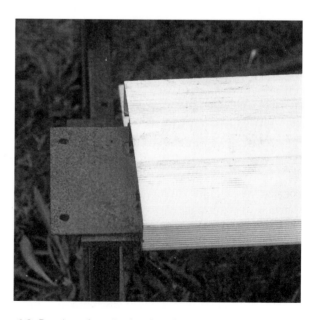

Figure 1.3. Regular safety checks of equipment can foresee the possibility of injury. Dangerous or hazardous bleachers should be repaired or replaced immediately.

Table 1.4. Strategies to Avoid Litigation

All personnel should be properly licensed and practicing within the laws
of the state, particularly in providing athletic training services

Establish strict rules for supervision and use of the facility

Have an established preparticipation plan including:

   Annual preparticipation health examination
   Insurance verification
   Medical data information cards
   Physician's clearance to participate

Hold a preseason/preparticipation meeting to:

   Inform participants and parents of the risks involved in sport
      participation
   Obtain written informed consent from the parents of minor children
      before participation

Establish a primary sports medicine team to:

   Record equipment purchases, reconditioning, and repairs
   Identify staff responsibilities during emergency situations
   Obtain adequate health insurance for participants and liability
      insurance for the staff
   Establish a communication system at each field or gymnasium
      station
   Develop standard injury documentation and referral forms
   Identify criteria to return an injured player to participation
   Select and purchase quality safety equipment from a reputable
      dealer
   Inspect safety equipment and supervise proper fitting, adjusting, and
      repair of equipment
   Inspect equipment, facilities, and fields for hazards and prohibit their
      use if found to be dangerous
   Establish policies for documentation, confidentiality, and storage of
      medical records

Post signs on and around equipment to describe proper use of the
   equipment

Require participants to wear protective equipment regularly, including
   protective eyewear in designated racquet sports

Issue only those helmets that meet standards established by the
   National Operating Commission on Standards for Athletic Equipment
   (NOCSAE)

Provide continuing education for coaches, sport supervisors, and athletic
   trainers through in-service workshops and programs

Act as a reasonably prudent professional in caring for all sport
   participants

---

cian. In many cases, schools and professional teams have the athlete give consent that all medical information can be shared between the athletic trainers and the supervising physician (9). Information provided to coaches and parents should be on a need-to-know basis only. This information should be given with the full knowledge and consent of the athlete, supervising physician, and the athletic trainer. This standard of confidentiality should also extend to all medical records kept within the confines of the athletic training room. For an individual under 18 years of age, parents or legal guardians must provide consent for the dissemination of this information.

Preventing Litigation

All members of the sports medicine team should be aware of their duty of care consistent with existing state laws, and complete that duty of care within established policies and standards of practice. Several steps can be taken to reduce the risk of subsequent litigation. Many of these steps are listed in **Table 1.4**.

The athletic trainer should have informed the coach of the physician's instructions immediately after the initial visit, and documented any subsequent care of the athlete. In addition, the athletic trainer should document the circumstances surrounding the second injury and inform the athletic director of the coach's actions should any questions arise from the athlete's parents or family physician. The athletic director may wish to speak directly with the coach concerning his/her disregard for the athlete's health and discuss how this action may now jeopardize the athletic program, and more importantly, the athlete's health.

> All members of the sports medicine team should be aware of their duty of care and complete that duty within established policies and standards of practice

MEDICAL RECORDS AND RECORD KEEPING

A individual received a severe blow to the anterior part of the right leg, which resulted in rapid swelling. The athletic trainer applied ice to limit swelling and told the individual to see a physician that day. The individual decided not to see the physician and returned home to ice the leg. Three days later, swelling was still present and the individual was unable to dorsiflex the foot. If litigation occurs as a result of this incident, what should have been done to protect against possible legal action?

> Accurate records are a major defense in litigation and serve to improve communication between all members of the primary sports medicine team

An important responsibility for athletic trainers is to develop and implement a comprehensive record-keeping system. Accurate records are critical in litigation and serve to improve communication between all members of the primary sports medicine team. Although the specific nature of record keeping will vary with the needs and function of the facility, several records should always be maintained. Documented information concerning preparticipation exams, insurance forms, personal data information cards, accident reports, daily treatments, rehabilitation programs, progress charts, and clearance for participation will document that personnel are providing their duty of care.

Preparticipation Exams

> Preparticipation exams should focus on the individual's medical history and include a physical examination of the musculoskeletal and cardiovascular systems

Preparticipation screening can determine the general health, maturity, and fitness level of an individual, detect those at risk for injury or those who may have conditions that may limit participation; identify individuals who may need counseling on health-related issues; and meet legal and insurance requirements (10,11). This screening is usually done 4 to 6 weeks prior to participation, and should be performed in the physician's office, where a more thorough and comprehensive assessment can be completed.

Although many states require annual evaluations for sport participation, many authorities now recommend complete screening examinations at the beginning of a new level of competition (junior high, high school, college), with abbreviated examinations at the start of a new sport season. The initial screening should focus on the individual's medical history and physical examination of the musculoskeletal and cardiovascular systems. Annual re-evaluations should focus on medical history and a limited physical examination, including maturity assessment; height, weight, and blood pressure measurements; cardiovascular assessment; skin examination; vision; and assessment of any new problems or evaluation of rehabilitation progress from old injuries (11).

The medical history form documents past injuries or illness, and should include specific questions for the female participant, such as menstrual or vaginal irregularities, eating habits, urinary tract disorders, and use of birth control pills or hormones (12). Medical history information should be confirmed by the parents of minor children to ensure accuracy.

The physical examination includes a general assessment of the body (**Field Strategy 1.1**) and an orthopedic assessment for muscle strength, joint laxity, posture, and cardiovascular fitness (**Field Strategy 1.2**). An example of a large station-type mass screening format to conduct multiple physical examinations can be seen in **Field Strategy 1.3**.

After the prescreening exam, the physician must determine the individual's eligibility to participate in sport. Although there are no universal standards regarding sport participation, **Table 1.5** provides a suggested list of disqualifying conditions for sport participation.

> The orthopedic exam should assess muscle strength, joint laxity, posture, and cardiovascular fitness

Medical Data Information Cards

In school programs, personal data information cards can document the individual's address and phone number, parent's address and phone number, who to contact in case of an emergency, and may also list pertinent health information, such as past injuries, medic alert conditions, and the health insurance carrier and policy number (**Fig. 1.4**). These cards should be easily accessible and carried when competitions are held at a site away from home.

Accident Reports

Accident reports document an injury, the immediate care, and instructions for follow-up care. These forms should be completed whenever an individual has to be removed from sport participation to be treated, or if the injury or illness affects participation. For example, if an individual injures an ankle during participation and

> Sport injuries should be documented if the individual has to be removed from participation or if the injury affects participation

Field Strategy 1.1. Physical Examination Record

Name _____ Date _____ Age _____ Birth date _____

Height _____ Vision: R ___ / ___ corrected _____ uncorrected _____
Weight _____   L ___ / ___ corrected _____ uncorrected _____
Pulse _____ Blood pressure _____ Percent body fat (optional) _____

	Normal	Abnormal Findings	Initials
1. Eyes			
2. Ears, nose, throat			
3. Mouth, teeth			
4. Neck			
5. Cardiovascular			
6. Chest, lungs			
7. Abdomen			
8. Skin			
9. Genitalia: hernia (male)			
10. Musculoskeletal: ROM, strength, etc			
a. neck			
b. spine			
c. shoulders			
d. arms, hands			
e. hips			
f. thighs			
g. knees			
h. ankles			
i. feet			
11. Neuromuscular			

12. Physical maturity (Tanner stage) 1   2   3   4   5

Comments re abnormal findings: _____
_____
_____
_____

Participation Recommendations
1. No participation in: _____
_____

2. Limited participation in: _____
_____

3. Requires: _____
_____

4. Full participation in: _____
_____

Physician Signature _____
Telephone number _____ Address _____
_____

Field Strategy 1.2. The Two-minute Orthopedic Scan Exam*

The athletic trainer should observe general symmetry; congenital abnormalities; hypertrophy or atrophy of the muscles; fluid joint motion; and note any discoloration, joint effusion, soft tissue edema, or deformity. Special attention should focus on joints previously injured or of special importance for the particular sport being played.

Muscular Actions	Observations and Joint Motion
Look at the ceiling, floor, over both shoulders, touch ears to shoulder	Cervical spine motion
Scapular elevation (shoulder shrugs), protraction (jut shoulders forward), and retraction (pull shoulders back)	Scapular-thoracic motion
Fully abduct and adduct shoulder	Shoulder motion
Fully rotate arms (medial and lateral)	Shoulder motion
Flex and extend elbows	Elbow motion
With arms at side and elbows flexed 90°, pronate and supinate forearm	Radial-ulnar motion
Flex and extend wrist; ulnar and radial deviation	Wrist motion
Flex and extend fingers; spread fingers; make fist	Finger motion
Raise straight leg forward, backward, to the sides	Hip motion
Flex and extend knees	Knee motion
"Duck walk" four to five steps away from examiner	Hip, knee, and ankle motion, possible knee pathology
With knees extended, touch toes	Hip motion, hamstring tightness, scoliosis
Raise up on toes	Calf symmetry, lower leg strength
Walk on heels and toes	Ankle motion

*Strength can be further assessed by adding mild resistance throughout the full range of motion.

is removed for the rest of practice to ice the region, this should be documented. If the individual injures the ankle in an unrelated sport accident and cannot participate in an activity the next day, the circumstance of injury should also be documented. This provides a record of the initial injury and lays the foundation for follow-up care. The accident report should include information such as that found in **Table 1.6**.

In litigation, these reports can document that duty of care was provided in a responsible manner. Litigation may be brought years after an injury. A statute of limitations can vary from 3 to 7 years, depending on state law. Check statutes in your state and keep all medical records in a safe, secure location for the designated time.

Accident reports document an injury, the immediate care, instructions for follow-up care, and can provide supportive evidence that duty of care was given

Field Strategy 1.3. Mass Station Screening Exam

Station	Additional Points	Personnel
1. Sign in, height, weight, vital signs, vision, body fat analysis	Blood pressure, pulse, heart (rhythm, rate, size, murmurs), visual acuity, paired eyes, equal size of pupils, protective eyewear	Trainer, nurse, or physician
2. Medical history	Personal, orthopedic, and family medical history	Trainer or nurse
3. Medical examination	Skin analysis, abdominal masses, genitalia (hernia), single organs, cardiovascular, urine analysis	Physician
4. Orthopedic examination	Postural assessment, range of motion, and muscular strength	Trainer or physician
5. Anaerobic assessment	Shuttle run, sit-ups, 40-yard dash, vertical jump	Trainer or coach
6. Aerobic assessment	Step test, timed mile run	Trainer or coach
7. Check out	Review records to determine level of participation (full, limited, no participation)	Physician

Injury Management, Rehabilitation, and Progress Charts

The physician and athletic trainer should work together to develop goals and objectives to return the injured individual to full activity. Documentation of records may include day-to-day treatment logs **(Fig. 1.5)** that record strapping or taping, therapeutic exercise logs, education or counseling provided to the individual, rehabilitation charts that detail the therapeutic exercise program, and progress notes to record the individual's movement toward attaining the goals. These documents and a final functional evaluation can help the physician determine when the individual is ready to return to full competition. All records and the physician's clearance for full participation may also be used to document duty of care and should be stored in a safe, secure location.

In administering immediate care to the individual who received a direct blow to the anterior leg, did you determine that an injury report should be completed documenting the injury and the need to see a physician? The individual should have been

All treatment and rehabilitation records, including the physician's clearance for participation, should be kept on file in a safe, secure location

Table 1.5. Disqualifying Conditions for Sport Participation

Physical Condition	Contact/ Collision	Limited Contact/ Impact	Noncontact— Strenuous	Noncontact— Moderately Strenuous	Noncontact— Nonstrenuous
Atlantoaxial instability	No	No	Yes; in swimming, no butterfly, breast stroke or diving starts	Yes	Yes
Acute illness	Requires individual assessment (e.g., contagiousness, exacerbation of illness)				
Cardiovascular					
Carditis	No	No	No	No	No
Hypertension					
Mild	Yes	Yes	Yes	Yes	Yes
Moderate	Requires individual assessment				
Severe	Requires individual assessment				
Congenital heart disease	Patients with mild forms can be allowed a full range of physical activities; patients with moderate or severe forms or those who are postoperative should be evaluated by a cardiologist before athletic participation				
Absence or loss of function in one eye	Eye guards may allow the athlete to participate in most sports, but this must be judged on an individual basis				
Detached retina	Consult an ophthalmologist				
Inguinal hernia	Yes	Yes	Yes	Yes	Yes
Absence of one kidney	No	Yes	Yes	Yes	Yes
Enlarged liver	No	No	Yes	Yes	Yes
Musculoskeletal disorders	Requires individual assessment				
History of serious head or spine trauma, repeated concussions or craniotomy	Requires individual assessment	Yes	Yes	Yes	
Convulsion disorder					
Poorly controlled	Yes	Yes	Yes	Yes	Yes
Well controlled	No	No	Yes; no swimming or weight lifting	Yes	Yes; no archery or riflery
Absence of one ovary	Yes	Yes	Yes	Yes	Yes
Pulmonary insufficiency	May be allowed to compete if oxygenation remains satisfactory during a graded stress test				Yes
Asthma	Yes	Yes	Yes	Yes	Yes
Sickle cell trait	Yes	Yes	Yes	Yes	Yes
Skin: boils, herpes, impetigo, scabies	While contagious, no contact sports or gymnastics using mats	Yes	Yes	Yes	
Enlarged spleen	No	No	No	Yes	Yes
Absent or undescended testicle	Yes; certain sports may require a protective cup	Yes	Yes	Yes	

Reproduced by permission of American Academy of Pediatrics Committee on Sports Medicine. 1988. Pediatrics, 81:737–739.

Medical Data Information Card

Name _____Age _____Gender_____ID# _____
Activity _____Sport _____

Home Address _____Phone_____
City _____State_____Zip_____

Parents/Guardian _____
Home Address _____Phone_____
City _____State_____Zip_____

In case of emergency contact: [if different than above.]
Name _____Relationship _____
Home Address _____Phone_____
City _____State_____Zip_____

Insurance carrier_____Policy number _____

Past injuries/illnesses that affected participation & dates: _____
_____

Special medic alerts or health concerns: _____
_____

Figure 1.4. Medical data information cards document pertinent personal and medical information on the individual, the contact in case of an emergency, and the current health insurance carrier and policy number.

Table 1.6. Information Needed on an Accident Report

Who was injured?
What activity was the individual participating in?
What body part was injured?
Where did the injury occur?
When did the injury occur (date and time)?
Was the individual wearing any protective equipment at the time of injury?
How did the injury occur (mechanism)?
What did you do to assess and manage the injury, including:

  History of the injury
  Observation and inspection of the injury site
  Palpation of soft and bony tissue for possible fracture
  Injury assessment and severity
  Immediate first aid care provided

What recommendation for referral to a physician was made?
Was determination of eligibility for continued participation made?
If referred to a physician, this determination should be completed by the physician and documented on the report

State College
Sports Medicine
Daily Treatments

Date _____

Name	Injury Area	Sport	Ice	Ice Massage	Ice Soak	Cold Pack	Cold Whirlpool	Contrast	Warm Whirlpool	Hydroculator	Ultrasound	Sound-Stim Come	EMS	FITRON/BIKE	BAPS Board	Multi-Axial	Cybex-Orthotron	Proprioception	Flexibility EX	Achilles Slant	Rehabilitation	Wound Cleansing	Padding	Wrap	Tape	Other	Trainer Initials

Figure 1.5. Daily treatment logs record strapping and taping, therapeutic exercise, use of modalities, and education or counseling of the individual.

instructed to have the physician complete and return the form to the athletic trainer to document the physician's orders for further care and eligibility for participation.

CAREER OPPORTUNITIES IN ATHLETIC TRAINING

Career opportunities for athletic trainers are available in both the public and private sectors. Envision yourself 10 years from now as an athletic trainer. Where would you like to be working at that time?

Today, athletic training is an excellent career choice for many women and men who want to work with interscholastic, intercollegiate, recreational, and professional athletes in a health-care environment. This allied health profession provides a challenging and valuable service needed at all levels of sport participation. Athletic trainers are generally employed in secondary school, intercollegiate, or professional athletic programs, sports medicine clinics, clinical and industrial health care programs, health and fitness clubs, or a combination of any of the above. The more common employment sites will be discussed.

High School and Collegiate Settings

High school and collegiate settings are often referred to as traditional athletic training settings. In high schools, the athletic trainer is often hired as a faculty member and given a reduced teaching load, or paid additional monies for athletic training duties. The individual begins work 2 to 3 weeks prior to the start of school with preseason practice sessions and provides health care coverage to athletes throughout the school year.

At the college level, athletic training responsibilities vary. At most colleges, the athletic trainer is hired to provide services only to athletes. In smaller schools the athletic trainer may teach part-time in the physical education or health department and provide athletic training services to athletes. The athletic trainers may also be asked to work in the campus health center supervising rehabilitation programs or educating students on health issues.

> High school and collegiate settings are often referred to as traditional athletic training sites

An advantage to working at a school site is seeing a variety of injuries, and having the satisfaction in helping competitive athletes stay healthy

Working in a school setting allows the athletic trainer to see a variety of injuries and illnesses and often contributes to general satisfaction in helping competitive athletes stay healthy. Depending on the number of athletic trainers working at the school, however, long work hours and excessive travel responsibilities can lead to premature burnout.

Sports Medicine Clinics

Privately-owned sports medicine clinics and related clinics provide a variety of job opportunities for athletic trainers (**Fig. 1.6**). Patients vary in age and level of performance and have a wider variety of conditions needing treatment. Some clinics specialize in only sport-related injuries, others deal in cardiac rehabilitation, exercise physiology, biomechanical analysis, workman's compensation injuries, or they may serve the general population. Athletic trainers working in a sports medicine clinic can expect to work a standardized work day; however, in some states, direct billing or licensure standards may restrict them from providing certain services, such as initial patient evaluation or using electrical modalities.

Dual High School/Clinic Athletic Trainer

Many sports medicine clinics hire athletic trainers to work in the clinic in the mornings and in local high schools in the afternoon

Many sports medicine clinics are subcontracting athletic training services to area high schools. The clinic hires the athletic trainer full-time, but splits the athletic trainer's time between the clinic in the morning and high school in the afternoon or evening. As

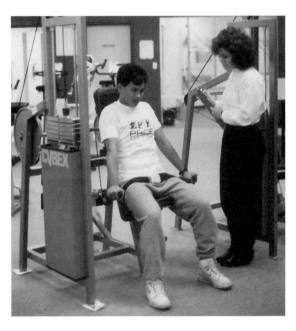

Figure 1.6. Patients at a sports medicine clinic vary in age, level of performance, and have a wider variety of conditions needing treatment.

mentioned earlier, direct billing or licensure laws may restrict some services provided by the athletic trainer in a clinic setting. This arrangement is growing in popularity throughout the United States, as evidenced in recent NATA studies (13). As licensure laws begin to adapt to the changing athletic training profession, the clinical setting may provide an excellent career option.

Industrial Health Care Programs

Many companies hire athletic trainers to provide employees with in-house athletic training services. Working under the direction of a physician, the athletic trainer can perform injury assessment, management, and rehabilitation; develop wellness and fitness programs; and provide education and counseling for employees. Not only is this cost-effective, it is also time efficient, as employees do not need to leave work for these services.

> Industries hire athletic trainers to provide employees with cost-effective in-house athletic training services

Professional Sport Teams

Athletic trainers for professional sport teams are usually hired by a single sport team to perform athletic training services throughout the year. During the competitive season the athletic trainer will concentrate on traditional duties, but during the remainder of the year, the athletic trainer may be asked to develop and supervise general conditioning programs, recruit players, do scouting, manage equipment, or make travel arrangements for the team. Salaries vary considerably, depending on the length of the playing season, revenues from television, and potential monies from playoffs and championships.

Have you determined what setting you would like to be working in as an athletic trainer? What advantages and disadvantages exist in each setting?

SUMMARY

Sports medicine applies medical and scientific knowledge to improve sport performance. The primary sports medicine team provides on-site supervision to prevent injury and deliver immediate health care. The athletic trainer, coach, sport supervisor, team physician, primary care physician, and sport participant are all members of this team. Athletic trainers are the essential link between the sport program and medical community. Working under the direction of a physician, athletic trainers are responsible for the prevention and care of athletic injuries. In addition, they are intimately involved in health care administration and continued professional development.

Standards of professional practice are ethical judgments that guide your actions and promote high standards of conduct and integrity. For an athletic trainer, NATA certification and state licensure can help meet one's duty of care in providing health care to sport participants. Decisions concerning whether or not an individual should participate in an activity should be made by the physician based on sound medical consideration. Should litigation occur, the injured person must prove that there was a duty of care, there was a breach of that duty, and there was harm caused by that breach. The athletic trainer can reduce the risk of injury and subsequent litigation by obtaining informed consent, recognizing the potential for injury and correcting it, warning participants of the risk of injury, hiring qualified personnel, and having a well-organized emergency care system.

Accurate records are a major defense in litigation and serve to improve communication between all members of the primary sports medicine team. Direct communication concerning preparticipation exams, accident reports, daily treatment or status reports, rehabilitation programs and progress charts, and clearance for participation will document that personnel are providing their duty of care.

Athletic trainers are generally employed in secondary school, intercollegiate, or professional athletic programs; sports medicine clinics; and industrial health care programs, at research facilities, health clubs, or a combination of any of the above. Each setting provides positive attributes for the athletic trainer who wants to work with athletes in a health care environment.

REFERENCES

1. Herbert DL. Legal aspects of sports medicine. Canton, OH: Professional Reports Corporation, 1990.
2. Mellion MB, and Walsh WM. The team physician. In *Sports medicine secrets*, edited by MB Mellion. Philadelphia: Hanley & Belfus, 1994.
3. NATA Board of Certification, Inc. Role Delineation Study, prepared by Columbia Assessment Services. Philadelphia: FA Davis, 1995.
4. National Athletic Trainers' Association. 1992. New NATA code of ethics approved. NATA News 4(7):15–16.
5. National Athletic Trainers' Association. 1992. Governmental affairs. NATA News 4(3):25.
6. Clement A. Law in sport and physical activity. Indianapolis: Benchmark Press, 1988.
7. Leverenz LJ, and Helms LB. 1990. Suing athletic trainers: part I, a review of the case law involving athletic trainers. Ath Train (JNATA) 25(3):212–216.
8. Leverenz LJ, and Helms LB. 1990. Suing athletic trainers: part II, implications for the NATA competencies. Ath Train (JNATA) 25(3):219–226.
9. Arendt E. 1996. What every health care professional should know. NATA News Jan:20–21.
10. Lambardo JA, Robinson JB, and Smith DM. Preparticipation physical evaluation (Monograph). Kansas City: American Academy of Family Physicians, American Academy of Pediatricians, American Medical Society for Sports Medicine, American Orthopedic Society for Sports Medicine, American Osteopathic Academy of Sports Medicine, 1992.
11. Tucker AM. The preparticipation evaluation. In *Sports medicine secrets*, edited by MB Mellion. Philadelphia: Hanley & Belfus, 1994.
12. Koester MC. 1995. Refocusing the adolescent preparticipation physical evaluation toward preventive health care. J Ath Tr 30(4):352–360.
13. NATA Professional Education Committee. 1996. Annual placement survey of graduates from athletic training educational programs. NATA News March:12–14.

The Mechanics of Tissue Injury and Healing

After completing this chapter, you should be able to:

- Define compression, tension, shear, stress, strain, bending, and torsion, and explain how each can play a role in injury to biological tissues

- Explain how the material constituents and structural organization of skin, tendon, ligament, muscle, and bone affect the ability of these structures to withstand the mechanical loads to which each is subjected

- List and describe common injuries to the skin, tendons, ligaments, muscles, and bone

- Describe the processes by which tissue healing occurs in skin, tendons, ligaments, muscles, and bone

- Explain the mechanisms by which nerves are injured and the processes by which nerves can heal

- Discuss the types of altered sensation that can result from nerve injury

- Describe how nutrition can enhance the healing process

Key Terms:

Adhesions	Cortical tissue
Afferent nerves	Cramp
Amenorrheic	Dermatomes
Anisotropic	Ecchymosis
Axial force	Edema
Ballistic stretch	Efferent nerves
Bending	Elastic limit
Bursitis	Failure
Calcific tendinitis	Fasciitis
Callus	Fracture
Cancellous tissue	Hematoma
Chemosensitive	Hypoxia
Compressive force	Interstitial tissue
Contusion	Mechanosensitive

Myositis	Strain
Myositis ossificans	Stress
Necrosis	Stress fracture
Neuroma	Tendinitis
Nociceptors	Tenosynovitis
Osteopenia	Tensile force
Referred pain	Torsion
Shear force	Viscoelastic
Spasm	Zone of primary injury
Static stretch	Zone of secondary injury

Human movement during sport and exercise is typically faster and/or produces greater force than is normally the case during activities of daily living. As a result, the potential for injury is also heightened. Understanding the different ways that forces act upon the body is necessary for understanding how to best prevent injuries. Likewise, understanding the material and structural properties of skin, tendon, ligament, muscle, bone, and nerve is essential for understanding how these tissues respond to applied forces.

This chapter begins with a general discussion of injury mechanisms, including descriptions of force and torque and their effects. Next are sections on soft tissues, bone, and nerve that address the mechanical characteristics of these tissues, the types of sport injury to which each can be subjected, and the processes by which the tissues heal. Finally, information will be provided on the essential nutrients needed to enhance the healing process.

INJURY MECHANISMS

Athletes routinely sustain larger than usual forces during both training and competition. What factors determine whether a given force results in injury?

Analyzing the mechanics of injuries to the human body is complicated by several factors. First, potentially injurious forces applied to the body act at different angles, over different surface areas, and over different periods of time. Second, the human body is composed of many different types of tissue, which respond differently to applied forces. Finally, injury to the human body is not an all or none phenomenon. That is, injuries range in severity. This section introduces the types of mechanical loading that can cause injury and describes the basic mechanical responses of biological tissues to these forms of loading.

Force and Its Effects

Force may be thought of as a push or a pull acting on a body. A multitude of forces act on the body routinely during day to day activities. The forces of gravity and friction enable an individual to move about in predictable ways when internal forces are produced by muscles. During sport participation, athletes can apply a force to a ball, bat, racquet, or club and, conversely, absorb forces from impact with a ball, the ground or floor, and an opponent.

When a force acts, there are two potential effects on the target object. The first is acceleration, or change in velocity, and the second is deformation, or change in shape. For example, when a racquetball is struck with a racquet, the ball is both accelerated (put in motion in the direction of the racquet swing) and deformed (flattened on the side struck). The greater the stiffness of the material to which a force is applied, the greater the likelihood that the deformation will be too small to be seen easily. The more elastic the material to which a force is applied, the greater the likelihood that the deformation will be temporary, with the body springing back to regain its original shape.

When a force is sustained by the tissues of the human body, two primary factors help to determine whether injury results. The first is the size, or magnitude of the force, and the second is the material properties of the involved tissues. When a relatively small force is applied, the response of the loaded structure is elastic, meaning that when the load is removed the material will return to its original size and shape. The greater the stiffness of the loaded structure, the smaller the deformation, or change in shape, in response to a given applied force. When an applied force is large enough to exceed the material's **elastic limit**, however, the structure is unable to elastically rebound to its original shape and some amount of permanent deformation results. Larger applied forces that exceed the material's ultimate failure limit produce mechanical **failure** of the structure, which translates to fracturing of bone or rupturing of soft tissues.

The direction that force is applied to biological materials also has important implications for injury potential. Many tissues are **anisotropic**, meaning that the structure is stronger in resisting force from some directions than from others. The anatomic properties of many of the joints of the human body also make them more susceptible to injury from a given direction. For example, lateral ankle sprains are much more common than medial ankle sprains because ligamentous support of the ankle is much stronger on the medial side. Consequently, in discussing injury mechanisms, force is commonly categorized according to the direction from which the force acts on the affected structure.

Force acting along the long axis of a structure is termed **axial force**. When the opponent in fencing is touched with the foil, the foil is loaded axially. When the human body is in an upright standing position, body weight creates axial loads on the femur and the tibia, the major weight-bearing bones of the lower extremity.

Axial loading that produces a squeezing or crushing effect is termed **compressive force** or compression (**Fig. 2.1**). The weight of the human body constantly produces compression on the bones that support it. The fifth lumbar vertebra must support the weight

Force produces acceleration and deformation of the object acted upon

Elastic limit
The maximum load that a material can sustain without permanent deformation

Failure
Loss of continuity; rupturing of soft tissue or fracture of bone

Anisotropic
Having different strengths in response to loads from different directions

Axial force
Force acting along the long axis of a structure

Compressive force
Axial loading that produces a squeezing or crushing effect on a structure

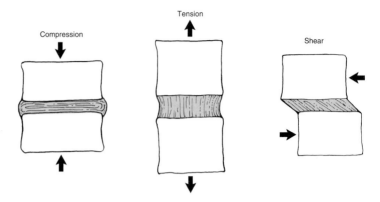

Figure 2.1. Compression and tension are directed along the longitudinal axis of a structure, whereas shear acts parallel to a surface.

of the head, trunk, and arms when the body is erect, producing compression on the intervertebral disc below it. When a football player is sandwiched between two tacklers, the force acting on the player is compressive. In the absence of sufficient padding, compressive forces sustained during contact sports often result in bruises or contusions.

Axial loading in the direction opposite that of compression is called **tensile force** or **tension (Fig. 2.1)**. Tension is a pulling force that stretches the object to which it is applied. Muscle contraction produces tensile force on the attached bone, enabling movement of that bone. When the foot and ankle are inverted or rotated excessively, the tensile forces applied to the ligaments may result in an ankle sprain.

Whereas compressive and tensile forces are directed toward and away from an object, a third category of force, termed shear, acts parallel or tangent to a plane passing through the object **(Fig. 2.1)**. **Shear force** tends to cause one part of the object to slide, displace, or shear with respect to another part of the object. Shear forces acting on the spine can cause spondylolisthesis, a condition involving anterior slippage of a vertebra with respect to the vertebra below it.

When force is sustained by the human body, another important factor related to the likelihood of injury is the magnitude of the **stress** produced by that force. Mechanical stress is defined as force divided by the surface area over which the force is applied **(Fig. 2.2)**. When a given force is distributed over a large area, the resulting stress is less than if the force were distributed over a smaller area. Alternatively, if a force is concentrated over a small area, the mechanical stress is relatively high. It is a high magnitude of stress, rather than a high magnitude of force, that tends to result in injury to biological tissues. One of the reasons that football and ice hockey players wear pads is that a pad distributes any

Tensile force
Axial loading that is opposite that of compressive force; a pulling force that tends to stretch the object to which it is applied

Shear force
A force that acts parallel or tangent to a plane passing through an object

Stress
The distribution of force within a body; quantified as force divided by the area over which the force acts

It is a high magnitude of stress rather than a high magnitude of force that causes injury

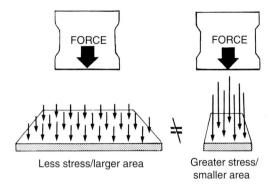

Figure 2.2. The stress produced by a force depends on the area over which the force is spread.

force sustained across the entire pad, thereby reducing the stress acting on the player.

Strain may be thought of as the amount of deformation an object undergoes in response to an applied force. Application of compressive force to an object produces shortening and widening of the structure, whereas tensile force produces lengthening and narrowing of the structure. Shear results in internal changes in the structure acted upon. The ultimate strength of biological tissues determines the amount of strain that a structure can withstand without fracturing or rupturing.

Injury to biological tissues can result from a single traumatic force of relatively large magnitude, or from repeated forces of relatively small magnitude. When a single force produces an injury, the injury is called an acute injury and the causative force is termed macrotrauma. An acute injury, such as a ruptured anterior cruciate ligament or a fractured humerus, is characterized by a definitive moment of onset followed by a relatively predictable process of healing. When repeated or chronic loading over a period of time produces an injury, the injury is called a chronic injury or a stress injury, and the causative mechanism is termed microtrauma. A chronic injury, such as glenohumeral bursitis or a metatarsal stress fracture, develops and worsens gradually over a period of time, typically culminating in a threshold episode in which pain and inflammation become evident. Chronic injuries may persist for months or years.

Many biological tissues, including tendon, ligament, muscle, and bone, tend to respond to gradually increased mechanical stress by becoming larger and stronger. When a runner's training protocol incorporates progressively increasing mileage, it is important that this occur in a gradual fashion so the body can adapt to the increased mechanical stress to prevent a stress-related injury. Overuse syndromes and stress fractures result from the body's inability to adapt to an increased training regimen.

Strain
Amount of deformation with respect to the original dimensions of the structure

Acute injuries are caused by a single force called macrotrauma

Stress injuries are caused by repeated loading called microtrauma

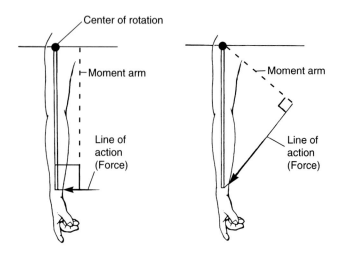

Figure 2.3. Torque created at the hinges of a door is the product of force and the force's moment arm.

Torque and Its Effects

Consider what happens when a swinging door is opened. A hand applies force to the door, causing it to rotate on its hinges (**Fig. 2.3**). Two factors influence whether the door will swing in response to the force. One factor is the force's magnitude. Equally important, however, is the force's moment arm. The moment arm is the perpendicular distance from the force's line of action to the axis of rotation. The product of a force and its moment arm is called torque, or moment. Torque may be thought of as rotary force. It is the amount of torque that determines whether a rotating structure will move.

In the human body, it is torque that produces rotation of a body segment about a joint. When a muscle develops tension it produces torque at the joint that it crosses. The amount of torque produced is the product of muscle force and the muscle's moment arm with respect to the joint center (**Fig. 2.4**). For example, the torque produced by the biceps brachii is the product of the tension developed by the muscle and the distance between its attachment on the radius and the center of rotation at the elbow.

Excessive torques can produce injury. Such torques are usually generated by forces external to the body rather than by the muscles. The simultaneous application of forces from opposite directions at different points along a structure, such as a long bone, generate a torque known as a bending moment, which can cause **bending** and, ultimately, can fracture a bone (**Fig. 2.5**). If a football player's leg is anchored to the ground and he is tackled on that leg from the front, while being pushed into the tackle from behind, a bending moment is created on the leg. When bending is present, the structure is loaded in tension on one side

Bending
Loading that produces tension on one side of an object and compression on the other side

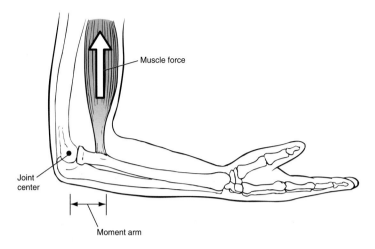

Figure 2.4. The torque produced at a joint is the product of the magnitude of muscle force and the muscle's moment arm (perpendicular distance of the muscle's line of action to the axis of rotation at the joint center).

and in compression on the opposite side **(Fig. 2.5)**. Because bone is stronger resisting compression than tension, the side of the bone loaded in tension will fracture if the bending moment is sufficiently large.

The application of torque about the long axis of a structure, such as a long bone, can cause **torsion**, or twisting of the structure **(Fig. 2.5)**. Torsion results in the creation of shear stress throughout the structure. In skiing accidents where one boot and ski are firmly planted and the skier rotates during a fall, torsional loads can cause a spiral fracture of the tibia.

When a bone bends, the side loaded in tension will fracture first

Torsion
Twisting of a structure around its longitudinal axis

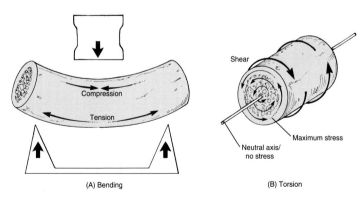

Figure 2.5. A, B. Bones loaded in bending are subject to compression on one side and to tension on the other. Bones loaded in torsion develop internal shear stress with maximal stress at the periphery and no stress at the neutral axis, as shown.

Chapter 2 The Mechanics of Tissue Injury and Healing **37**

Factors that influence the likelihood of injury when a force is sustained include force magnitude and direction, the area over which the force acts, the force's moment arm (which determines the amount of torque generated), and the type(s) of tissue affected.

SOFT TISSUE INJURIES

Tendon and ligament are both collagenous connective tissues, yet they are somewhat different in both structure and function. Based on these differences, what are the implications for injury?

Skin, tendon, ligament, and muscle are soft (non-bony) tissues that behave in characteristic ways when subjected to different forms of loading. Anatomical structure and material composition influence the mechanical behavior of each tissue.

Anatomical Properties of Soft Tissue

Skin, tendon, and ligament are named collagenous tissues after their major building block, collagen. Collagen is a protein that is strong in resisting tension. Collagen fibers have a wavy configuration in a tissue that is not in tension (**Fig. 2.6**). This enables collagenous tissues to stretch slightly under tensile loading as these fibers straighten. Thus, collagen fibers provide strength and

> Collagen resists tension and provides strength and flexibility to tissues, but is relatively inelastic

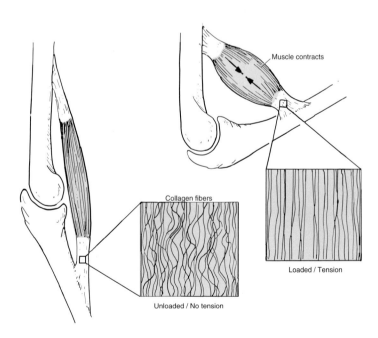

Muscle contracts

Collagen fibers

Loaded / Tension

Unloaded / No tension

Figure 2.6. Collagen fibers are wavy in configuration when unloaded and straightened when loaded in tension.

flexibility to tissues, but are relatively inelastic. Elastin, another protein, provides added elasticity to some connective tissue structures, such as the ligamentum flavum of the spine.

Skin

The skin is composed of two major regions. The outer region, the epidermis, has multiple layers containing the pigment melanin, along with the hair, nails, sebaceous glands, and sweat glands (**Fig. 2.7**). Beneath the epidermis is the dermis, containing blood vessels, nerve endings, hair follicles, sebaceous glands, and sweat glands.

The epidermis and dermis are the outer and inner layers of skin

The dermis is composed of dense irregular connective tissue, characterized by a loose, multidirectional arrangement of collagen fibers. This fiber arrangement enables the resistance of multidirectional loads, including compression, tension, and shear. This type of tissue also forms the fascia, fibrous sheets of connective tissue that surround the muscles. Dense irregular connective tissue also covers internal structures such as the liver, lymph nodes, bones, cartilages, and nerves.

Tendons, Ligaments, and Aponeuroses

Tendons connect muscle to bone, whereas ligaments connect bone to bone. Both structures are composed of dense regular connective tissue, consisting of tightly packed bundles of unidirectional collagen fibers. In tendons, the collagen fibers are arranged in a parallel pattern, enabling resistance of high, unidirectional tensile loads

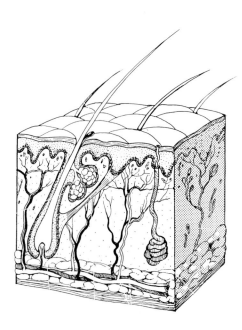

Figure 2.7. Skin. The structures contained in the epidermis and dermis.

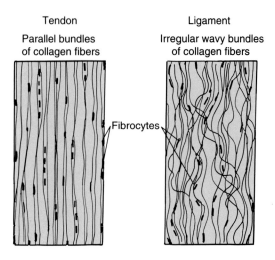

Tendon — Parallel bundles of collagen fibers

Ligament — Irregular wavy bundles of collagen fibers

Fibrocytes

Figure 2.8. Collagen arrangements in tendon and ligament.

The arrangements of collagen fibers in tendons and ligaments provide strength against the loads to which the tissues are subjected

Viscoelastic
Responding to loading over time with changing rates of deformation

Extensibility is the ability to be stretched, whereas elasticity is the ability to return to normal length after extension or shortening has taken place

Static stretch
Slow, sustained muscle stretching used to increase flexibility

Muscle is stretched more effectively by long static stretches than by short ballistic stretches

Ballistic stretch
Increasing flexibility by utilizing repetitive bouncing motions at the end of the available range of motion

when the attached muscle contracts (**Fig. 2.8**). In ligaments, the collagen fibers are largely parallel, but also interwoven among each other (**Fig. 2.8**). This arrangement is well-suited to ligament function, enabling resistance of large tensile loads along the long axis of the ligament, but also providing resistance to smaller tensile loads from other directions.

Ligaments contain more elastin than tendons, and so, are somewhat more elastic than tendons. From a functional standpoint, this is appropriate, since both ends of the ligaments are connected to bones, while tendons attach on one end to muscle, a tissue with some elasticity.

The aponeuroses are another set of structures formed by dense regular connective tissue. These are strong, flat, sheet-like tissues that attach muscles to other muscles or to bones.

Muscle

Muscle is a highly organized structure. Each muscle cell, or fiber, is surrounded by a sheath known as the endomysium. Small numbers of fibers are bound up into fascicles by a dense connective tissue sheath called the perimysium. A muscle is composed of a number of fascicles surrounded by the epimysium (**Fig. 2.9**).

The structure and composition of muscle enable it to function in a **viscoelastic** fashion—that is, muscle is characterized by both time-dependent extensibility and elasticity. Extensibility is the ability to be stretched or to increase in length, whereas elasticity is the ability to return to normal length after either lengthening or shortening has taken place. The viscoelastic aspect of muscle extensibility enables muscle to stretch to greater lengths over time in response to a sustained tensile force. This means that a **static stretch** maintained over a period of 30 seconds is more effective in increasing muscle length than a series of short **ballistic stretches**.

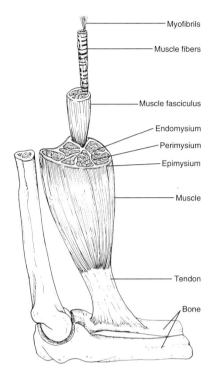

Myofibrils

Muscle fibers

Muscle fasciculus

Endomysium

Perimysium

Epimysium

Muscle

Tendon

Bone

Figure 2.9. Muscle tissue.

Another of muscle's characteristic properties, irritability, is the ability to respond to a stimulus. Stimuli affecting muscles can be either electrochemical, such as an action potential from the attaching nerve, or mechanical, as with an external blow to the muscle. If the stimulus is of sufficient magnitude, muscle responds by developing tension.

The ability to develop tension is a property unique to muscle. Although some sources refer to this ability as *contractility*, a muscle may or may not contract (shorten) when tension is developed. For example, isometric "contraction" involves no joint movement and no change in muscle length, and eccentric "contraction" actually involves lengthening of the muscle developing tension. Only when a muscle develops tension concentrically does it also shorten. When a stimulated muscle develops tension, the amount of tension present is the same throughout the muscle and tendon and at the site of the tendon attachment to bone.

Skin Injury Classifications

Forces applied to the body in different ways and from different directions result in different types of injury. Since the skin is the body's first layer of defense against injury, it is the most frequently injured body tissue.

Abrasions are common minor skin injuries caused by shear when the skin is scraped with sufficient force, usually in one direction, against a rough surface. The greater the applied force, the more layers of skin that are scraped away.

Blisters are minor skin injuries caused by repeated application of shear in one or more directions, as happens when a shoe rubs back and forth against the foot. The result is the formation of a pocket of fluid between the multiple layers of the epidermis, or between the epidermis and dermis, as fluid migrates to the site of injury.

Skin bruises are injuries resulting from compression sustained during a blow. Damage to the underlying capillaries causes the accumulation of blood within the skin.

Common minor skin injuries include abrasions, blisters, skin bruises, incisions, lacerations, avulsions, and puncture wounds

Incisions, lacerations, avulsions, and punctures are breaks in the skin resulting from injury. An incision is clean cut, produced by the application of a tensile force to the skin as it is stretched along a sharp edge. A laceration is an irregular tear in the skin that typically results from a combination of tension and shear. An avulsion is a severe laceration that results in complete separation of the skin from the underlying tissues. A puncture wound is formed when a sharp object, such as a shoe spike or nail, penetrates the skin and underlying tissues with tensile loading. The care of skin wounds with bleeding present is discussed in Chapter 3.

Other Soft Tissue Injury Classifications

Injuries to the soft tissues below the skin are also dependent upon the nature of the causative force. Other factors of relevance are the location (superficial vs. deep) and the material properties of the involved tissues.

Contusion
Compression injury involving accumulation of blood and lymph within a muscle; a bruise

Muscle **contusions**, or bruises, result from compression sustained from heavier blows. Such injuries vary in severity in accordance with the area and depth over which blood vessels are ruptured. **Ecchymosis**, or tissue discoloration, may be present if the hemorrhage is superficial. As blood and lymph flow into the damaged area, swelling occurs, often resulting in the formation of a hard mass composed of blood and dead tissue called a **hematoma**. This mass may restrict body segment range of motion. Nerve compression usually accompanies such injuries, leading to pain and sometimes temporary paralysis.

Ecchymosis
Superficial tissue discoloration

Hematoma
Localized mass of blood and lymph confined within a space or tissue

Muscle contusions are rated in accordance with the extent to which associated joint range of motion is impaired. A first degree contusion causes little to no range of movement restriction, a second degree contusion causes a noticeable reduction in range of motion, and a third degree contusion causes severe restriction of motion. With a third degree contusion, the fascia surrounding the muscle may also be ruptured, causing swollen muscle tissues to protrude.

Strains and sprains are tension injuries to tendons and ligaments, respectively

Muscle and tendon strains and ligament sprains are caused by an abnormally high tensile force that produces rupturing of the tissue and subsequent hemorrhage and swelling. The likelihood of strains and sprains depends on the magnitude of the force acting and the structure's cross-sectional area. The greater the cross-sectional area of a muscle, the greater its strength, meaning the more force it can produce and the more force is translated to the attached tendon. However, the larger the cross-sectional area of the tendon, the greater the force that it can withstand, since an increased cross-sectional area translates to reduced stress. It is almost always the muscle portion of the musculotendinous unit that ruptures first, since tendons, by virtue of their collagenous composition, are about twice as strong as the muscles to which they attach (1).

Tendons are about twice as strong as the muscles to which they are attached

Strains and sprains are categorized as first, second, and third degree. First degree strains or sprains are accompanied by some pain, but may involve only microtearing of the collagen fibers, with no readily observable symptoms. There may be mild discomfort, local tenderness, mild swelling, and ecchymosis, but no loss of function. Second degree tensile injuries of these tissues are characterized by more severe pain, more extensive rupturing of the tissue, detectable joint instability, and/or muscle weakness and limited joint range of motion. Third degree injuries of this nature produce severe pain, a major loss of tissue continuity, loss of range of motion, and complete instability of the joint (2).

Although typically not associated with injury, muscle **cramps** and **spasms** are painful involuntary muscle contractions common to the sport setting. A cramp is a painful involuntary contraction that may be clonic, with alternating contraction and relaxation, or tonic, with continued contraction over a period of time. Cramps appear to be brought on by a biochemical imbalance, sometimes associated with muscle fatigue. A muscle spasm is an involuntary contraction of short duration caused by reflex action that can be biochemically derived or initiated by a mechanical blow to a nerve or muscle.

Myositis and **fasciitis** refer, respectively, to inflammation of a muscle's connective tissues and inflammation of the sheaths of fascia surrounding portions of muscle. These are chronic conditions that develop over time as the result of repeated body movements that irritate these tissues.

Tendinitis and **tenosynovitis** are inflammation of a tendon or the tendon sheath. Tendinitis is a chronic condition characterized by pain and swelling with tendon movement. Tenosynovitis may be either acute or chronic. Acute tenosynovitis is characterized by a snapping sound with movement, inflammation, and local swelling. Chronic tenosynovitis has the added symptom of nodule formation in the tendon sheath.

Prolonged chronic inflammation of muscle or tendon can result in the accumulation of mineral deposits resembling bone in the affected tissues, known as ectopic calcification. Accumulation of mineral deposits in muscle tissue is known as **myositis ossificans**. A common site is the quadriceps region. In tendons, the condition is called **calcific tendinitis**.

Cramp
Painful involuntary muscle contractions, either tonic or clonic

Spasm
Transitory muscle contractions

Myositis
Inflammation of connective tissues within a muscle

Fasciitis
Inflammation of the fascia surrounding portions of a muscle

Tendinitis
Inflammation of a tendon

Tenosynovitis
Inflammation of a tendon sheath

Myositis ossificans
Accumulation of mineral deposits in muscle tissue

Calcific tendinitis
Accumulation of mineral deposits in a tendon

Bursitis
Inflammation of one or more bursae

Bursitis involves irritation of one or more bursae, the fluid-filled sacs that serve to reduce friction in the tissues surrounding joints. Bursitis may also be acute or chronic, brought on by either a single traumatic compression force or by repeated compressions associated with overuse of the joint.

Soft Tissue Healing

Stages of healing and repair are a) acute response (reaction phase), b) repair and regeneration, and c) remodeling

After an athletic injury has occurred, proper care involves immediate and follow-up treatments and rehabilitation. Because the normal healing process takes place in a regular and predictable fashion, the knowledgeable athletic trainer or sport supervisor can follow the various signs and symptoms exhibited at the injury site to monitor how healing is progressing. Healing of soft tissues is a three-phase process involving acute response, repair and regeneration, and remodeling. Knowing when it is appropriate to begin rehabilitation and when it is acceptable to return an athlete to practice and competition require knowledge and understanding of the healing process.

The acute phase of inflammation begins with local vasoconstriction

The immediate response to injury is the acute inflammatory phase, also known as the reaction phase, which lasts for the first several days following an injury. The characteristics of inflammation include redness, local heat, swelling, pain, and, in severe cases, loss of function. The beginning of the acute phase involves local blood vessel constriction lasting from a few seconds to as long as 10 minutes. This vasoconstriction curtails loss of blood and enables the initiation of clotting. However, the same vasoconstriction can also result in **hypoxia** and tissue **necrosis** caused by lack of oxygen to the area. Following the vasoconstriction phase, vasodilation is brought on by the presence of heparin and other chemical mediators. In conjunction with this, there is an increased blood flow to the region, causing swelling. Blood from the broken vessels and damaged local tissues form a hematoma, which, in conjunction with necrotic tissue, forms the **zone of primary injury**.

Hypoxia
Having a reduced concentration of oxygen in air, blood, or tissue; less severe than anoxia

Necrosis
Death of a tissue due to deprivation of a blood supply

Zone of primary injury
Initial region of injured tissue composed of blood and necrotic tissue

Swelling, or **edema**, occurs as the vascular walls become more permeable and increased pressure within the vessels forces plasma out into the **interstitial tissues (Fig. 2.10)**. These processes speed the arrival of several types of specialized cells that ingest dead cells and any foreign material or infectious agents, provide an anticoagulant, dilate the blood vessels and increase blood vessel permeability, and stimulate nerve endings to cause pain. This chain of chemical activity produces the **zone of secondary injury**, which includes all of the tissues affected by inflammation, edema, and hypoxia.

Zone of secondary injury
Region of damaged tissue following vasodilation

Edema
Swelling resulting from collection of exuded lymph fluid in the interstitial tissues

Interstitial tissues
Relating to spaces within a tissue or organ

Repair and regeneration of injured tissue takes place from approximately 2 days following the injury through the next 6 to 8 weeks, overlapping the later part of the acute inflammation phase. This stage begins when the hematoma is sufficiently diminished in size to allow room for the growth of new tissue. Although

Repair and regeneration overlaps the acute phase and lasts 2 days through the next 6 to 8 weeks

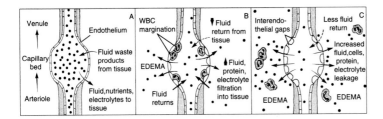

Figure 2.10. Edema forms when histochemical agents open the pores in the vascular walls, allowing plasma to migrate into the interstitial space.

the skin has the ability to regenerate new skin tissue, the other soft tissues replace damaged cells with scar tissue.

Healing through scar formation begins with the accumulation of exuded fluid containing a large concentration of protein and damaged cellular tissues. This accumulation forms the foundation for a highly vascularized mass of immature connective tissues that include fibroblasts, cells capable of generating collagen. The fibroblasts begin to produce immature collagen through a process known as fibroplasia. By the fourth or fifth day following the injury, a weak, vascular connective tissue has been produced over the injury. Over the next 2 to 4 weeks, this scar tissue increases in tensile strength and decreases in vascularity. As less new collagen is required, the number of fibroblasts at the site is reduced.

Because scar tissue is fibrous, inelastic, and nonvascular, it is less strong and less functional than the original tissues. Scar formation can reduce the structure's tensile strength by as much as 30% compared with pre-injury strength. The development of the scar also typically causes the wound to shrink in size, resulting in decreased flexibility of the affected tissues following the injury.

The final phase of injury recovery is known as the remodeling phase. This period involves maturation of the newly formed tissue, decreased fibroblast activity, increased organization of the extracellular matrix, and a return to normal histochemical activity. In soft tissue the process begins about 3 weeks post-injury, overlapping the repair and regeneration phase. It continues for a year or more as collagen fibers become oriented along the lines of mechanical stress to which the tissue is usually subjected.

Muscle fibers are permanent cells that do not reproduce in response to injury or training. However, there are reserve cells in the basement membrane of each muscle fiber that are able to regenerate muscle fiber following injury (3). Severe muscle injury can result in scarring or the formation of **adhesions** within the muscle, which inhibits muscle fiber regeneration. Following severe injury, muscle may regain only about 50% of its pre-injury strength (3). This factor has major implications toward early return to competition prior to completing a full rehabilitation program.

Since tendons and ligaments have few reparative cells, healing of these structures may take more than a year. If these tissues undergo abnormally high tensile stress before scar formation is

By the 4th or 5th day following injury, a weak, vascular connective tissue has been produced over the injury

Scar tissue is fibrous, inelastic, and nonvascular, making it less strong and less functional than the original tissues

Adhesions
Tissues that bind the healing tissue to adjacent structures, such as other ligaments or bone

complete, the newly formed tissues can be elongated. In ligaments, this may result in joint instability.

Since tendons, ligaments, and muscles hypertrophy and atrophy in response to levels of mechanical stress, complete immobilization of the injury leads to atrophy, loss of strength, and decreased rate of healing in these tissues. The amount of atrophy is generally proportional to the time of immobilization. Thus, although immobilization may be necessary to protect the injured tissues during the early stages of recovery, strengthening exercises should be implemented as soon as is appropriate during rehabilitation of the injury. The sport participant is at increased risk for reinjury as long as the affected tissues are below pre-injury strength.

💡 *Because tendons are stronger than the muscles to which they attach, the muscle, rather than the tendon, typically ruptures when the musculotendinous unit is overloaded. Although ligaments have more elasticity than tendons, because they attach at both ends to bone, they tend to rupture and/or be permanently stretched when bones displace at a joint.*

BONE INJURIES

❓ *A distance runner complains of localized pain around the head of the second metatarsal that increases after training sessions. The pain has been present for three weeks and is progressively getting worse. What injury should be suspected? What implications does this hold for the athlete's continued training?*

Bone behaves predictably in response to stress, in keeping with its material constituents and structural organization. The composition and structure of bone render a material that is quite strong for its relatively light weight.

Anatomical Properties of Bone

The primary constituents of bone are calcium carbonate, calcium phosphate, collagen, and water. The minerals, making up 60 to 70% of bone weight, provide stiffness and strength in resisting compression. Collagen provides bone with some degree of flexibility and strength in resisting tension. There is a progressive loss of collagen and an increase in bone brittleness with aging. Thus, the bones of children are more pliable than the bones of adults.

As bones develop, longitudinal bone growth continues only as long as the bone's epiphyseal plates, or growth plates, continue to exist (**Fig. 2.11**). Epiphyseal plates are cartilaginous discs found near the ends of the long bones. These are the sites where longitudinal bone growth takes place on the diaphysis (central) side of the plates. During, or shortly following, adolescence, the plate disappears and the bone fuses, terminating longitudinal growth. Most epiphyses close around age 18, although some may be present until about age 25.

Although the most rapid bone growth occurs prior to adulthood, bones continue to grow in diameter throughout most of the life-

High tensile stress before scar formation is complete can cause elongation of the new, formative tissues

Complete immobilization of an injury leads to atrophy, loss of strength, and decreased rate of healing

Collagen provides bone with some degree of flexibility and strength in resisting tension

Most epiphyses close around age 18, although some may be present until about age 25

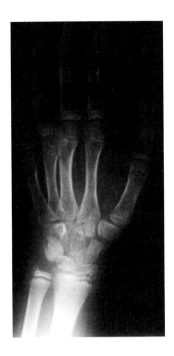

Figure 2.11. The distal epiphyseal growth plates of the radius and ulna are clearing visible on this radiograph.

span. The internal layer of the periosteum builds new concentric layers of bone tissue on top of the existing ones. At the same time, bone is resorbed or eliminated around the sides of the medullary cavity, so that the diameter of the cavity is continually enlarged. The bone cells that form new bone tissue are called osteoblasts, and those that resorb bone are known as osteoclasts. In healthy adult bone, the activity of osteoblasts and osteoclasts, referred to as bone turn-over, is largely balanced. The total amount of bone remains approximately constant until about the time that women reach their forties and men reach their sixties, when a gradual decline in bone mass begins. Sport participants past these ages may be at increased risk for bone fractures. Regular participation in weight-bearing exercise, however, has been shown to be effective in reducing age-related bone loss.

No matter what the athlete's age, some bones are more prone to fracture as a result of their internal composition. Bone tissue is categorized as either **cortical**, if the porosity is low—with 5 to 30% nonmineralized tissue—or as **cancellous**, if the porosity is high—with 30 to over 90% of nonmineralized tissue (**Fig. 2.12**). Most human bones have outer shells of cortical bone, with cancellous bone beneath. Cortical bone is stiffer, which means that it can withstand greater stress, but less strain than cancellous bone. Cancellous bone, however, has the advantage of being spongier than cortical bone, which means that it can undergo more strain before fracturing. The mineralization of cancellous bone varies with the individual's age, and location of the bone within the body. Both cortical and cancellous bone are anisotropic, which means that they exhibit different strength and stiffness in response to

Osteoblasts form new bone tissue, whereas osteoclasts resorb bone

Regular participation in weight bearing exercise has been shown to be effective to some extent in mediating age-related bone loss

Cortical
Bone tissue of relatively high density

Cancellous
Bone tissue of relatively low density

Because cortical bone is stiffer than cancellous bone, it can withstand greater stress, but less strain

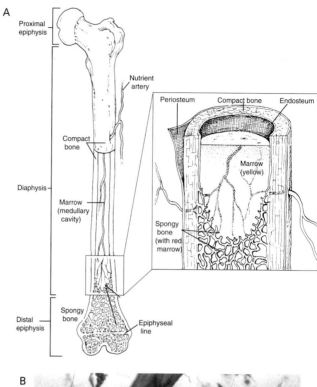

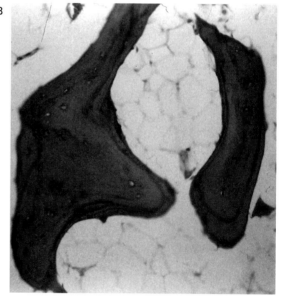

Figure 2.12. Bone macrostructure. Note the epiphyseal growth lines at either end of the bone (**A**). The cortical bone surrounds the cancellous bone and medullary cavity. Cancellous bone is more porous than cortical bone, as can be seen in the electron micrograph photo above (**B, C**).

C

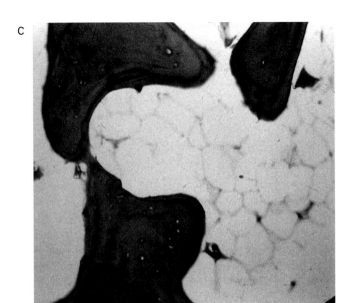

Figure 2.12. *(continued).*

forces applied from different directions. Bone is strongest in resisting compressive stress and weakest in resisting shear stress.

Bone size and shape also influence the likelihood of fracture. The shape and size of a bone is largely determined by the direction and magnitude of forces to which they are habitually subjected. The direction in which new bone tissue is formed has been found to be adapted to best resist the loads encountered, particularly in regions of high stress, such as the femoral neck. The mineralization and girth of bone increase in response to increased stress levels. For example, the bones of the dominant arm of professional tennis players and professional baseball players have been found to be larger and stronger than the bones of their nondominant arms (4,5).

Bone Injury Classifications

A **fracture** is a disruption in the continuity of a bone (**Fig. 2.13**). The type of fracture sustained depends on the type of excessive mechanical loading, as well as the health and maturity of the bone at the time of injury. Fractures are said to be simple when the bone ends remain intact within the surrounding soft tissues and compound when one or both bone ends protrude from the skin.

Since bone is stronger in resisting compression than both tension and shear, acute compression fractures of bone are rare. Under combined loading, however, a fracture resulting from a torsional load may be impacted by the presence of a compressive load. An impacted fracture is one in which the opposite sides of the fracture are compressed together. Fractures that result in

Bone is strongest in resisting compression and weakest in resisting shear

The mineralization and girth of bone increase in response to increased stress levels

Fracture
A disruption in the continuity of a bone

Fractures are simple when the bone ends remain intact within the surrounding soft tissues and compound when one or both bone ends protrude from the skin

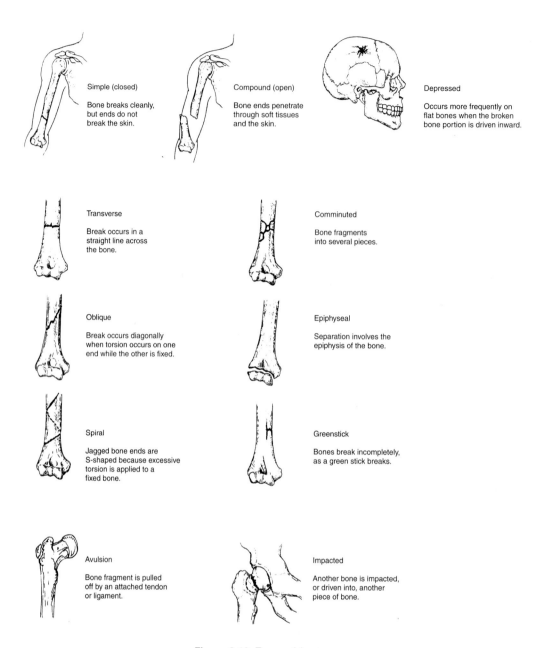

Simple (closed)

Bone breaks cleanly, but ends do not break the skin.

Compound (open)

Bone ends penetrate through soft tissues and the skin.

Depressed

Occurs more frequently on flat bones when the broken bone portion is driven inward.

Transverse

Break occurs in a straight line across the bone.

Comminuted

Bone fragments into several pieces.

Oblique

Break occurs diagonally when torsion occurs on one end while the other is fixed.

Epiphyseal

Separation involves the epiphysis of the bone.

Spiral

Jagged bone ends are S-shaped because excessive torsion is applied to a fixed bone.

Greenstick

Bones break incompletely, as a green stick breaks.

Avulsion

Bone fragment is pulled off by an attached tendon or ligament.

Impacted

Another bone is impacted, or driven into, another piece of bone.

Figure 2.13. Types of fractures.

depression of bone fragments into the underlying tissues are termed depressed.

Since the bones of children contain larger relative amounts of collagen than adult bones, they are more flexible and resistant to fracture than adult bones. Consequently, greenstick fractures, or incomplete fractures, are more common in children than in adults, and are typically caused by bending or torsional loads.

Avulsions are another type of fracture caused by tensile loading; they involve a tendon or ligament pulling a small chip of bone

Greenstick fractures are more common in children than adults

away from the rest of the bone. Explosive throwing and jumping movements may result in avulsion fractures. When loading is very rapid, a fracture is more likely to be comminuted, containing multiple fragments.

Stress fractures result from repeated low-magnitude forces and differ from acute fractures, in that they worsen over time. These overuse fractures begin as a small disruption in the continuity of the outer layers of cortical bone and eventually result in complete cortical fracture with possible displacement of the bone ends. Stress fractures of the metatarsals, the femoral neck, and the pubis have been reported among runners who have apparently overtrained. Stress fractures of the pars interarticularis region of the lumbar vertebrae have also been reported to occur in higher than normal frequencies among female gymnasts and football linemen (6).

Osteopenia, a condition of reduced bone mineral density, predisposes the athlete to fractures of all kinds, but particularly to stress fractures. The condition is primarily found among adolescent female athletes, especially distance runners, who are **amenorrheic**. Although amenorrhea among this group is not well understood, it appears to be related to low percent body fat and/or high training mileage. The link between cessation of menses and osteopenia is also not well understood. Possible contributing factors include hyperactivity of osteoclasts, hypoactivity of osteoblasts, hormonal factors, and insufficiencies of dietary calcium or other minerals or nutrients.

> When loading is very rapid, the fracture is more likely to contain multiple fragments

Stress fracture
Fracture resulting from repeated loading with relatively lower magnitude forces

Osteopenia
Condition of reduced bone mineral density that predisposes the individual to fractures

Amenorrheic
Having an absence or abnormal cessation of menstruation

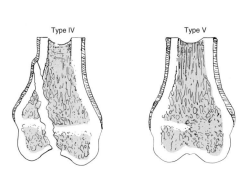

Figure 2.14. Epiphyseal injuries.

Epiphyseal Injury Classifications

The bones of children and adolescents are more prone to growth-plate injuries and avulsion fractures, rather than ligament and muscle-tendon injuries, which are more commonly seen in adults. These epiphyseal injuries may involve the cartilaginous epiphyseal plate, articular cartilage, or apophysis (**Fig. 2.14**). The apophyses are sites where a major tendon attaches onto a growing bony prominence. The bone shape is influenced by the tensile loads produced by the contracting musculotendinous unit. The epiphyses of long bones are known as pressure epiphyses, the apophyses are known as traction epiphyses, after the types of physiological loading present at these sites. Both acute and repetitive loading can injure the growth plate, potentially resulting in premature closure of the epiphyseal junction and termination of bone growth. "Little league elbow," or medial epicondylitis, for example, is a stress injury to the medial epicondylar epiphysis of the humerus.

> Both acute and repetitive loading can injure the growth plate, potentially causing premature closure of the epiphyseal junction and termination of bone growth

Salter (7) has categorized acute epiphyseal injuries as follows:

Type I   Complete separation of the epiphysis from the metaphysis with no fracture to the bone
Type II   Separation of the epiphysis and a small portion of the metaphysis
Type III Fracture of the epiphysis
Type IV   Fracture of a part of the epiphysis and metaphysis
Type V   Compression of the epiphysis without fracture, resulting in compromised epiphyseal function

Another category of epiphyseal injuries is referred to collectively as osteochondrosis. Osteochondrosis results from a disruption of the blood supply to an epiphysis, with associated tissue necrosis and potential deformation of the epiphysis. Osteochondrosis occurs more commonly between the ages of 3 and 10 and is more prevalent among boys than girls (7). Specific disease names have been given to osteochondrosis at the sites of most common occurrence. For example, Legg-Calvé-Perthes' disease is osteochondrosis of the femoral head and is discussed later in the text.

> Disruption of blood supply to an epiphysis produces osteochondrosis

The apophyses are also subject to osteochondrosis, particularly among adolescent athletes. These conditions, referred to as apophysitis, may be idiopathic and are often associated with traumatic avulsion-type fractures. Common apophyseal injuries and their sites include Sever's disease (posterior calcaneus), Osgood-Schlatter disease (tibial tuberosity), Larsen-Johansson syndrome (inferior patella), medial epicondylitis (medial epicondyle of humerus), and apophysitis of the hip (iliac crest, ischial tuberosity) (8). These conditions will be discussed later in the text.

Bony Tissue Healing

Healing of acute bone fractures is a three phase process, just as with soft tissue healing. The acute inflammatory phase lasts approximately 4 days. Damage to the periosteum and surrounding soft tissues results in the formation of a hematoma in the medullary canal and surrounding tissues. The ensuing inflammatory response

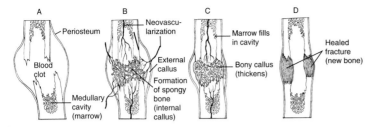

Figure 2.15. The process of enchondral bone healing through callus formation.

involves vasodilation, edema formation, and histochemical changes associated with soft tissue inflammation.

In the repair and regeneration phase, osteoclasts resorb damaged bone tissues, while osteoblasts build new bone. Between the fractured bone ends, a fibrous vascularized tissue known as a **callus** is formed (**Fig. 2.15**). The callus contains weak, immature bone tissue that strengthens with time through bone remodeling. The process of callus formation is known as enchondral bone healing. An alternative process, known as direct bone healing, can occur when the fractured bone ends are immobilized in direct contact with one another. This enables new, interwoven bone tissue to be deposited without the formation of a callus. Unless a fracture is surgically fixed by metal plates, screen, rods, or screws, healing normally takes place through the enchondral process (3). Because noninvasive treatment is generally preferred, a fixation device is only implanted when it appears unlikely that the fracture will heal acceptably without one.

Remodeling of bone tissue involves osteoblast activity on the concave side of the fracture, which is loaded in compression, and osteoclast activity on the convex side of the fracture, which is loaded in tension. The process continues until normal shape is restored and bone strength is commensurate with the loads to which the bone is routinely subjected.

Because stress fractures continue to worsen as long as the site is overloaded, it is important to recognize these injuries as early as possible. Elimination or reduction of the repetitive mechanical stress causing the fracture is the primary factor necessary for healing. This allows a gradual restoration of the proper balance of osteoblast and osteoclast activity present in the bone.

💡 *Pain localized around the second metatarsal head in a runner's foot is a classic symptom of a stress injury. The runner should be referred to a physician. If a fracture is present, activity should be curtailed until the injury has healed and the athlete has been cleared for participation by the supervising physician.*

NERVE INJURIES

❓ *A football lineman is complaining of pain radiating down the posterior aspect of the left leg. What condition might be suspected because of the radiating pain? Is medical referral necessary for this type of injury?*

Callus
Fibrous tissue containing immature bone tissue that forms at fracture sites during repair and regeneration

Fracture healing normally involves callus formation

It is important to recognize stress injuries as early as possible because they tend to worsen with time

The nervous system is divided into the central nervous system, consisting of the brain and spinal cord, and the peripheral nervous system, which includes 12 pairs of cranial nerves and 30 pairs of spinal nerves, along with their branches **(Fig. 2.16)**. Injuries to any of these nerves can be devastating to the individual and may lead to temporary or permanent disability.

Anatomical Properties of Nerves

Each spinal nerve is formed from anterior and posterior roots on the spinal cord that unite at the intervertebral foramen. The posterior branches are the **afferent** (sensory) **nerves** that transmit information from sensory receptors in the skin, tendons, ligaments, and muscles to the central nervous system. The anterior branches are the **efferent** (motor) **nerves** that transmit control signals to the muscles. The nerve fibers are heavily vascularized and are encased in a multi-layered protective sheath of connective tissue.

Nerve Injury Classifications

Nerves are most commonly injured by tensile or compressive forces. Tensile injuries of nerves typically occur during severe high-speed accidents, such as automobile accidents or high-speed impact collisions in contact sports (9). When a nerve is loaded in tension, the nerve fibers tend to rupture prior to the rupturing

Afferent nerves
Nerves carrying sensory input from receptors in the skin, muscles, tendons, and ligaments to the central nervous system

Efferent nerve
Nerves carrying stimuli from the central nervous system to the muscles

Both tensile and compressive forces can injure nerves

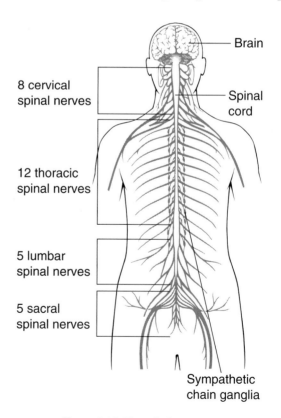

8 cervical
spinal nerves

12 thoracic
spinal nerves

5 lumbar
spinal nerves

5 sacral
spinal nerves

Brain

Spinal
cord

Sympathetic
chain ganglia

Figure 2.16. The spinal nerves.

of the surrounding connective tissue sheath (10). Because the nerve roots on the spinal cord are not protected by connective tissue, they are particularly susceptible to tensile injury, especially stretching of the brachial plexus or cervical nerve roots.

Compressive injuries of nerves are more complex because their severity depends on the magnitude and duration of loading and whether the applied pressure is direct or indirect (9). Since nerve function is highly dependent on oxygen provided by the associated blood vessels, damage to the blood supply caused by a compressive injury results in damage to the nerve.

Nerve injuries can result in a range of afferent symptoms, from complete loss of sensation to severe pain. Terms used to describe altered sensation include hypoesthesia, a reduction in sensation; hyperesthesia, heightened sensation; and paresthesia, a sense of numbness, prickling, or tingling. Pinching of a nerve can result in a sharp wave of pain that is transmitted through a body segment. Irritation or inflammation of a nerve can result in chronic pain along the nerve's path.

Pinching of a nerve can result in a sharp wave of pain or burning sensation that is transmitted through a body segment

Nerve Healing

When a nerve is completely severed, healing does not occur and loss of function is typically permanent. Unless such injuries are surgically repaired, random regrowth of the nerve occurs, resulting in the formation of a **neuroma**, or nerve tumor.

When nerve fibers are ruptured in a tensile injury, but the surrounding myelin sheath remains intact, it is sometimes possible for a nerve to regenerate along the pathway provided by the sheath during healing. Such regeneration is relatively slow, however, proceeding at a rate of less than 1 mm per day or about 2.5 cm per month (3).

Neuroma
A nerve tumor

💡 *Pain radiating down the posterior aspect of a leg is symptomatic of sciatic nerve injury or impingement and may indicate a herniated disc. The athlete should be referred immediately to a physician for evaluation.*

PAID

❓ *Two teammates each sprain an ankle at about the same time and damage similar structures. While rehabilitating the ankles, one athlete shirks exercises because of excessive pain, and the other performs workouts without complaint. What variables may be at work here?*

Pain is a universal symptom common to most injuries. It is important to recognize that the individual's perception of pain is influenced by a host of physical, chemical, social, and psychological factors.

Neurological Basis of Pain

Pain is brought about by stimulation of specialized afferent nerve endings called **nociceptors**. With most acute sport-related injuries, pain is initiated by **mechanosensitive** nociceptors responding

Nociceptors
Specialized nerve endings that transduce pain

Mechanosensitive
Sensitive to mechanical stimulation

Chemosensitive
Sensitive to chemical
stimulation

to the traumatic force that caused the injury. With chronic injuries and during the early stages of healing of acute injuries, pain persists due to the activation of **chemosensitive** nociceptors.

Small-diameter, slow transmission nerves carry pain impulses; large-diameter, fast transmission nerves carry other sensations, such as touch, temperature, and proprioception. Both types of fibers communicate with the spinal cord through the substantia gelatinosa (SG) of the cord's dorsal horn. Specialized T cells then transmit impulses from all of the afferent fibers up the spinal cord to the brain, with each T cell carrying a single impulse.

The substantia gelinosa of the dorsal spinal cord is believed to function as a gatekeeper for pain impulses entering the central nervous system

In the gate control theory of pain, the SG acts as a gate keeper to allow either a pain response or one of the other afferent sensations to be transported by each T cell (11). The theory is substantiated by the observation that increased sensory input can reduce the sensation of pain. For example, extreme cold can often numb pain. Because hundreds or thousands of "gates" are in operation, however, it is more common that added sensory input reduces, rather than eliminates, the feeling of pain since pain impulses get through to some of the T cells.

Factors That Mediate Pain

The body produces pain-killing chemicals similar to morphine called beta-endorphin and methionine enkephalin. Both work by blocking neural receptor sites that transmit pain. Several different sites in the brain produce endorphins. Stressors, such as physical exercise, mental stress, and electrical stimulation, provoke the release of endorphins into the cerebrospinal fluid. A phenomenon called "runner's high," a feeling of euphoria that occurs among long-distance runners, has been attributed to endorphin release. The brain stem and pituitary gland produce enkephalins. Enkephalins block pain neurotransmitters in the dorsal horn of the spinal cord.

Morphine-like chemicals called endorphins and enkephalins are produced naturally by the body in response to stressors

The central nervous system also imposes a set of cognitive and affective filters on both the perception of pain and the subsequent expression of perceived pain. Social and cultural factors can be powerful influences on pain tolerance level. In American society, for example, it is much more acceptable for females than for males to express feelings of pain. Individual personality and a state of mental preoccupation can also be significant mediators of pain.

Referred Pain and Radiating Pain

Referred pain
Pain felt in a region of the body other than where the source or actual cause of the pain is located

Referred pain is pain that is perceived at a location remote from the injured site. One possible explanation is that neurons carrying pain impulses split into several branches within the spinal cord. Although some of these branches connect with other pain transmitting fibers, some also connect with afferent nerve pathways from the skin. This cross-branching can cause the brain to misinterpret the true location of the pain (12).

In at least some instances, referred pain behaves in a logical and predictable fashion. For example, pain from the internal organs is typically projected outward to corresponding **dermatomes** of the skin, as is the case with a heart attack or a ruptured spleen or kidney.

Referred pain should not be confused with radiating pain, which is pain that is felt both at its source and along a nerve. Pinching of the sciatic nerve at its root may cause pain to radiate along the length of the nerve as it travels down the posterior aspect of the leg.

Differences in pain perception and tolerance can be caused by differences in chemical, social, and psychological influences, as well as by differences in the severity of the original injury and the progression of the healing process.

Dermatomes
A region of skin supplied by a single afferent neuron

Radiating pain is felt both at its source and along a nerve

NUTRITION

Think for a minute or two about how nutrition can influence the repair and healing process of damaged tissue. Can an individual return to peak performance without the necessary energy sources?

Proper nutrition for an active individual is essential to provide the necessary nutrients to perform work. In addition, extended inactivity can result in a slight weight gain, placing additional stress on injured joint structures. As such, cardiovascular endurance activities should be initiated as soon as possible to simply burn calories.

Carbohydrates are the main energy fuel for the body. In addition, the brain uses blood glucose almost exclusively as its fuel and does not have a stored supply of this nutrient. Although fat does provide a large store of potential energy and serves as a cushion to protect the vital organs and provide thermal insulation, it has little function in wound healing. Proteins serve a vital role in the maintenance, repair, and growth of body tissues. When carbohydrate reserves are low, the synthesis of glucose will draw upon protein, thus further draining the body's protein "stores," especially muscle protein. In extreme conditions, this can lead to a reduction in lean tissue and place an excessive load on the kidneys as they excrete the nitrogen-containing by-products of protein breakdown (13). Without an adequate carbohydrate and protein intake, repair and healing of damaged tissues will be prolonged.

Vitamins also play an important role in wound healing. Riboflavin (vitamin B_2), pyridoxine (vitamin B_6), pantothenic acid, folacin, and vitamin B_{12} all aid in energy metabolism. Vitamin C maintains the intercellular matrix of cartilage, bone, and dentine, and is required for collagen secretion. A lack of vitamin C can result in deficient wound healing, evident in inferior vascularization and scanty collagen deposition. Vitamin A is necessary to maintain epithelial tissue and vitamin D promotes growth and mineralization of bones and aids in the absorption of calcium. Vitamin E

Food Guide Pyramid
A Guide to Daily Food Choices

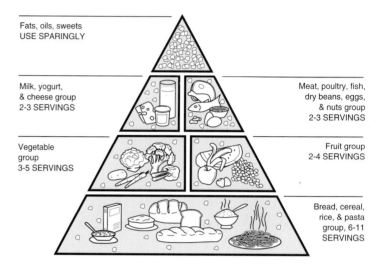

Figure 2.17. The US Department of Agriculture (USDA) now recommends a diet high in fruits, vegetables, and grains and a low intake of fat and sugar.

prevents cell membrane damage, and vitamin K is essential in blood clotting (13).

Calcium aids in blood clotting and, coupled with sodium, is necessary for proper nerve function. Zinc is known to promote faster healing. Water is essential to transport nutrients, control thermoregulation, and aid in metabolic reactions (13).

The food guide pyramid now recommends that a diet should be high in fruits, vegetables, and grains and low in fat and sugar **(Fig. 2.17)**. Under normal circumstances, this diet should provide an adequate source of carbohydrates, protein, fat, vitamins, minerals, and water to promote wound healing and prevent unnecessary weight gain. Dietary supplements are not necessary if the individual's diet is nutritionally balanced.

An injured individual must have an adequate diet that provides the nutrients necessary to enhance wound healing. In addition, a diet high in carbohydrates should supply the energy necessary to compete on a highly competitive level.

SUMMARY

The nature of a sports-related injury depends on the magnitude, direction, and point of application of the applied force(s), as well as on the health and strength of the affected tissues. When the force acting on a structure exceeds the structure's ultimate failure limit, failure occurs. This translates to fracturing of bone and rupturing of soft tissues. Biological tissues are strongest in resisting the form of loading to which they are most commonly subjected. The material compositions of skin, tendon, ligament, and muscle make them particularly strong in resisting tension, whereas bone is strongest in resisting compression.

The body's response to injury is a well-ordered, predictable process. The initial reaction is known as the acute inflammatory phase, which lasts for approximately the first 4 days following injury. During this phase, subcellular agents are rushed to the site to remove the damaged tissue. From about 2 days through the next 6 weeks following the injury, the repair and regeneration phase sets in. In this phase, fibroblasts produce a scar over soft tissue ruptures and osteoblasts produce a callus across most bone fractures. The final phase, known as the remodeling or maturation phase, begins about 3 weeks post-injury and lasts a year or more as the tissues strengthen and become reoriented along lines of mechanical stress.

The pain associated with injuries is caused by mechanical and/ or chemical insult to the nerves. Nerves can be injured through both tensile and compressive overloads. Only when the protective sheath surrounding the nerve remains intact can nerve regeneration occur following an injury.

REFERENCES

1. Elliott DH. 1967. The biomechanical properties of tendon in relation to muscular strength. Ann Phys Med 9:1.
2. Carlstedt CA, Nordin M. Biomechanics of tendons and ligaments. In *Basic biomechanics of the musculoskeletal system*, edited by M Nordin and VH Frankel. Philadelphia: Lea & Febiger, 1989.
3. American Academy of Orthopaedic Surgeons. *Athletic training and sports medicine*. Park Ridge, IL: American Academy of Orthopaedic Surgeons, 1991.
4. Jones HH, et al. 1977. Humeral hypertrophy in response to exercise. J Bone Joint Surg 59A:204–208.
5. Watson RC. Bone growth and physical activity. In *International conference on bone measurements*, edited by RB Mazess. DHEW Pub No NIH 75-683, Washington, DC, 1973.
6. Jackson DW, Wiltse LL, and Cirincione RJ. 1976. Spondylolysis in the female gymnast. Clin Orthop Rel Res 117:68–73.
7. Salter RB. *Textbook of disorders and injuries of the musculoskeletal system*. Baltimore: Williams & Wilkins, 1983.
8. Peck DM. 1995. Apophyseal injuries in the young athlete. Am Fam Phys 51(8):1891–1898.
9. Rydevik B, Lundborg G, and Skalak R. Biomechanics of peripheral nerves. In *Basic biomechanics of the musculoskeletal system*, edited by M Nordin and VH Frankel. Philadelphia: Lea & Febiger, 1989.
10. Sunderland S. *Nerves and nerve injuries*. Edinburgh: Churchill Living-stone, 1978.
11. Newton RA. Contemporary views on pain and the role played by thermal agents in managing pain symptoms. In *Thermal agents in rehabilitation*, edited by S Michlovitz. Philadelphia: FA Davis, 1990.
12. Ottoson D, and Lundberg T. *Pain treatment by transcutaneous electrical nerve stimulation: A practical manual*. New York: Springer-Verlag, 1988.
13. McArdle WD, Katch FI, and Katch VL. *Exercise physiology: energy, nutrition, and human performance*. Philadelphia: Lea & Febiger, 1993.

Sports Injury Management

Chapter 3: **Emergency Procedures**

Chapter 4: **Sports Injury Assessment**

Chapter 5: **Therapeutic Exercise and Therapeutic Modalities**

Chapter 6: **Protective Equipment**

Chapter 7: **Protective Taping and Wraps**

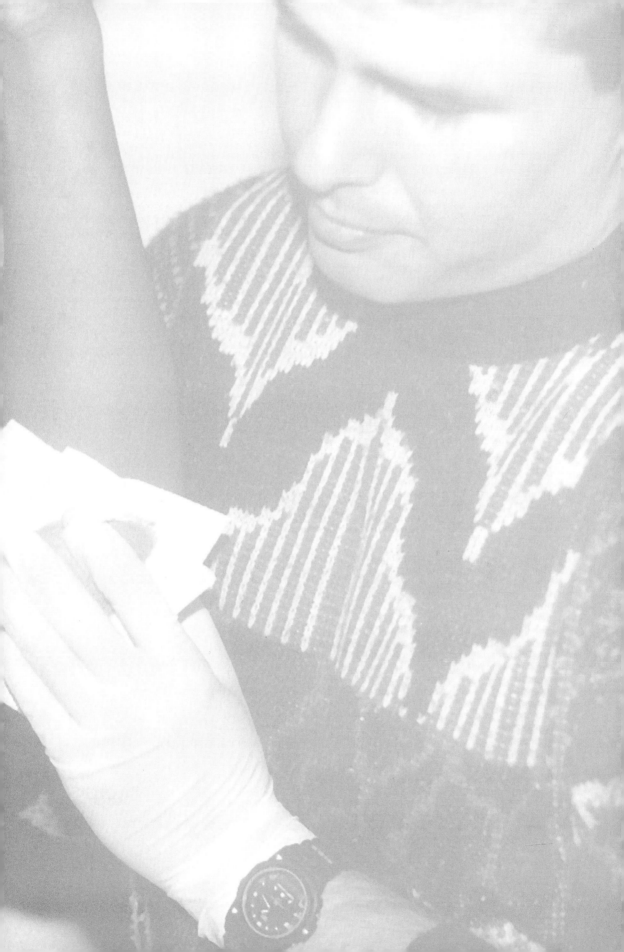

Kathy Fox, MA, ATC, PT, SCS

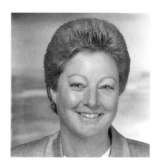

Like many people in athletic training, I got interested in the profession after an injury. As a result, I went to the State University of New York at Cortland for an undergraduate degree in education with emphasis in athletic training, then went right into graduate school at Miami University in Ohio. Although I currently work at Braintree Hospital in the outpatient physical therapy clinic, I administer the entire sports medicine program for the hospital and its 35 satellite clinics.

As an administrator, I am responsible for the budget, hiring, and evaluation of the athletic trainers, procuring high school contracts, marketing and public relations for the program, and serving as a sounding board and ombudsman for the staff. I love the administrative part of this job, especially working with the public to advance the visibility of the athletic training profession. As an advocate for the profession, I require my entire staff to do community service presentations 3 to 4 times each year. At first, some were reluctant to do public speaking; however, many now present regularly at the state athletic training meetings, annual physical education, recreation, and dance conventions, and participate in regular workshops and seminars for C.E.U. credit for area NATA-certified athletic trainers.

The athletic trainers who work in the clinic really have a limited role. They serve mainly as clinical aides and perform tasks such as applying superficial heat and cold, supervising an established strengthening program, assisting in setting up the treatment area, and making sure the facility is clean and neat. Unfortunately, in our state, these trainers are not being utilized to their fullest potential because of the current licensure law and third-party billing policies.

All of the trainers split their time between the clinic and an area high school or college. The workload averages about 40 hours per week and, as such, there is less burnout among our employees. We provide a full-time salary and health benefits, and pay the trainers for their travel time and mileage to the school. A dual position provides a unique opportunity to maintain skills in two separate environments, treat a more diverse clientele over a wider age range, and see a broader array of orthopedic injuries and conditions.

Although area schools could benefit more from a full-time trainer on staff to supervise on-site rehabilitation and follow the athlete through the entire injury healing process, we provide a community service that is unequaled in the area. We provide on-site health care for the athletic program, immediate access to any medical specialist in the field, a comprehensive rehabilitation team, and an array of professional consultants who work with area communities to provide a holistic health care system for their children. From a business perspective, the hospital loses out because the athletic trainers are locked into a morning schedule in the clinic to accommodate the schools in the afternoon, evenings, and weekends. In the summer, however, the athletic trainers are in the clinic 40 hours a week. While there, they cannot practice to the full potential of their license in the nontraditional setting. This is really unfortunate. To my knowledge, only one state, Missouri, has taken a leadership role in changing this dilemma.

If you are interested in working in a clinic in a dual role, I would suggest getting dual certification as a physical therapy assistant or physical therapist, just because of the third-party billing situation. I also think it's imperative that people in athletic training be committed to teaching athletic training in one way or another. This doesn't necessarily have to be in a classroom setting, but it means being an advocate for the profession by taking knowledge and respecting it enough to share it with others. It implies that you are committed to your profession and to improving that profession. That's what really identifies great athletic trainers.

Kathy Fox is a vocal advocate for the athletic training profession. In her dual role as an athletic trainer and physical therapist, she has worked extensively in sports medicine clinics and in area high schools. She is now the Director of the Sports Medicine Program for the Braintree Hospital Rehabilitation Network in Braintree, Massachusetts.

Emergency Procedures

After completing this chapter, you should be able to:

- Describe the signs, symptoms, and management of potentially life-threatening conditions

- Identify preventative measures to reduce the risk of life-threatening conditions

- Indicate major components of an emergency procedures plan

- Describe the procedures and techniques used in a primary and secondary injury assessment

- Identify emergency conditions that warrant immediate action by emergency medical services (EMS)

- Describe proper procedures to transport a seriously injured individual

Key Terms:

Acclimatization	Primary survey
Crepitus	Pupillary light reflex
Cyanosis	Rubor
Diastole	Secondary survey
Diplopia	Sign
Emergency plan	Symptom
Heat cramps	Systole
Hyperthermia	Total airway obstruction
Hypothermia	Triage
Pallor	Unconsciousness
Partial airway obstruction	Vital signs

Serious injuries can be frightening, particularly when breathing or circulation is impaired or the individual is unconscious. As the first person on the scene, you are expected to evaluate the situation, assess the extent and seriousness of injury, recognize life-threatening conditions, provide immediate emergency care, and initiate any emergency procedures to provide follow-up medical care. Although few sport-related injuries are serious enough to impair breathing or circulation, these injuries do occur.

In this chapter you will first learn what conditions may pose a threat to an individual's life. Next, the importance of developing an emergency care plan by facility personnel and local emergency medical services (EMS) will be introduced. You will then move step by step through a primary and secondary survey to determine if an emergency exists and EMS should be summoned. Finally, after summoning EMS, you will learn how to assist the emergency medical team to secure a seriously injured individual to a stretcher in preparation to transport the individual to a nearby medical facility.

EMERGENCY SITUATIONS

? *Think for a minute or two about what injuries or conditions might become life threatening to an individual. Although these injuries or conditions may occur during sport participation, they may not be directly related to the actual participation. As such, an understanding of these conditions can aid in early recognition and treatment.*

Injuries or conditions that impair, or have the potential to impair, vital function of the central nervous system and cardio-respiratory system are considered emergency situations. Many serious injuries are clearly evident and recognizable, such as lack of breathing or absence of a pulse. These conditions are identified by checking the **ABCs**: **A**irway, **B**reathing, **C**irculation, and **s**evere arterial bleeding. This immediate **primary survey** determines unresponsiveness, recognizes and identifies immediate life-threatening situations, and dictates what action is needed to care for the individual. Other conditions, however, such as internal bleeding, shock, or heat stress, may cause the individual's condition to slowly deteriorate. A **secondary survey** involves a more detailed, hands-on, head-to-toe assessment to detect conditions that may not, in themselves, pose an immediate threat to life, but if left unrecognized and untreated, could lead to serious complications.

To recognize an injury, symptoms and diagnostic signs are gathered. A **symptom** is information provided by the injured individual regarding their perception of the problem. These conditions, or subjective feelings, include blurred vision, ringing in the ears, fatigue, dizziness, nausea, headache, pain, weakness, or an inability to move a body part. A diagnostic **sign** is a measurable physical finding regarding the individual's condition that the athletic trainer sees, feels, hears, or smells when assessing the individual. Interpreting the symptoms and signs is the foundation used to recognize and identify the injury or condition. In sport injuries, the secondary survey comprises the largest portion of the total injury assessment process. Emergency conditions that will be discussed include:

1. Obstructed airway emergencies
2. Cardiopulmonary emergencies
3. Unconscious athlete
4. Hemorrhage
5. Fractures
6. Shock

Always check the ABCs: **A**irway, **B**reathing, **C**irculation, and **s**evere arterial bleeding

Primary survey
Immediate assessment to determine unresponsiveness and status of the ABCs

Secondary survey
Detailed head-to-toe assessment to detect medical and injury-related problems that, if unrecognized and untreated, could become life-threatening

Symptom
Subjective information provided by an individual regarding their perception of the problem

Sign
Objective measurable physical findings that you hear, feel, see, or smell during the assessment

7. Hyperthermia (heat stress)
8. Hypothermia (cold stress)

Where appropriate, the mechanism of injury, signs and symptoms, prevention, and treatment of the conditions will be discussed. Assessment is presented in the primary and secondary survey sections.

OBSTRUCTED AIRWAY

? *During a field hockey game, a player suddenly stops running, grabs the throat with both hands, and appears to be choking. Think for a minute or two about what has occurred and what you need to do to immediately handle this situation.*

The airway can become partially or totally blocked by a solid foreign object (mouth guard, bridgework, chewing gum, chaw of tobacco, or mud), fluids (blood clots from head injuries or vomitus), swelling in the throat caused by allergic reactions, or, more commonly, the back of the tongue (due to unconsciousness). An obstructed airway prevents adequate oxygen from being exchanged in the lungs and can lead to **cyanosis** and death.

The airway can become blocked by a solid foreign object, fluids, swelling in the throat, or the back of the tongue

Cyanosis
A dark blue or purple tinge to the skin due to insufficient oxygen in the blood

Partial Airway Obstruction

When a person has a **partial airway obstruction**, there is still some air exchange in the lungs and the individual will be able to cough. The individual will typically grasp the throat in the universal distress signal for choking **(Fig. 3.1)**. If the individual is able to cough forcefully, do not interfere. Stand beside the person and

Partial airway obstruction
Choking in which the individual has some air exchange in the lungs and is able to cough

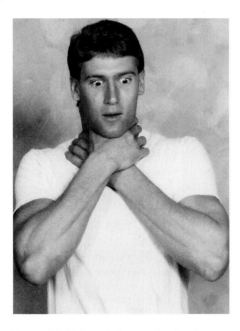

Figure 3.1. Universal distress sign for choking.

encourage them to continue coughing in an attempt to dislodge the obstruction. An ineffective cough or a high pitched noise during breathing indicates poor air exchange and should be treated as a total airway obstruction.

Total Airway Obstruction

Total airway obstruction
Choking in which the individual has no air passing through the vocal cords and is unable to speak or cough

In a **total airway obstruction**, no air is passing through the vocal cords, so the individual is unable to speak, breathe, or cough. The universal distress signal is almost always apparent. The athletic trainer must react quickly to clear the airway and stimulate the breathing process. Protocol for clearing the airway and restoring respirations is explained in the primary survey section.

The field hockey player is giving the universal distress sign, but is coughing, indicating only a partial airway obstruction. Did you determine that you should not interfere, but instead should encourage the individual to cough in an attempt to dislodge the mouth guard? If so, you are correct.

CARDIOPULMONARY EMERGENCIES

During a soccer game, a spectator standing behind you suddenly grabs the chest, staggers, then collapses. Think for a minute or two about what has occurred and what you may need to do to provide emergency care in this situation.

Cardiac arrest may result from strenuous physical activity, direct trauma, electrical shock, excessive alcohol or other chemical substance abuse, suffocation, drowning, or heart anomalies. Signs and symptoms include pain originating behind the sternum and radiating into either or both arms (usually the left), into the neck, jaw, teeth, upper back, or superior middle abdomen. Shortness of breath, nausea, and a feeling of impending doom are also present. Cardiopulmonary resuscitation (CPR) combines ventilation and heart compression to artificially pump oxygenated blood to the brain, heart, and other vital organs to sustain life until advanced medical care can be obtained. CPR protocol is explained in the primary survey.

The individual clutched the chest and collapsed. This may signal a possible heart attack. Tell someone to call an ambulance while you initiate the primary survey to determine if breathing and circulation are impaired.

UNCONSCIOUS ATHLETE

Two soccer players attempted to head a ball, but inadvertently struck heads. Both went down on the turf. One got up shaking his head, but the other player does not appear to be moving. As you approach this player, what actions should be completed first?

Head injuries are the leading cause of loss of consciousness in sport activity. Consciousness is defined on a continuum that grades levels of behavior in response to verbal and sensory stimuli, and

Table 3.1. Glasgow Coma Scale

Eyes	Open	Spontaneously	4
		To verbal command	3
		To pain	2
		No response	1
Best motor response	To verbal commands	Obeys	6
	To painful stimulus[b]	Localizes pain	5
		Flexion–withdrawal	4
		Flexion–abnormal	3
		Extension–abnormal	2
		No response	1
Best verbal response[c]		Oriented and converses	5
		Disoriented and converses	4
		Inappropriate words	3
		Incomprehensible sounds	2
		No response	1
Total			3–15

[a] The Glasgow Coma Scale is based on eye opening, motor, and verbal response and is used to monitor changes in level of consciousness. If response on the scale is given a number, then responsiveness of the injured party can be expressed by totalling the figures. Lowest score is 3; highest is 15. A score of 12 or greater is considered to be a mild injury, 9 to 11 is a moderate injury, and 8 or less is a severe head injury
[b] Squeeze trapezius, pinch soft tissue between thumb and forefinger or in the axilla, knuckle to sternum; observe arms
[c] Arouse injured party with painful stimulus if necessary

is measured with the Glasgow Coma Scale (**Table 3.1**). Being fully alert implies that the individual is aware of the surroundings and can respond to questions. **Unconsciousness** identifies an individual who lacks conscious awareness and is unable to respond to superficial sensory stimuli, such as pinching in the arm pit or the rapping of knuckles on the sternum. Coma, the most depressed state of consciousness, occurs when the individual cannot be aroused even by stimuli as powerful as pin pricks.

Try to communicate by calling the individual's name. You may have to shout loudly to get a response. Pinch the soft tissue in the armpit or rap your knuckles on the sternum and observe any painful withdrawal. If the individual does not respond, immediately check the ABCs. If the individual is unconscious but breathing, proceed to the secondary survey for a more thorough head-to-toe assessment. A more detailed assessment of consciousness can be found in Chapter 14, in the section on assessment of cranial injuries.

Did you call the individual's name and try to arouse the person through sensory stimulation? Make sure breathing and circulation are not impaired before moving on to the secondary survey.

> Consciousness is determined through verbal and sensory stimuli using the Glasgow Coma Scale

> **Unconsciousness**
> Impairment of brain function wherein the individual lacks conscious awareness and is unable to respond to superficial sensory stimuli

> Coma occurs when an individual cannot be aroused even by stimuli as powerful as pin pricks

? *A second baseman collided with a runner and was cleated across the front of the shin and is now bleeding. Think for a minute or two about how you will control hemorrhage to limit blood loss and risk of infection.*

Severe hemorrhage causes a decrease in blood volume and blood pressure. To compensate for this factor, the heart's pumping action must increase. Because there is less blood in the system, however, the strength of the pumping action is weakened, resulting in a characteristic rapid, weak pulse. Severity of bleeding is dependent upon age, weight, general physical condition, whether bleeding is arterial or venous bleeding, where bleeding originated, if blood is flowing freely externally or internally into a body cavity, and whether the bleeding is a threat to respiration.

Arterial bleeding from an oxygen-rich vessel is characterized by a spurting, bright red color. Major arteries, when completely severed, often constrict and seal themselves for a short period. If the artery is only punctured or partially severed, however, bleeding can be severe. Venous bleeding from an oxygen-depleted vessel appears as a dark bluish-red, almost maroon color. The continuous steady loss of blood can be heavy. Most superficial veins collapse if they are cut, but bleeding from deep veins can be as profuse and as difficult to control as arterial bleeding. Capillary bleeding is usually very slow and often described as oozing. The blood is red but a duller shade than arterial blood. This type of bleeding clots easily.

External Bleeding

External bleeding is the result of an exposed skin wound. Large exposed wounds carry a higher threat of infection than smaller ones. Complications from infection may include bacterial inoculation (the spread of bacteria into the underlying tissues), increased tissue damage, and foreign body contamination (1). Universal safety precautions should always be followed when dealing with external hemorrhage and body fluids (**Table 3.2**).

Control of Hemorrhage

> External bleeding is best controlled with direct pressure and elevation

External bleeding is best controlled with direct pressure and elevation. Pressure is applied directly over the wound with a sterile gauze pad, compressing the region against the underlying bone. Elevation utilizes gravity to reduce blood pressure, and thus aids blood clotting. In more severe bleeding, indirect pressure points can also help control hemorrhage, but should not be used if a fracture is suspected because of possible movement of the fractured bone ends.

Wound Cleansing

Each wound should be thoroughly cleansed with saline water to prevent infection, debride wound material and tissue, and cleanse

Table 3.2. Universal Safety Precautions in Treating Wounds

Whenever a wound is present in which oozing or bleeding occurs, the sporting activity should be stopped as soon as possible. The individual should be removed for treatment and should not be returned to participation until cleared by appropriate medical personnel

Wash hands with germicide soap before and after using latex gloves

Wear gloves for all routine procedures, such as:

Caring for wounds (abrasions, lacerations, avulsions, blisters, pustules or boils, and aspiration of a bursa or hematoma)

Being in contact with contaminated material containing blood or bodily fluids (bandages, ace wraps, urine samples, towels)

On-the-field evaluations where bleeding must be controlled (lacerations, bloody nose, open fracture)

Change gloves after each treatment. Discard gloves that are torn, cut, or punctured into a biohazard container

Wear a protective face mask and eyewear if a procedure may generate droplets of fluid that may spray into the practitioner's mouth, nose, or eyes

Sterilize instruments thoroughly and handle with care. Dispose of used needles, scalpel blades, and other "sharp" sticks into a biohazard container. Needles, once used, should never be recapped nor removed from disposable syringes by hand. Any needle pricks or cuts should be reported to the supervising physician so that appropriate supportive therapy may be instituted

Clean all tables and counters regularly with a 10:1 bleach solution. Wash all slightly blood-stained towels and linens in hot water and bleach. Heavily stained towels and linens should be placed in an appropriate green cloth bag and disposed of with other biohazard waste

Have a well-marked, designated, red biohazard container easily accessible in the training room. Materials that should be disposed of include used scalpel blades, needles, soiled gauze and bandages, soiled latex gloves, and towels soiled with blood or potentially hazardous body fluids

Use an approved pocket mask shield when giving artificial respiration

Health-care workers with open lesions should refrain from direct contact with individuals until the lesions have healed

Inoculations for hepatitis should be required for all staff and student athletic trainers

Educate staff, coaches, athletes, and student athletic trainers about the risks for contacting and spreading contagious diseases

For confidential information, referrals, and educational materials on HIV, hepatitis, and other communicable diseases, call the CDC National Hotline at 1-800-342-2437.

the surrounding intact skin. Because of its antibacterial effects, mild Ivory soap may be used to cleanse the wound, and Betadine or a similar solution may be used to cleanse the surrounding normal skin (1). Ointments, such as Neosporin, Bacitracin, or Johnson & Johnson First Aid Cream, may then be applied to prevent further bacterial inoculation.

Wound Dressing

After initial cleaning, debridement, and antiseptic procedures are completed, the wound should be covered with an occlusive dressing to prevent further risk of infection. Occlusive dressings retain moisture next to the wound and have been shown to enhance healing and reduce pain associated with the wound (2). Three main types of occlusive dressings include semipermeable films, hydrogels, and hydrocolloids. Semipermeable films, such as Bioclusive, Tegaderm, and Opsite, are permeable to water vapor, oxygen, and other gases, but are impermeable to water and bacteria. The films are waterproof, conform to body contours, and do not require frequent changes. Hydrogels, such as Spenco 2nd Skin and Vigilon, are transparent substances whose composition is more than 90% water. These dressings can absorb excess exudate from the wound, and are often used in treating blisters, minor lacerations, and burns. Hydrocolloids, such as DuoDERM, Comfeel, and Tegasorb, are the most widely used absorbent polymers. When applied to a wound, any exudate is absorbed into the inner gel lining and conforms to the wound contours until removed. These dressings are also waterproof and can be left in place for several days (2). Use of an occlusive dressing allows the wound to remain soft and pliable, preventing re-injury during athletic competition. **Field Strategy 3.1** explains the immediate control of hemorrhage and proper disposal of blood-soaked materials.

Internal Hemorrhage

Internal bleeding can result from blunt trauma or certain fractures (such as those of the pelvis, rib, or skull). Because internal hemorrhage is not visible, it can be overlooked, which can lead to shock. The history of injury (i.e., a fall, a deceleration injury, or severe blunt trauma), coupled with signs and symptoms of shock, should indicate that possible internal bleeding exists. **Field Strategy 3.2** lists the signs and symptoms that indicate possible internal bleeding and explains emergency management.

After applying latex gloves, control hemorrhage on the baseball player by using direct compression and elevation. When bleeding has stopped, cleanse the wound with a saline solution and cover it with an sterile occlusive dressing. Discard the gloves and any gauze pads containing blood in a properly identified biohazard bag. Refer the individual to a physician if suturing is needed.

FRACTURES

A football player was tackled resulting in a possible lower leg tibial fracture. To prevent unnecessary pain that may lead to shock, how should the leg be immobilized?

A fracture is a break in the continuity of a bone and is classified as open or closed, depending on whether the skin surface is pene-

Internal bleeding can result from blunt trauma or certain fractures

Field Strategy 3.1. Management of External Hemorrhage

Put on latex or rubber gloves before you attempt to control hemorrhage

Apply direct pressure

Place sterile gauze dressing directly over the wound, compressing the tissues and blood vessels against the underlying bone

If bleeding stops, cleanse the wound with a normal saline solution. Betadine or a similar solution may be used to cleanse the surrounding skin

Apply an antiseptic ointment, such as Bacitracin, Neosporin, or Johnson & Johnson First Aid Cream

Secure a sterile occlusive dressing over the wound. *Never* remove a dressing that becomes blood soaked

Place another dressing on top of the previous one and hold both in place

Elevate the injured area

Place the limb above the heart to slow the flow of blood and speed clotting

Elevation is contraindicated in cervical injuries, internal injuries, impaled objects, and in fractures or dislocations because movement may cause further damage or intensify the bleeding

Apply indirect digital pressure

Pressure points are places where an artery is close to a bony surface, and can be compressed against the underlying bone to reduce blood flow to the distal injury site. The two most common are the brachial artery in the upper arm and the femoral artery in the anterior hip

Hold the pressure point only as long as is necessary to stop the bleeding. Reapply the pressure if bleeding recurs

Discard all blood soaked gauze pads in a properly labeled red biohazard bag. *Do not* throw them into a wastebasket

To remove soiled gloves, use the dominant hand to reach to the opposite hand and grasp the wrist band of the soiled glove. Pull the wrist band away from the wrist and distal to the palm of the hand so the soiled portion of the glove is enveloped by the glove itself. Once removed, that glove is now placed in the palm of the remaining gloved hand. The process is repeated. Both gloves are then discarded in a biohazard receptacle. The hands should then be washed with soap and water

If you are away from the training room, place the pads and soiled gloves in a plastic bag and discard that bag in the red biohazard bag when you return to the training room. The biohazard bag is then disposed of according to the facility's procedures for disposal of biohazard waste. (For information on proper disposal of biohazard waste, contact your local hospital.)

trated. Because of infection, open fractures are more serious than closed fractures. Signs of fracture include swelling and bruising (discoloration), deformity and/or shortening of the limb, point tenderness, grating or **crepitus**, guarding or disability, or exposed bone ends. Assessment and recognition is confirmed through the use of palpation, percussion, vibration, compression, and distrac-

> Signs of fracture include swelling, discoloration, deformity and/or shortening of the limb, point tenderness, grating or crepitus, guarding or disability, or exposed bone ends

Crepitus
Cracking or grating sound heard during palpation that indicates a possible fracture

Field Strategy 3.2. Management of Internal Bleeding

Signs and symptoms

Bleeding from the mouth, rectum, or other body openings; bloody fluid from the nose or ears
Low blood pressure, usually 90/60 mm Hg or lower, with a rapid, weak pulse
Severe respiratory distress; rapid breathing, possibly becoming shallow
Pale, cold, and clammy skin with profuse sweating
Feeling of impending doom, restlessness, or anxiety
Dull eyes, dilated pupils that are slow to respond to light
Nausea and vomiting blood; the blood may look like used coffee grounds
Rigidity or spasms of the abdominal wall muscles

Emergency management

Maintain an open airway
Activate EMS as quickly as possible
Loosen any restrictive equipment or padding at the neck and waist
Monitor the vital signs and check for possible fractures. Splint if appropriate
Treat for shock and keep the individual quiet
Anticipate vomiting; in the absence of a spinal injury, place the individual on their side with the head pointing downward to allow for drainage
Continue to monitor vital signs until the ambulance arrives

---

tion. These techniques are discussed in the secondary survey (See **Figure 3.16**).

A suspected fracture should be splinted before the individual is moved to avoid damage to surrounding ligaments, tendons, blood vessels, or nerves. Damaged blood vessels may impair circulation to distal body parts. If nerves are damaged, sensation or muscle movement may become impaired. Fractures of the femur and fractures resulting in no distal pulse are considered to be emergencies requiring immediate transportation to the nearest medical facility.

Splints are used to support, immobilize, and protect a possible fracture site (**Fig. 3.2**). *If in doubt, always immobilize the joint above and below the suspected fracture site.* The more common rigid splints are made of wood, wires, aluminum, or cardboard. Soft splints include pillows, blankets, towels, and dressings, such as the sling and swathe. Pneumatic (air) splints are easy to apply and can be left on for x-rays. Air splints, however, should not be used in an open fracture or in a fracture with deformity, as the bone ends may move during application. Traction splints are used for long-bone fractures. By using a pump to remove air from the splint encircling the fractured limb, vacuum splints allow the limb to remain in the exact position it was found.

Because fingers and toes may be covered in any splint, be sure to check circulatory impairment by observing bilateral skin color, temperature, and capillary refill. Capillary refill is checked by

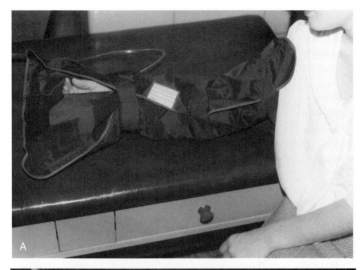

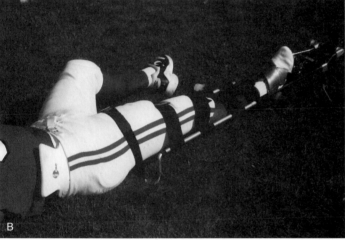

Figure 3.2. Fractures may be immobilized with a vacuum splint (**A**) or traction splint (**B**).

blanching the nails and watching for a rapid return of the normal pink color under the nail. **Field Strategy 3.3** summarizes general principles used to splint fractures (3).

Because the joints above and below the tibia must be immobilized, it is best to use a traction splint or vacuum splint. The leg should then be elevated to prevent the onset of shock. For the athlete's comfort and safety, an ambulance should be summoned to transport this individual to the nearest medical facility.

SHOCK

The leg has been immobilized in a traction splint and elevated above the heart to prevent the onset of shock until the ambulance arrives. What other measures can be taken to reduce the risk of shock?

Field Strategy 3.3. Principles of Emergency Splinting for Suspected Fractures

Establish an open airway and complete the primary survey

Remove any clothing and jewelry around the injury site. Clothing should be cut away with scissors to avoid unnecessarily moving the injured area

Check the distal pulse beyond the fracture site. If it is weak, check for internal hemorrhage

Cover all wounds, including open fractures, with sterile dressings and secure them. Do not attempt to push the bone ends back underneath the skin

Apply minimal in-line traction and maintain it until the splint is in place and secured. Immobilize the joint above and below the fracture site. Severely angulated fractures should not be straightened—immobilize the limb in the position you find it

Splint firmly, but not too tightly to impair circulation. Recheck distal pulse. Check vital signs and arrange for transportation to the nearest medical facility

---

> Shock can occur in any injury involving pain, bleeding, internal trauma, fracture, or with spinal injuries

Shock can occur to some degree in any injury involving pain, bleeding, internal trauma, fracture, or spinal injury. This condition occurs when the heart is unable to exert adequate pressure to circulate enough oxygenated blood to the vital organs. Reasons may stem from a damaged heart that fails to pump properly, low blood volume from blood loss or dehydration, or dilated blood vessels, leading to blood pooling in larger vessels away from vital areas (**Fig. 3.3**). The heart pumps faster, but, due to reduced volume, pulse rate is weakened and blood pressure drops (hypotension). This rapid, weak pulse is the most prominent sign of shock. As the individual's condition deteriorates, breathing becomes rapid and shallow. Vital body fluids pass through the weakened capillaries, leading to further circulatory distress. If not corrected, circulatory collapse can lead to unconsciousness and death.

The severity of shock depends on age, physical condition, pain tolerance, fatigue, dehydration, presence of any disease, extreme cold or heat exposure, or improper handling or movement of an injured area (4). **Field Strategy 3.4** summarizes the signs and symptoms and immediate management of shock.

💡 *To minimize the risk of shock, the properly immobilized limb has been elevated above the heart. Keep any spectators away from the area and keep the individual quiet and warm, to maintain body heat until the ambulance arrives.*

HYPERTHERMIA

❓ *A runner has just completed a half-marathon on a warm sunny day. Think for a minute about how the body dissipates internal heat generated during exercise. Under what circumstances would the environment alter thermal regulation in the body?*

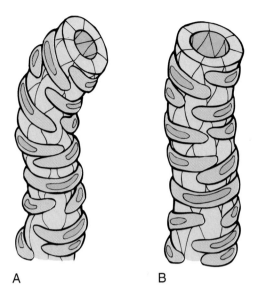

A   B

Figure 3.3. A. The diameter of an arteriole blood vessel is controlled by circular layers of smooth muscles that either constrict or relax to regulate peripheral blood flow. **B**. During shock, blood vessels vasodilate. This action increases the size of the vascular bed and decreases resistance to blood flow, resulting in blood pooling in larger vessels, depriving the brain and vital organs of needed oxygen. As a result, heart rate increases, giving the characteristic rapid, weak pulse that is often the first sign of shock.

Hyperthermia, or elevated body temperature, occurs when internal heat production is no longer in balance with external heat loss **(Fig. 3.4)**. The hypothalamus initiates cooling or heat retention mechanisms to maintain a relatively constant body core (skull, thoracic, and abdominal regions) temperature between 36.1° and 37.8°C (97° to 100°F).

Hyperthermia
Elevated body temperature

Internal Heat Regulation

Internal heat is generated during muscular activity through energy metabolism. As exercise begins, heart rate and cardiac output increase, while superficial venous and arterial blood vessels dilate to divert warm blood to the skin surface. Heat is dissipated when the warm blood flushes into skin capillaries and is evident when the face becomes flushed and reddened on a hot day or after exercise.

At rest, with air temperature below 30.6°C (87°F), about two-thirds of the body's normal heat loss occurs as a result of conduction (via direct contact with a cooler object), convection (via air or water flow), and radiation (via infrared waves) **(Fig. 3.5)** (5). As air temperature approaches skin temperature and exceeds 30.6°C (87°F), evaporation becomes the predominant means of heat dissipation. Usually, body heat is warmer than the environment and heat energy is dissipated through the air or into surrounding cooler

As air temperature approaches skin temperature and exceeds 30.6°C (87°F), evaporation becomes the predominant means of heat dissipation

Field Strategy 3.4. Management of Shock

Signs and symptoms

Restlessness, anxiety, disorientation, or dizziness
Cold, clammy, moist skin; initially chalklike, but later may appear cyanotic
Profuse sweating and extreme thirst
Eyes are dull, sunken, with pupils dilated
Nausea and/or vomiting
Shallow, irregular breathing, but may also be labored, rapid or gasping
Pulse is rapid and weak

Management of shock

Activate EMS. Secure and maintain an open airway
Control any major bleeding and splint any fractures. This will reduce shock
    by slowing bleeding and will help ease the pain. If the individual has a
    leg fracture, keep the leg level while splinting the fracture. Raise the leg
    only after it has been properly immobilized
If you do not suspect a head or neck injury or a leg fracture, elevate the
    feet and legs 8 to 12 inches. If there are breathing difficulties, the
    individual might be more comfortable with the head and shoulders
    raised in a semi-reclining position. With a head injury, elevate the head
    and shoulders to reduce pressure on the brain. In a suspected neck
    injury, keep the individual lying flat.
If the individual vomits or is unconscious, place them on their side to
    avoid blocking the airway with any fluids. This allows the fluids to drain
    from the mouth
Maintain body heat by keeping the individual warm, but do not overheat.
    Remove any wet clothing if possible and cover the individual with a
    blanket. Keep the individual quiet and still. Avoid any rough or excessive
    handling
Do not give the individual anything by mouth, in case surgery is indicated
Monitor vital signs every 2 to 5 minutes until the ambulance arrives

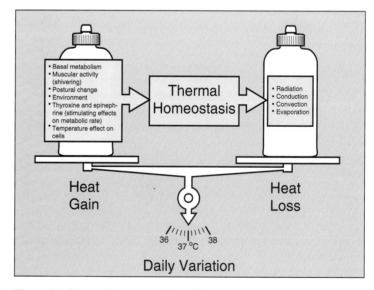

Figure 3.4. Thermal homeostasis is achieved when internal heat production and heat loss are properly balanced to maintain a relatively constant
body core temperature.

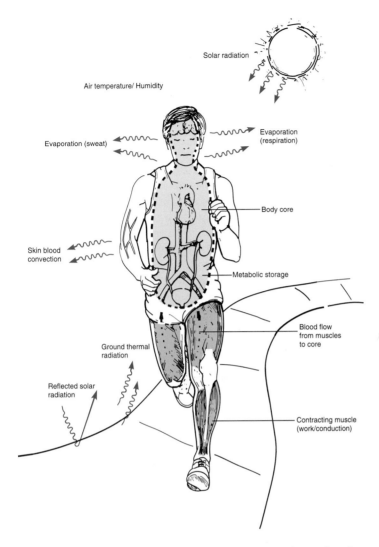

Figure 3.5. Heat production from within working muscles is transferred to the body core and skin. During exercise, body heat is dissipated into the surrounding environment by radiation, conduction, convection, and evaporation.

objects. When the temperature of the surrounding air or objects in the environment, such as the sun or hot artificial turf, exceeds skin temperature, heat can be absorbed.

A person exercising in heat may sweat two to three liters (L) of body water in 1 hour and up to 15 L per day, depending on their physical condition (6). Sweating itself does not cool the body; evaporation of the sweat cools the body. Furthermore, about 350 mL of water seeps through the skin every day and another 300 mL of water is vaporized from mucous membranes in the respiratory passages. It is not uncommon for sport participants to lose 1.5 to 2.5 L/hr of water during exercise. When dehydrated, delivery of oxygen to working muscles is reduced, resulting in early fatigue.

Mild dehydration of 2 to 3% can reduce work capacity by 15 to 20% (6). Although an individual may continually drink water throughout an exercise bout, less than 50% of fluid lost will be replenished (7).

Measuring the Heat Stress Index

The heat stress index is a measure of ambient air temperature, humidity, and solar radiant energy. Of these, relative humidity is the most important factor that determines the effectiveness of evaporative heat loss. Relative humidity is the ratio of water in the air to the total quantity of moisture that can be carried in air at a particular temperature and is expressed as a percentage. For example, 65% relative humidity means that ambient air contains 65% of the air's moisture-carrying capabilities at the specific temperature. A sling psychrometer is commonly used to measure heat stress by exposing a dry-bulb and wet-bulb thermometer to rapid air flow. General guidelines for safe participation in hot, humid environments, using a sling psychrometer are listed in **Table 3.3**.

> Relative humidity is the most important factor that determines the effectiveness of evaporative heat loss

Preventing Heat Emergencies

Several steps can be taken to reduce the risk of heat injury:

Identify individuals at risk. Healthy individuals at risk for heat injuries include those poorly acclimatized or conditioned, individuals inexperienced with heat injuries, individuals with a large muscle mass, overweight individuals, large athletes, children, and the elderly. Also at risk are individuals with congenital heart disease, diabetes, or anorexia nervosa (8).

Acclimatization. Exercising moderately during repeated heat exposure can result in a physiological adaptation to a new environment, which can improve performance and heat tolerance. This process, called **acclimatization**, is one of the most effective measures to prevent heat stress. In general, gradual participation over 7 to 10 days for approximately 1.5 to 2 hours/day is sufficient to acclimate the body to the environment. Furthermore, exercise

Acclimatization
Physiologic adaptations of an individual to a different environment, especially climate or altitude

Table 3.3. Participation Guidelines Using Wet-Bulb Temperature (WBT) Range

°F	°C	Recommendations
60	15.5	No prevention necessary
61 to 65	16.2 to 18.4	Alert persons to symptoms of heat stress and the importance of adequate hydration
66 to 70	18.8 to 21.1	Insist that adequate water be ingested
71 to 75	21.6 to 23.8	Rest periods and water breaks every 20 to 30 minutes; place limits on intense activity
76 to 79	24.5 to 26.1	Modify practice considerably and curtail activity for unacclimated individuals
80	26.5	Cancel practice

intensity and duration should gradually increase over several weeks until it is comparable to competitive levels (9).

Clothing. Light-colored, lightweight, porous clothing is preferred. Evaporative heat loss occurs only when clothing is thoroughly wet and sweat can vaporize. Therefore, changing into a dry shirt may hinder heat dissipation (6,7). Heavy sweat suits or rubberized plastic suits produce high relative humidity close to the skin and retard evaporation, increasing the risk of heat illness (5).

Even with loose-fitting porous jerseys, wrappings or protective pads, and football helmets can seal off 50% of the body surface and severely limit evaporative cooling. Increased metabolic rate needed to carry the weight of the equipment and increased temperatures on artificial surfaces also increase the risk for heat-related illnesses. To counter this, football players should initially practice in short-sleeved tee shirts, shorts, and low-cut socks. On hot, humid days, uniforms should not be worn, and, if possible, shoulder pads and helmets should be removed often to allow for radiation and evaporative cooling.

Fluid hydration. Ten to 20 minutes prior to exercise, participants should consume 13 to 20 ounces of cold water (5°C; 41°F) and should have unlimited access to water at all times during exercise. Cold liquids, especially water, empty from the stomach and small intestines into the blood stream faster than warm liquids (6,7,10). Although electrolyte solutions are unnecessary for individuals with a normal diet, evidence suggests that in prolonged activity exceeding 60 to 90 minutes, beverages containing 4 to 8% carbohydrates should be consumed to maintain a sufficient concentration of blood glucose for the working muscles (10,11).

Weight charts. Losing 2% of body weight can impair temperature regulation. Furthermore, a 4% decrease in body weight translates into a 6% decrease in maximal aerobic capacity and a 12% reduction in exercise time (9). As a rule of thumb, for every pound of water lost, 1 pint of water (16 oz) must be consumed.

Temperature/humidity. A sling psychrometer should be used on questionable days to determine safe participation before activity begins. Follow the guidelines outlined in **Table 3.3**, with water breaks scheduled every 20 to 30 minutes.

Practice schedules. On hot, humid days, schedule workouts in the morning or evening to avoid the worst heat of the day. Allow frequent water breaks (10 minutes every half hour), shorten the practice, and lessen the intensity. Whenever possible, get the players out of the sun and remove any restrictive equipment, pads, and helmets.

Heat Cramps

Heat cramps are painful, involuntary muscle spasms caused by excessive water and electrolyte loss, particularly sodium, during and after intense exercise in heat. Paradoxically, the condition more frequently occurs in a well-conditioned, acclimated athlete who has overexerted in hot weather or rehydrated with only water

> Heavy sweat suits and rubberized plastic suits produce high relative humidity close to the skin and retard evaporation

> On hot, humid days, reschedule activities during the morning or evening to avoid the worst heat of the day

Heat cramps
Painful, involuntary muscle spasms caused by excessive water and electrolyte loss

Factors that place
individuals at risk for heat
cramps include lack of
acclimatization, use of
diuretics, and sodium
depletion in the diet

(5). Cramps commonly occur in the calf and abdominal muscles, but may involve the upper extremity muscles. Risk factors include lack of acclimatization, use of diuretics, and sodium depletion in the normal diet. Body temperature is not usually elevated and the skin remains moist and cool (5). Pulse and respiration may be normal, or slightly elevated, and dizziness may be present.

Heat Exhaustion

Heat exhaustion usually occurs in unacclimatized people early in the summer or during the first hard training sessions. Individuals who wear protective equipment or heavy uniforms are also at risk, as evaporation through the material may be retarded. The individual may appear ashen and gray. Other symptoms include fatigue; weakness; uncoordinated gait; dizziness; a small urine output; headache; rapid and shallow respirations; and a rapid, weak pulse **(Fig. 3.6)**. Sweating mechanisms are generally working profusely, making the skin wet, cool, and clammy. Sweating, however, may be reduced if the person is dehydrated. An elevated core temperature generally does not exceed 39.5°C (103°F) (7).

Heat Stroke

Heat stroke is the least common, but most serious, heat-related illness. In football, heat stroke is second only to head injuries as the most frequent cause of death. Also seen in distance runners

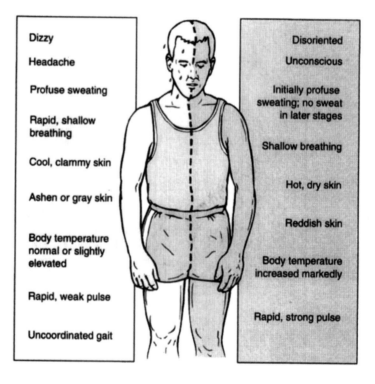

Dizzy

Headache

Profuse sweating

Rapid, shallow breathing

Cool, clammy skin

Ashen or gray skin

Body temperature normal or slightly elevated

Rapid, weak pulse

Uncoordinated gait

Disoriented

Unconscious

Initially profuse sweating; no sweat in later stages

Shallow breathing

Hot, dry skin

Reddish skin

Body temperature increased markedly

Rapid, strong pulse

Figure 3.6. Comparison of the signs and symptoms associated with heat exhaustion and heat stroke.

and wrestlers dehydrated through weight loss, it is almost always preceded by prolonged, strenuous physical exercise. During exercise, the thermoregulatory system can become overloaded and the body's cooling mechanisms fail to dissipate the rising core temperature. The hypothalamus shuts down all heat-control mechanisms, including the sweat glands, to conserve water loss. As a result, a vicious circle is created: as core temperature increases, metabolic rate increases, which, in turn, increases heat production. As temperature continues to elevate, permanent brain damage may occur. Core temperature can rise to 105°F and has been known to reach 107° to 108°F (12). If untreated, death is imminent.

Initial symptoms include a feeling of burning up, deep breathing, irritability, profuse sweating, and an unsteady gait. As the condition deteriorates, sweating ceases and the skin is hot and dry, and appears reddened or flushed (**Fig. 3.6**). As core temperature rises, the pulse becomes rapid and strong, as high as 150 to 170 beats per minute. Tissue damage by excessive body heat leads to vasomotor collapse, shallow breathing, decreased blood pressure, and a rapid and weak pulse. Muscle twitching or seizures may occur just before the individual lapses into coma (5,12).

> Heat stroke is usually preceded by prolonged strenuous physical exercise in individuals who are poorly acclimated, dehydrated, or when evaporation of sweat is inhibited

> During heat stroke, as core temperature rises, the pulse becomes rapid and strong, as high as 150 to 170 beats per minute

Emergency Care for Heat Stress

Treatment for all heat conditions involves immediately moving the person to a cool place, removing all equipment and unnecessary clothing, and cooling the body. Place the individual supine (face up), with the feet elevated above the heart to maintain blood pressure and circulation to the brain. Cool fluids with a diluted electrolyte solution may be administered unless the individual is unconscious. With heat cramps, static stretching and ice massage over the affected area are helpful. This individual should be watched carefully as this condition may precipitate heat exhaustion or heatstroke.

In suspected heat exhaustion and heat stroke, activate EMS. Fluid replacement and rapid cooling of the body is a priority, particularly over the major blood vessels in the armpit, groin, and neck regions. **Field Strategy 3.5** lists the signs, symptoms, and immediate care for heat-related conditions. Physical activity should not be resumed until the individual has returned to the predehydrated state and has been cleared by a physician.

> Fluid replacement and rapid cooling of the major blood vessels in the armpits, groin, and neck are a priority

During the half-marathon, the runner's body heat was dissipated through radiation, conduction, convection, and evaporation. Environmental stresses, such as high temperature, relative humidity, radiation, and wind velocity, can overload the heat-dissipating mechanisms leading to hyperthermia.

HYPOTHERMIA

Think for a minute or two about how the body maintains heat in cold weather. How can an individual prevent heat loss during adverse weather conditions?

Field Strategy 3.5. Management of Heat-related Conditions

Condition	Signs and Symptoms	Treatment
Heat cramps	Involuntary muscle spasms or cramps; normal pulse and respirations; profuse sweating and dizziness	Rest in cool place; massage cramps with ice and do static stretching; drink cool water with diluted electrolyte solution
Heat exhaustion	Weakness; confusion; headache; profuse sweating; skin is wet, cool, clammy, and may appear ashen gray; breathing is rapid and shallow; pulse is weak	Rest in cool room; remove equipment and clothing; execute rapid cooling of body; sponge or towel the individual with cool water; individual may need IV fluids; discontinue activity until well recovered
Heat stroke	Irritability progresses to apathy; unsteady gait and disorientation; pulse is rapid and strong; skin is hot and dry and appears red or flushed; blood pressure falls; may have convulsions, seizures, or slip into coma	ACTIVATE EMS! Rest in cool room; rapidly cool the body with ice on the major blood vessels or use wet compresses; treat for shock; and transport immediately to trauma center

Hypothermia
Decreased body temperature

Hypothermia, or reduced body temperature, occurs when the body is unable to maintain a constant core temperature. With cold weather or decreased circulating blood temperature, the body attempts to maintain normal core temperature by vasoconstricting surface blood vessels to prevent blood from shunting to the skin. In addition, certain chemicals are released that increase metabolic activity and heat production in the heart, liver, brain, and endocrine organs. If these two actions are insufficient to maintain core temperature, shivering begins. With this mechanism, heat is produced through involuntary contractions in skeletal muscles, as long as energy supplies last.

Cold emergencies may occur in two ways. In one, the core temperature remains relatively constant, but the shell temperature decreases. This leads to localized injuries from frostbite. The other occurs when both core temperature and shell temperature decrease, leading to general body cooling. All body processes slow down and systemic hypothermia occurs. If left unabated, death is imminent.

Shivering can produce heat through involuntary muscle contractions only as long as energy supplies last

Preventing Cold-related Injuries

Body heat is lost through respiration, radiation, conduction, convection, and evaporation. Inadequate insulation from the cold or

Field Strategy 3.6. Reducing the Risk for Cold Injuries

Check weather conditions and take into account possible deterioration

Watch individuals around you who may be susceptible to cold for signs of frostbite

Dress in several light layers instead one heavy layer. Wear windproof, dry, well-insulated mittens, gloves, and garments (pants and jacket) that will allow water vapor to escape. Wool is excellent. Wear a ski cap, face mask, and neck warmer to protect the face and ears. Keep the feet dry and insulated from the cold

Stay dry by wearing appropriate rain gear or protective clothing. If you get wet, change as soon as you can into dry clothing

Breathe through the nose, rather than the mouth, to minimize heat and fluid loss. Avoid dehydration by drinking water. Do not drink alcoholic beverages or snow because this will worsen hypothermia

Carry nutritious snacks that contain carbohydrates and sugars for quick energy during exercise. Eat small amounts of food often

Keep your back to the wind. Do not stand in one position for an extended period. Keep wriggling your toes to bring warm blood to the foot area. Do not touch any metal with bare skin

---

wind, restrictive clothing, use of alcohol or tobacco products, age (young or old), poor diet lacking adequate glycogen and fat, and decreased circulation predispose an individual to cold-related injuries. Several steps can be taken to prevent heat loss and are summarized in **Field Strategy 3.6**. Although "layered" clothing allows for several thin layers of insulation, the insulating ability of clothing can be decreased as much as 90% when saturated through either external moisture or condensation from sweating (5). If conditions are bad enough, it might be better to cancel the practice or event for the day.

> The insulating ability of clothing can be decreased by as much as 90% when saturated through either external moisture or condensation from sweating

Frostbite Injuries

Frostbite is caused when soft tissue freezes. Superficial frostbite involves the skin and underlying superficial tissue. The area may feel firm to the touch, but the tissue beneath is soft and resilient. Deep frostbite involves the tissues deep to the skin and subcutaneous layers and may result in complete destruction of the injured tissue. The skin feels hard because it is actually frozen tissue. Damage depends on the depth and penetration of cold resulting from varying degrees of duration, temperature of exposure, and wind velocity (13).

> Tissue damage is dependent on the depth and penetration of the cold resulting from varying degrees of duration, temperature of exposure, and wind velocity

Areas commonly affected are the fingertips, toes (especially in constricting footwear), earlobes, and tip of the nose. The skin initially appears red and swollen and the individual will complain of diffuse numbness that may or may not be preceded by a itchy or prickly sensation. The area then turns white with a yellow or blue tint that looks "waxy" (12,13).

The person should be taken indoors, protected from any further

> In frostbite, the skin initially appears red and swollen, and the individual will complain of diffuse numbness that may or may not be preceded by a itchy or prickly sensation

Field Strategy 3.7. Management of Frostbite

Signs and symptoms

1°   Initially, skin appears red then white and is usually painless, but soft to the touch. The condition is typically seen by friends first

2°   Skin appears red and swollen and may have an itchy or prickly sensation. Condition progresses to white or waxy skin color with diffuse numbness. Skin is firm, but tissue beneath is soft

3°   Skin appears blotchy white to yellow-gray or blue-gray. Skin is hard the entire depth and totally numb

Management

Take the person indoors to protect the area from any further refreezing. Remove any clothing, jewelry, or rings, and immerse the injured area in water heated 40° to 42°C (104° to 108°F) for 30 to 45 minutes. Avoid hot water, as this may burn the person

As the area thaws, swelling may occur due to capillary damage and plasma may leak into surrounding tissues

When completely rewarmed, gently dry the affected area and apply a sterile dressing. If fingers or toes are being rewarmed, place sterile dressings between the digits before covering the entire area with towels or a blanket to keep it warm

Transport the individual to the nearest trauma center with the limb slightly elevated

refreezing, and subjected to careful, rapid rewarming of the area. **Field Strategy 3.7** identifies the signs and symptoms of frostbite and the immediate management.

Systemic Body Cooling

Normal skin temperature in cool weather ranges between 32° to 34°C (90° to 93°F) and can drop as low as 21° to 23°C (70° to 73°F) before the body core begins to cool. At 4.4°C (40°F), over half the body's generated heat can be lost from an uncovered head. Air movement produces a wind chill factor that increases heat loss.

When core temperature falls below 34.4°C (94°F), heart and respirations slow down, cardiac output and blood pressure fall, and, as the skin and muscles cool, shivering increases violently. Numbness sets in and even the simplest task becomes difficult to perform. If core temperature continues to drop below 32°C (90°F), shivering ceases and muscles become cold and stiff. If intervention is not initiated, death is imminent. **Table 3.4** further highlights the stages of systemic hypothermia, or general body cooling.

Treatment involves maintenance of the ABCs and rapid rewarming of the entire body. Activate EMS because advanced life support is often necessary. If the individual is conscious, warm fluids may be given; however, alcohol and caffeine should be avoided.

At 4.4°C (40°F) over 50% of the body's heat can be lost from an uncovered head

Table 3.4. Stages of Systemic Hypothermia

Core Temperature (°F)	Symptoms
96 to 99	Intense, uncontrollable shivering is present
91 to 95	Violent shivering persists. If conscious, it may be difficult to speak
86 to 90	Shivering decreases and is replaced by strong muscular rigidity. Muscle coordination deteriorates to jerky erratic movements. Thinking is clouded and the person may have total amnesia
81 to 85	Person becomes irrational, loses awareness of the surroundings, and drifts into a stuporous state. Muscular rigidity continues and heart rate and respirations slow. Cardiac arrhythmias may be present
78 to 80	Person becomes unconscious and cannot respond to spoken word. Reflexes cease to function and the heartbeat becomes erratic
Below 78	Cardiac and respiratory centers in the brain fail. Edema and hemorrhage occurs in the lungs, leading to death

The body maintains heat through vasoconstriction of blood vessels, stimulation of metabolic activity, and shivering. Localized and systemic cold injuries can be prevented by covering exposed skin, wearing a hat, and dressing in layers to conserve body heat.

EMERGENCY PLAN

A gymnast slipped off the springboard on an approach to a vault and collided full force into the vaulting horse. The individual is now lying on the floor and does not appear to be moving. Think for a minute or two about what you should do to provide immediate care to this person and how should additional help be summoned?

An **emergency plan** is a well-developed process that activates the emergency health care services of the facility and community to provide immediate health care to an injured individual. In essence, should an accident occur, it is a pre-established plan to determine:

who will render emergency care and control the situation
what care will be provided
who will call Emergency Medical Services (EMS)
who will supervise the other activity areas if supervisors must leave those areas to assist at the accident scene
the procedures for proper use and disposal of items and equipment exposed to blood or bodily fluids

Emergency plan
A process that activates emergency health care services of the facility and community

Field Strategy 3.8. Developing an Emergency Care Plan

Are all supervisors currently certified in emergency first aid and CPR? Is one individual identified as the medical liaison, or "captain"? Does this person have advanced first aid training?

When an emergency occurs, who will activate EMS? If the medical liaison must summon additional staff to help control the situation, who will supervise the other activity areas and do crowd control?

Who has access to locked gates or doors? Who will direct the ambulance to the accident scene?

Has the facility invited representatives from EMS to become familiar with the floor plan of the facility? Does the facility regularly have announced and unannounced mock emergency drills to practice the procedures? Is EMS involved in these drills?

Have all sport participants been medically cleared to participate? Are appropriate documents completed (i.e., physical examination, permission to participate, informed consent, and emergency information)? Have the athletic trainers and supervisors been informed of any orthopedic or health problems that might affect participation?

Do you have emergency cards for each participant, with family phone numbers, physicians names and numbers, special instruction/ considerations, and who to contact when parents/guardians are unavailable?

Does everyone know the location and have easy access to first-aid kits, splints, stretchers, fire extinguishers, and a phone? Are emergency numbers posted near each phone (i.e., EMS, hospital, training room, school nurse, facility medical liaison, fire and police departments)?

What information will be provided over the telephone?
  Type of emergency situation
  Possible injury/condition
  Current status of the injured party
  Assistance being given to the injured party
  Exact location of the facility or injured individual (give cross streets to assist EMS) and specific point of entry to the facility
  Telephone number of phone being used

Do you have different emergency procedures for the various facilities (pool, gymnasia, weight room, training room, and fields)?

Who will be responsible for informing the individual's parents/guardians that an emergency has occurred?

Are proper injury records completed after the injury and kept on file in a central, secure location?

At least once each year the primary sports medicine team and related individuals should meet with representatives from EMS to discuss, develop, and evaluate the emergency plan. A written plan should be developed for each activity site. It is critical during emergencies that everyone work together to ensure medical attention is not delayed. **Field Strategy 3.8** lists several important issues and questions to address in developing an emergency plan. *As the first person on the scene, you should initiate the facility's emergency plan, do a primary survey, and summon help from colleagues, one of whom should call the local EMS.*

PRIMARY INJURY ASSESSMENT

The gymnast is lying motionless on the mat after colliding with the vaulting horse. In initiating the facility's emergency procedures plan, what priorities do you need to assess to determine if breathing or circulation are impaired?

The primary injury assessment, or primary survey, should establish the level of unresponsiveness and initiate or maintain adequate breathing and circulation until help arrives. Assessment of all injuries, no matter how minor, should always include a primary assessment. In most cases, this is completed quickly when approaching the injured individual and observing them moving or talking. As such, one can proceed immediately to the secondary injury assessment. If the person, however, is not moving or is unresponsive, initiate the primary survey. Occasionally collisions occur in sport activities and more than one player is injured. **Triage** refers to assessing all injured individuals quickly, then returning to the most seriously injured and giving immediate treatment to that person.

When approaching the individual, check the surrounding area to see if any equipment or apparatus may have contributed to the injury. Scan the individual and note body position and any noticeable deformities. In severe brain injuries, a neurological sign called posturing of the extremities may occur (**Fig. 3.7**). When posturing is evident, an emergency exists and medical assistance should be summoned immediately. Unless a possible spinal injury has been totally ruled out, always assume one is present and stabilize the head and neck before proceeding. The following information is provided as a guide in performing a primary assess-

Triage
Assessing all injured individuals to determine priority of care

As you approach an individual, check the surrounding area to see if any equipment or apparatus may have contributed to the injury

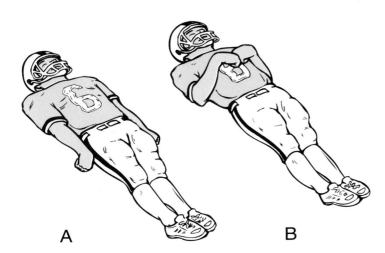

A   B

Figure 3.7. Body posturing may occur as (**A**) decerebrate rigidity, which is characterized by extension in all four extremities, or (**B**) decorticate rigidity, which is characterized by extension of the legs and flexion of the elbows, wrist, and fingers. Both conditions indicate a severe brain injury.

ment and in no way should be substituted for formal instruction and certification in the current standards of cardiopulmonary resuscitation offered through the American Red Cross or American Heart Association.

Assess Unresponsiveness

Without moving the individual, tap the shoulder or arm while calling the individual's name. You may have to shout to get a response. Look at the facial expression and any eye movement. Does the individual respond to your voice by opening the eyes, moving a body part, or answering a question? Do they withdraw from painful stimuli (i.e., knuckle to the sternum or being pinched)? If the individual cannot open the eyes on verbal command or does not demonstrate withdrawal from painful stimulus, activate EMS and proceed to check the ABCs. This step should take 5 to 10 seconds.

Open the Airway

In a supine position, the tongue may slide posteriorly to close the epiglottis over the windpipe. By moving the jaw forward, the tongue is lifted away from the epiglottis to open the airway. This may be all that is necessary for spontaneous breathing to return. If breathing does not recur, a foreign object may be obstructing the airway. If the individual has a helmet on, *under no circumstances should the helmet be removed unless special circumstances are present (i.e., the screws securing the face mask are stripped and the individual is in respiratory distress, or you are unable to assess the airway)* (14). In either case, helmet removal should be performed only by personnel trained in the procedure.

If a spinal injury is suspected, it is not necessary to remove the face mask. A pocket mask can be slid between the chin and the lowest portion of the face mask or through the eye hole of the face mask, then placed into position over the mouth and nose. Research has shown that this method allows faster activation of rescue breathing or CPR and limits extraneous cervical spine motion that may occur with other face mask removal techniques (15). If, however, a pocket mask is not available, the entire face mask must be removed to have clear access to the airway. It is critical to stabilize the head and neck while another individual removes the face mask with a manual or power screwdriver, or a Trainer's Angel. There are two methods to open the airway when no obstruction is present: head tilt/chin lift method and jaw thrust method. If the airway is obstructed by a foreign object, the Heimlich maneuver, abdominal thrusts, and a finger sweep may be used to clear the airway.

If the airway is obstructed by a foreign object, the Heimlich maneuver, abdominal thrusts, and a finger sweep may be used to clear the airway

Head Tilt/Chin Lift Method

Open the airway by placing the tips of your fingers under the jaw. Lift forward while simultaneously pushing down on the individu-

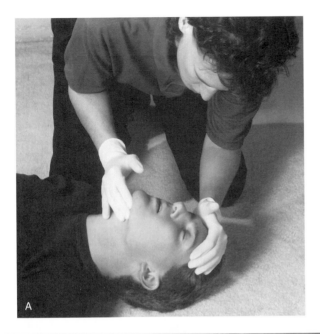

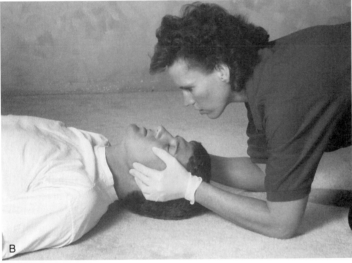

Figure 3.8. A. Head tilt/chin lift method. **B**. Jaw thrust method.

al's head. Avoid any excessive force **(Fig. 3.8A)**. Keep the mouth slightly open. This method is recommended except when a head or neck injury is suspected.

If you suspect a head or neck injury, do not move the individual's head or neck. Try first to lift the chin without tilting the head back. If this maneuver is unsuccessful, slowly and gently tilt the head until breaths can go in. It is unlikely that tilting the head slightly will further damage the neck and one must remember that a nonbreathing individual's greatest need is for air.

Jaw Thrust Method

If the head tilt method is unsuccessful because of a helmet or shoulder pads, the jaw thrust technique may be used. While maintaining the head in a fixed position, rest your elbows on either side of the individual's head. Grasp the individual's lower jaw and lift forward with both hands, keeping the mouth slightly open **(Fig. 3.8B)**. This technique can be used with a pocket mask. As rescue breathing begins, a third rescuer can remove the screws holding the face mask clips to the helmet. When the clips are removed, the face mask can be carefully rotated out of position with very little cervical spine motion being exerted (15).

Heimlich Maneuver

Stand behind the individual and wrap your arms around their waist. Make a fist with one of your hands and place the thumb side of the fist halfway between the navel and lower tip of the sternum (xiphoid process) **(Fig. 3.9A)**. Grasp the fist with the other hand. Keeping the elbows out, press the fist into the individual's abdomen with 5 quick, upward thrusts. Each thrust should be a separate, distinct movement. The action of the thrust pushes up on the diaphragm, compressing air in the lungs, and creates a forceful pressure against the blockage, thus expelling or exploding the object from the airway. Recheck the individual after every 5 thrusts. Repeat the thrusts until the obstruction is cleared or the individual becomes unconsciousness.

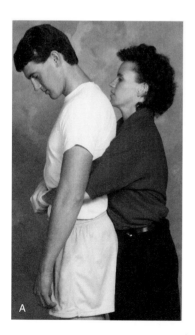
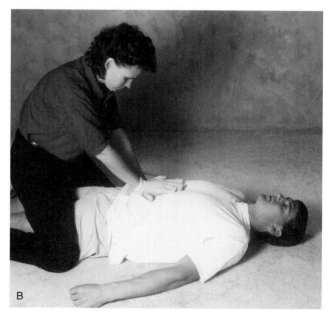

Figure 3.9. A. Heimlich maneuver. **B**. Abdominal thrusts in an unconscious individual.

Abdominal Thrusts

When unconscious, position the individual's head and open the airway to check for breathlessness. Straddle the thighs, keeping your weight centered over your knees. Place the heel of one hand midway between the individual's navel and lower tip of the sternum (**Fig. 3.9B**). Place the other hand directly on top of the first hand. Press into the abdomen up to 5 times with quick, upward thrusts.

Finger Sweep

If a foreign object is lodged in the back of the throat and is visible, you may be able to remove the object. Be careful not to drive the object farther into the throat. With the hand closest to the victim's feet, open the mouth by grasping both the tongue and lower jaw between your thumb and fingers. Insert the index finger from the other hand into the mouth along the far cheek, extending deep into the throat to the base of the tongue (**Fig. 3.10**). Using a hooking motion, dislodge the object and move it into the mouth for removal. **Field Strategy 3.9** lists protocol used to clear an obstructed airway.

Establish Breathing

Breathing is assessed with the look, listen, feel principle: *look* to see if the chest is rising or falling; *listen* for air exchange through the mouth or nose, or both; *feel* with a cheek to determine if there is air exchanged (**Fig. 3.11**). The depth of respirations indicates the volume of air being exchanged. Take 3 to 5 seconds to assess

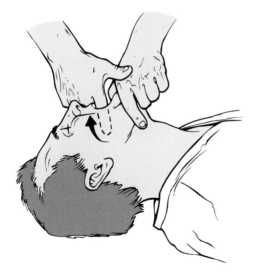

Figure 3.10. Use the index finger to sweep away any visible foreign matter that may be obstructing the airway.

Field Strategy 3.9. Management of an Obstructed Airway

Ask, "Are you choking? Can you speak?" Look for the universal distress sign or nodding of the head. Reassure the individual you are there to help

Perform several Heimlich maneuver thrusts. Ask, "Are you still choking?" Repeat abdominal thrusts until the object is dislodged or the individual collapses. *If* they collapse, then—

> Position the head. Give 2 full breaths, each breath lasting from 1 to 1½ seconds. If your breath is unable to enter into the individual's mouth, then—
>
> Reposition the individual's head and give 2 more breaths. *If* you are still unable to breathe into the individual, then—
>
> Tell someone to call for an ambulance; say, "Airway is obstructed, call 911" (or your local emergency number or the telephone operator)

Perform 6 to 10 abdominal thrusts

Do a finger sweep. If the object is visible, attempt to remove it, but use caution not to lodge the object in farther

Give 2 full breaths again. If you are unable to breathe air into the individual, then repeat the full sequence until the airway is cleared or the ambulance arrives. The total sequence for an unconscious individual is: 6 to 10 abdominal thrusts, finger sweep, and 2 breaths

---

the presence of breathing. If breathing is absent, send someone to activate EMS while you perform the following steps.

1. Using the hand placed on the forehead, pinch the nostrils closed. Take a deep breath. Place your mouth over the individual's mouth to establish an airtight seal and give two slow breaths, each lasting 1½ to 2 seconds (take a breath after each breath). The chest should rise. **NOTE: To avoid contact with blood-borne pathogens, use a disposable physical barrier, such as a pocket mask, before doing mouth to mouth resuscitation.**

2. Remove your mouth to allow air to escape from the injured person's mouth and do the look, listen, feel technique to note air exchange.

3. Check the pulse at the carotid artery. Locate the Adam's apple with the index and middle finger. Slide the fingers to the side of the neck closest to you between the large neck muscle and windpipe (**Fig. 3.12**). Do not use the thumb, as it has its own pulse. Very little pressure is needed to detect the pulse. Take 5 to 10 seconds to establish the presence of a pulse.

4. If a pulse is present but the individual does not resume breathing, continue giving a breath every 5 seconds (12 breaths per minute) for an adult, or every 4 seconds (15 breaths per minute) for a child. After 10 to 12 breaths, recheck the pulse to ensure the heart is still beating. Continue give breaths until help arrives.

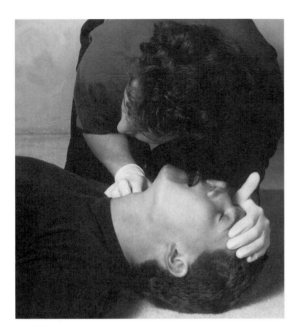

Figure 3.11. To assess respirations: Look to see if the chest is rising, listen for air exchange through the mouth or nose, and feel on your cheek if there is air exchanged.

5. If no pulse is present, proceed with cardiopulmonary resuscitation (CPR).

Establish Circulation

Each heart beat circulates blood to the vital organs. Combined with oxygen, minimal life support is sustained until advanced emergency care can be provided by trained emergency personnel. Circulation is maintained through chest compressions.

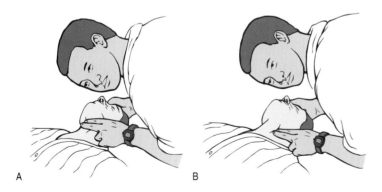

A   B

Figure 3.12. A, B. To take a carotid pulse, place two fingers on the larynx (Adam's apple), then gently slide the fingers into the groove between the larynx and sternocleidomastoid muscle on the side closest to you.

1. Locate the substernal notch with the hand closest to the individual's feet. Place the middle finger in the notch and index finger on the sternum.
2. Place the other hand (base hand) on the midline of the sternum with the thumb against the index finger of the distal hand.
3. Place the other hand on top of the base hand and bring your shoulders directly over the individual's sternum. Interlace the fingers to hold them off the chest wall and begin a cycle of 15 chest compressions and 2 breaths for an adult **(Fig. 3.13)**. The sternum should be compressed 1½ to 2 inches at a rate of 80 times per minute. In a child the ratio is 5 chest compressions to 1 breath. The heel of one hand is used to compress the midsternum 1 to 1½ inches.
4. After four continuous cycles, which should take about 1 minute, take another pulse for about 5 seconds.
5. If the individual's pulse does return, check and maintain breathing. If breathing does not return, begin rescue breathing and continue to monitor the pulse.
6. If breathing returns, monitor the ABC's and proceed with a secondary assessment.
7. If the pulse does not return, continue CPR until the ambulance arrives.

Never interrupt CPR for more than 5 seconds, because blood flow will drop to zero. **Field Strategy 3.10** demonstrates a full

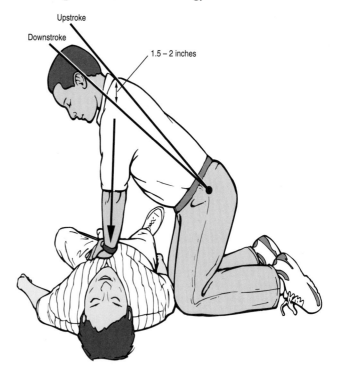

Figure 3.13. To perform CPR, keep your arms straight and fingers interlaced. Compress the sternum downward 1½ to 2 inches.

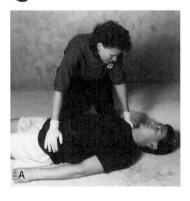

Establish unresponsiveness

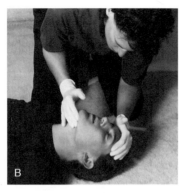

Open Airway

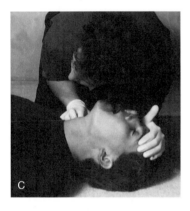

Breathing: Look, Listen, Feel
Note breathing rate and depth

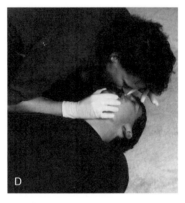

Give two breaths

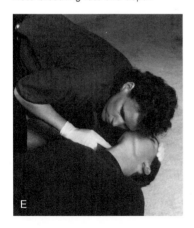

Check the carotid pulse
Note pulse rate and strength

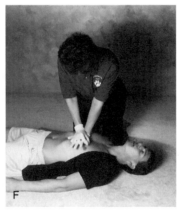

Locate proper hand position
Do chest compressions
(15 compressions; 2 ventilations)

Table 3.5. Flow Chart for the Primary Survey

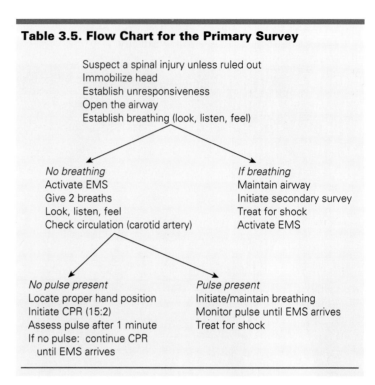

Suspect a spinal injury unless ruled out
Immobilize head
Establish unresponsiveness
Open the airway
Establish breathing (look, listen, feel)

No breathing
Activate EMS
Give 2 breaths
Look, listen, feel
Check circulation (carotid artery)

If breathing
Maintain airway
Initiate secondary survey
Treat for shock
Activate EMS

No pulse present
Locate proper hand position
Initiate CPR (15:2)
Assess pulse after 1 minute
If no pulse: continue CPR
   until EMS arrives

Pulse present
Initiate/maintain breathing
Monitor pulse until EMS arrives
Treat for shock

primary survey without an obstructed airway. **Table 3.5** is a flow chart that outlines the various action steps taken during a primary survey.

The gymnast was not moving as you approached. Upon arrival, however, the athlete groaned and moved an arm, verifying that breathing and circulation is present. Proceed to the secondary survey, but continue to monitor the ABCs in case shock occurs.

SECONDARY INJURY ASSESSMENT

The gymnast is somewhat lethargic but does respond to verbal commands. Breathing is shallow but pulse is normal. Think for a minute or two about how you will proceed to determine the seriousness of injury.

A secondary injury assessment involves a detailed hands-on, head-to-toe assessment to detect conditions that may not, in themselves, pose an immediate threat to life, but, if left unrecognized and untreated, could lead to serious complications. If the individual is moving and speaking or if the individual is unconscious and ABCs are adequate, begin the secondary injury assessment. In nearly all cases, an individual will regain consciousness in a short period of time and can then respond to your questions.

Many athletic trainers and other medical personnel begin the secondary survey with an assessment of **vital signs**, including pulse, respiration, blood pressure, and skin temperature. Although not vital signs, skin color, pupillary response to light, and eye movement should also be documented. Each of these factors will be discussed in the appropriate sections of the secondary assessment process. **Table 3.6** lists what abnormal vital signs may indicate.

A popular methodical process used extensively in sports injury assessment is the **HOPS** format and is used throughout the text. HOPS is an acronym for:

History of the injury.
Observation and inspection
Palpation
Special tests

The HOPS format uses both subjective information (history of the injury) and objective information (observation and inspection, palpation, and special tests) to recognize and identify problems contributing to the condition. In emergency situations, HOPS assessment includes an overall scan of the entire body. In a non-emergency sport injury, HOPS assessment focuses on a specific injury and associated structures and is discussed in detail in Chapter 4.

History of the Injury

An accurate history of the injury can help determine the extent and seriousness of injury. The individual's response, or lack of response, to verbal commands can also determine the level of consciousness. In a semiconscious or unconsciousness individual, information can be gathered from other players, officials, or by-standers. Remember, however, that an individual who is not fully responsive may have a head or neck injury. As such, stabilization of the head and neck must be maintained throughout the entire secondary survey. Ask the conscious individual to describe their perception of the problem, including the primary complaint, mechanism of injury, site and severity of pain, and any weakness or disability resulting from the injury.

Position yourself close to the individual and speak in a calm, confident manner. Tell the individual not to move the head or neck for any reason. Reassure the individual you are there to help. Questions should be open-ended to allow the person to provide as much information as possible about their perception of the problem. Listen attentively for clues that may indicate the nature of the injury. **Field Strategy 3.11** lists several questions to determine a history of the injury.

Vital signs
Objective measurements of pulse, respiration, blood pressure, and skin temperature, indicating normal body function

HOPS sports injury assessment:
    History of the injury
    Observation and inspection
    Palpation
    Special tests

Table 3.6. Abnormal Vital Signs and What They May Indicate

Pulse

Rapid, weak	Shock, internal hemorrhage, diabetic coma, or heat exhaustion
Rapid, bounding	Heat stroke, fright, fever, hypertension, or apprehension
Slow, bounding	Skull fracture, stroke, drug use (barbiturates and narcotics), certain cardiac problems, or some poisons
No pulse	Blocked artery, low blood pressure, or cardiac arrest

Respiration

Shallow breathing	Shock, heat exhaustion, insulin shock, chest injury, or cardiac problems
Irregular breathing	Airway obstruction, chest injury, diabetic coma, asthma, or cardiac problems
Rapid, deep	Diabetic coma, hyperventilation, or some lung diseases
Frothy blood	Lung damage, such as a puncture wound to the lung from a fractured rib or other penetrating object
Slowed breathing	Stroke, head injury, chest injury, or use of certain drugs
Wheezing	Asthma
Crowing	Spasms of the larynx
Apnea	Hypoxia (lack of oxygen), congestive heart failure, or head injuries
No breathing	Cardiac arrest, poisoning, drug abuse, drowning, head injury, or intrathoracic injuries with death imminent

Blood Pressure

Systolic is <100 mm	Hypotension caused by shock, hemorrhage, heart attack, internal injury, or poor nutrition
Systolic is >135 mm	Hypertension

Skin Temperature

Dry, cool	Exposure to cold or cervical, thoracic, or lumbar spine injuries
Cool, clammy	Shock, internal hemorrhage, trauma, or heat exhaustion
Hot, dry	Disease, infection, high fever, heat stroke, or overexposure to environmental heat
Hot moist	High fever
Isolated hot spot	Localized infection
Cold appendage	Circulatory problem
"Goose pimples"	Communicable disease, exposure to cold, pain, or fear

Table 3.6. (continued)

Skin Color

Red	Fever, hypertension, heat stroke, carbon monoxide poisoning, diabetic coma, alcohol abuse, infectious disease, inflammation, or allergy
White or ashen	Emotional stress (fright, anger, etc.), anemia, shock, heart attack, hypotension, heat exhaustion, insulin shock, or insufficient circulation
Blue or cyanotic	Heart failure, some respiratory disorders, and poisoning. In dark-skinned individuals, a bluish cast can be seen in the mucous membranes, the lips, and nail beds
Yellow	Liver disease or jaundice

Pupils

Constricted	Individual is using opiate-based drug or has ingested some poisons
Unequal	Head injury or stroke
Dilated	Shock, hemorrhage, heat stroke, coma, cardiac arrest, death, or use of a stimulant drug

Observation

In approaching the individual, observe body position for posturing and noticeable deformities that may indicate a fracture or dislocation. Is the individual breathing normally or in respiratory distress? Can the individual focus on your face and respond to commands? Is the person alert, restless, lethargic, or nonresponsive? Do they moan, groan, or mumble? Do the pupils of the eyes appear normal or dilated? Is there redness, bruising, or discoloration in the facial area or behind the ears? Note any clear fluid or bloody discharge from the ears or nose. This could be cerebrospinal fluid leaking from the cranial area as a result of a skull fracture. Is there visible swelling or deformity in the muscle(s) or joint? Always do bilateral comparison whenever possible.

Observe body position for noticeable deformities that may indicate a fracture or dislocation

Respiration

Breathing rate varies with the gender and age of an individual, but averages 12 to 20 breaths per minute in an adult and 20 to 28 breaths per minute in a child. Breathing rate is assessed by doubling the number of respirations in a 30-second period. Shallow breathing may indicate shock, heat exhaustion, chest injury, or a cardiac condition. Frothy blood during respirations may indicate lung damage due to a fractured rib.

Field Strategy 3.11. Determining the History of Injury and Level of Consciousness

Stabilize the head and neck; there may be a spinal injury!!

If unconscious:

Call the person's name loudly and gently tap the sternum or touch the arm. If no response, rap the sternum more forcibly or pinch the soft tissue in the armpit and note any withdrawal from the painful stimuli. If no response, immediately initiate the primary survey

If ABCs are adequate, proceed to the secondary survey. If you did not see what happened, question other players, officials, and bystanders. Ask:

What happened?

Did you see the individual get hit or did they just collapse?

How long has the individual been unconscious? Was it immediate or gradual? If gradual, did anyone talk to the individual before you arrived? What did the person say? Was it coherent? Did the person moan, groan, or mumble?

Has this ever happened before to this individual?

If conscious, ask:

What happened? If lying down, find out if they were knocked down, fell, or rolled voluntarily into that position

Did you hear any sounds or any unusual sensations when the injury occurred? Are they alert and aware of the surroundings or do they have any short- or long-term memory loss?

Do you have a headache? Where is the pain? Can you point to the area? Is the pain getting worse or better? If there is more than one painful area, ask which area hurts the most

Can you describe the pain? Is it localized or does it radiate into other areas?

Have you ever injured this body part before or experienced a similar injury? When did this happen?

How are you feeling now? Are you nauseous or sick to your stomach? Are you dizzy? Can you see clearly?

Are you taking any medication (prescription, over-the-counter, vitamins, birth control pills, etc)?

Are you allergic to anything?

Do not lead the individual. Let them describe what happened, and listen attentively for clues that will indicate the nature of the injury. Be professional and reassuring

Skin Color

Rubor
Reddish skin

Pallor
Ashen or pale skin

Skin color can indicate abnormal blood flow and low blood oxygen concentration in a particular body part or area. Three colors are commonly used in light-skinned individuals: red, white or ashen, and blue. A reddish skin color, or **rubor**, may indicate dilated capillary vessels from an increased blood flow, indicating fever, hypertension, or heat stroke. **Pallor**, ashen, or white skin color is caused by vasoconstriction of the capillaries resulting in decreased blood flow. This may indicate shock, heart attack, or hypotension. Skin that is bluish indicates cyanosis due to a possible heart failure, a respiratory disorder, or an obstructed airway. In dark-skinned individuals, skin pigments mask cyanosis. However, a bluish cast can be seen in mucous membranes (mouth, tongue, and inner eyelids), the lips, and nail beds. Fever in these individuals can be seen by a red flush color at the tips of the ears.

Pupils

Rapid constriction of pupils when the eyes are exposed to intense light is called the **pupillary light reflex**. Upon examination with a small bright light source, such as a pen light, the eyes may appear normal, constricted, unequal, or dilated **(Fig. 3.14)**. Unequal pupils indicate a possible head injury or stroke. Dilated pupils indicate shock, hemorrhage, cardiac arrest, coma, or death.

To test eye movement, ask the individual to focus on a single object. If the individual sees two images instead of one, it is called **diplopia**, or double vision. This condition occurs when the external eye muscles fail to work in a coordinated manner. Ask the individual to watch your fingers move to various positions. Test the individual's depth perception by placing a finger several inches in front of the individual and ask the person to reach out and touch the finger. Move the finger to several different locations and repeat the touch.

Pupillary light reflex
Rapid constriction of pupils when exposed to intense light

Diplopia
Double vision

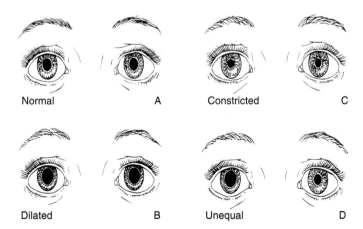

Normal   A   Constricted   C

Dilated   B   Unequal   D

Figure 3.14. Pupil size. **A**. Normal pupil size. **B**. Dilated pupils. **C**. Constricted pupils. **D**. Unequal pupils.

Palpation

Palpate for temperature, swelling, point tenderness, crepitus, deformity, muscle spasm, cutaneous sensation, and pulse

Palpation involves using the pads of the fingers in small circular or side-to-side motions to detect anomalies in bony and soft tissue structures. Palpations can detect eight different physical findings: pulse, temperature, swelling, point tenderness, crepitus, deformity, muscle spasm, and cutaneous sensation. Palpations begin at the head and move methodically down to the feet. **Field Strategy 3.12** lists the process commonly used in a head-to-toe assessment.

Pulse

Factors such as age, gender, aerobic physical condition, degree of physical exertion, medications or chemical substances being taken, blood loss, and stress all influence pulse rate and strength (3). Pulse is usually taken at the carotid artery because it is not normally obstructed by clothing, equipment, or strappings. Normal adult resting rates range between 60 and 80 beats a minute; aerobically conditioned athletes may be as low as 44 to 50 beats a minute. Normal rates for children range from 80 to 150 beats. Pulse is assessed during the secondary survey by doubling the pulse rate during a 30-second period. A rapid, weak pulse indicates shock. A slow, bounding pulse indicates a possible skull fracture, stroke, or cardiac problem.

Temperature

Core temperature is measured by a thermometer placed under the tongue, in the armpit, ear, or rectum. Rectal temperatures, usually 0.5°F higher than oral temperatures, are considered to be a more accurate measurement of temperature in the body's core (skull, thoracic, and abdominal regions) (5). Body temperature can also be reflected in the skin. Normally the skin is dry, but certain conditions, such as cold, shock, or fever, can alter surface blood vessels indicating a serious problem. Skin temperature is assessed by placing the back of the hand against the individual's forehead or by palpating appendages bilaterally (**Fig. 3.15**).

Bony Palpations

Possible fractures can be detected with palpation, percussion, vibration, compression, and distraction (**Fig. 3.16**). Palpation can detect deformity, crepitus, swelling, or increased pain at the fracture site. Percussion utilizes a tapping motion of the finger over a bony structure. A tuning fork sends vibrations through the bone in a similar manner and typically causes increased pain at a fracture site. For example, if an upper arm (humerus) fracture is suspected, tap lightly on the inside bony prominence at the elbow (medial epicondyle of the humerus). If the individual complains of pain in a specific region on the humerus, suspect a possible fracture. Compression is performed by gently compressing the distal end of the bone toward the proximal end, or by encircling the body

Field Strategy 3.12. Protocol for Head-to-toe Palpations

Stabilize the head and neck until a spinal injury is ruled out

Palpate the scalp and facial area for lacerations, deformities, or depressions. Discoloration over the mastoid process behind the ear (Battle's sign) or around the eyes (raccoon eyes) or presence of blood or cerebrospinal fluid from the ears or nose may indicate a skull fracture

Check the eyes for any injury, presence of contact lenses, pupil size, equality, and pupillary response to light. Both pupils may appear slightly dilated in an unconscious athlete. If the individual is conscious, check eye movement and tracking

Check the mouth for a mouthguard, dentures, broken teeth, or blood that may have caused or could cause a possible airway obstruction. Sniff for any odd breath odor, such as a fruity smell (diabetic coma) or alcohol

Palpate the cervical spine for point tenderness or obvious deformity. Check the anterior neck for indications of impact or bruising

Inspect and palpate the chest for possible wounds, discoloration, deformities, and chest expansion upon breathing. If the patient is unconscious, rap on the sternum to see if the individual withdraws from the touch. With conscious patients, use sternal or lateral rib compression to determine a possible rib fracture

Inspect and palpate the abdomen for tenderness, rigidity, distention, spasms, or pulsations. Palpate the lower back for deformity and point tenderness. Do not move the individual

Inspect and palpate the upper extremities for deformity, point tenderness, swelling, muscle spasm, and discoloration. Pinch in the armpit. Touch the fingers and ask if the individual can feel it. Does it feel the same on both hands? Can the individual move the fingers and squeeze your hand? Is there bilateral grip strength? Take a radial pulse and feel for skin temperature. Do not move the limbs or change body position

Inspect and palpate the pelvis and lower extremities for deformity, point tenderness, swelling, muscle spasms, and discoloration. Take a distal pulse at both the medial ankle (posterior tibial artery) and dorsum of the foot (dosalis pedis). Feel for skin temperature. Squeeze the gastrocnemius and pinch the top of the foot. Touch the toes and ask if the individual can feel it. Does it feel the same on both feet? Have the individual wiggle the toes and move the feet. Do not move the limbs or change body position

Recheck vital signs every 2 to 5 minutes until the ambulance arrives

Remember: **Do no harm to the individual.** If in doubt, assume the worse and treat accordingly

---

part, such as a foot or hand, and gently squeezing, thereby compressing the heads of the bones together. Again, if a fracture is present, pain will increase at the fracture site. Distraction employs a tensile force, whereby the application of traction to both ends of the fractured bone will help relieve pain.

> Distraction employs a tensile force, whereby pain should be relieved if a fracture is present

Soft Tissue Palpation

Deformity, such as an indentation, may indicate a rupture in a musculotendinous unit. A protruding, firm bulge may indicate a joint dislocation, ruptured bursa, or hematoma. Swelling may indicate diffuse hemorrhage or inflammation in a muscle, liga-

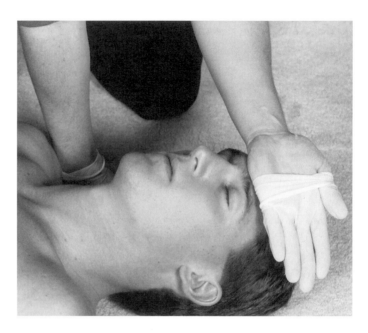

Figure 3.15. To assess skin temperature, place the back side of the hand against the individual's forehead, or compare appendages bilaterally by palpation and blanching of the nails.

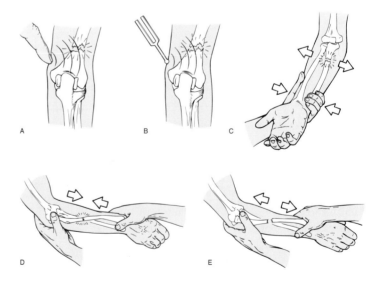

Figure 3.16. Determining a possible fracture. **A**. Percussion. **B**. Vibration using a tuning fork. **C, D**. Compression. **E**. Distraction. If the bone is fractured, pain will increase with percussion, vibration, and compression, but will decrease with distraction.

ment, bursa, or joint capsule. Note where point tenderness is elicited, as this may indicate the injured structure.

Cutaneous Sensation

Run your fingernails along both sides of the arms and legs, and ask the individual if it feels the same on both sides of the body part. Pain perception can also be tested by applying a sharp and dull point to the skin. Note whether the individual can distinguish the difference.

Special Tests

In an emergency, special tests are usually limited to determining whether a spinal injury is present. This can be assessed by the individual's response to verbal and motor commands. In a semiconscious or conscious individual, the inability to move a body part may indicate serious nerve damage to the central nervous system. Although initial assessment of unresponsiveness will be completed in the primary survey, further assessment of muscular movement should be completed before moving the individual.

Muscular Movement

In evaluating muscle movement, avoid any unnecessary movement of the individual. Ask the individual to wiggle the fingers and toes on both hands and feet. If this task is completed, place your fingers in both of their hands and ask the person to squeeze the fingers. Compare grip strength in both hands. Then have the individual dorsiflex and plantarflex both feet and compare bilateral strength.

In an unconscious individual, a verbal or motor response is not possible. Painful stimulation, however, may produce a reaction movement. For example, pinching the soft tissue in the person's armpit or striking the sternum with a knuckle may produce an eyelid flutter or involuntary movement away from the stimulus. Always remember, however, that slight traction should always be applied to the head of an unconscious individual to stabilize the head and neck region in case an involuntary reaction movement occurs. If there is no reaction, this indicates either a serious head or neck injury or that the individual is in a coma. This individual should not be moved until emergency personnel arrive. Monitor the ABCs, recheck the vital signs, and treat for shock.

Blood Pressure

Blood pressure is the force per unit area exerted on the walls of a blood vessel, generally the aorta. As one of the most important vital signs, blood pressure reflects the effectiveness of the circulatory system. Changes in blood pressure are very significant. **Systolic blood pressure** is measured when the left ventricle contracts and expels blood into the aorta. It is approximately 120 mm Hg for the healthy adult. **Diastolic blood pressure** is the residual

Systole
Pressure in aorta when left ventricle contracts

Diastole
Residual pressure in aorta between heart beats

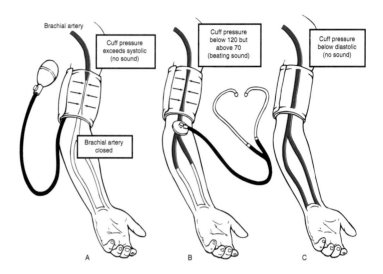

Figure 3.17. To measure blood pressure, apply the cuff snugly around the arm just proximal to the elbow (**A**). Inflate until the pressure gauge registers about 200 mm Hg. Blood flow is occluded and the brachial artery can no longer be palpated in the cubital fossa. Place the stethoscope over the brachial artery in the cubital fossa (**B**). Slowly deflate the cuff and listen for the first soft beating sounds (systolic pressure). As pressure is reduced still further, the sound will become louder and more distinct, but will gradually disappear as blood no longer becomes constricted. The pressure at which the sound disappears is the diastolic pressure (**C**).

pressure present in the aorta between heart beats and averages 70 to 80 mm Hg in healthy adults. Blood pressure may be affected by gender, weight, race, lifestyle, and diet. Blood pressure is measured in the brachial artery with a sphygmomanometer and stethoscope and is illustrated in **Figure 3.17**. Abnormal blood pressure values or low blood pressure may indicate shock, hemorrhage, or heart attack.

The gymnast reported pain on the left side of the chest that increased during deep inhalations. Discoloration is present on the lower left side of the anterior chest wall. Palpation elicited pain in the region of the 9th and 10th ribs on the lateral side and increased with compression on the sternum. Muscle strength and sensation in the hands and feet appear normal.

DETERMINATION OF FINDINGS

You have completed the emergency assessment of the gymnast. Pain is present in the thoracic region and deep respirations are inhibited and painful. Should you activate EMS to transport this individual to the nearest trauma center?

After completing the secondary assessment, a decision must be made on how best to handle the situation. If EMS has already been activated, control hemorrhage, splint suspected fractures, treat for shock, reassess vital signs every 2 to 5 minutes, and wait for the ambulance to arrive before moving the individual. As a general rule, an individual should be referred to the nearest trauma center if any life-threatening situation is present or if any loss of normal function occurs. Conditions that warrant activation of EMS and referral to a physician are listed in **Table 3.7**. If in doubt, always refer.

An individual should be referred to the nearest trauma center if there is a loss of function or a life-threatening situation present

This individual has painful, limited respirations; palpable pain; and discoloration in the thoracic region over the 9th and 10th ribs. EMS should be activated to transport this individual to the nearest trauma center for further assessment and treatment.

MOVING THE INJURED PARTICIPANT

How should this individual be transported to avoid additional pain and to keep the condition from getting worse?

The safest manner to move an individual is with a stretcher. Ideally, five trained individuals should roll, lift, and carry an injured person. The captain (the most medically-trained individual) will stabilize the head and give commands for each person to slowly lift the injured individual onto the stretcher. The individual is then secured on the stretcher. On command, the stretcher is raised to waist level. The individual should be carried feet first so the captain can constantly monitor the individual's condition. **Field Strategy 3.13** describes how to secure and move an individual on a stretcher.

When referring an individual to a trauma facility, document information, including the mechanism of injury, symptoms and vital signs, and any weakness, change of sensation, or disability as

Table 3.7. Emergency Conditions That Should be Referred to the Nearest Trauma Center or Physician

Medical emergencies that require activation of EMS (911)

Respiratory arrest or any irregularity in breathing
Severe chest or abdominal pains
Excessive bleeding from a major artery or a significant loss of blood
Suspected spinal injury
Head injury with loss of consciousness
Open fractures and fractures involving the femur, pelvis, or several ribs
Joint fracture or dislocation with no distal pulse
Severe signs of shock or possible internal hemorrhage

Injuries that require immediate referral to a physician

Eye injuries
Dental injuries when a tooth has been knocked loose or knocked out
Minor or simple fractures
Lacerations that may require suturing
Injuries in which a functional deficit is noticeable
Loss of normal sensation, diminished or absent reflexes
Noticeable muscular weakness in the extremities
Any injury where you may have doubts about its severity or nature

Field Strategy 3.13. Transporting an Injured Individual on a Stretcher

A. *Unless ruled out, assume that a spinal injury is present.* Place all extremities in an axial alignment. If the individual is lying face down, roll the individual supine. Four or five people are required to "log roll" the individual. The "captain" of the team (the most medically trained individual) stabilizes the head and neck in the position as they were found, regardless of the angle. The captain should position the arms in the cross-arm technique, so that, during the log roll, the arms will end in the proper position.

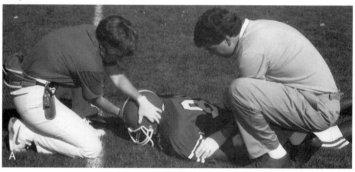

B. Place the spine board as close as possible beside the individual. Each person is responsible for one body segment: one at the shoulder, one at the hip, one at the knees, and, if needed, one at the feet. On command, roll the individual onto the board in a single motion.

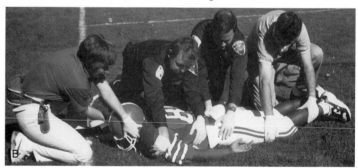

C. Once on the board, the captain continues to stabilize the head and neck, and, if not done previously, another person applies support around the cervical region. The chest is secured to the board first, then the feet. With a football player, do not remove the helmet.

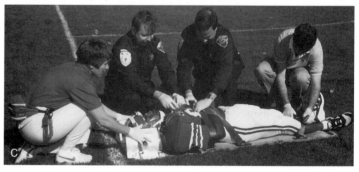

D. When secured to the board, four people lift the stretcher while the captain continues to monitor the individual's condition. Transport the individual feet first.

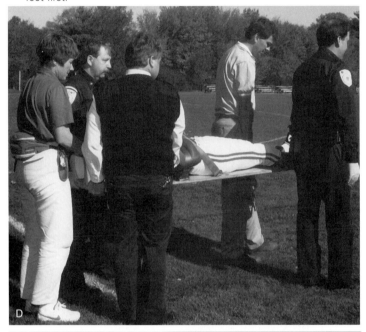

a result of the injury. Relay this information, and what actions were taken, to the appropriate individual (EMT, paramedic, or physician). A competitive school athlete seen by a physician should provide the school athletic trainer or coach with a written report from the physician stating the diagnosis and status of the athlete relative to return to sport participation. The athlete should not be allowed to return to competition until clearance is provided in writing by the supervising physician.

The injured gymnast should be transported on a stretcher by EMTs. The athletic trainer should provide the EMTs with information on the history of the injury, symptoms, vital signs, and any weakness, change of sensation, or disability as a result of the injury. In addition, any on-the-scene management of the situation and the results should be provided to the EMTs.

SUMMARY

Athletic trainers, coaches, and sport supervisors must know emergency procedures to recognize and assess life-threatening conditions. These emergencies may involve obstructed airway, cardiopulmonary emergencies, unconscious athlete, serious hemorrhage, fractures, shock, hyperthermia, and hypothermia. The facility should develop and implement an emergency procedures plan in consultation with local EMS to address these emergency situations.

Assessment of all injuries, no matter how minor, should always include a primary injury assessment. Primary injury assessment determines unresponsiveness and assesses the ABCs: Airway, Breathing, Circulation, and serious bleeding. The secondary survey includes a hands-on, head-to-toe assessment to detect medical and injury-related problems that do not pose an immediate life-threatening situation, but may do so if left untreated. The HOPS format uses both subjective information (history of the injury) and objective information (observation and inspection, palpation, and special tests) to recognize and identify problems contributing to the condition.

As a general rule, refer an individual to the nearest trauma center if any life-threatening situation is present or if the injury results in loss of normal function. In moving a seriously injured or unconscious individual, always suspect a possible head, neck, or spinal injury, and never move that individual unless qualified emergency medical personnel are present. If in doubt, suspect the worst and activate EMS for assistance.

REFERENCES

1. Foster DT, Rowedder LJ, and Reese SK. 1995. Management of sports-induced skin wounds. J Ath Tr 30(2):135–140.
2. Rheinecker SB. 1995. Wound management: the occlusive dressing. J Ath Tr 30(2):143–146.
3. Grant HD, Murray RH, and Bergeron JD. *Brady emergency care*. Englewood Cliffs, NJ: Prentice Hall, 1990.
4. Hafen BQ, and Karren KJ. *First aid and emergency care workbook*. Englewood, CO: Morton, 1990.
5. Ryan AJ. Heat stress. In *Prevention of athletic injuries: the role of the sports medicine team*, edited by FO Mueller and AJ Ryan. Philadelphia: FA Davis, 1991.
6. Leski MJ. Thermoregulation and safe exercise in the heat. In *Sports medicine secrets*, edited by MB Mellion. Philadelphia: Hanley & Belfus, 1994.
7. McArdle WD, Katch FI, and Katch VL. *Exercise physiology: energy, nutrition and human performance*. Philadelphia: Lea & Febiger, 1991.
8. Gutierrez G. 1995. Solar injury and heat illness: treatment and prevention in children. Phys Sportsmed 23(7):43–48.
9. American College of Sports Medicine. *ACSM's guidelines for exercise testing and prescription*. Baltimore: Williams & Wilkins, 1995.
10. Harrelson GL. 1986. Factors affecting the gastric emptying of athletic drinks. J Ath Tr 21(1):20–21.
11. Coyle EF. 1994. Fluid and carbohydrate replacement during exercise: how much and why? Spts Sci Exch 7(3):50.
12. Mellion MB, and Shelton GL. Safe exercise in the heat and heat injuries. In *The team physician's handbook*, edited by MB Mellion, WM Walsh, and GL Shelton. Philadelphia: Hanley & Belfus, 1990.
13. Fritz RL, and Perrin DH. Cold exposure injuries: prevention and treatment. In *Clinics in sports medicine*, edited by RL Ray, Vol. 8, no. 1. Philadelphia: WB Saunders, 1989.

14. Segan RD, Cassidy C, and Bentkowski J. 1993. A discussion of the issue of football helmet removal in suspected cervical spine injuries. J Ath Tr 28(4):294–305.
15. Ray R, Luchies C, Bazuin D, and Farrell RN. 1995. Airway preparation techniques for the cervical spine-injured football player. J Ath Tr 30(30):217–221.

Sports Injury Assessment

After completing this chapter, you should be able to:

- Identify the two main body segments and demonstrate anatomical position

- Define terms relative to direction, regions, and joint motion

- Describe the HOPS injury assessment process and the specific components in each portion of the process

- Differentiate between injury recognition and diagnosis

- Describe the components of SOAP notes and identify information recorded in each section

Key Terms:

Active movement	**Hypoesthesia**
Acute injury	**Indication**
Anatomical position	**Inspection**
Anesthesia	**Modalities**
Antalgic gait	**Muscle spindle**
Appendicular segment	**Myotome**
Atrophy	**Nerve root**
Axial segment	**Observation**
Chronic injury	**Painful arc**
Congenital	**Paresthesia**
Contraindication	**Passive movement**
Dermatome	**Prognosis**
Diagnosis	**Proprioceptors**
Ecchymosis	**Referred pain**
Effusion	**Resisted movement**
Goniometer	**Somatic pain**
Hyperesthesia	**Static position**
Hypertrophy	**Visceral pain**

With a sport-related injury, the athletic trainer is expected to evaluate the situation, assess the extent and seriousness of injury, and determine if referral to a physician is necessary (**Fig. 4.1**). This vital component in sports injury management is called injury assessment. Injury assessment allows for accurate recognition of the problem, determines appropriate and immediate treatment, and provides the foundation to develop a comprehensive rehabili-

> Injury assessment allows for accurate recognition of the problem, determines an appropriate and immediate treatment, and serves as a foundation to develop a comprehensive rehabilitation program

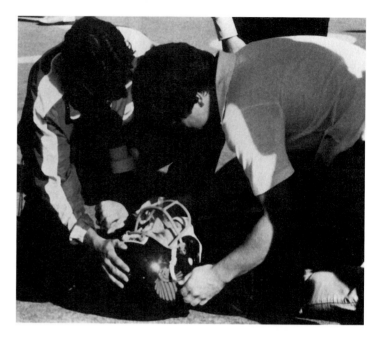

Figure 4.1. As the first person on the scene, you are expected to evaluate the situation, assess the extent and seriousness of injury, manage the injury, and determine if referral to the physician is necessary.

tation program. Without an accurate assessment, an injury may be neglected, leading to possible permanent deformity or disability. This role is essential in providing immediate health care.

This chapter focuses on key components in injury assessment using the HOPS format. First, a review of body regions, anatomical directions, and terms used to describe injuries or illnesses will be discussed. Then, beginning with an actual injury scenario, each section of the chapter will move step-by-step through the injury assessment process, describing terms and general techniques used to recognize and identify the injury.

ANATOMICAL FOUNDATIONS

? *A soccer player fell on an outstretched arm. You suspect a fracture above the elbow and have called the team physician. How will you present information so the physician can visualize the exact location of injury in order to assist you in taking appropriate action?*

Using correct terminology is crucial when communicating with members of the medical community. Anatomical terms, such as superior and inferior, medial and lateral, or thoracic and abdominal, help pinpoint the exact location on which to focus. Medical terms are used to describe the site, severity, and level of disability resulting from an injury. A brief overview of body segments and anatomical position, and terms related to directions, regions, and joint movements, will be discussed.

Body Segments and Anatomical Position

The human body is separated into two main segments: the axial and appendicular (**Fig. 4.2**). The **axial segment** relates to the head and trunk, and includes the chest and abdomen. The abdomen is further delineated into four quadrants (**Fig. 4.3**). The **appendicular segment** relates to the extremities. Direction or position on the body is based on the **anatomical position**. In this position the body is erect, facing forward, with the arms at the side of the body, palms facing forward.

Axial segment
Central part of the body, including the head and trunk

Appendicular segment
Relates to the extremities of the body, including the arms and legs

Anatomical position
Standardized position with the body erect, facing forward, with the arms at the sides, palms facing forward

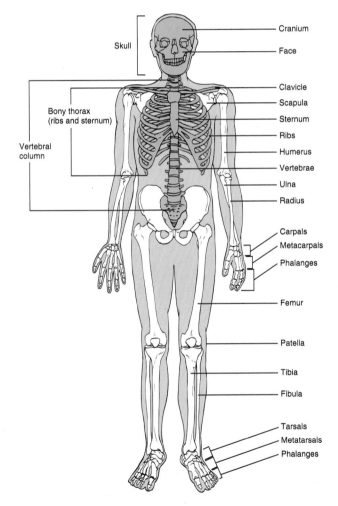

Figure 4.2. The human body is separated into two main regions. The axial region, shaded in red, includes the head and trunk. The appendicular region, shown in black and white, includes the extremities.

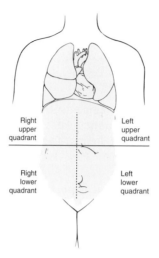

Right upper quadrant

Left upper quadrant

Right lower quadrant

Left lower quadrant

Figure 4.3. The abdomen and pelvic cavity is divided into four quadrants.

Directional Terms

Directional terms describe where one body part is relative to another

Directional terms are used to describe where one body part is relative to another. For example, the elbow is superior to the wrist, the chest is on the anterior thorax, and the big toe is on the medial side of the foot. These terms are always used relative to anatomical position, regardless of the body's actual position. In speaking with the team physician, the athletic trainer might report that pain is on the distal humerus, or just superior to the elbow. In this manner, the physician can better visualize where the pain is located. Common directional terms used in injury assessment are defined and illustrated in **Table 4.1**.

Table 4.1. Directional Terms

Term	Definition	Illustration	Example
Superior (cranial)	Toward the head or cranium		The heart is superior to the abdomen
Inferior (caudal)	Toward the lower part of the body		The pelvic cavity is inferior to the thoracic cavity
Anterior	Toward the front of the body		The quadriceps muscles lie anterior to the femur

Table 4.1. (continued)

Term	Definition	Illustration	Example
Posterior	Toward the back of the body		The buttock muscles lie posterior to the pelvis
Proximal	Closest to a reference point		The shoulder is proximal to the elbow
Distal	Farthest from a reference point		The wrist is distal to the elbow
Medial	Toward or at the midline of the body		The little finger is medial to the thumb
Lateral	Away from the midline of the body		The thumb is lateral to the little finger
Bilateral	Pertaining to both sides of the outer body		The ears are bilateral on the skull
Superficial	Toward or at the body surface		The skin is superficial to the muscles
Deep	Away from the body surface		The femur is deep to the skin

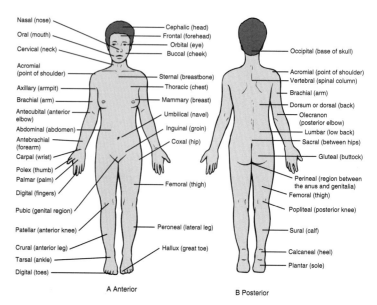

Figure 4.4. Regional terms are used to depict specific body areas.

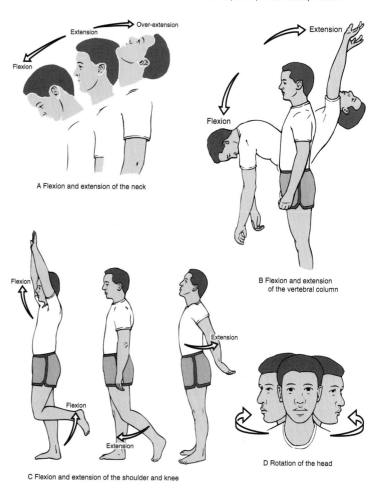

A Flexion and extension of the neck

B Flexion and extension of the vertebral column

C Flexion and extension of the shoulder and knee

D Rotation of the head

Figure 4.5. Movements allowed at synovial joints.

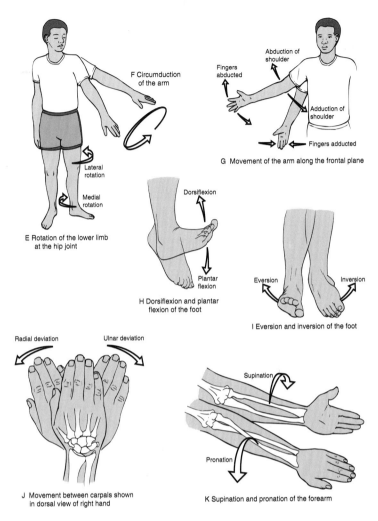

F Circumduction of the arm

Lateral rotation

Medial rotation

E Rotation of the lower limb at the hip joint

Abduction of shoulder

Fingers abducted

Adduction of shoulder

Fingers adducted

G Movement of the arm along the frontal plane

Dorsiflexion

Plantar flexion

H Dorsiflexion and plantar flexion of the foot

Eversion

Inversion

I Eversion and inversion of the foot

Radial deviation

Ulnar deviation

J Movement between carpals shown in dorsal view of right hand

Supination

Pronation

K Supination and pronation of the forearm

Figure 4.5. (continued)

Regional Terms

Regional terms are used to specify a general area of the body, such as the nasal, thoracic, abdominal, axillary, or popliteal region. Regional terms are illustrated in **Figure 4.4**.

> Regional terms specify a general area of the body

Joint Movement Terms

Injury assessment typically focuses on freely moveable joints. Although a specific joint can perform an isolated single motion, many activities, such as throwing or kicking a ball, require several simultaneous movements. In injury assessment, a single movement, such as abduction or flexion, is used to assess range of motion and muscle weakness at a specific joint. The various individual motions are defined and illustrated in **Figure 4.5**. Specific joint motions are discussed in the appropriate chapters.

The soccer player fell on an outstretched arm and you sus-pected a possible fracture. In explaining the site of pain, you might report that extreme pain is present two inches proximal to the elbow joint, particularly on the medial aspect of the humerus.

ASSESSING AN INJURY

A high school football player is complaining of an sharp, aching pain in the posterior ankle region. It is particularly bothersome when he goes up on his toes, during sprints, or when he explodes upward from his crouched stance. Think for a minute or two about what information should be gathered from this indi-vidual to help identify factors that may have caused the injury.

Emergency situations are evaluated using a primary and sec-ondary survey to determine injuries or conditions that might pose a threat to life. In a specific sport-related injury, the HOPS format, introduced in Chapter 3, is used extensively to assess an injury in a consistent, systematic process. HOPS is an acronym for:

History of the injury
Observation and inspection
Palpation
Special tests

The HOPS format uses both subjective information (history of the injury) and objective information (observation and inspection, palpation, and special tests) to recognize and identify the condi-tion. These steps are followed in all injury assessments.

On-the-field vs. Off-the-field Assessment

Ideally, injury assessment should be conducted in a physician's office or training room where some amount of privacy exists. In addition, pressure to complete a thorough exam is not usually a factor in these locations. Realistically, however, this may not be possible.

Many injury assessments occur on the field during competition, where environmental conditions, such as rain, mud, or snow, may complicate the process. Officials, coaches, or parents may put pressure on the athletic trainer to assess the injury quickly to determine the playing status of the injured individual. After the primary survey is completed, the "on-the-field" assessment ascer-tains if a moderate or serious injury is present (i.e., fracture, dislocation, unstable joint, severe bleeding, rupture of the muscu-lotendinous unit, or nerve damage). If so, appropriate immobiliza-tion and transportation should be utilized in removing the individ-ual from the field or court. Once off the field or court, a more thorough exam can be conducted. Decisions on the extent of injury, treatment, and playing status must be based on sound medical assessment despite external influencing factors. Regard-less of where the assessment occurs, all protocols should contain the same basic components that are relevant, accurate, and mea-surable.

Field Strategy 4.1. Injury Assessment Protocol

History of the Injury

Primary complaint
   Nature, location, and onset of the condition
Mechanism of injury
   Cause of stress, position of limb, and direction of force
   Changes in running surface, shoes, equipment, techniques, or
   conditioning modes
Characteristics of the symptoms
   Nature, location, severity, and duration of symptoms
   Disability resulting from the injury
Related medical history
Past musculoskeletal injuries, congenital abnormalities, and family history

Observation and Inspection

Observation should analyze
   Symmetry and appearance
   Motor function
Inspection at the injury site
   Observe for deformity, swelling, discoloration, scars, and general skin
     condition

Palpation

Bony structures; determine a possible fracture
Soft tissue structures
Palpate for skin temperature, swelling, deformity, crepitus, point
   tenderness, muscle spasm, cutaneous sensation, and pulse

Special Tests

Joint range of motion
Resisted manual muscle testing
Neurologic testing
   Motor testing
   Sensory testing
   Reflex testing
Stress tests
Functional testing in sport-specific skills

At this level of understanding, sections on assessment throughout the text will be limited to basic concepts and skills. Students wishing to learn more advanced assessment and rehabilitation skills should enroll in an upper level athletic training class. Using the scenario listed above, each component of the assessment process will be described. At the end of each section, symptoms and signs will be provided to help recognize and identify the injury. A brief outline of the steps can be seen in **Field Strategy 4.1**.

HISTORY OF THE INJURY

The football player complained of a sharp, aching pain on the posterior aspect of the ankle that increased when the foot was plantar flexed. Think for a minute or two about what questions

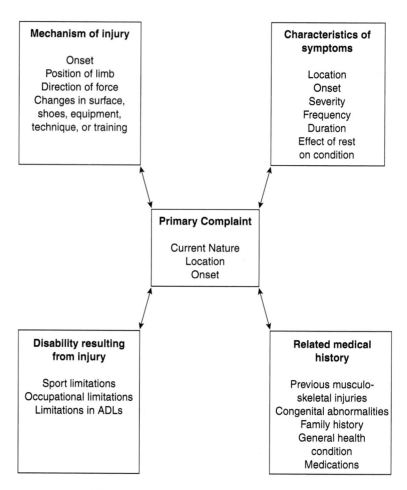

Figure 4.6. The components of a history of an injury.

should be asked to help identify the cause and extent of the condition.

Identifying the history of the injury can be the most important step in injury assessment. A complete history includes information on the primary complaint, cause or mechanism of injury, extent of pain or disability due to the injury, previous injuries to the area, and family history, all of which may have a bearing on this specific condition. This information can identify reasons for the weakness or pain and may indicate possible injured structures prior to initiating the physical evaluation. These topics are summarized in **Figure 4.6**.

History taking requires a great deal of patience and practice in asking the right questions. In an on-the-field assessment, it is imperative to focus on only vital information. Present yourself in a competent professional manner. Listen attentively and maintain eye contact. This establishes rapport with the injured athlete and may lead to more accurate responses to the questions and instructions.

A complete history includes information on the
Primary complaint
Cause or mechanism of injury
Extent of pain or disability
Previous injuries to the area
Family history

Listen attentively and maintain eye contact

Primary Complaint

The primary complaint focuses on what the injured individual believes may be the current injury. Questions should be phrased to allow the individual to describe the current nature, location, and onset of the condition (1). For example, ask: What is the problem? Where does it hurt? Did you hear any sounds like a snap or pop? What activities or motions are weak or painful? Realize, however, that the individual may not wish to carry on a lengthy discussion about the injury or may trivialize the extent of pain or disability. Be patient and keep questions simple. Pay close attention to words and gestures used to describe the condition, as they may provide clues to the quality or intensity of the symptoms.

Mechanism of Injury

After listening to the primary complaint, determine the mechanism of injury. This is probably the most important information gained in taking a history. Ask how the condition occurred: Did you fall? In what position did you land? Were you struck by an object or another individual? In what position was the involved body part, and what direction was the force? If the condition developed over time, ask when the injured person first became aware of the problem. Have there been recent changes in running surface, shoes, equipment, techniques, or conditioning modes? These factors may lead to abnormal stress on joints or body parts and may account for blisters, stress fractures, medial tibial stress syndrome, or chronic pain from overuse injuries. It is important to visualize how the injury occurred to determine possible damaged structures. This helps direct the objective evaluation.

Characteristics of the Symptoms

The primary complaint must be explored in detail to discover the evolution of symptoms, including the nature, location, severity, and duration of pain or disability. The individual's pain perception, for example, can indicate what structures may be injured. There are two categories of pain: somatic and visceral. **Somatic pain** arises from the skin, ligaments, muscles, bones, or joints, and is the most common type of pain encountered in sport injuries. **Visceral pain** results from disease or injury to an organ in the thoracic or abdominal cavity, such as compression, tension, or distension of the viscera. **Referred pain** is a type of visceral pain that travels along the same nerve pathways as somatic pain and is perceived by the brain as somatic in origin. Referred pain, for example, occurs when an individual has a heart attack. The individual feels pain in the chest, the left arm, and sometimes the neck. **Figure 4.7** demonstrates cutaneous areas where pain from visceral organs can be referred.

Pain can travel up or down the length of any nerve and be referred to another region. For example, an individual who has a low back problem can feel the pain down the gluteal region into

> Allow the individual to describe the current nature, location, and onset of the condition

> The individual's pain perception can indicate what structures may be injured

Somatic pain
Pain originating in the skin, ligaments, muscles, bones, or joints

Visceral pain
Pain resulting from injury or disease to an organ in the thoracic or abdominal cavity

Referred pain
Pain felt in a region of the body other than where the source or actual cause of the pain is located

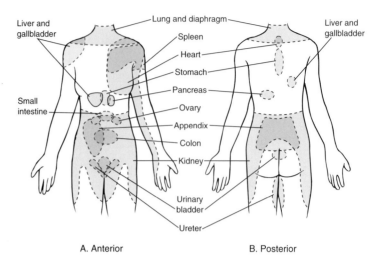

Liver and gallbladder
Lung and diaphragm
Spleen
Heart
Stomach
Pancreas
Small intestine
Ovary
Appendix
Colon
Kidney
Liver and gallbladder
Urinary bladder
Ureter

A. Anterior   B. Posterior

Figure 4.7. A, B. Certain visceral organs can refer pain to specific cutaneous areas. Keep this in mind if all special tests are negative, yet the individual continues to feel pain at a specific site.

> If a nerve is injured, pain or a change in sensation, such as a numbing or burning sensation, can be felt along the length of the nerve

the back of the leg. If a nerve is injured, pain or a change in sensation, such as a numbing or burning sensation, can be felt along the length of the nerve.

To assess the condition, ask detailed questions about the location, onset, severity, frequency, and duration of the individual's symptoms. For example, ask the football player: Where does it hurt the most? Can you point to a specific spot? Is the pain limited to that area or does it radiate into other parts of the leg or foot? When does the pain set in (early morning, during exertion, or at night)? On a scale from 1 to 10, with 10 most severe, how bad is the pain? How long does the pain last? What activities aggravate or alleviate the symptoms? How long has the condition been present? Has the pain changed or stayed the same? What medications, treatments, or exercise programs have improved the situation in the past?

If pain is localized, limited bony or soft tissue structures are involved. Diffuse pain around the entire joint indicates that several structures are injured, or the joint is inflamed. These answers can also determine if the individual has an **acute injury** resulting from a specific event leading to a sudden onset of symptoms, or a **chronic injury** characterized by a slow, sustained development of symptoms that culminate in a painful inflammatory condition.

> **Acute injury**
> Injury from a specific event leading to a sudden onset of symptoms
>
> **Chronic injury**
> Injury characterized by a slow, sustained development of symptoms that culminates in a painful inflammatory condition

Disability Resulting From the Injury

> Limitation in activities should include limitations in work and daily activities

Determine what the individual is unable to do because of pain, weakness, or disability from the injury. Questions should not be limited to sport participation, but should include occupational limitations and limitations in daily activities. Activities of daily living (ADLs) are actions most people perform without thinking, such as combing the hair, brushing the teeth, or walking up or down stairs. In questioning the football player, ask what activities are limited because of the injury. Has the injury affected his job, school work, or ADLs?

Related Medical History

Obtain information regarding other problems or conditions that might have affected this injury. Information extrapolated from the individual's preseason physical examination may verify past childhood diseases or medical problems: allergies; use of contact lenses or prosthetic devices; and past episodes of infectious diseases, loss of consciousness, recurrent headaches, heat stroke, seizures, or eating disorders. Previous musculoskeletal injuries or congenital abnormalities may place additional stress on joints predisposing the individual to certain injuries. Ask if the individual is on any prescribed or over-the-counter medication. The type, frequency, dosage, and effect may mask some symptoms.

A common method used to elicit information on the history of an injury is to group five categories of questions, and is remembered with the acronym **PQRST**:

Provocative—**P**alliative—**P**ast injuries
Quality—**Q**uantity
Region—**R**adiation
Severity scale
Timing

Examples of questions that may be used in each category may be found in **Field Strategy 4.2**. These are only provided as a guide and are not listed in any specific order.

💡 *The varsity football player is 17 years old. His primary complaint is a sharp, aching pain on the posterior aspect of the ankle in the region of the Achilles tendon. He rates the pain as a 6 on the 10 point scale when he is walking and a 9 when he does wind sprints or explodes upward from his crouched stance. Pain is reduced when he ices the region after practice. He cannot recall injuring the ankle, but the pain has been present for 3 weeks and does not seem to be improving. A physician has not been consulted about this injury.*

OBSERVATION AND INSPECTION

❓ *A significant amount of information has been gathered from the football player. The next step is to observe the individual and inspect the injury site. What observable factors might indicate the seriousness of injury?*

Observation and inspection begins the objective evaluation in an injury assessment. Although explained as a separate step, observation begins the moment the injured person is seen and continues throughout the assessment. **Observation** refers to the visual analysis of overall appearance and symmetry and general motor function **(Fig. 4.8)** (2). **Inspection** refers to factors seen at the actual injury site, such as redness, bruising, swelling, cuts, or scars.

Observation
Visual analysis of overall appearance, symmetry, general motor function, posture, and gait

Inspection
Refers to factors seen at the actual injury site, such as redness, swelling, bruising, cuts, or scars

Field Strategy 4.2. Developing a History of the Injury

Determine the (a) primary complaint; (b) mechanism of injury; (c) characteristics of the symptoms; (d) functional deficits relative to ADLs (Activity of Daily Living); and (e) related medical history. ASK:

Provocative—Palliative—Past Injuries or Conditions

What is the problem? Do you recall how it happened?
Do you remember what position the limb was in, and the direction of force?
What activities aggravate or alleviate the symptoms?
What have you done for it? Has this helped?
What different activities have you been doing in the last week? (Ask about changes in shoes, equipment, running surfaces, or conditioning modes, such as frequency, duration, intensity, type, or technique.)
Have you ever injured this area before? Who evaluated the injury? What did you do for it then? Did it help?
Have you had any medical problems recently? (Look for problems that may refer pain from visceral organs, heart, and lungs.) Do you have any allergies? Are you on any medication?
Do you have any musculoskeletal problems elsewhere in the body? (These may result in changes in gait or technique that transfer abnormal forces to other structures.)
Has anyone in your family had a similar problem?

Quality—Quantity

Can you describe the pain (dull ache, throbbing, sharp, intermittent, red-hot, or burning)?
Did you hear any sounds during the incident? Any snaps, pops, or cracks? (This may indicate the tissues involved in the injury.)
Did you notice any swelling or discoloration at the time of the injury?
Have you had any muscle spasms or numbness with the injury?

Region—Radiation

Where is the pain or weakness located?
Is the pain localized in one area? Can you point to the most painful site?
Does the pain or numbness radiate up or down the limb?

Severity Scale

On a scale of 1 to 10, with 10 being very severe, how would you rate your pain or weakness?
Is the pain worse in the morning, during activity, after activity, or at night? When the pain sets in, how long does it last? Is it the same type of pain that you are experiencing now?
Are there certain activities you are unable to perform because of the pain? Which ones?

Timing

Did the pain come on gradually (overuse problem) or suddenly (acute problem)?
When the pain sets in, how long does it last?
Was the pain greatest when the injury first occurred, or did it get worse the second or third day?
How long has this injury been a problem?
How old are you? (Many chronic problems are age-related.)

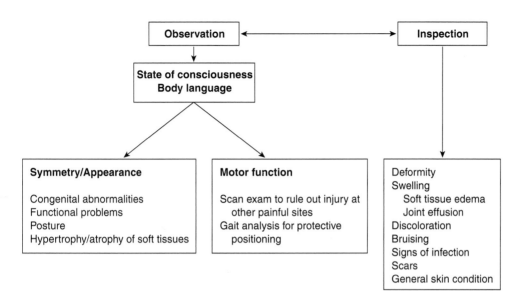

Figure 4.8. The components of observation and inspection.

Observation

Often the athletic trainer sees an acute injury happen. In many instances, however, the individual will come to the sideline or training room complaining of pain or discomfort. Immediately assess the individual's state of consciousness and body language that may indicate pain, disability, fracture, dislocation, or respiratory distress. Note the individual's general posture, willingness and ability to move, ease in motion, and general overall attitude (2). Using discretion in safeguarding the athlete's privacy, the injured area should be fully exposed. This may involve the removal of protective equipment and clothing.

Note the individual's willingness and ability to move, general posture, consistency in limitations of motion, and general overall attitude

Symmetry and Appearance

Visually scan the body to detect **congenital** or functional problems that may be contributing to the injury. Observe any abnormalities in the spinal curves, general symmetry of the various body parts, and general attitude of the body from an anterior, lateral, and posterior view. For example, does the individual naturally stand with the back straight, shoulders back, and head in a straight and level position? Does the body look symmetrical? Visually scan soft tissue for **hypertrophy** or **atrophy**. **Field Strategy 4.3** provides a more detailed assessment of general symmetry and appearance in a standing position.

Congenital
Existing since birth

Hypertrophy
Increase in general bulk or size of an individual tissue, such as a muscle, not due to tumor formation

Atrophy
A wasting away or deterioration of tissue due to disease, disuse, or malnutrition

Motor Function

Many individuals use a scan exam and gait analysis to assess general motor function. The scan exam rules out injury at other joints that may be overlooked due to intense pain or discomfort at the

Many individuals use a scan exam and gait analysis to assess general motor function

Field Strategy 4.3. Assessment of General Appearance and Symmetry

Anterior View

Is the head and neck in the midline of the body? Does the facial region appear well-shaped and normal?

The slope of the shoulder muscles should appear bilaterally equal and well-rounded with no prominent bony structures. The level of the shoulder on the dominant side will usually be lower than the nondominant side.

Note any scars or muscular atrophy that may be present.

Is the space between the arms and body the same on both sides?

Are both hands held in the same position?

Does the rib cage look symmetrical, with no bony protrusions?

Are the folds of the waist at the same height?

Are the kneecaps (patellae) level and facing forward?

Are the distal bony prominences of the lower leg bilaterally level? Are arches present on both feet? Do the feet angle equally?

Side View

Can you draw an imaginary straight plumb line from the ear through the middle of the shoulder, hip, knee, and ankle?

Does the back have any excessive curves?

Are the elbows held near full extension?

Does the pelvis appear to be level?

Are the knees straight, flexed, or hyperextended? Normally they should be slightly flexed.

Posterior View

Does the spine appear to be straight? Note any abnormal prominence of any bony structures or muscle atrophy.

Are the scapulae at the same height and resting at the same angle? Do they lie flat against the rib cage?

Are the waist folds level? Are the posterior gluteal folds level?

Are the skin creases on the posterior knee level?

Do both Achilles tendons descend straight to the floor? Are the heels straight, angled in (varus), or angled out (valgus)?

---

primary injury site. The injured person is observed doing gross motor movements in the neck, trunk, and extremities. Note if there is any hesitation to move a body part or if the individual prefers to use one side over another. Gross motor movements may include looking up at the ceiling; rotating the head sideways in both directions; bending forward to touch the toes; rotating the trunk; bringing the palms together above the head and behind the back; doing a straight leg raise forward, backward, and sideways; bending the knees; and walking on the heels and toes.

When not **contraindicated**, observe the normal swing of the individual's arms and legs while the individual walks several yards. Stand behind, in front, and to the side of the individual to observe from all angles. A shoulder injury may be evident in a limited arm swing or by holding the arm close to the body in a splinted position.

Indication
A condition that could benefit from a specific action

Contraindication
A condition adversely affected by a specific action

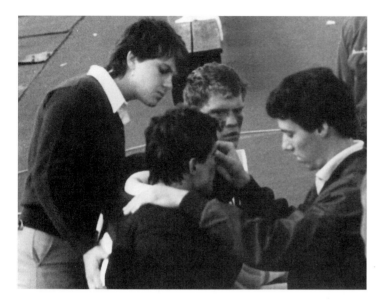

Figure 4.9. Inspect for any deformities, swelling, discoloration, scars, and general skin condition.

A lower extremity injury may produce a noticeable limp, or **antalgic gait**.

Inspection of the Injury Site

Inspect the localized injury site for any deformity, swelling (edema or joint effusion), discoloration (redness, bruising, or ecchymosis), signs of infection (redness, swelling, pus, or red streaks), scars that might indicate previous surgery, and general skin condition (oily, dry, blotchy red spots, sores, or hives) **(Fig. 4.9)**. Swelling inside the joint is called localized intra-articular swelling, or joint **effusion**, and makes the joint appear enlarged, red, and puffy. **Ecchymosis** is discoloration or swelling outside the joint in the surrounding soft tissue due to a bruise or injury under the skin. Always compare the injured area to the opposite side if possible. This bilateral comparison helps to establish what is normal for this individual.

Although the football player appeared to have good body symmetry, he was unable to raise up on his toes or walk without a noticeable limp. Visual inspection of the Achilles tendon demonstrated redness and slight swelling on the posterior aspect of the tendon.

PALPATION

The Achilles tendon is red, swollen, and painful. How can the area be palpated to determine the extent and severity of injury without causing additional pain?

Antalgic gait
Walking with a limp to avoid pain

Localized inspection of the site should detect any deformities, discoloration, edema, scars, and general skin condition

Effusion
The escape of fluid from the blood vessels into a cavity or joint

Ecchymosis
Superficial tissue discoloration

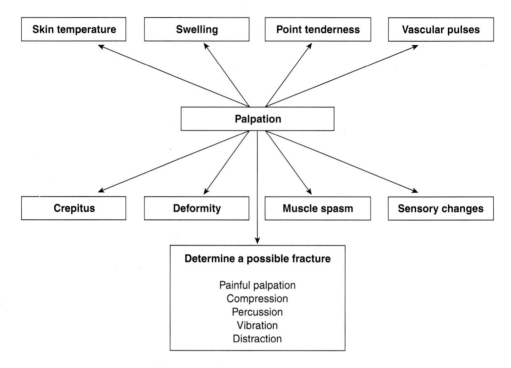

Figure 4.10. The components of palpation.

Bilateral palpation of paired anatomical structures can detect eight physical findings: temperature, swelling, point tenderness, crepitus, deformity, muscle spasm, cutaneous sensation, and pulse (**Fig. 4.10**). Before touching the individual, make sure your hands are clean and warm. Always wear latex examination gloves as a universal precaution against disease and infection to protect both yourself and the athlete. Begin palpation with gentle circular pressure followed by gradual deeper pressure (**Fig. 4.11**). Always begin palpation on structures away from the injury site and progress toward the injured area. Palpate the painful area last to avoid any carryover of pain into noninjured areas.

When the fingers first touch the skin, note skin temperature. Increased temperature at the injury site could indicate inflammation or infection, whereas decreased temperature could indicate a reduction in circulation. Swelling can be localized in a small area, or diffuse. If swelling is inside the joint, motion will often be limited because of congestion caused by extra fluid. Point tenderness and crepitus indicate damage to bony or soft tissue structures and should be palpated with as little pressure as possible. Cutaneous sensation can be tested by running the fingers along both sides of the body part and asking the individual if it feels the same on both sides. This technique will determine possible nerve involvement, particularly if the individual has numbness or tingling in the body limb. Peripheral pulses are taken distal to an injury to rule out damage to a major artery. Common sites are

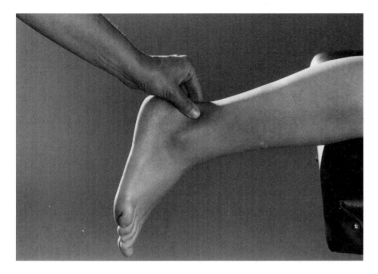

Figure 4.11. Begin palpation with gentle circular pressure, followed by gradual deeper pressure. Feel for skin temperature, swelling, point tenderness, crepitus, deformity, muscle spasm, cutaneous sensation, and pulse.

the radial pulse at the wrist and dorsalis pedis on the dorsum of the foot (**Fig. 4.12**) .

Palpation of bones determines the possibility of fractures, crepitus, and loose bony or cartilaginous fragments. Possible fractures can be assessed by palpating around the entire limb, with percussion, vibration through the use of a tuning fork, compression, and

Palpation of bones determines the possibility of fractures, crepitus, and loose bony or cartilaginous fragments

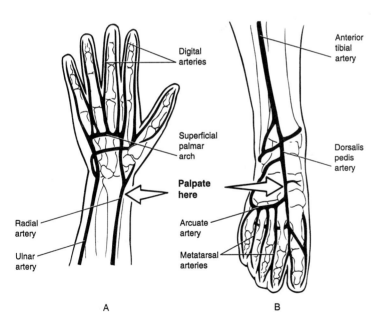

Figure 4.12. Pulses can be taken at the radial pulse in the wrist (**A**) or at the dorsalis pedis on the dorsum of the foot (**B**).

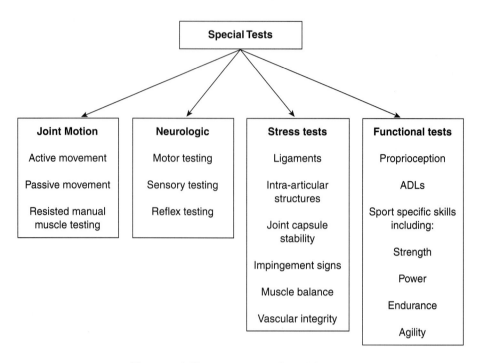

Figure 4.13. The components of special tests.

distraction (see **Figure 3.16**). If test results indicate a possible fracture, assume one is present and immobilize the region.

💡 *Palpation revealed warmth and slight swelling over the distal Achilles tendon. Sharp pain was elicited directly over the tendon, approximately one inch proximal to its distal insertion into the calcaneus. All fracture tests were negative.*

SPECIAL TESTS

❓ *There is little risk of a fracture present. How will you proceed to test the integrity of the soft tissue structures to determine the extent and severity of injury? What factors might limit range of motion at the joint?*

After fractures and/or dislocations have been ruled out, soft tissue structures, such as muscles, ligaments, the joint capsule, and bursae, are assessed using special tests. Although a more extensive explanation will be given in the individual chapters, general principles will be discussed here. Special tests assess joint motion, muscle strength, neurologic integrity, joint stability, and coordination and balance in functional skills (**Fig. 4.13**).

> Special tests assess joint motion, muscle strength, neurologic integrity, joint stability, and coordination and balance in functional skills

Joint Range of Motion

Active movement is joint motion performed voluntarily by the individual through muscular contraction, and is typically called

> **Active movement**
> Joint motion performed voluntarily by the individual through muscular contraction

active range of motion (AROM). In contrast, **passive range of motion** (PROM) occurs when the injured limb or body part is moved with no assistance from the injured individual. When resistance is added to the motion, it is called **resisted movement**.

AROM determines possible damage to contractile tissue (musculotendinous unit), and measures muscle strength and movement coordination. PROM distinguishes injury to noncontractile tissues (bone, ligaments, bursae, joint capsule, and neurovascular structures).

To measure range of motion, ask the individual to actively move the injured body part through the various joint motions and compare each motion with the uninjured body part. For example, ask the football player to bilaterally move the top of both feet toward the shin, away from the shin, bring the soles of the feet together, and move the soles of the feet away from the midline of the body. Compare the fluidity and extent of movement in both feet to see if they are bilaterally equal.

Limitation in motion may be due to pain, swelling, muscle spasm, muscle tightness, joint contractures, nerve damage, or mechanical blocks, such as a loose body. Ask if the motion causes pain and at what point in the motion the pain occurs. Does the pain appear only in a limited range of motion (painful arc)? Is the pain the same type of pain associated with the primary complaint? Perform any painful movements last, because this will avoid any carryover of pain from testing one motion to the next. If no pain is present during passive motion but is present during active motion, the musculotendinous unit is involved. If noncontractile tissue is injured, passive movement is painful and limitation of movement may be seen.

Joint range of motion can be measured quantitatively with a **goniometer (Fig. 4.14)**. The instrument is a protractor with two rigid arms that intersect at a hinge joint, and can measure both joint position and available joint motion (3). This measurement can determine when the individual has regained normal motion at a joint and is ready to return to participation.

Resisted Manual Muscle Testing

To measure muscle strength or to detect an injury to the nervous system, an overload pressure may be applied in a stationary or **static position**, or throughout the full range of motion. Muscle weakness and pain indicate a muscular strain. Muscle weakness in the absence of pain may indicate nerve damage.

In a static position, overload pressure is done in a neutral or relaxed position to relax joint structures and reduce joint stress. As such, muscles and their tendons are stressed more. In a fixed position, the individual is asked to elicit a maximal contraction while the body part is stabilized to prevent little or no joint movement. For example, to test strength in the ankle dorsiflexors, flex the ankle at 90° and apply downward overpressure on the dorsum

Passive movement
A limb or body part is moved through the range of motion with no assistance from the individual

Resisted movement
Any form of active motion in which a dynamic or static muscular contraction is resisted by an outside force applied manually or mechanically

If pain is present during active motion but not during passive motion, the musculotendinous unit has been injured

If pain is present during passive motion and active motion, the noncontractile tissues around the joint have been injured

Goniometer
Protractor used to measure joint position and available joint motion (range of motion)

Static position
Stationary position in which no motion occurs

Resisted manual muscle testing can assess muscle strength after an injury or surgery, and detect injury to the nervous system

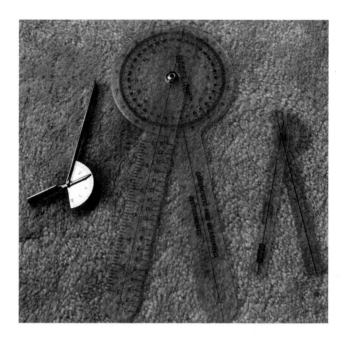

Figure 4.14. Goniometers come in a variety of sizes for the different body joints. Each is a protractor with two rigid arms that can measure joint position and range of motion.

of the foot and tell the individual not to let the foot move **(Fig. 4.15)**. Contractions are held at least 5 seconds and repeated 5 to 6 times, to indicate muscle weakening and the presence or absence of pain (4).

Two advantages of testing throughout the full range of motion are: 1) a better overall assessment of weakness can be determined,

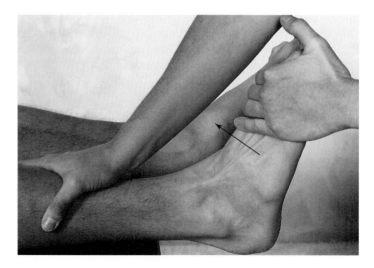

Figure 4.15. To test muscle strength at the ankle in a static position, stabilize the lower leg with one hand. Apply a downward overpressure on the dorsum of the foot and ask the individual to prevent any movement.

and 2) a **painful arc** of motion can be located that might go undetected if the test is only performed in the midrange. The muscle(s) to be tested is placed on stretch in an elongated position, with the body segment stabilized, to isolate the muscle movement. This position prevents other muscles in the area from performing the movement. Manual pressure is exerted throughout the full range of motion and is repeated several times to reveal weakness or pain. Ask if the motion causes pain. In this manner, both subjective information (what the individual feels) and objective information (weakness) is gathered.

Neurologic Testing

A segmental nerve is the portion of a nerve that originates in the spinal cord and is referred to as a **nerve root**. Each nerve root is named by its point of departure from the spinal cord. In nearly all instances, each nerve root supplies nerve impulses to, or innervates, a series of muscles and an area of skin. The motor component of the nerve innervates muscle, called a **myotome**, and the sensory component of the nerve innervates skin, called a **dermatome**. Nerve roots leave the spinal cord to travel distally throughout the body. Several nerves may combine to form a plexus, such as the brachial plexus that innervates the upper extremity. As the nerve roots travel distally, two or more consecutive segmental nerve roots may combine to form a peripheral nerve. Nerves are more commonly injured by tensile or compressive forces and will be reflected in both motor and sensory deficits.

Motor Testing

Nearly all muscles receive segmental innervation from 2 or more nerve roots; however, selected motions may be innervated predominantly by a single nerve root (myotome). Muscle weakness or paralysis identified through resisted manual muscle testing should be referred to a physician to rule out a serious nerve injury.

Sensory Testing

To assess sensory perception, touch the person with a cotton ball, a paper clip, pads of the fingers, and fingernails. Ask the individual if it feels sharp or dull. Does the sensation feel the same on the injured body segment as it does on the uninjured body segment? Abnormal responses may include decreased tactile sensation (**hypoesthesia**), excessive tactile sensation (**hyperesthesia**), or loss of sensation (**anesthesia**). **Paresthesia** is another abnormal sensation characterized by a numbness, tingling, or burning sensation. **Figure 4.16** illustrates cutaneous sensation patterns for the segmental and peripheral nerves.

Reflex Testing

Damage to the central nervous system can also be detected by the reflexes. Exaggerated, distorted, or absent reflexes indicate

Painful arc
Pain located within a limited number of degrees in the range of motion

Testing throughout the full range of motion provides a better overall assessment of muscle weakness and can detect a painful arc of motion

Nerve root
The portion of a nerve associated with its origin in the spinal cord, such as C_6 or L_5

Myotome
A group of muscles primarily innervated by a single nerve root

Dermatome
A region of skin supplied by a single afferent neuron

Nerves are more commonly injured by tensile or compressive forces, and will be reflected in both motor and sensory deficits

Hypoesthesia
Decreased tactile sensation

Hyperesthesia
Excessive tactile sensation

Anesthesia
Partial or total loss of sensation

Paresthesia
Abnormal sensations, such as numbness, tingling, itching, or burning

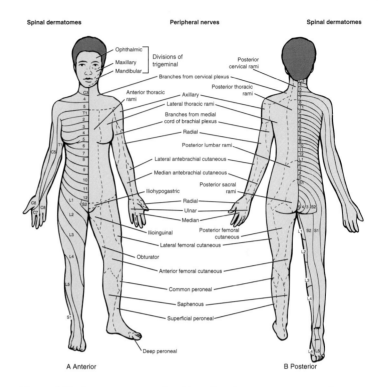

Spinal dermatomes   Peripheral nerves   Spinal dermatomes

A Anterior   B Posterior

Figure 4.16. Cutaneous sensation. Note that the cutaneous sensation patterns of the spinal nerves (**dermatomes**) differ from the patterns innervated by the peripheral nerves.

degeneration or injury in specific regions of the nervous system, often before other signs are apparent. The most familiar reflex is the patellar, or knee jerk, reflex that is elicited by striking the patellar tendon with a reflex hammer, causing a rapid contraction of the quadriceps muscle (**Fig. 4.17**). **Table 4.2** lists common deep tendon reflexes and the spinal segments tested.

Stress Tests

Each body segment has a series of stress tests to assess joint function and integrity of joint structures. These tests assess liga-

Table 4.2. Commonly Tested Deep Tendon Reflexes

Deep Tendon Reflexes	Segmental Levels
Biceps	Cervical **5**, 6
Brachioradialis	Cervical 5, **6**
Triceps	Cervical **7**, 8
Patellar	Lumbar 2, **3**, 4
Achilles	Sacral **1**

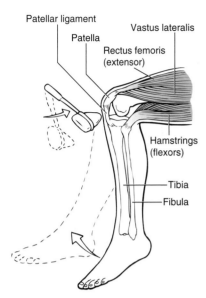

Figure 4.17. Reflexes can indicate if there is nerve root damage. The most familiar stretch reflex is the knee jerk, or patellar reflex, performed by tapping the patellar tendon with a reflex hammer, causing involuntary knee extension.

ments, intra-articular structures, joint capsule stability, impingement signs, muscle balance, and vascular integrity. For example, **Figure 4.18** demonstrates a drawer test on the ankle joint to assess the integrity of the joint collateral ligaments. During an on-the-field assessment, tests to determine a possible fracture and major ligament damage at a joint should always be performed before moving an injured individual. Only the specific tests deemed necessary for the injury should be used. Because of the focus of this text, a limited number of stress tests will be discussed within the individual chapters.

> Stress tests assess ligaments, intra-articular structures, joint capsule stability, impingement signs, muscle balance, and vascular integrity

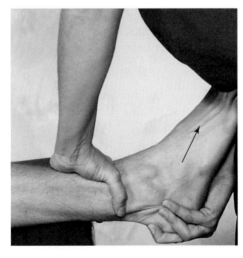

Figure 4.18. Applying an anterior tensile force at the ankle in a neutral position can assess the integrity of the joint collateral ligaments.

Functional Testing

Before permitting an individual to return to sport participation after an injury, it is imperative the individual's condition be fully evaluated so risk of reinjury is minimal. Functional testing includes assessment of motor coordination or proprioception and sport specific skill performance.

Proprioceptors are specialized deep sensory nerve cells sensitive to stretch, tension, and pressure. These cells detect minute changes in muscle dynamics and limb movement, and can instantaneously modify motor behavior to prevent injury. For example, by stepping in a hole, the ankle inverts. **Muscle spindles** in the peroneal muscles respond to stretch on the muscles and, through reflex action, initiate a strong contraction to prevent excessive inversion, thus preventing damage to the supporting joint ligaments. Alterations in proprioceptive input due to injury alter balance, reaction time, and motor control, placing the individual at a higher risk for reinjury. For an active sport participant, small changes can be significant. An individual's balance can be tested by performing tasks with the eyes closed, such as walking a straight line on the toes and heels, balancing on a wobble board, or walking sideways on the hands while in a push-up position.

Sport-specific tests are active movements performed by the individual during sport participation. In the rehabilitation process, the individual generally performs these skills at low intensity; as the individual's condition improves, intensity is increased. With a lower leg injury, the individual might begin by walking or jogging, then running forward and backward. If these skills are performed pain-free and without a limp, the individual might then be asked to run in a figure-8 pattern or a zigzag pattern. Again, each test must be performed pain-free and without a limp.

Functional tests should be sport-specific and demonstrate fluid, pain-free motion. These tests assess strength, agility, flexibility, joint stability, endurance, coordination, and proprioception. Any individual who has been discharged from a rehabilitation program should also pass the functional tests and be cleared by a physician for participation.

Stress tests were completed on the football player. Active plantar flexion and passive dorsiflexion at the ankle were limited and painful. Resisted plantar flexion was weak and caused sharp pain in the distal Achilles tendon area. Joint stability tests were negative and did not produce an increase in pain. The individual has normal bilateral sensation on the feet. At this point in the assessment, have you determined what possible condition may be present?

INJURY RECOGNITION

The football player complained of a sharp, aching pain over the Achilles tendon area during activity. The painful site was isolated and all stress tests were negative. Passive dorsiflexion was

Proprioceptors
Specialized deep sensory nerve cells in joints, ligaments, muscles, and tendons sensitive to stretch, tension, and pressure, which are responsible for position and movement

Muscle spindle
Encapsulated receptor found in muscle tissue sensitive to stretch

Alterations in proprioceptive input due to injury may alter balance, reaction time, and motor control

Functional tests assess strength, agility, flexibility, joint stability, endurance, coordination, and proprioception

uncomfortable, but active and resisted plantar flexion was weak and very painful. Think for a minute about what this positive test indicates. Does the individual need to see a physician?

Injury recognition is the final step in assessment. A fine line is drawn between recognition of a sport-related injury and a diagnosis. A **diagnosis** is the definitive determination of the nature of the injury or illness and can be done only by medical professionals. Athletic trainers recognize a possible injury or illness based on their assessment and, as needed, may refer the individual for a diagnosis. With professional preparation and practice, your skills, as well as the ability to recognize injuries, will improve.

A systematic and thorough assessment can determine the extent and seriousness of injury. The final decision in any injury assessment is often very difficult. Subjective and objective information gathered during the assessment must be analyzed and decisions must be made on what is best for the injured individual. Can the situation be handled on-site or should the individual be referred to a physician? A course of action must be determined to minimize pain and discomfort for the injured party. The athletic trainer must decide:

1. If an ambulance should be summoned to transport the injured individual to the nearest trauma facility.
2. If the individual should be referred to the family's primary-care physician, team physician, or outpatient clinic for follow-up care.
3. If the condition can be managed on-site, with the intent to refer the individual if signs and symptoms fail to improve in a timely manner.
4. The best mode of transportation to move the injured individual to the sideline, bench, training room, hospital, or physician's office.

As a general rule, the individual should always be referred to the nearest trauma center or emergency clinic if any life-threatening situation is present or if the injury results in loss of normal function. For example, if the individual is unable to walk without a limp, referral to a physician is warranted. Conditions necessitating immediate referral to a trauma center are listed in **Table 3.12**. If in doubt, always refer to the appropriate individual (i.e., head athletic trainer, team physician, emergency room, or primary care physician).

If the injured individual is referred to a physician or trauma facility, document the information gathered during the injury assessment, including the mechanism of injury, primary complaint, signs and symptoms, and any action taken. Relay this information to the appropriate individual (EMT, paramedic, or physician). A competitive school athlete seen by a physician should provide the school athletic trainer or coach with the physician's written report stating the diagnosis and if the athlete can return to sport participation, and when. Should the injury be managed on-site, re-evaluate

Diagnosis
Definitive determination of the nature of the injury or illness made only by physicians

An individual should always be referred to the nearest trauma center if any life-threatening situation is present, or if the injury results in loss of normal function

the injury daily to ensure satisfactory improvement. If no improvement is seen, modification in protection, treatment, activity level, and the need for referral to a physician may need to be implemented.

If you recognized the injury as Achilles tendinitis, you are correct. Significant pain and weakness are present, and, therefore, this individual should be referred to a physician to develop an appropriate treatment and rehabilitation plan.

SOAP NOTES

Many athletic trainers find employment in a sports medicine or physical therapy clinic. Why is it important for each employee of the clinic to be consistent and thorough in all injury assessments and keep accurate records?

SOAP notes provide another organized structure for decision making and problem solving in sports injury management. Used in many physical therapy clinics, sports medicine clinics, and athletic training rooms, these notes document patient care and serve as a vehicle of communication between the on-site clinicians and other health-care professionals. The records provide information to avoid duplication of services and state the present status and tolerance of that individual to the care being rendered by a given health care provider.

SOAP is an acronym of the separate components used in documentation:

Subjective evaluation
Objective evaluation
Assessment
Plan

The supervising physician determines the diagnosis of the patient and may then refer the individual to an athletic trainer or physical therapist to determine an appropriate treatment and rehabilitation program. There are four separate sections of SOAP notes.

Subjective Evaluation

The subjective evaluation (history of the injury) includes the primary complaint, mechanism of injury, location, onset and behavior of symptoms, functional impairments, pain perception, previous injuries to the area, and family history (5). This information is from the individual and reflects their attitude, mental condition, and perceived physical state.

Objective Evaluation

The objective evaluation (observation and inspection, palpation, and special tests) provides appropriate, measurable documentation relative to the individual's condition. This information can be

SOAP is an acronym for:
   Subjective evaluation
   Objective evaluation
   Assessment
   Plan

Subjective evaluation includes information on the primary complaint, mechanism of injury, location, onset and behavior of symptoms, functional impairments, pain perception, previous injuries to the area, and family history

repeatedly measured to track progress from the initial evaluation through the final clearance for discharge and return to sport participation. Measurable factors may include edema, ecchymosis, atrophy, range of motion, strength, joint instability, functional disability, motor and sensory function, and cardiovascular endurance. A detailed postural assessment and gait analysis may also be documented in this section.

Objective assessment measures edema, ecchymosis, atrophy, range of motion, strength, joint instability, functional disability, motor and sensory function, and cardiovascular endurance

Assessment

After the objective evaluation, the clinician will analyze and assess the individual's status and **prognosis**. Long-term goals are then established to accurately reflect the individual's status after rehabilitation. These long-term goals might include pain-free range of motion, bilateral strength, power and muscular endurance, cardiovascular endurance, and return to full functional status. Short-term goals are then developed to outline the expected progress within a week or two of the initial injury. These might include immediate protection of the injured area and control of inflammation, hemorrhage, muscle spasm, or pain. Short-term goals are updated with each progress note. Progress notes may be written weekly or biweekly to document progress.

Prognosis
Probable course or progress of an injury or disease

Assessment includes long-term and short-term goals

Plan

The final section of the note lists the **modalities**, therapeutic exercises, educational consultations, and functional activities utilized to achieve the short-term goals (5). The written plan includes the following information:

1. The immediate treatment given to handle any acute problem
2. The frequency and duration of treatments, rehabilitation exercises, and evaluation standards to determine progress toward the goals
3. On-going patient education
4. Criteria for discharge

Modalities
Therapeutic physical agents that promote optimal healing, such as thermotherapy, cryotherapy, electrotherapy, or manual therapy, while reducing pain and disability

The treatment plan lists the modalities, therapeutic exercises, educational consultations, and functional activities used to achieve the short-term goals

As the short-term goals are achieved and updated, periodic "in-house review" of the individual's records permit the clinicians to evaluate patient progress. As the individual progresses in the treatment plan, gradual return to activity may help motivate them to work even harder to return to full functional status. When it is determined the individual can be discharged and cleared for participation, a discharge note is written to close the file. All information included within the file is confidential and cannot be released to anyone without written approval from the patient.

Health care facilities should uniformly document specific services rendered, record patient evaluation, progress, and assessment, particularly when numerous individuals are involved in the patient's rehabilitation program. SOAP notes are commonly used to keep comprehensive, concise, and accurate records.

SUMMARY

Sports injury assessment is a problem-solving process of an injury that incorporates subjective and objective information that is reliable, accurate, and measurable. The HOPS format is used in injury assessment and includes history, observation and inspection, palpation, and special tests. Utilizing the HOPS format, subjective information (history) is gathered from the individual regarding their perception of the problem. This information may include:

1. The primary complaint
2. Mechanism of injury
3. Perception of pain and related symptoms
4. Disabilities resulting from the injury
5. Related medical history

To confirm information gathered in the subjective evaluation, an objective assessment is performed to discover the source of the individual's primary complaint. This segment of the assessment process includes:

1. Observation, including general body symmetry and appearance, motor function, and inspection at the injury site
2. Bony and soft tissue palpations to determine a possible fracture or dislocation, and abnormal temperature, swelling, point tenderness, crepitus, deformity, muscle spasm, cutaneous sensation, and pulse
3. Range of motion testing to distinguish injuries to contractile tissue versus noncontractile tissue
4. Neurological testing through motor function and sensory perception
5. Stress tests for specific joints or structures

Documented information gathered during assessment establishes a baseline of information used to recognize and identify a possible cause of injury. This information can help the supervising physician accurately diagnosis the problem and provides a basis for treatment and rehabilitation programs.

SOAP notes are used in many sports medicine facilities to document the injury evaluation, assess the individual's status and prognosis, and outline the treatment plan. The treatment plan should delineate the frequency and duration of treatments, rehabilitation exercises, on-going patient education, evaluation standards to determine progress, and criteria for discharge. These notes serve as a vehicle of communication between the various health-care providers and help an injured individual return safely to sport participation.

REFERENCES

1. Urberg MM, and Scott NC. 1988. A self-scored medical history teaching technique. Fam Med 20(6):458–460.
2. Fitzgerald MA. 1991. Perfecting the art: the physical exam. RN 54(11):34–38.

3. Clarkson HM, and Gilewich GB. *Musculoskeletal assessment: joint range of motion and manual muscle strength*. Baltimore: Williams & Wilkins, 1989.
4. Magee DJ. *Orthopedic physical assessment*. Philadelphia: WB Saunders, 1992.
5. Saunders HD. Evaluation of a musculoskeletal disorder. In *Orthopaedic and sports physical therapy*, edited by JA Gould and GJ Davies. St. Louis: Mosby, 1989.

Therapeutic Exercise and Therapeutic Modalities

After completing this chapter, you should be able to:

- Identify the factors that influence how an individual reacts to, and recovers from, a disabling injury

- Identify and describe the process of designing a therapeutic exercise program

- Explain the four phases of a therapeutic exercise program, goals, and methodology of implementation

- List the criteria used to clear an individual to return to full participation in sport

- Identify the principles of cryotherapy and thermotherapy, indications and contraindications for their use, and their application to manage inflammation and promote healing

- Describe other medications and electrical modalities that may be used in the management of sports injuries

Key Terms:

Active inhibition	Iontophoresis
Analgesic effect	Muscular endurance
Antipyresis	Muscular power
Ballistic stretching	Open-chain exercises
Cardiovascular endurance	Overload principle
Closed-chain exercises	Phonophoresis
Cold allergies	Plyometric training
Contracture	Proprioceptive neuro-
Contraindication	muscular facilitation
Coordination	(PNF)
Cryokinetics	Raynaud's phenomenon
Cryotherapy	Static stretching
Flexibility	Sticking point
Hypermobility	Strength
Hypomobility	Therapeutic drugs
Indication	Thermotherapy

The ultimate goal of therapeutic exercise is to return the injured sport participant to full activity, pain-free and fully functional. To do this, attention must focus on controlling inflammation and regaining normal joint range of motion, flexibility, muscular strength, muscular endurance, coordination, and power. Furthermore, cardiovascular endurance and strength in the unaffected limbs must also be maintained. Each component should be addressed within an individualized exercise program. Therapeutic modalities and medications may also be utilized throughout the exercise program to enhance repair and healing of damaged tissues.

In this chapter you will first learn about the emotional stages an individual may experience after injury. Second, you will learn how to develop a basic therapeutic exercise program, including criteria used to determine when an individual is ready to progress in the program and, ultimately, return to sport activity. Finally, common therapeutic modalities and medications used to control inflammation and pain will be discussed. The material covered in this chapter will be elaborated on in Chapters 8 to 16 for the various body segments.

PSYCHOLOGY AND THE INJURED PARTICIPANT

How would you feel if you had trained very hard for a specific sport and were suddenly unable to participate because of an injury? What impact would these feelings have on your motivation to participate in a daily rehabilitation program?

To an individual who enjoys sport participation, an injury can be devastating. For many, the development and maintenance of a physically fit body provides a focal point for social and economic success important for self-esteem and identity. An individual's coping mechanisms are based on several factors, including their personality, coping resources, history of past stressors (e.g., previous injuries, academics, family life), and previous intervention strategies (1). These factors lay the foundation used to address recovery from an athletic injury.

Likewise, recovery from an injury is dependent on several personal and situational elements, such as self-esteem, self-motivation, relationship with the coach and team members, characteristics of the injury (e.g., severity, history, and type), timing of the injury (e.g., preseason, in-season, play-offs), level and intensity of the player, and role on the team (1). All of these factors interact with the cognitive, emotional, and behavioral responses of the athlete in a cyclical pattern to impact the success or failure of a therapeutic exercise program.

The cognitive, or knowledge, appraisal and response to injury is influenced by the individual's recognition of the injury, understanding of the goal adjustments, and their belief that they directly impact the success of the exercise program. It has been found that athletes who perceive some control over their rehabilitation

> Coping mechanisms are based on personality, coping resources, a history of past stressors, and the success of previous intervention strategies

outcomes demonstrate a higher perceived self-efficacy and perform better on their exercise program than those who perceive less control (2). The clinician, however, must not negate the emotional responses that will be exhibited throughout the exercise program. Seriously injured individuals may fear social isolation or loss of income, or potential scholarships as a result of the injury. This fear of the unknown may lead to increased tension, anger, and depression during the exercise period. If the individual does not perceive a gradual rate of recovery, frustration and boredom may deter a successful outcome. The clinician should encourage the injured athlete to develop a positive attitude by utilizing social supportive networks and psychological skills to manage pain, thus directing the individual's energies into compliance with the treatment protocols. Positive encouragement may allow the athlete to feel better about pushing themselves to a higher intensity despite discomfort, fatigue, or pain (1).

It is critical that the sports medicine team include the athlete as an integral part of the rehabilitation process. This is especially important when goals are established that direct the exercise program. They must be realistic and provide some means of measurement so the athlete can perceive a gradual rate of recovery. Whenever possible, the rehabilitation program should mirror the individual's regular training program, including the level of intensity, frequency, and duration. With activity modification and creativity, the competitive athlete may be able to do limited exercise with the team. This may reduce the feeling of isolation and being left out of daily interaction with the coach and other players. Using graphs or charts to document progress can also help the individual see improvement. The clinician must develop a positive professional relationship with the athlete to assist them in recovering physically and psychologically from their injuries.

An individual's emotional state will have a direct impact on success of an exercise program. Charts, graphs, and activity modification that directly mirror regular training will help motivate the individual to progress through the exercise program.

DEVELOPING A THERAPEUTIC EXERCISE PROGRAM

In Chapter 4, you determined the problem was Achilles tendinitis. What long-term goals might you and the athlete establish for the therapeutic exercise program? How will you measure progress?

In designing an individualized therapeutic exercise program, several sequential steps help identify the needs and treatment goals of the patient (**Fig. 5.1**). First, the patient's present level of function is assessed, including range of motion, muscle strength, neurologic integrity, joint stability, and quality of functional activities. Secondly, the assessment is interpreted to identify structural or functional deficits. From these deficits, long- and short-term goals are established to return the athlete safely to participation.

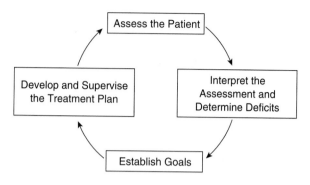

Figure 5.1. An individualized therapeutic exercise program is developed and maintained through continuous identification of the needs and treatment goals of the patient.

Finally, in conjunction with a physician, a treatment plan is developed and implemented to attain those goals. This process is on-going and is based on constant supervision and reassessment of the program. If progress is not seen, the individual should be referred back to the supervising physician for re-evaluation and adaptations should accordingly be made to the program.

Therapeutic exercise and modalities are used throughout the treatment plan to facilitate the rehabilitation process. In addition, the physician may also prescribe medications. To return the individual safely to participation, the therapeutic exercise program is divided into four phases. The termination of one phase and initiation of the next phase may overlap. Each phase, however, has a specific role. In phase one, the inflammatory response, pain, swelling, and ecchymosis are controlled. Phase two regains any deficits in range of motion at the affected joint and begins to restore proprioception. Phase three regains muscle strength, endurance, and power in the affected limb. Phase four prepares the individual to return to activity and includes sport-specific skill training, regaining coordination, and improving cardiovascular conditioning. Each phase and expected outcomes are discussed in more detail later in the chapter. **Table 5.1** lists the various phases of a therapeutic exercise program.

Long-term goals for the football player might include: pain-free bilateral range of motion, increased flexibility in the Achilles tendon, bilateral muscle strength, endurance, power, maintenance of cardiovascular endurance, increased proprioception and kinesthetic awareness, and pain-free unlimited motion in sport-specific skills.

PHASE ONE: CONTROLLING INFLAMMATION

The football player has pain and tenderness on the Achilles tendon and weakness in plantar flexion. What modalities might you use to control inflammation? Would you include any exercises during this phase?

Table 5.1. Therapeutic Exercise Program

Phase One: Controlling Inflammation

Control inflammatory stage and minimize edema using **PRICE** principles
  (**P**rotect, **R**estrict activity, **I**ce, **C**ompression, and **E**levation)
Maintain range of motion, joint flexibility, strength, endurance, and
  power in the unaffected body parts
Maintain cardiovascular endurance

Phase Two: Restoration of Motion

Restore range of motion to within 80% of normal in the unaffected limb
Restore joint flexibility as observed in the unaffected limb
Begin proprioceptive stimulation through closed-chain exercises
Begin pain-free isometric strengthening exercises on the affected limb
Begin unresisted pain-free functional patterns of sport-specific motions
Maintain muscular strength, endurance, and power in unaffected
  muscles
Maintain cardiovascular endurance

**Phase Three: Developing Muscular Strength, Power,
  and Endurance**

Restore full range of motion in the affected limb
Restore muscular strength, endurance, and power using resisted
  exercise
Restore proprioception
Maintain cardiovascular endurance
Initiate minimal to moderate resistance in sport-specific functional
  patterns

Phase Four: Return to Sport Activity

Analyze skill performance and correct biomechanical inefficiencies in
  motion
Improve muscular strength, endurance, and power
Restore coordination and balance
Improve cardiovascular endurance
Increase sport-specific functional patterns and return to protected
  activity, as tolerated

Phase one of the exercise program begins immediately after injury assessment. The primary goal is to control inflammation by limiting hemorrhage, edema, muscle spasm, and pain. The individual can move into phase two when the following criteria have been attained:

> The primary goal of phase one is to limit hemorrhage, edema, muscle spasm, and pain

Control of inflammation, with minimal edema, swelling, muscle
  spasm, and pain
Range of motion, joint flexibility, muscular strength, endurance,
  and power are maintained in the general body
Cardiovascular fitness is maintained at the preinjury level

Collagenous scar formation, a natural component of the repair and regeneration of injured tissue, is less efficient and tolerant of tensile forces than the original mature tissue. The length of the inflammatory response is a key factor that influences the ultimate

The longer the inflammatory process, the more likely the resulting scar tissue will be less dense and weaker in yielding to applied stress

stability and function of scar tissue. The longer the inflammatory process progresses, the more likely the resulting scar tissue will be less dense and weaker in yielding to applied stress. Furthermore, immobilization for more than 2 weeks may lead to joint adhesions that inhibit muscle fiber regeneration (3). **PRICE** is a well known acronym for **p**rotect, **r**estrict activity, **i**ce, **c**ompression, and **e**levation, and is used to combat the inflammatory process.

Control of Inflammation

In Chapter 2, you learned that hemorrhage and edema cause a pooling of tissue fluids and blood products that increases pain and muscle spasm. For this reason, cryotherapy (cold application) is preferred during the acute inflammatory phase. Cold application leads to vasoconstriction, decreased circulation and capillary permeability, and limits secondary hypoxic injury. Nerve impulses and conduction velocities are diminished, leading to an **analgesic effect** and a reduction in muscle spasm. An elastic compression wrap can assist in decreasing edema formation and reduce the swelling by promoting reabsorption of the fluid, yet can allow for some expansion in cases of extreme swelling. It is recommended that compression be applied within minutes and should remain for a minimum of 24 hours (4). Elevation reduces capillary hydrostatic pressure and, therefore, decreases the amount of fluid forced out of the capillaries into the surrounding tissue spaces. The end result is less edema formation. **Field Strategy 5.1** explains acute care of soft tissue injuries using the PRICE principle.

Analgesic effect
Condition whereby pain is not perceived; a numbing or sedative effect

Protect and Restrict Activity

Early protected motion and the loading and unloading of joints through partial weight-bearing exercise maintain joint lubrication to nourish articular cartilage, meniscus, and ligaments, leading to an optimal environment for proper collagen fibril formation. The type of protection selected and the length of activity modification depend on injury severity, structures damaged, and the philosophy of the supervising physician. Several materials can be used to protect the area, including elastic wraps, tape, pads, slings, braces, splints, and casts. Many of these techniques are illustrated in Chapters 6 and 7. If an individual limps or cannot walk without pain, crutches should be recommended. Proper crutch fitting and use are summarized in **Field Strategy 5.2**.

Restricted activity does not imply cessation of activity, but simply means "relative rest," that is, decreasing activity to a level below that required in sport, but tolerated by the recently-injured tissue or joint. Strengthening exercises can be alternated with cardiovascular exercises, such as swimming, use of a stationary bike, or upper body ergometer (UBE), as long as the injured area is not irritated or inflamed.

Restricted activity implies decreasing activity to a level below that required to participate in sport, but tolerated by the injured tissue or joint

Field Strategy 5.1. Acute Care of Soft Tissue Injuries

Ice Application

Apply ice for 20 to 30 minutes directly to the skin

Ice applications should be repeated every 1½ to 2 hours when awake and may extend from 1 to 72+ hours postinjury

Skin temperature can determine when acute swelling has subsided. For example, if the area (compared bilaterally) feels warm to the touch, swelling continues. If in doubt, it is better to extend the application of cold

Compression

On an extremity, apply the wrap in a distal to proximal direction to prevent extracellular fluid from moving into the distal digits

Take a distal pulse to ensure the wrap is not overly tight

Horseshoe pads of felt may be placed around the malleolus, in combination with an elastic wrap or tape, to prevent or limit ankle swelling

Maintain compression continuously on the injury for the first 24 hours

Elevation

Elevate the body part above the heart

While sleeping, place a hard suitcase between the mattress and boxspring or place the extremity on a series of pillows

Restrict Activity and Protect the Area

If the individual is unable to walk without a limp, fit the person for crutches and apply an appropriate protective device to limit unnecessary movement of the injured joint

If the individual has an upper extremity injury and is unable to move the limb without pain, fit the person with an appropriate sling or brace

Did you determine that the application of ice, compression, elevation, and protected movement can control pain and inflammation in the injured Achilles tendon? If so, you are correct. Early pain-free range-of-motion and flexibility exercises and general strength and cardiovascular exercises may be included as long as the injury is not irritated.

PHASE TWO: RESTORATION OF MOTION

The acute inflammatory symptoms have been controlled using the PRICE principles. What exercises can restore range of motion and enhance healing?

Phase two restores range of motion and flexibility, while maintaining general body strength and cardiovascular endurance. If the individual is in an immobilizer or splint, remove the splint for treatment and exercise. The splint can then be replaced to support

Field Strategy 5.2. Fitting and Using Crutches and Canes

Fitting Crutches

Have the individual stand erect in flat shoes
Place the tip of the crutch slightly in front of, and to the side of, the involved leg
Adjust the length so the axillary pad is approximately 1 to 1½ inches (2 to 3 finger widths) below the axilla, to avoid undue pressure on the neurovascular structures
Adjust the hand grip so the elbow is flexed at about 30°, and is at the level of the greater trochanter

Fitting for a Cane

Place the individual in the same position as above. Adjust the hand grip so the elbow is flexed at about 30°

For Nonweight-bearing on One Limb

Stand on the uninvolved leg. Lean forward and place both crutches and the involved leg approximately 12 inches in front of the body
Body weight should rest on the hands, not the axillary pads
With the good leg, step through the crutches as if taking a normal step. Repeat the process
If possible, the involved leg should be extended while swinging forward to prevent atrophy of the quadriceps muscles

Going Up and Down Stairs

Place both crutches under the arm opposite the handrail
To go **up** the stairs, step **up with the good leg** while leaning on the rail
To go **down** the stairs, place the crutches down to the next step and step **down with the involved leg**

Progressing to Partial Weight Bearing

As tolerated, place as much body weight onto the involved leg, taking the rest of the weight on the hands
Make sure a good heel-toe technique is used, whereby the heel strikes first, then the weight is shifted to the ball of the foot

Using One Crutch or Cane

One crutch or cane is placed on the uninvolved side and moves forward with the involved leg
The individual should not lean heavily on the crutch or cane

and protect the injured site. The individual can move into phase three when the following criteria have been completed:

Inflammation and pain are under control
Range of motion is within 80% of normal in the unaffected limb
Bilateral joint flexibility is restored and proprioception is maintained
Cardiovascular endurance and general body strength is maintained at the preinjury level

Several factors can limit joint motion, including a bony block, joint adhesions, muscle tightness, tight skin or an inelastic dense scar tissue, swelling, pain, or the presence of fat or other soft tissues that block normal motion. In addition, prolonged immobilization can lead to muscles losing their flexibility and assuming a shortened position, called a **contracture**. Connective tissue around joints has no contractile properties. Although connective tissue is somewhat supple and will elongate slowly with a sustained stretch, like muscle tissue, it will adaptively shorten when immobilized. This state of limited range of motion is called **hypomobility**. Connective tissue and muscles can be lengthened through stretching and proprioceptive neuromuscular facilitation exercises. **Hypermobility**, or excessive motion (joint laxity), however, should be avoided, as this condition cannot be reversed.

Joint Range of Motion

Full pain-free range of motion need not be achieved before strength exercises are initiated, but certain skills requiring full functional motion, such as throwing, squats, or certain agility drills, must wait until proper joint mechanics are restored. Exercises should be relatively pain-free and may be facilitated during early stages by completing the exercises in a warm or hot whirlpool, to provide an analgesic effect and relieve the stress of gravity on sensitive structures.

Range-of-motion exercises may be done passively or actively. With passive range of motion, the individual is placed in a comfortable position, with the joint supported, such as lying on a table or having the body segment supported in one of your hands (**Fig. 5.2**). The limb is then moved through the range of motion by the athletic trainer. Active range-of-motion exercises can enhance circulation through a pumping action during muscular contraction and relaxation. Examples of range-of-motion exercises can be seen in **Field Strategy 5.3**.

Flexibility

Flexibility is the total range of motion at a joint that occurs pain-free and is a combination of normal joint mechanics, soft tissue mobility, and muscle extensibility. Flexibility can be increased through ballistic or static stretching techniques. **Ballistic stretching** uses repetitive bouncing motions at the end of the available range of motion. Because generated momentum may carry the body part beyond normal range of motion, the muscles being stretched often remain contracted to prevent overstretching, leading to microscopic tears in the musculotendinous unit. In a **static stretch**, movement is slow and deliberate. The muscle is stretched to the point at which a mild burn is felt, is maintained in that position for about 15 seconds, and is repeated several times. **Field Strategy 5.4** explains how static stretching is used to improve flexibility.

Limited joint motion may be caused by a bony block, joint adhesions, muscle tightness, tight skin or an inelastic dense scar tissue, swelling, pain, or the presence of fat or other soft tissues that block normal motion

Contracture
Adhesions occurring in an immobilized muscle, leading to a shortened contractile state

Hypomobility
Decreased motion at a joint

Hypermobility
Increased motion at a joint; joint laxity

Painful exercises can be facilitated by using a warm or hot whirlpool to provide an analgesic effect and relieve the stress of gravity on sensitive structures

Flexibility
Total range of motion at a joint dependent on normal joint mechanics, mobility of soft tissues, and muscle extensibility

Ballistic stretching
Increasing flexibility by utilizing repetitive bouncing motions at the end of the available range of motion

Static stretching
Slow, sustained muscle stretching used to increase flexibility

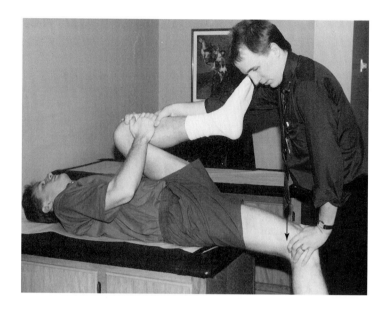

Figure 5.2. To passively stretch a muscle group, stabilize the proximal body segment and apply a gentle slow, sustained movement of the distal body part through the available range of motion (indicated by the arrow) until tension is felt. Then apply a slight overpressure. Do not bounce the extremity at the end of the range of motion. In the stretched position, the patient should feel slight tension or tightness of the structures being stretched, but no pain.

Proprioceptive neuromuscular facilitation (PNF)
Exercises that stimulate proprioceptors in muscles, tendons, and joints to improve flexibility and strength

Active inhibition
Technique whereby an individual consciously relaxes a muscle prior to stretching

Proprioceptive neuromuscular facilitation (PNF) exercises promote and hasten the response of the neuromuscular system through stimulation of the proprioceptors. These exercises increase flexibility in one muscle group (agonist), while simultaneously improving strength in another muscle group (antagonist). If instituted early in the program, PNF stretches can aid in elongating scar tissue. One technique utilizes **active inhibition**, whereby the muscle group reflexively relaxes prior to the stretching maneuver. The athletic trainer stabilizes the limb to be exercised. Resisted contractions, held for 3, 6, or 10 seconds, are alternated with passive stretching of the muscle group **(Fig. 5.3)**.

When range of motion has been achieved, repetition of motion through actual skill movements can improve coordination and joint mechanics as the athlete progresses into phase three of the program. For example, a pitcher may begin throwing without resistance in front of a mirror to visualize the action. This can also motivate the individual to continue to progress in the therapeutic exercise program.

In phase two, did you determine what range-of-motion exercises should be conducted at the ankle? Cryotherapy or thermotherapy may also be used during this phase.

Field Strategy 5.3. Range-of-motion Exercises for the Lower and Upper Extremity

A. Ankle. Write out the letters of the alphabet using sweeping capital letters. Do all letters three times

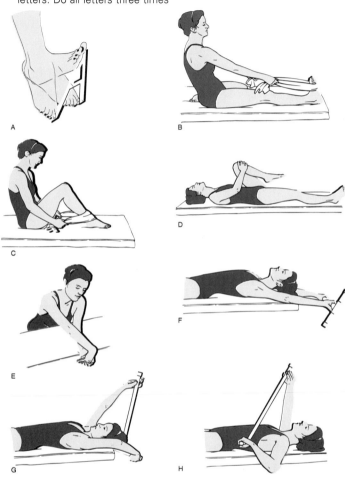

B. Achilles tendon. In a seated position, wrap a towel around the forefoot and slowly stretch the Achilles tendon
C. Knee. In a seated position with the knee slightly bent, wrap a towel around the lower leg and slowly bring the lower leg toward the buttocks
D. Hip. Lying down, bring one knee toward the chest. Repeat with the other knee
E. Wrist or elbow. Using the unaffected hand, slowly stretch the affected hand or forearm in flexion and extension
F. Shoulder flexion. Using a wand or cane, use the unaffected arm to slowly raise the wand high above the head
G. Shoulder lateral (external) rotation. Using a wand or cane, use the unaffected arm to slowly do lateral (external) rotation of the glenohumeral joint
H. Shoulder medial (internal) rotation. Using a wand or cane, use the unaffected arm to slowly do medial (internal) rotation of the glenohumeral joint

Avoid vigorous stretching of tissues in the following conditions:
   After a recent fracture
   After prolonged immobilization
   With acute inflammation or infection in or around the joint
   With a bony block that limits motion
   With muscle contractures or joint adhesions that limit motion
   With acute pain occurring during stretching
Stretching is facilitated by warm body tissues. Therefore, a brief warm-up
   period is recommended. If it is not possible to jog lightly, stretching
   could be performed after a superficial heat treatment
In the designated stretch position, position yourself so a sensation of
   tension is felt, but without discomfort
Do not bounce; hold the stretch for 10 to 30 seconds until a sense of
   relaxation occurs. Be aware of the feeling of relaxation, or "letting go."
   Repeat the stretch 6 to 8 times
Breathe rhythmically and slowly. Exhale during the stretch
Do not be overly aggressive in stretching. Increased flexibility may not be
   noticed for 4 to 6 weeks
If an area is particularly resistant to stretching, partner stretching or
   proprioceptive neuromuscular facilitation (PNF) stretching may be used

PHASE THREE: DEVELOPING MUSCULAR STRENGTH, ENDURANCE, AND POWER

> **?** *The football player has regained normal range of motion at the ankle and wants to return to practice. Is this a good idea? Will reinjury occur? Why?*

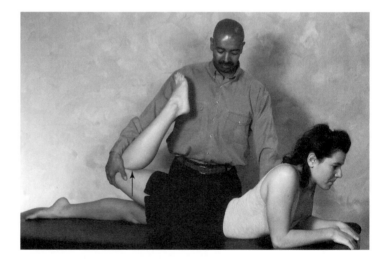

Figure 5.3. In performing proprioceptive neuromuscular facilitation stretching, the athletic trainer passively stretches a muscle group. In this photo, the hip flexors are being stretched. When slight tension is felt, the athlete contracts the muscle group against resistance for 3, 6, or 10 seconds. The muscle is then passively stretched again. This process is repeated four to five times.

Phase three focuses on developing muscular strength, endurance, and power in the injured extremity as compared to the uninjured extremity. The individual can move into phase four when the following criteria have been completed:

Bilateral range of motion and joint flexibility are restored
Muscular strength, endurance, and power in the affected limb are equal or near equal to the unaffected limb
Cardiovascular endurance and general body strength are at, or better than the preinjury level
Sport-specific functional patterns should be completed using mild to moderate resistance

Muscular Strength

Strength is the ability of a muscle or group of muscles to produce resulting force in one maximal effort. This is done through isometric, isotonic, or isokinetic exercises (**Fig. 5.4**). Strength increases via the **overload principle**, whereby physiological improvements occur only when an individual physically demands more of their muscles than is normally required. This theory, based on the specific **a**daptations to **i**mposed **d**emands (SAID) principle, states that the body responds to a given demand with a specific and predictable adaptation (3). Overload is achieved by manipulating frequency, intensity, or duration of the exercise program. Frequency refers to the number of exercise sessions per day or week. Intensity reflects both the caloric cost of the work and specific energy systems activated. Duration refers to the length of a single exercise session. Strength gains depend primarily on the intensity of the overload and not the specific training method. Muscular strength is improved with a minimum 3 days per week of training that include 12 to 15 repetitions/bout of 8 to 10 exercises for the major muscle groups (5).

Knight's **d**aily **a**djusted **p**rogressive **r**esistance **e**xercise (DAPRE) is an objective method of increasing resistance as the individual's strength increases or decreases (6). A fixed percent of the maximum weight for a single repetition (1 RM) is lifted during the first and second set. Maximum repetitions of the resistance maximum (RM) are lifted in the third set. Adaptations to the amount of weight lifted are then increased or decreased accordingly in the fourth set and in the first set of the next session. Guidelines for the DAPRE method are listed in **Table 5.2**.

Isometric Training

Isometric training measures a muscle's maximum potential to produce static force. The muscle is at a constant tension, whereas muscle length and joint angle remain the same. Isometric exercise is useful in the first two phases of the exercise program: (a) when motion is contraindicated by pathology or bracing, (b) when motion is limited because of muscle weakness at a particular angle,

Muscle strength
The ability of a muscle to produce resulting force in one maximal effort, either statically or dynamically

Overload principle
Physiologic improvements occur only when an individual physically demands more of the muscle than is normally required

Overload is achieved by manipulating frequency, intensity, or duration of the exercise program

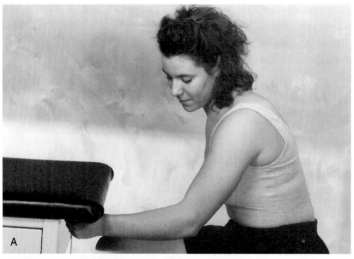

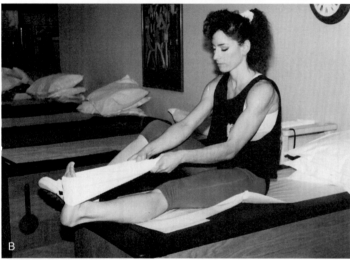

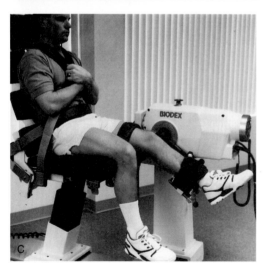

Figure 5.4. Muscle strength may be gained through (**A**) isometric exercise, (**B**) isotonic exercise, or (**C**) isokinetic exercise.

called a **sticking point**, or (c) when a painful arc is present. Isometric strength exercises are the least effective training method, as gains are isolated to a range of 10° on either side of the joint angle.

Sticking point
Insufficient strength to move a body segment through a particular angle

Isotonic Training (Variable Speed/Fixed Resistance)

In isotonic exercise, a maximal muscle contraction generates a force to move a constant load throughout the range of motion at a variable speed (7). This method is readily available with free weights, elastic tubing, and weight machines. This training method permits exercise of multiple joints simultaneously, allows for both eccentric and concentric contractions, and permits weight-bearing closed kinetic chain exercises. A disadvantage is that when a load is applied, the muscle can only move that load through the range of motion with as much force as the muscle provides at its weakest point.

In isotonic training, a maximal muscle contraction generates a force to move a constant load through the range of motion at a variable speed

Isokinetic Training (Fixed Speed/Variable Resistance)

Isokinetic training, or accommodating resistance, allows an individual to provide muscular overload and angular movement to rotate a lever arm at a controlled velocity or fixed speed. Cybex, Biodex, or KinCom are examples of this strength training method. Two advantages to isokinetic training are that a muscle group can be exercised to its maximum potential throughout the full range of motion, and the resistance mechanism essentially disengages when pain is experienced by the patient (8). The machines are, however, quite expensive (ranging from $25,000 to $60,000).

Table 5.2. Daily Adjusted Progressive Resistance Exercise (DAPRE) Program

Set	Weight	Repetitions
1	50% of RM	10
2	75% of RM	6
3	100% of RM	Maximum
4	Adjusted[a]	Maximum

Number of Reps During Set 3	Adjusted Working Weight During Set 4	Next Day Exercise Session[b]
0 to 2	Decrease by 5–10 lb and repeat set	
3 to 4	Decrease by 0–5 lb	Keep the same
5 to 7	Keep the same	Increase by 5–10 lb
8 to 12	Increase by 5–10 lb	Increase by 5–15 lb
13+	Increase by 10–15 lb	Increase by 10–20 lb

[a] Adjusted work weight is gauged on individual differences completed in Set 3.
[b] Adjusted work weight for the next day is gauged on individual differences completed in Set 4.

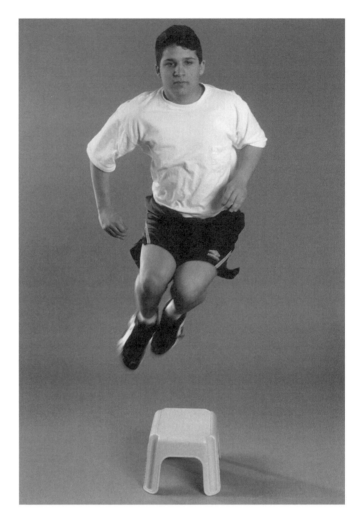

Figure 5.5. An example of plyometric exercise is the lateral jump over an object. In this exercise, the athlete jumps vertically and pushes sideways off the ground. The knees are brought up to the chest to clear the object.

Muscular Endurance

Muscular endurance
The ability of muscles to exert tension over an extended period

Muscular endurance is the ability of muscle tissue to exert repetitive tension over an extended period. The more rapidly the muscle fatigues, the less endurance it has. Increases in muscle endurance may influence strength gains; however, strength development has not been shown to increase muscle endurance. Muscular endurance is gained by lifting low weights at a faster contractile velocity, with more repetitions in the exercise session, or with use of stationary bikes, aquatic therapy, Stair Master, Nordic Track, or a Slide Board (3).

Muscular Power

Muscular power
The ability of muscles to produce force at a given time

Muscular power is the ability of muscle to produce force in a given time. Power training is started after the injured limb has

Field Strategy 5.5. Power and Strength Exercises

Stairs

Use a "low" walking stance and vigorously swing the arms
Triple stairs: Walk only. One repetition is a round trip from the bottom of
  the stairwell to the top and back down. Use the walk down as recovery
Double stairs: Emphasize technique
Single stairs: Emphasize speed

Bounding

Involves one foot take off and landing for 30 to 40 yards. Swing the arms
  vigorously to provide a strong movement
Run-Run-Bound: Establish number of bounds (repetitions) and the number
  of sets
Distance: Establish the number of bounds in a given distance

**Hops (Can Be Performed One-legged or Two-legged for
  Established Distance)**

Singles goal: 40 to 50 yards
Double goal: Sequence of 10 hops in each of 3 sets

Uphill Running

Decrease the stride length and make sure foot strike is underneath the
  body rather than in front
Land on the forefoot/toes, not on the heels

Bench Steps with Barbells

Step up, up, down, down. Begin with a light weight and add 1 minute
  daily until consecutive step-ups can be done for a pre-set period of time

regained at least 80% of the muscle strength in the unaffected limb. Regaining power involves weight training at higher contractile velocities or using plyometric exercises. **Plyometric training** employs the inherent stretch–recoil characteristics of skeletal muscle through an initial rapid eccentric (loading) stretch of a muscle to produce tension prior to initiating an explosive concentric contraction of the muscle (**Fig. 5.5**). The greater the stretch from the muscle's resting length, the greater the force the muscle can lift or overcome. Injury, however, can result if the individual does not have full range of motion, flexibility, and near normal strength before beginning these exercises. These exercises should be performed every 3 days to allow the muscles to recover from fatigue. **Field Strategy 5.5** lists examples of exercises for developing muscular power and strength.

Plyometric training
Exercises that employ explosive movements to develop muscular power

Open- vs. Closed-chain Exercises

In rehabilitation, a common error is to forget that injury and subsequent immobilization affects the proprioceptors in the skeletal muscles, tendons, and joints. Nonweight-bearing exercises, called **open-chain exercises**, produce great gains in peak force

Open-chain exercises
Nonweight-bearing exercises in which the distal joints function independently of the other joints

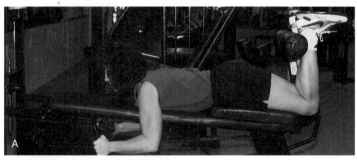

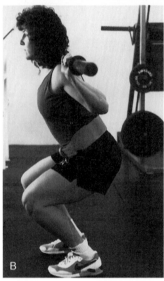

Figure 5.6. A. Open-chain exercise for the hamstrings. **B**. Closed-chain exercise for the hip and knee extensors.

Closed-chain exercises
Weight-bearing exercises in which movement at one joint will produce predictable motion at another joint

production; however, the exercises are usually limited to one joint in a single plane, have greater potential for joint shear, have limited functional application, and have limited eccentric and proprioceptive retraining (**Fig. 5.6A**). In contrast, **closed-chain exercises** (weight-bearing) can retrain joint dynamics and muscle proprioceptors to respond more effectively (**Fig. 5.6B**). Closed-chain exercises are recommended for several reasons: 1) some exercises can be initiated early in the rehabilitation process, 2) multiple joints are exercised through weight-bearing and muscular coconstractions, 3) velocity and torque are more controlled, 4) shear forces are reduced, 5) proprioceptors are reeducated, 6) postural and stabilization mechanics are facilitated, and 7) exercises can work in spiral or diagonal movement patterns (2).

Should the football player resume playing after full range of motion is attained? If you determined that muscle strength, endurance, and power need to be developed prior to allowing gradual return to activity, you are correct.

PHASE FOUR: RETURN TO SPORT ACTIVITY

? *The football player has regained near normal strength in the affected limb as compared to the unaffected limb, and maintained cardiovascular endurance by riding a stationary bike. What additional factors need to be considered to prepare this individual to return to full activity?*

The individual should be returned to their sport activity as soon as possible after muscle strength, endurance, and power are restored. During phase four, the individual should correct any biomechanical inefficiencies in motion, restore coordination in performing sport-specific skills, and improve cardiovascular endurance. The individual may be returned to activity if the following goals are attained:

Coordination and balance are normal

Sport-specific functional patterns are restored in the injured extremity

Muscle strength, endurance, and power in the affected limb is equal to that of the unaffected limb

Cardiovascular endurance is at, or greater than, the preinjury level

If needed, the individual wears appropriate taping, padding, braces, or protective devices to prevent reinjury

The individual receives clearance to return to participation by the supervising physician

Coordination

Coordination refers to the body's ability to execute smooth, fluid, accurate, and controlled movements. Simple movement, such as throwing a ball, involves a complex muscular interaction utilizing the appropriate speed, distance, direction, rhythm, and muscle tension to execute the task (9). Coordination is divided into two categories: gross motor movements involving large muscle groups, and fine motor movements utilizing small muscle groups. Gross motor movements involve activities such as standing, walking, skipping, and running. Fine motor movements are precision actions, particularly with the fingers, such as picking up a coin, clutching an opponent's jersey, or picking up a ground ball with a glove.

Coordination and proprioception are directly linked. Closed-chain activities, performed in the early stages of rehabilitation, help restore proprioceptive input and improve coordination. Constant repetition of motor activities, using sensory cues (tactile, visual, or proprioceptive), or increasing the speed of the activity over time can continue to develop coordination in phase four (9). A wobble board, biomechanical ankle platform system (BAPS) board, and ProFitter are often used to improve sensory cues and balance in the lower extremity. PNF patterns and the ProFitter

Coordination
The body's ability to execute smooth, fluid, accurate, and controlled movements

Coordination is divided into gross motor movements involving large muscle groups, and fine motor movements utilizing small muscle groups

Coordination can be restored with constant repetition of motor activities, using sensory cues, or increasing the speed of the activity over time

Field Strategy 5.6. Lower Extremity Exercises to Improve Balance and Proprioception

Flat Foot Balance Exercises

Stand on one foot (stork stand) and maintain balance for 3 to 5 minutes
Stand on one foot with the toes off the floor and maintain balance for 3 to 5 minutes
Stand on one foot and maintain balance while dribbling a ball

Balancing on the Toes

Balance on the toes/forefoot using both feet for 3 to 5 minutes, then use only one foot
Balance on the toes and dribble a ball

ProFitter Exercises

In a location with a sturdy hand rail, stand on the ProFitter with the feet perpendicular to the long axis of the rails. Gently slide side-to-side, placing pressure first on the toes, then on the heels
Progress to more rapid movement. When you feel comfortable, do the sliding motion without hand support. Keep track of the repetitions and sets

BAPS Board Exercises

Begin, in a seated position, by rotating the foot clockwise and counterclockwise
Stand and perform the exercises while holding onto a sturdy support
Progress to a free-standing position and control the board through the range of motion
Progress to dribbling a ball while balancing on the board

may also be used to improve sensory cues in the upper and lower extremities. **Field Strategy 5.6** lists several lower extremity exercises used to improve coordination and balance.

Sport-specific Skill Conditioning

Therapeutic exercise should progress to the load and speed expected of the individual's sport. A baseball player, for example, performs skills at different speeds and intensities than a football lineman. Therefore, exercises must be coupled with functional training, or specificity of training, related to the physical demands of the sport. A baseball pitcher may have begun to move the injured arm through the throwing pattern with mild to moderate resistance in the early phases of rehabilitation. In the final phase, the individual should increase resistance and speed of motion in a pain-free functional pattern. Initially, short throws with low intensity can be used, progressing to longer throws and low intensity. As the player feels more comfortable with the action, the number of throws and intensity are increased. Similar programs can be developed for other sports.

Specificity of training relates to the physical demands of the sport

Cardiovascular Endurance

Cardiovascular endurance, commonly called aerobic capacity, is the body's ability to sustain submaximal exercise over an extended period of time and depends on the efficiency of the pulmonary and cardiovascular systems. When injured, or when an individual chooses to stop aerobic training, detraining occurs within 1 to 2 weeks (4). If the individual returns to activity without high cardiovascular endurance, fatigue sets in quickly, placing the individual at risk for reinjury.

Like strength training, maintaining and improving cardiovascular endurance are influenced by frequency, duration, and intensity. Aerobic training should occur 3 to 5 days per week lasting longer than 20 minutes, at an intensity of 60% to 90% of maximal heart rate (10). Nonweight-bearing exercises, such as swimming, rowing, biking, or use of the UBE can be helpful early in the therapeutic program, particularly if the individual has a lower extremity injury. Walking, cross-country skiing, jumping rope, or running can be performed as the condition improves. **Field Strategy 5.7** lists several cardiovascular conditioning exercises.

> *In addition to regaining the physical properties in the rehabilitation process, the football player must pass all functional skills pain-free and have a doctor's medical clearance. He may also be required to wear appropriate taping or pads to ensure safe return. Remember that all written documentation of the exercise program and written medical clearance should be placed in the individual's file and stored in a safe, secure location for 3 to 5 years.*

THERAPEUTIC MODALITIES AND MEDICATIONS

> *In developing the treatment plan for the injured football player, your first task was to control inflammation. What therapeutic modalities might be used in the other phases to enhance the healing process?*

Therapeutic modalities can create an optimal environment for injury repair by limiting the inflammatory process and breaking the pain–spasm cycle. Modality use is dependent on the supervising physician's exercise prescription, injury site, type, and severity of injury. An **indication** is a condition that could benefit from a specific modality, whereas a **contraindication** is a condition that could be adversely affected if a particular modality is used. Modalities may be indicated and contraindicated for the same condition. For example, thermotherapy (heat therapy) may be contraindicated for tendinitis during phase one of the exercise program. Once acute inflammation is controlled, however, heat therapy may be indicated. Frequent assessment of the condition will indicate if the appropriate modality is being used.

Several categories of modalities are available:

1. Cryotherapy/cryokinetics includes ice massage, ice and contoured cryo packs, ice immersion and cold whirlpools, commercial cold-gel and chemical packs, and vapocoolant sprays

---

Cardiovascular endurance
The body's ability to sustain submaximal exercise over an extended period of time

---

Cardiovascular endurance training should include activity 3 to 5 days per week, lasting over 20 minutes, at an intensity of 60% to 90% of maximal heart rate

---

Modality use is dependent on the supervising physician's exercise prescription, injury site, and type and severity of injury

Indication
A condition that could benefit from a specific action

Contraindication
A condition adversely affected by a specific action

Field Strategy 5.7. Cardiovascular Conditioning Exercises

Jumping Rope. The rope should pass from one armpit, under the feet, to the other armpit. Jump with the forearms near the ribs at a 45° angle. Rotation occurs at the hand and wrist. Jump with minimal ground clearance

Two-footed jumps
Two feet. Bounce on the balls of the feet
Tap heel of one foot to toe of other foot on one jump
Pepper
Arm crossovers and foot crossovers

One-footed jumps
One foot hop
Rocker step. Rock forward and backward with feet in a forward straddle
Heel strikes and toe taps
Jogging steps

Stair Master. 20 minutes is recommended 3 to 4 times a week
Beginner level
Manual or Pike's Peak mode at Level 2 for 3 for 5 minutes
Increase time to 8, 10, 15, and 20 minutes
Advanced level
When 20 minutes are comfortable, decrease time to 5 to 8 minutes, and increase level intensity for 5 to 8 minutes, then increase time again. As intensity increases, include warm-up and cool-down periods

Treadmill
Beginner level
Begin with a ground level (0° incline) for 5 minutes at about 2.5 mph, increasing to 8, 10, 15, and 20 minutes
Intermediate level
When 20 minutes is comfortable, increase speed to 3 to 5.0 mph, and progress to 8, 10, 15, and 20 minutes. Allow for warm-up and cool-down periods
For example: warm-up at 2.5 mph for 5 min
increase speed to 4.0 to 5.0 mph for 10 min
cool-down at 2.5 mph for 5 min
total workout = 20 min
Advanced level
Increase incline during warm-up and decrease incline during cool-down

Upper Body Ergometer (UBE)
Beginner level
Start at 120 RPM for 4 minutes, alternating directions; 2 minutes forward—2 minutes backward
Intermediate level
Progress to 90 RPM and increase time to 6, 8, and 10 minutes
Advanced level
Alternate directions as tolerated. Duration should not exceed 12 minutes
For example: warm-up at 90 RPM for 2.5 minutes
workout at 60 RPM for 5 minutes
cool-down at 120 RPM for 2.5 minutes

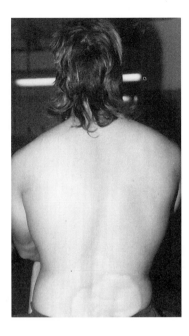

Figure 5.7. A slightly raised white or red irritation may appear shortly after cold application in individuals who are sensitive to cold or who have cold allergies.

2. Thermotherapy includes whirlpools, hydrocollator packs, paraffin baths, contrast baths, diathermy, ultrasound, and phonophoresis
3. Neuromuscular electrical stimulation includes electrical muscle stimulation (EMS) units, iontophoresis, and transcutaneous electrical nerve stimulation (TENS)
4. Intermittent compression
5. Continuous passive motion
6. Massage
7. Medications

Because of the nature of this text, only a general overview of the basic modalities will be provided. Individuals who wish to have detailed information on advanced electrical modalities should enroll in a specialized class on this topic.

Cryotherapy

Cryotherapy is an umbrella term that describes multiple types of cold application. The immediate response of cold application is tissue cooling, which decreases circulation and cell metabolism, thus limiting secondary hypoxic injury. Cold also decreases muscle spasm and pain. Therefore, cryotherapy is the modality of choice during phase one of the therapeutic exercise program. Cryotherapy, however, is contraindicated in individuals with **Raynaud's phenomenon**, **cold allergies (Fig. 5.7)**, or high blood pressure. It is also contraindicated over areas that have a compromised circulatory supply or anesthetized skin.

Depth of cold penetration can reach 5 cm and depends on the amount of subcutaneous insulation, vascular response to skin

Cryotherapy
Cold or ice application

Raynaud's phenomenon
Intermittent bilateral attacks of ischemia in the digits, marked by severe pallor, burning, and pain brought on by cold

Cold allergies
Hypersensitivity to cold, leading to superficial vascular reaction manifested by transient itching, erythema, hives, or whitish swellings (wheals)

Table 5.3. Cryotherapy Application

Indications	Contraindications
Acute or chronic pain	Decreased cold sensitivity and/or hypersensitivity
Acute or chronic muscle spasm/guarding	Cold allergy
Acute inflammation or injury	Circulatory impairment
Postsurgical pain and edema	Raynaud's phenomenon
Superficial first degree burns	Hypertension
Used with exercises to:	Anesthetized skin
Facilitate mobilization	Arthritis
Relieve pain	Possible frostbite
Decrease muscle spasticity	Cardiac or respiratory disorders
Increase ROM	Nerve palsy

cooling, limb circumference, and temperature and duration of application (11). **Table 5.3** lists indications and contraindications for cryotherapy application.

Cryotherapy is usually applied for 15 to 30 minutes per treatment and can be applied hourly during the first 24 to 72 hours after injury. Studies show that a wet wrap applied between the skin and ice bag insulates against the full effects of the cold and limits the effectiveness of the treatment. If used less than 30 to 60 minutes, frostbite should not occur (4). In addition, certain methods of cryotherapy may be used prior to range-of-motion exercises and at the conclusion of an exercise bout. Use of cold treatments prior to exercise is called **cryokinetics**. With each method of cold application, the individual will experience four progressive sensations: cold, burning, aching, and finally analgesia.

> If ice is applied directly to skin for less than 30 to 60 minutes, frostbite should not occur

Cryokinetics
Use of cold treatments prior to an exercise session

> Ice massage is commonly used prior to range-of-motion exercises and friction massage when treating chronic tendinitis and muscle strains

Ice Massage

Ice massage is particularly useful for its analgesic effect in relieving pain that may inhibit stretching of a muscle and has been shown to decrease muscle soreness when combined with stretching (12). It is commonly used prior to range-of-motion exercises and friction massage when treating chronic tendinitis and muscle strains. Treatment consists of water frozen in a cup, then rubbed over the skin in small circular motions for 7 to 10 minutes. A wooden tongue depressor frozen in the cup provides a handle for easy application.

Ice Packs and Contoured Cryo Cuffs

Ice packs made of flaked ice or small cubes can be safely applied to the skin for 20 to 30 minutes without danger of frostbite. Furthermore, ice packs can be molded to the body's contours, held in place by a cold compression wrap, and elevated above the heart to minimize swelling and pooling of fluids in the interstitial tissue spaces.

Contoured cryo cuffs utilize ice water placed in an insulated thermos. When the thermos is raised above the body part, water

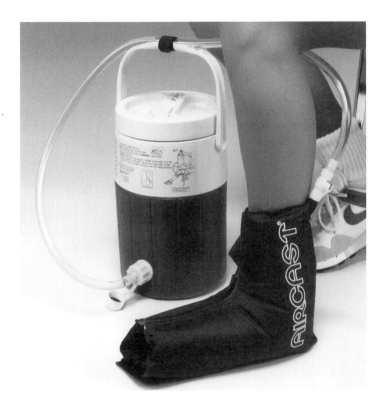

Figure 5.8. Contoured cryo cuffs are an effective means of cold application. When the thermos is raised above the body part, water flows into the cryo pack, maintaining cold compression for 5 to 7 hours.

flows into the cryo pack, maintaining cold compression for 5 to 7 hours (**Fig. 5.8**). Although more expensive, the devices combine ice and compression over a longer period of time without threat of frostbite (13).

Ice Immersion and Cold Whirlpools

Ice immersion and cold whirlpools are used to quickly reduce surface temperature of a distal extremity, i.e., forearm, hand, ankle, or foot. Because of the analgesic effect and buoyancy of water, both modalities are often used during the inflammatory phase and combined with range-of-motion exercises. Cold whirlpool baths also provide a hydromassaging effect by controlling the amount of air emitted through the electrical turbine.

A bucket or cold whirlpool is filled with water and ice and maintained at a temperature between 10 and 15° C (49 and 59° F) (4). The lower the temperature range, the shorter the duration of immersion. Treatment lasts from 5 to 15 minutes. When pain is relieved, the part is removed from the water and functional movement patterns are performed. As pain returns, the area is reimmersed. The cycle continues three to four times.

> Because of the analgesic effect and buoyancy in water, ice immersion and cold whirlpools are often used during the inflammatory phase with range-of-motion exercises

> The lower the temperature range, the shorter the duration of immersion

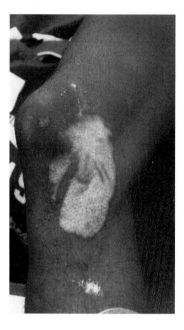

Figure 5.9. This intercollegiate soccer player fell asleep with a chemical ice bag on his leg, unaware of a small leak in the bag. The resulting irritation led to a second degree chemical burn to the skin.

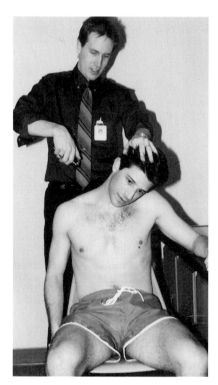

Figure 5.10. Vapocoolant sprays temporarily freeze superficial tissues and aid the clinician in reducing the pain-spasm cycle prior to stretching exercises.

Commercial Cold-gel and Chemical Packs

A commercial cold-gel pack has a gelatinous substance enclosed in a strong vinyl case, and can conform to the body's natural contours. Used with compression and elevation, it is an effective cold application. The packs are stored at a temperature of about −5° C for at least 2 hours prior to application (4,12). A wet towel is placed between the pack and skin to prevent frostbite and maintain a hygienic surface for the reusable packs. Treatment time is 15 to 20 minutes.

Chemical packs are convenient to carry in a training kit, are disposable after a single use, can conform to the body part, but can be expensive. The packs are activated by squeezing or hitting the pack against a hard area. The chemical reaction is at an alkaline pH and can cause skin burns if the package breaks open and the contents spill **(Fig. 5.9)**. As such, the packs should never be squeezed in front of the face, and if possible, should be placed inside another plastic bag. Treatment ranges from 15 to 20 minutes; however, as the pack warms, it becomes ineffective as a cold treatment.

A wet towel is placed between the pack and skin to prevent frostbite and maintain a hygienic surface for the reusable packs

Vapocoolant Sprays

Fluoromethane evaporates rapidly when applied to the skin, and as such, the effects are very superficial. This technique is often used to freeze the skin prior to stretching a muscle **(Fig. 5.10)**. The bottle of vapocoolant spray is inverted and sprayed in a unidirectional parallel sweeping pattern over the involved site. The clinician then stretches the body part as tolerated by the patient.

Thermotherapy

Thermotherapy, or heat application, is used after the acute inflammatory stage to increase blood flow and promote healing in the injured area. Heat has an analgesic, or sedative, effect and can increase circulation and cellular metabolism, and decrease muscle spasm and pain. Used prior to stretching exercises, thermotherapy can increase extensibility of connective tissue, leading to increased range of motion (14). Depth of penetration ranges from 2 cm, with superficial thermotherapy, to 2 to 5 cm, with penetrating thermotherapy (15). **Table 5.4** lists indications and contraindications for thermotherapy.

Thermotherapy
Heat application

Thermotherapy can increase extensibility of connective tissue, leading to increased range of motion

Whirlpools

Whirlpools combine warm or hot water with a hydromassaging effect to increase superficial skin temperature, decrease muscle spasm and pain, and facilitate range of motion exercises after prolonged immobilization **(Fig. 5.11)**. Treatment time ranges from 20 to 30 minutes. Only the body part being treated should be immersed. **Field Strategy 5.8** lists indications, contraindications, technique, and suggested temperatures.

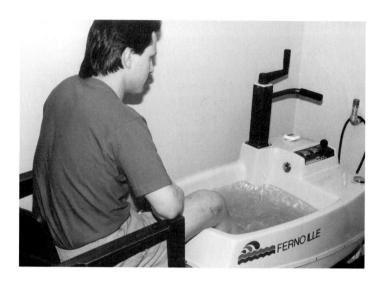

Figure 5.11. Hot whirlpools increase superficial skin temperatures, leading to an analgesic effect, which can reduce muscle spasm and pain, facilitate range-of-motion exercises, and promote healing.

Hydrocollator Packs

Hydrocollator packs provide superficial moist heat to a slightly deeper tissue level than a whirlpool (11,12). The packs consist of several silicone gel compartments encased in a canvas fabric stored in a hot water unit **(Fig. 5.12)**. The pack is wrapped in a commercial padded hot-pack cover and placed directly over the injury site for 20 minutes. The patient should never lie on top of the pack, as this may accelerate the rate of heat transfer leading to burns on sensitive skin. After 5 minutes of treatment, the area should be checked for any redness or signs of burning.

Paraffin Baths

Paraffin baths provide heat to contoured bony areas (feet, hands, or wrists). A paraffin and mineral oil mixture is heated in a unit at 47.0 to 54.4°C (125 to 130°F) (12). All jewelry is removed, and

Table 5.4. Thermotherapy Application

Indications	Contraindications

Subacute or chronic injuries to:
  Reduce swelling, edema, and ecchymosis
  Reduce muscle spasm/guarding
Increase blood flow to:
  Increase ROM prior to activity
  Resolve hematoma
  Increase tissue healing
Relieve joint contractures
Fight infection
	Acute inflammation or injuries
	Impaired or poor circulation
	Subacute or chronic pain
	Impaired or poor sensation
	Impaired thermal regulation
	Malignancy
	Patients, either elderly or infants, who cannot
	  report their reactions

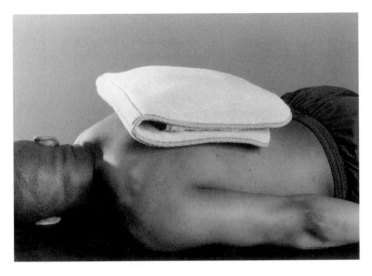

Figure 5.12. Moist heat treatments can produce burns to sensitive skin. To avoid this, place the hydrocollator pack in a commercial padded towel and periodically check the skin surface for any redness or signs of burning.

the body part is thoroughly cleansed, and then dipped into the bath several times (**Fig. 5.13**). When this process is completed, the body part is wrapped in a plastic bag and towel to maintain heat, then elevated for 15 to 20 minutes. The wax is then peeled

 Field Strategy 5.8. Techniques for Using a Whirlpool Bath

Indications	Contraindications
Subacute and chronic inflammation	Acute injuries
Peripheral nerve injuries	Fever (hot whirlpool)
Peripheral vascular injuries	Certain skin conditions
Increase range of motion	

Apply a povidone-iodine (Betadine) additive, or a 5% bleach solution to the water as an antibacterial agent, especially if anyone has an open wound
Recommended temperature and treatment times include:

Cold whirlpools	55 to 65° F	5 to 15 mins.
Hot whirlpools		
extremity	98 to 110° F	20 to 30 mins.
full body	98 to 102° F	10 to 12 mins.

Assist the patient into the water. Turn the turbine on and adjust the height to direct the water flow 6 to 8 inches away from the injury site
Instruct the patient to move the body part through the available range of motion to increase blood flow to the area, aid in removal of debris, and improve proprioception
Turn the turbine off and remove the patient from the water. Dry the treated area and assist the individual from the whirlpool area
Drain and cleanse the whirlpool tub after each use
Cultures for bacterial and fungal agents should be conducted monthly from water samples in the whirlpool turbine and drain

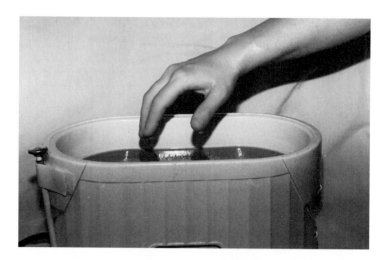

Figure 5.13. In a paraffin bath treatment, the limb is thoroughly cleansed, dipped several times into the solution, then wrapped in plastic and a towel to maintain heat.

off and returned to the bath, where it can be reused. The mineral oil in the wax keeps the skin soft and pliable during massage, when treating a variety of hand and foot conditions.

Contrast Baths

Contrast baths combine cryotherapy and thermotherapy in subacute or chronic injuries, to reduce edema and restore range of motion. Two whirlpools or containers are placed next to each other. One is filled with cold water and ice at 10 to 15°C (49 to 59°F), and the other is filled with hot water at 37 to 44°C (98.6 to 111°F) (12). The injured extremity is alternated between the two tubs at a 3:1 or 4:1 ratio (hot water to cold water) for approximately 20 minutes. The treatment begins and ends in cold water prior to starting therapeutic exercise, but, in chronic conditions, treatment is more often concluded in warm immersion.

> Contrast baths combine cryotherapy and thermotherapy in subacute or chronic injuries to reduce edema and restore range of motion

Diathermy

Diathermy uses electromagnetic energy to elicit deep penetrating thermal effects. The two forms of diathermy, shortwave and microwave, can decrease joint stiffness, pain, and muscle spasm, and facilitate healing of soft tissue injuries in the postacute stage. The depth of penetration and extent of heat production depends on wave frequency, the electrical properties of the tissues receiving the energy, and the type of applicator used (12).

> Diathermy can decrease joint stiffness, pain, and muscle spasm, and facilitate healing of soft tissue injuries in the postacute stage

Ultrasound

Ultrasound uses high frequency sound waves to elicit thermal and nonthermal effects in deep tissue (**Fig. 5.14**). Thermal effects

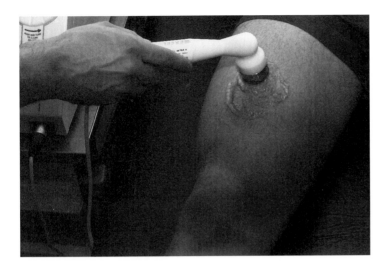

Figure 5.14. In an ultrasound treatment, a coupling agent is used between the transducer head and area being treated. The head is moved in small circles or longitudinal strokes to distribute the energy as evenly as possible and to prevent damage to the underlying tissues.

elevate tissue temperature and increase collagen tissue extensibility, blood flow, and sensory and motor nerve conduction velocity, and reduce muscle spasm and pain. Nonthermal effects increase cell membrane and vascular wall permeability, tissue regeneration, and protein synthesis, and reduce edema (12,15). Ultrasound is used to manage several soft tissue conditions, such as tendinitis, bursitis, muscle spasm, and calcium deposits in soft tissue, and to reduce joint contractures, pain, and scar tissue.

Phonophoresis

Phonophoresis is a technique whereby ultrasound is used to drive medication through the skin to the underlying tissues. An advantage of this modality is that the medication is delivered directly to the injury site. This technique is used in the postacute stage of conditions such as tendinitis, bursitis, arthritis, or contusions.

Phonophoresis
The introduction of medication through the skin with the use of ultrasound

Neuromuscular Electrical Stimulation

Neuromuscular electrical stimulation (NMES) is used to relieve pain; reduce swelling, muscle spasm, and atrophy; increase blood flow, range of motion, and muscle strength; enhance wound healing; reeducate muscle; and, through iontophoresis, introduce anti-inflammatory, analgesic, or anesthetic drugs to an injured area (13,16). Electrical stimulation can be used in the early stages of exercise when the muscle is at its weakest (**Fig. 5.15**).

Neuromuscular electrical stimulation (NMES) can relieve pain; reduce swelling, muscle spasm, and atrophy; increase blood flow, range of motion, and muscle strength; enhance wound healing; reeducate muscle; and, through iontophoresis, introduce anti-inflammatory, analgesic, or anesthetic drugs to an injured area

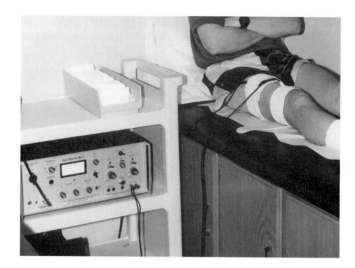

Figure 5.15. Electrical muscle stimulation can maintain muscle size and strength during immobilization, re-educate muscles, prevent muscle atrophy, and increase blood flow to tissues to decrease pain and spasm.

Iontophoresis

Iontophoresis uses a direct current to drive charged molecules from certain medications, such as anti-inflammatories (hydrocortisone), anesthetics (lidocaine), or analgesics (aspirin or acetaminophen) into damaged tissue. The medication is placed under the electrode with the same polarity and the molecules are pushed away from the electrode into the skin, toward the injured site.

Iontophoresis
Technique whereby direct current is used to drive charged molecules from certain medications into damaged tissue

Transcutaneous Electrical Nerve Stimulation (TENS)

TENS is used to produce analgesia and decrease acute and chronic pain. Also, it is often used continuously after surgery or in a 30- to 60-minute session several times a day (16). It is thought that TENS works to override the body's internal signals of pain (gate

TENS is used to produce analgesia and decrease acute and chronic pain

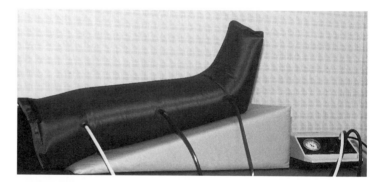

Figure 5.16. An air-filled boot or sleeve can provide pressure or intermittent compression to an injured area to reduce edema.

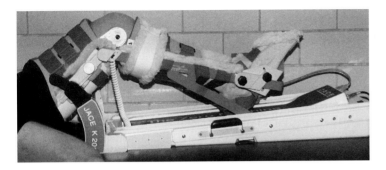

Figure 5.17. Continuous passive motion machines are often used postsurgically to apply an external force to move the joint through a limited range of motion.

theory of pain) and stimulates the release of endomorphins, a strong opiate-like substance produced by the body. Most units are small enough to be worn on a belt and are battery-powered. The electrodes are taped on the skin over or around the painful site or may be secured along the peripheral or spinal nerve pathways.

Intermittent Compression Units

Intermittent compression uses compression and elevation to decrease blood flow to an extremity and assist venous return, thus decreasing edema. A boot or sleeve is applied around the injured extremity. Compression is formed when air or cold water inflates and deflates the unit intermittently for 20 to 30 minutes, several times a day **(Fig. 5.16)**.

> Intermittent compression decreases blood flow to an extremity and assists in venous return, thus decreasing edema

Continuous Passive Motion (CPM)

Continuous passive motion units apply an external force to move the joint through a limited range of motion **(Fig. 5.17)**. It is primarily used postsurgically at the knee. The application is relatively pain free and has been shown to stimulate the intrinsic healing process; maintain articular cartilage nutrition; reduce disuse effects; retard joint stiffness and the pain-spasm cycle; and benefit collagen remodeling, joint dynamics, and pain reduction (15,17).

Massage

Soft tissue massage is an excellent means to increase cutaneous circulation, cell metabolism, and venous and lymphatic flow to assist in the removal of edema, stretch superficial scar tissue, and decrease neuromuscular excitability (15). To reduce friction between the patient's skin and hand, particularly over hairy areas, lubricants are often used, such as massage lotion, peanut oil, coconut oil, or powder. Massage over a larger area involves effleurage (stroking), pétrissage (kneading), tapotement (percussion), and vibration to treat muscle, tendon, and joint conditions.

> Massage can increase cutaneous circulation, cell metabolism, and venous and lymphatic flow to assist in removal of edema, stretch superficial scar tissue, and relax muscle tissue

Medications

Therapeutic drugs
Prescription or over-the-counter medications used to treat an injury or illness

Therapeutic drugs are either prescription or over-the-counter medications used to treat an injury or illness. Common drugs used to control pain, inflammation, and muscle spasm include anesthetics, analgesics, nonsteroidal anti-inflammatory drugs (NSAIDs), adrenocorticosteroids, and muscle relaxants.

Local anesthetics eliminate short-term pain in a specific body part and are identified by their "-caine" suffix (i.e., lidocaine, procaine, and benzocaine). The drugs may be topically applied to skin for minor irritations (burns, abrasions, mild inflammation), introduced into subcutaneous tissues via phonophoresis or iontophoresis (bursitis, tendinitis, contusions), injected by a physician into soft tissue around a laceration for surgical repair (suturing), or injected by a physician near a peripheral nerve to interrupt nerve transmission (nerve block) (18).

Analgesics and nonsteroidal anti-inflammatory drugs (NSAIDs) are used to decrease edema, relieve mild to moderate pain (analgesia), decrease body temperature associated with fever (**antipyresis**), increase collagen strength, and inhibit coagulation and blood clotting. NSAIDS are very effective during the early stages of healing; however, prolonged use (2 or more weeks) may actually retard the healing process. Examples of analgesics and NSAIDs include aspirin (acetylsalicylic acid), acetaminophen (Tylenol), ibuprofen (Advil, Nuprin, Motrin), Indocin, Feldene, and Clinoril.

Analgesics and NSAIDs decrease edema, relieve mild to moderate pain, decrease body temperature associated with a fever, increase collagen strength, and inhibit coagulation and blood clotting

Antipyresis
Action whereby body temperature associated with a fever is reduced

Acetaminophen reduces pain and fever, but does not have any appreciable anti-inflammatory or anticoagulant effects. Unlike aspirin, acetaminophen is not associated with gastrointestinal irritation. However, high doses can be toxic to the liver and may be fatal (18).

Aspirin is the most commonly used drug to relieve pain and inflammation. Because of its anticoagulation properties, it is not used during the acute phase. Aspirin is associated with a number of adverse side effects, including gastrointestinal irritation. With chronic use or high doses, renal problems, liver toxicity, congestive heart failure, hypertension, aspirin intoxication, or poisoning may occur (19).

Ibuprofen and the other NSAIDs are administered primarily for pain relief and anti-inflammatory effects. Although many are still associated with some stomach discomfort, they provide better effects in many patients. Taking the medication after a meal or with a glass of milk or water will greatly reduce stomach discomfort.

Adrenocorticosteroids are steroid hormones produced by the adrenal cortex. Examples of these drugs include cortisone, prednisone, and hydrocortisone. These drugs can be used to decrease edema, inflammation, erythema, and tenderness in a region, and can be topically applied, given orally, or injected by a physician into a specific area, such as a tendon or joint (18). Because many of these drugs can lead to breakdown and rupture of structures, long-term use is contraindicated.

Adenocorticosteroids decrease edema, inflammation, erythema, and tenderness in a region; they can be topically applied, given orally, or injected into a specific area

Skeletal muscle relaxants are used to relieve muscle spasms, which can result from certain musculoskeletal injuries or inflammation. These medications break the pain-spasm cycle by allowing more normal muscle excitability, which, in turn, decreases pain and improves motor function. Examples of muscle relaxants include Flexeril, Soma, and Dantrium.

After reading this section, did you determine that NSAIDs, cryotherapy, intermittent compression, EMS, and TENS can be used in the early phases of healing? Thermotherapy, cryotherapy, ultrasound, and EMS can be used in the later stages of repair. What can the football player do at home to assist treatments provided in the athletic training room?

SUMMARY

Rehabilitation begins immediately after injury assessment. The level of function and dysfunction is assessed, results are interpreted, a list of deficits is formulated, long- and short-term goals are established, and a course of action is developed, including therapeutic exercises, modalities, and medications. The program is then supervised and periodically reassessed with appropriate changes made.

Phase one of the therapeutic exercise program should focus on control of inflammation, muscle spasm, and pain. Phase two should regain any deficits in range of motion and proprioception at the affected joint as compared to the unaffected joint. Phase three should regain muscular strength, endurance, and power in the affected limb. Phase four prepares the individual to return to activity and includes analysis of motion, sport-specific skill training, regaining coordination, and cardiovascular conditioning. Throughout the total therapeutic exercise program, nutritional and psychological needs of the injured individual should be addressed.

Therapeutic modalities supplement the exercise program to control inflammation and enhance healing. At the conclusion of the exercise program, the supervising physician will determine if the individual is ready to return to full activity. This decision is based on the individual's range of motion, flexibility, muscular strength, endurance, power, biomechanical skill analysis, coordination, and cardiovascular endurance. If additional protective bracing, padding, or taping is necessary to enable the individual to return safely to activity, this should be documented in the individual's file. It should be stressed that use of any protective device should not replace a maintenance program of conditioning exercises. Year-round conditioning can prevent many injuries from recurring.

The athletic trainer should keep a watchful eye on the athlete when they return to activity. If the individual begins to show signs of pain, swelling, or discomfort, or if skill performance deteriorates, the individual should be re-evaluated to determine if activity should continue or if the therapeutic exercise program needs to be reinstituted.

REFERENCES

1. Wiese-Bjornstal DM, Smith AM, and LaMott EE. 1995. A model of psychologic response to athletic injury and rehabilitation. Ath Tr Spts Health Care Perspect 1(1):17–30.
2. Shaffer SM. 1992. Attributions and self-efficacy as predictors of rehabilitative success. Masters thesis. Champaign-Urbana: University of Illinois.
3. Harrelson GL. Introduction to rehabilitation. In *Physical rehabilitation of the injured athlete*, edited by JR Andrews and GL Harrelson. Philadelphia: WB Saunders, 1991.
4. Knight KL. *Cryotherapy in sport injury management*. Champaign: Human Kinetics, 1995.
5. McArdle WD, Katch FI, and Katch VL. *Exercise physiology: energy, nutrition, and human performance*. Baltimore: Williams & Wilkins, 1996.
6. Knight KL. 1979. Rehabilitating chondromalacia patellae. Phys Sportsmed 7(10):147–148.
7. IOC Medical Commission. 1991. Terminology and units of measurement for the description of exercise and sport. J Appl Spt Sci Res 5(2):108.
8. Perrin DH. *Isokinetic exercise and assessment*. Champaign, IL: Human Kinetics, 1993.
9. Schmitz TJ. Coordination assessment. In *Physical rehabilitation: assessment and treatment*, edited by SB O'Sullivan and TJ Schmitz. Philadelphia: FA Davis, 1988.
10. American College of Sports Medicine. 1990. The recommended quantity and quality of exercise for developing and maintaining cardiorespiratory and muscular fitness in healthy adults. Sports Med Bull 13(3):1–4.
11. Halvorson GA. 1990. Therapeutic heat and cold for athletic injuries. Phys Sportsmed 18(5):87–94.
12. Michlovitz SL. Cryotherapy: the use of cold as a therapeutic agent. In *Thermal agents in rehabilitation*, edited by SL Michlovitz. Philadelphia: FA Davis, 1990.
13. Cooper M. Use of modalities in rehabilitation. In *Physical rehabilitation of the injured athlete*, edited by JR Andrews and GL Harrelson. Philadelphia: WB Saunders, 1991.
14. Leadbetter WB, Buckwalter JA, and Gordon SL. *Sports-induced inflammation*. Park Ridge, IL: American Academy of Orthopaedic Surgeons, 1990.
15. Starkey C. *Therapeutic modalities for athletic trainers*. Philadelphia: FA Davis, 1993.
16. Windsor RE, Lester JP, and Herring SA. 1993. Electrical stimulation in clinical practice. Phys Sportsmed 21(2):85–93.
17. O'Donoghue PC, McCarthy MR, Gieck JH, and Yates CK. 1991. Clinical use of continuous passive motion in athletic training. Ath Tr (JNATA) 26(3):200–208.
18. Ciccone CD, and Wolf SL. *Pharmacology in rehabilitation*. Philadelphia: FA Davis, 1990.
19. Kisner C, and Colby LA. *Therapeutic exercise: foundations and techniques*. Philadelphia: FA Davis, 1990.

Protective Equipment

After completing this chapter, you should be able to:

- Identify the principles used to design protective equipment

- Explain the types of materials used in the development of padding

- List the organizations responsible for establishing standards for protective devices

- Fit selected equipment (i.e., football helmets, mouth guards, and shoulder pads)

- Identify and discuss common protective equipment for the head and face, torso, and the upper and lower body

Key Terms:

Diffuse injury

Focal injury

High-density material

Low-density material

Prophylactic

Resilience

Protective equipment, when properly used, can protect the sport participant from accidental or routine injuries associated with a particular sport. There are limitations, however, to its effectiveness. Today's players are faster, stronger, and more skilled. A natural outcome of wearing protective equipment is to feel more secure. Unfortunately, this often leads to more aggressive play, which can result in injury to the participant or an opponent. Protective equipment can only be effective if it meets minimum standards of protection, is in good condition, is clean, is properly fitted, is used regularly, and is used properly.

In this chapter, principles of protective equipment and materials used in the development of padding will be discussed first. Second, discussion of protective equipment for the head and face is followed by equipment commonly used to protect the upper body and lower body. Where appropriate, guidelines for fitting specific equipment are listed in field strategies. Although several commercial braces and support devices are illustrated, these are intended only to demonstrate a variety of products available to protect a body region.

Sport participants must be protected from high-velocity–low-mass forces and low-velocity–high-mass forces

Focal injury
Injury in a small, concentrated area, usually due to high-velocity–low-mass forces

Diffuse injury
Injury over a large body area, usually due to low-velocity–high-mass forces

Prophylactic
Preventative or protective

Design and selection of equipment should be based on the optimal level of impact intensity afforded by the given thickness, density, resilience, and temperature of energy-absorbing material

Low-density material
Materials that absorb energy from low-impact intensity levels

High-density material
Materials that absorb more energy from higher-impact intensity levels through deformation, thus transferring less stress to a body part

> *What type of energy-absorbing material can best protect a body region from a single blow? What material can best protect an area subjected to repeated blows?*

In contact and collision sports, the participant must be protected from high-velocity–low-mass forces, and low-velocity–high-mass forces. High-velocity–low-mass forces occur when an individual is struck by a ball, puck, bat, or hockey stick. The low mass and high speed of impact lead to forces concentrated in a smaller area, resulting in **focal injuries**. Low-velocity–high-mass forces occur when an individual falls on the ground or ice or is checked into the sideboards of an ice hockey rink, thereby absorbing the forces over a larger area leading to **diffuse injuries**. Techniques and equipment to prevent or protect an injury site are called **prophylactic** devices.

Sport-related injuries can result from a variety of factors, including:

Illegal play
Poor technique
Inadequate conditioning
Poorly matched player levels
A previously injured area that is now vulnerable to reinjury
Low tolerance of a player to injury
Inability to adequately protect an area without restricting motion
Poor quality, maintenance, or cleanliness of protective equipment

Protective equipment can protect an area from accidental or routine injuries through several means, many of which are listed in **Table 6.1** (1). Design and selection should be based on the optimal level of impact intensity afforded by the given thickness, density, and temperature of energy-absorbing material. Soft, **low-density material** is light and comfortable to wear, but is only effective at low levels of impact intensity. Examples of low-density material include gauze padding, foam, neoprene, Sorbothane, felt, and moleskin. In contrast, firmer, **higher-density material** of

---

Table 6.1. Equipment Design Factors that Can Reduce Potential Injury

Increase the impact area
Transfer or disperse the impact area to another body part
Limit the relative motion of a body part
Add mass to the body part to limit deformation and displacement
Reduce friction between contacting surfaces
Absorb energy
Use materials resistant to the absorption of bacteria, fungus, and viruses that can be easily cleaned and disinfected

---

the same thickness tends to be less comfortable, offers less cushioning of low-level impact, but can absorb more energy by deformation and, thus, transfers less stress to an area at higher impact intensity levels (1). Examples of high-density material include thermomoldable plastics, such as orthoplast and thermoplast, and casting materials, such as fiberglass or plaster. Many of these materials are shown in **Figure 6.1**.

Soft foam over a bruised area will not absorb high impact forces as effectively as a denser foam. To address this factor, many equipment designers layer material of varying density. Soft, low-density material is placed next to the skin, covered by increasingly more dense material away from the skin, to absorb and disperse high-intensity blows.

Another factor to consider in energy-absorbing material is its **resilience** or memory. Resilience is the ability of a material to regain its shape quickly after impact. Highly resilient materials are commonly used over areas subjected to repeated impact. Nonresilient or slow-recovery resilient material offers the best protection and is used over areas that are subjected to one-time or occasional impact. It is important to select equipment that will absorb impact forces and disperse it before injury occurs to the underlying body part.

Nonresilient or slow-recovery resilient materials are best for protecting a body region subjected to a one-time or occasional blow. Highly resilient materials are used over an area subjected to repeated blows. In addition, a laminated layering of soft, low-density material covered by a firmer, higher density material will absorb high-impact forces better.

Resilience
The ability to bounce or spring back into shape or position after being stretched, bent, or impacted

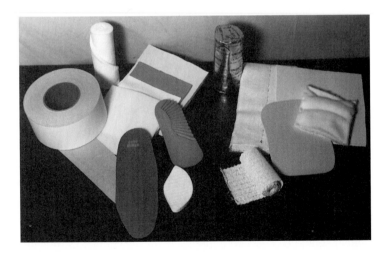

Figure 6.1. On the left are examples of low-density material used to cushion low-level impact forces. These include moleskin, gauze padding, foam materials, neoprene, Sorbothane, and felt. On the right are high-density materials, such as thermomoldable plastics and casting materials, that can absorb more energy by deformation and, thus, transfer less stress to an injured area.

? *Preseason football camp has just begun. What guidelines should be used to properly fit a football helmet?*

Many head and facial injuries can be prevented with regular use of properly fitted helmets and facial protection. Standards of protection have vastly improved through the combined efforts of athletic governing bodies, the American Society for Testing and Materials (ASTM), the National Operating Committee on Standards for Athletic Equipment (NOCSAE), and the Hockey Equipment Certification Council (HECC) of the Canadian Standards Association (CSA). NOCSAE has established safety standards for football, baseball, softball, and lacrosse helmets and face masks. The CSA governs ice hockey helmets; the ASTM establishes standards for bicycle helmets and material standards for other protective equipment.

Football Helmets

Football helmets are typically air- or fluid-filled, closed-cell padded, or a combination. The shells may be constructed of plastic or a polycarbonate alloy. Polycarbonate is a plastic used in making jet canopies and police riot gear and is lightweight and scratch- and impact-resistant. Helmets vary in life expectancy. The polycarbonate alloy shell has a 5-year warranty, the ABS plastic shell has a 2-year warranty, the AHI (Athletic Helmets, Inc.) helmet should be retired after 6 years, and Riddell recommends retiring their helmet after 10 years (2). All helmets must protect the cranium from low-velocity–high-mass impact forces that could conceivably fracture the skull, and must be NOCSAE approved. On all new and reconditioned helmets is a visible warning label that states:

> **Warning:** Do not strike an opponent with any part of this helmet or face mask. This is a violation of football rules and may cause you to suffer severe brain or neck injury, including paralysis or death. Severe brain or neck injury may also occur accidentally while playing football. NO HELMET CAN PREVENT ALL SUCH INJURIES. USE THIS HELMET AT YOUR OWN RISK.

Always follow manufacturer's guidelines when fitting a football helmet. Prior to fitting, the athletes should have haircuts in the style that will be worn during the athletic season and wet their heads to simulate game conditions. **Field Strategy 6.1** lists the general steps in fitting a padded football helmet. To inflate an air bladder helmet, hold the bulb with an arch in the hose and bulb; to deflate, hold the bulb in a straight position. Once fitted, the helmet should be checked periodically for several factors, including (2):

1. Proper fit that may be altered by hair length
2. Proper placement or deterioration of any foam padding
3. Loss of air from cells, especially if the team is traveling to a different altitude

All helmets must protect the cranium from low-velocity–high-mass impact forces that could conceivably fracture the skull

Field Strategy 6.1. Proper Fitting of a Padded Football Helmet

A. The player's haircut should be the style that will be worn during the competitive season and the player should wet the hair to simulate game conditions. The helmet should fit snugly on the player's head with the cheek pads snug against the sides of the face. The front straps of the chinstrap should be applied first, followed by the back straps. The chin pad should be an equal distance from each side of the helmet

B. The helmet should be one inch (one to two finger widths) above the player's eyebrows. The face mask should extend two to three finger widths away from the player's nose

C. The face mask should allow for complete field of vision

D. The back of the helmet should cover the base of the skull, and the ear holes should match up with the external auditory ear canal. With the chin strap secured, the helmet should not move when you pull the face guard up and down or side to side

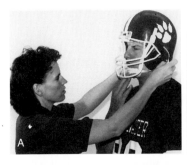
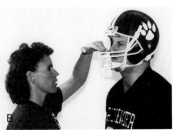
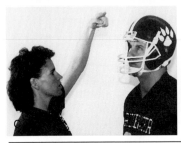
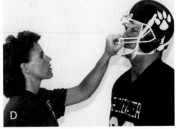

4. Cracks in the vinyl or rubber covering air, foam, or liquid padded helmets
5. All rivets, screws, Velcro, and snaps, to ensure that they are properly fastened and holding protective parts
6. Cracks in the shell, particularly noting any cracks around holes
7. Spread of the face mask

If any factors observed in the regular inspection indicate a need to repair and/or replace the helmet, this should be done immediately. In addition to replacing damaged helmets, helmets must be reconditioned every 2 years to maintain NOCSAE standards.

Ice Hockey Helmets

All ice hockey helmets are required to meet HECC standards and carry the stamp of approval from the CSA (**Fig. 6.2**). These helmets must absorb and disperse high-velocity–low-mass forces (high stick or puck), and low-velocity–high-mass forces (being checked into the sideboard or falling on the ice). As with a football helmet, proper fit is achieved when a snug-fitting helmet does not move in one direction when the head is turned in the other.

Batting Helmets

> On a baseball helmet, it is best to have a thick layer of foam between the primary energy absorber and the head, to allow the shell to move slightly and deform

Batting helmets used in baseball and softball require the NOCSAE mark and must be a double ear-flap design. It is best to have a thick layer of foam between the primary energy absorber and the head, to allow the shell to move slightly and deform. This maximizes its ability to absorb missile kinetic energy from a ball or bat and prevents excessive pressure on the cranium. The helmet should be snug enough so that it does not move or fall off during batting and running bases.

Other Helmets

> A stiffer shell on a bicycle helmet results in better diffusion and resilience to the impact

Lacrosse helmets are made of a high-resistant plastic or fiberglass shell and must meet NOCSAE standards. The helmet, wire face guard, and chin pad are secured with a four-point chin strap (**Fig. 6.3**). The helmet should not move in one direction when the head moves in another.

Bicycle helmets have a plastic or fiberglass rigid shell with a chin strap and an energy-absorbing foam liner (**Fig. 6.2**). A stiffer

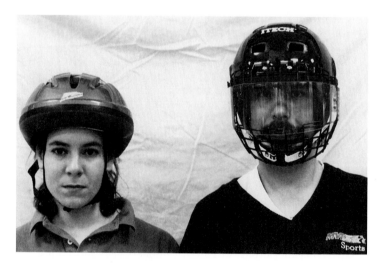

Figure 6.2. Bicycle helmets (left) can reduce the severity of head injuries and protect against serious upper facial injuries. Ice hockey helmets and face mask (right) can greatly reduce cranial and facial injuries.

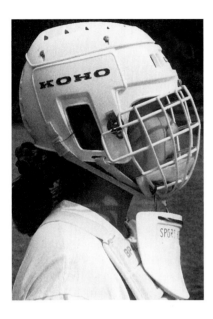

Figure 6.3. Lacrosse helmets provide full face and neck protection.

shell results in better diffusion and resilience to impact. A firm, dense foam liner is more effective at higher velocities, whereas a less stiff foam provides more protection at lower velocities. As in other helmets, a snug fit is necessary for a proper fit.

Face Guards

Football face guards are made of either a heavy-gauge, plastic-coated steel rod or a rigid, plastic-like material designed to withstand impacts from blunt surfaces, such as the turf or a player's knee or elbow. When properly fitted, the face mask should extend two finger-widths away from the forehead and allow for complete field of vision **(Field Strategy 6.1B)**. The effectiveness of a football face guard depends on the strength of the guard itself, the helmet attachments, and the four-point chin strap on the helmet.

Ice hockey face guards are made of clear plastic (polycarbonate), steel wire, or a combination of the two **(Fig. 6.2)**. The use of mandatory face guards in ice hockey has been shown to reduce the incidence of facial lacerations without increasing head and neck injuries (3). The guard stands approximately 1 to 1½ inches away from the nose. If a wire mesh is used, the holes should be small enough to prevent penetration of a hockey stick. The lacrosse face guard is a wire mesh guard that has a padded chin region in case the guard is driven back during a collision with another player **(Fig. 6.3)**. Face masks used by catchers and the home plate umpire in baseball and softball should fit snugly to the cheeks and forehead, but should not impair vision. Men's and women's fencing masks have an adjustable spring to prevent the mask from moving during competition.

An effective football face guard depends on the strength of the guard itself, the helmet attachments, and the four-point chin strap on the helmet

Mouth Guards

A mouth guard can prevent dental and oral soft tissue injuries and, to a lesser extent, jaw fractures, cerebral concussions, and TMJ injuries

Mouth guards should be durable, resilient, resistant to tear, inexpensive, easy to fabricate, tasteless, odorless, and clearly visible to officials

A properly fitted mouth guard can absorb energy, disperse the impact, cushion the contact between the upper and lower teeth, and keep the upper lip away from the incisal edges of the teeth (4). This action significantly reduces dental and oral soft tissue injuries and, to a lesser extent, jaw fractures, cerebral concussions, and temporomandibular joint (TMJ) injuries (4,5).

Mouth guards should be durable, resilient, resistant to tear, inexpensive, easy to fabricate, tasteless, odorless, and clearly visible to officials (4,6). The athlete should cut down the mouth guard only if the device extends beyond the posterior molars. Athletes who cut the device to a size that only covers the front four teeth will void the product's injury prevention warranty and doing this could lead to an unexpected airway obstruction (2). Although players may complain that a mouth guard interferes with speech, the benefits of preventing oral injuries far outweigh the disadvantages. Mouth guards are available in three basic types: stock (ready-made), mouth-formed, and custom-made from a model of an impression of the athlete's maxillary arch.

Stock mouth guards are usually made of latex rubber or plastic and are available in small, medium, and large sizes. Because they are not formed around the teeth, constant pressure must be exerted to hold the mouth guard in place. Due to their bulky size, they often interfere with speech and breathing and are easily ejected from the mouth. As such, this type is the least favored among sport participants (4).

The most popular type is the thermal-set, mouth-formed mouth guard (**Fig. 6.4**). This guard is readily available, inexpensive, and has a loop strap for attachment to a face mask. The loop strap has two advantages: it prevents individuals from choking on the mouth guard in an emergency; and it prevents the individual from losing the mouth guard when ejected from the mouth. The guard consists of a firm outer shell fitted with a softer inner material. The softer material is thermally or chemically set after being molded to the player's teeth. **Field Strategy 6.2** demonstrates how to fit a thermoplastic mouth-formed mouth guard.

The most effective type of mouth protector is the custom-made mouth guard. These protectors require fabrication by a dentist,

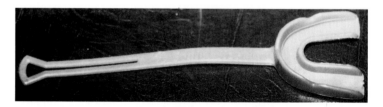

Figure 6.4. The thermal-set, mouth-formed mouth guard is very popular because it is inexpensive, readily available, and has a loop strap for attachment to a face mask.

Field Strategy 6.2. Fitting Mouth-formed Mouth Guards

A. Submerge the mouth guard only, not the loop strap, in boiling water for 20 to 25 seconds, or until soft and pliable. Shake off any excess water, but do not rinse the mouth guard in cold water, as this decreases pliability

B. Place the mouth guard directly in the mouth over the upper dental arch. Center the mouth guard with your thumbs using the loop strap as a guide

C. Close the mouth, but do not bring the teeth together or bite down on the mouth guard. Place the tongue on the roof of the mouth and suck as hard as possible for 15 to 25 seconds. The sucking mechanism acts as a vacuum to mold the mouth guard around the teeth and gums

D. Rinse the mouth guard in cold water to harden the material. Check the finished product for any significant indentations on the bottom surface and be sure it is centered correctly. If any imperfections or errors are noted, do not reheat the mouth guard because this decreases its effectiveness. Select a new mouth guard and repeat the process

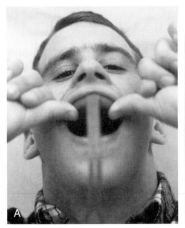
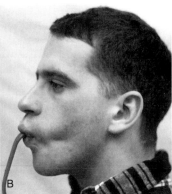

making them more expensive. The dentist takes an impression of the maxillary teeth of each player and makes a model. Over this model, a material, such as thermoplastic vinyl, is then vacuum-adapted. Another type of custom-made mouth protector is the bimaxiallary mouth guard that covers both upper and lower dental arches. The mandible is opened to a predetermined position, such as the position of heavy breathing. This guard does not interfere with breathing, provides protection for the lower teeth and upper teeth, and stabilizes the mandible to the head to reduce mandibulocranial force transmission (4).

Eye Wear

Glass lenses, ordinary plastic lenses, and open eye guards do not provide adequate eye protection and, in many situations, can increase the risk and severity of injury. Several types of approved eye protectors are commercially available for the sport participant

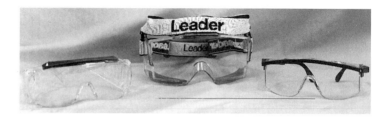

Figure 6.5. Eye protectors should be made from polycarbonate, which is lightweight, and scratch- and impact-resistant.

Polycarbonate is lightweight, scratch- and impact-resistant, and can have an antifog and ultraviolet inhibitor incorporated into the lens

(Fig. 6.5). These protectors may be made from plastic or polycarbonate, both of which can be incorporated with prescription lenses. As mentioned early, polycarbonate is lightweight, scratch- and impact-resistant, and can have an antifog and ultraviolet inhibitor incorporated into the lens (7). The frame should be constructed of a resilient plastic, with reinforced temples, hinges, and nose piece. Adequate cushioning should protect the eyebrow and nasal bridge from sharp edges. Lenses should be 3 mm thick. A sweatband can be worn to keep sweat out of the eye guard, but it should be removed when not participating.

Any person with good vision in only one eye should consult an ophthalmologist on whether or not to participate in a given sport. One-eyed athletes have reduced visual fields and depth perception. If a decision is made to participate, the individual should wear maximum eye protection during all practices and competitions.

Contact lenses improve peripheral vision, astigmatism, and do not normally cloud during temperature changes. However, they do not protect against eye injury

Although sport participants often wear contact lenses because they improve peripheral vision, and astigmatism, and do not normally cloud during temperature changes, they do not protect against eye injury. Hard contact lenses often dislodge and dust may get underneath the lens and damage the cornea, or the cornea may be scratched while inserting or removing the lens. Soft contact lenses, although more comfortable, should not replace more effective eye protection.

Ear Wear

With the exception of boxing, wrestling, and water polo, few sports have specialized ear protection **(Fig. 6.6).** Repeated friction and trauma to the ear can lead to a permanent deformity, called hematoma auris, or cauliflower ear (see Chapter 14). Comfort and fit are determined by the individual; however, the head gear should not move during contact with another player or compress the external ear.

Throat and Neck Protectors

Blows to the anterior throat can cause serious airway compromise. Catchers in baseball and softball wear a built-in or attachable throat guard on their masks, as do fencing, field hockey, lacrosse,

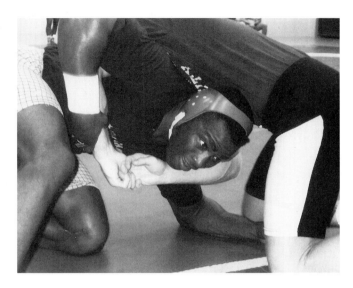

Figure 6.6. Ear wear can prevent friction and trauma to the ear that may led to permanent deformity.

and ice hockey players. In addition, specialized padded neck collars may be worn by ice hockey or field hockey players.

Cervical neck rolls are designed to limit motion of the cervical spine and have been shown to be effective in protecting players with a history of repetitive burners or stingers (8). A high, thick, and stiff posterolateral pad at the base of the neck provides some fixation of the cervical spine **(Fig. 6.7)**. Cervical collars and neck rolls, however, do not decrease axial loading on the cervical spine when the neck is flexed during a tackle.

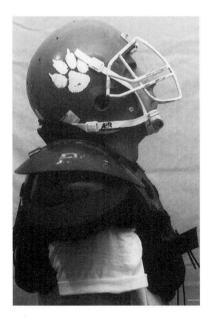

Figure 6.7. A high, thick stiff posterolateral pad at the base of the neck can provide added protection to the cervical spine, but cannot reduce axial loading during a tackle when the head is lowered.

In fitting a football helmet, the helmet should be snug enough to prevent movement of the helmet in one direction when the head moves in another. Proper fit may be altered by hair length, deterioration of internal padding, loss of air from cells, and spread of the face mask, necessitating periodic checks for proper fit.

PROTECTIVE EQUIPMENT FOR THE UPPER BODY

You have successfully fitted the football player with a helmet. What guidelines are used to properly fit the shoulder pads for the player?

In the upper body, special pads and braces are often used to protect the shoulder region, ribs, thorax, breasts, arm, elbow, wrist, and hands. Depending on the sport, special design modifications are needed to allow maximum protection while providing maximal performance.

Shoulder Protection

Shoulder pads should protect the soft and bony tissue structures in the chest, upper back, and shoulder, particularly the acromion process. When used with a neck guard, motion in the midcervical spinal region may be inhibited, reducing the risk of brachial plexus nerve injuries (9). Football shoulder pads come in two general types; flat and cantilevered. Flat shoulders pads, often worn by quarterbacks and receivers, provide less protection to the shoulder region, but allow more motion at the glenohumeral joint. Cantilevered pads, worn by linemen and linebackers, limit motion at the glenohumeral joint, but provide better protection against high-impact forces. Commercial football shoulder pads can be supplemented with other pads to protect the cervical spine, upper extremity, abdomen, ribs, flank, and back. For example, ice hockey shoulder pads can fit under the football pads to further protect the acromion process. Detachable shoulder pad extensions and biceps pads protect the deltoid and upper arm region, respectively. **Field Strategy 6.3** lists the general steps used in fitting football shoulder pads.

Shoulder pads do not protect the glenohumeral joint from excessive motion. As a result, sprains to the glenohumeral joint may occur. Tape restraints or commercial protective braces, such as the one shown in **Figure 6.8**, can be used to limit abduction of the glenohumeral joint.

Elbow, Forearm, Wrist, and Hand Protection

The entire arm is constantly subjected to compressive and shearing forces, such as those seen in overuse throwing injuries at the elbow, blocking and tackling an opponent, deflecting projectiles,

Field Strategy 6.3. Fitting Football Shoulder Pads

A. Determine the player's chest size by measuring circumference at the nipple line. Select pads for the player's position. Place the pads on the shoulders and tighten all straps and laces. The straps should be snug enough to prevent no more than a two-finger-width distance between the pads and body. The laces should be centered over the sternum and the entire clavicle should be covered

B. The acromioclavicular joint and deltoid should be adequately covered and protected by the upper portion of the arch and deltoid padding

C. The entire scapula should be covered with the lower pad arch extending below the inferior angle of the scapula

D. With the arms abducted, the neck opening should not be uncomfortable or pinch the neck

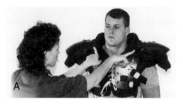
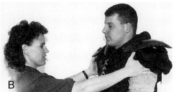
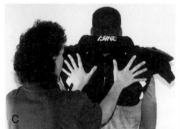
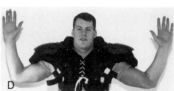

pushing opponents away to prevent collisions, or to break a fall. Examples of several specialized pads and braces for the elbow, forearm, wrist, and hand can be seen in **Figure 6.9**. In more recent years, silicone rubber and thermomoldable foam have been used to customize protective pads for the forearm, wrist, and hand (**Fig. 6.10**).

Thorax, Rib, and Abdominal Protection

Many collision and contact sports require special protection of the thorax, rib, and abdominal areas. Catchers in baseball and softball wear full thorax and abdominal protectors to prevent high-speed blows from a bat or ball. Individuals in fencing and goalies in many sports also wear full thorax protectors (**Fig. 6.11A**). Quarterbacks and wide receivers in football may wear rib protectors composed of air-inflated, interconnected cylinders to absorb impact forces caused during tackling (**Fig. 6.11B**). Rib protectors should be fitted according to the manufacturer's instructions.

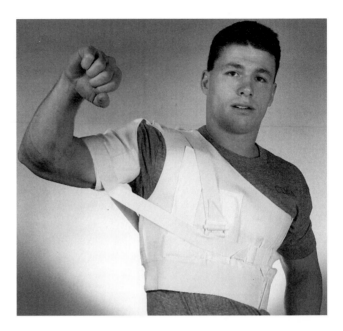

Figure 6.8. The Sawa shoulder brace can limit glenohumeral motion in chronic shoulder injuries.

Sport Bras

Sport bras prevent excessive vertical and horizontal breast motion during exercise, and fall into three styles (10):

1. Bras made from nonelastic material with wide shoulder straps and wide bands under the breasts to provide upward support **(Fig. 6.12A)**. Waist-length designs can prevent cutting in below the breasts
2. Compressive bras that bind the breasts to the chest wall **(Fig. 6.12B)**. Women with medium-sized breasts prefer this type
3. Bras with minor modifications, usually with less elasticity. These are not considered true sport bras, although they are marketed as such

Girls and women with small breasts may not need a special bra. Women with a size C cup or larger need a firm, supportive-type bra. The bra should have nonslip straps and no irritative seams or fasteners next to the skin and it should be firm and durable. Choice of fabric will depend on the intensity of activity, support needs, sensitivity to fiber, and climatic and seasonal conditions (10). A cotton/poly/lycra fabric is a popular blend seen in many sport bras. In hot weather, an additional outer layer of textured nylon mesh can promote natural cooling of the skin. In sports requiring significant overhead motion, bra straps should stretch to prevent the bra from riding up over the breasts. In activities where overhead motion is not a significant part of the activity, nonstretch straps connected directly to a nonelastic cup are preferable.

> Girls and women with a bra size C cup or larger need a firm, supportive-type bra

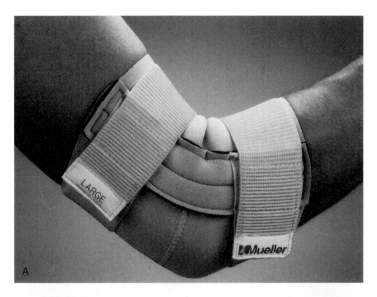

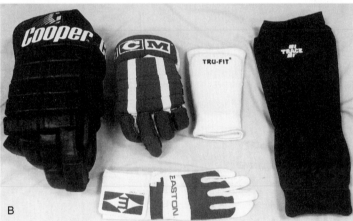

Figure 6.9. Specialized braces, pads, and gloves can protect the elbow (**A**), and forearm, wrist, and hand from injury (**B**).

Lumbar/Sacral Protection

Lumbar/sacral protection includes weight-training belts used during heavy weightlifting, abdominal binders, and other similar supportive devices (**Fig. 6.13**). Each should support the low back in a more vertical lifting posture, stabilize the trunk, and prevent spinal deformity or damage during heavy lifting (11). Use of belts or binders can significantly increase intra-abdominal pressure to reduce compressive forces in the vertebral bodies and lessen the risk of low back trauma.

 In fitting the shoulder pads, did you adequately protect the acromion process, deltoid musculature, pectoral, and scapular region? When the player raised his arms, was the neck opening comfortable and nonconstrictive. If so, the pads are fitted correctly.

Use of weight-training belts or abdominal binders can significantly increase intra-abdominal pressure to reduce compressive forces in the vertebral bodies and lessen the risk of lower back trauma

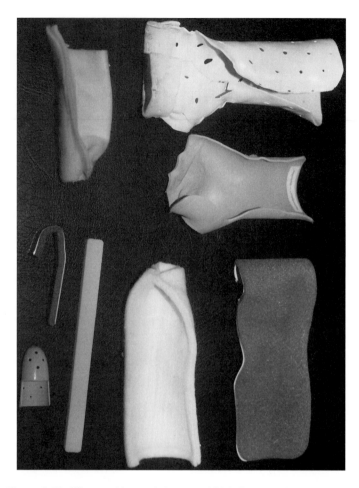

Figure 6.10. Silicone rubber and thermomoldable foam can be used to customize protective pads for the forearm, wrist, and hand.

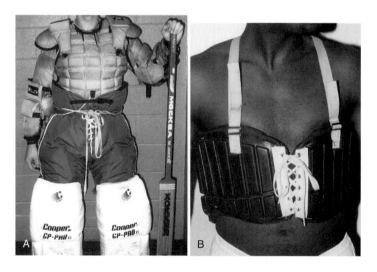

Figure 6.11. Ice hockey requires extensive chest protection (**A**). In other sports, ribs protectors may be used (**B**).

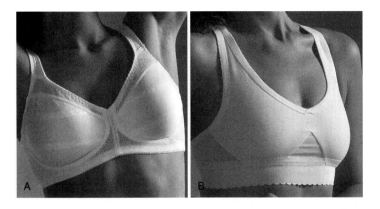

Figure 6.12. Sport bras may be made of nonelastic material with wide shoulder straps and bands under the breasts for larger breasted girls and women (**A**), or can be made of an elastic material to compress or bind the breasts to the chest wall (**B**).

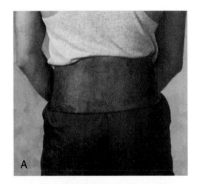

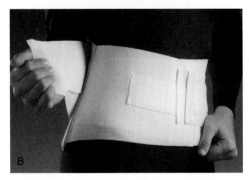

Figure 6.13. Weight-training belts (**A**), abdominal binders (**B**), and other lumbar supportive devices support the abdominal contents, stabilize the trunk, and prevent spinal deformity or damage.

? *A baseball player has a chronic lateral ankle sprain that requires external support. What method of support can provide a higher level of protection for this player?*

In the lower body, commercial braces are commonly used to protect the knee and ankle. In addition, special pads are used to protect bony and soft tissue structures in the hip and thigh region. Depending on the sport, special design modifications are needed to allow maximum protection while providing maximum performance.

Hip and Buttock Protection

In collision and contact sports, the hip and buttock region require special pads typically composed of hard polyethylene covered with layers of Ensolite to protect the iliac crest, sacrum and coccyx, and genital region (**Fig. 6.14A**). A girdle with special pockets can effectively hold the pads in place. Hip spica braces (see Chapter 7) are used to limit excessive hip abduction after a muscular groin strain. The male genital region is best protected by a protective cup placed in the athletic supporter (**Fig. 6.14B**).

Thigh Protection

The thigh and upper leg pads, such as those illustrated in **Figure 6.14A**, slip into ready-made pockets in the girdle to prevent injury to the quadriceps area, and can be used in other sports to prevent a quadriceps contusion (12). Thigh pads should be placed over the quadriceps muscle group, approximately 6 to 7 inches proximal to the patella. When using asymmetrical thigh pads, the larger flare should be placed on the lateral aspect of the thigh to avoid injury to the genitalia (2). In addition to thigh pads, neoprene sleeves can provide uniform compression, therapeutic warmth, and support for a quadriceps or hamstring strain.

Knee and Patella Protection

The knee is second only to the ankle and foot in incidence of injury. Knee pads can protect the area from impact during a collision or fall and, in wrestling, protect the prepatellar and infrapatellar bursa from friction injuries. In football, knee pads reduce contusions and abrasions when falling on turf.

Knee braces fall into three broad groups: prophylactic or preventative, functional, and rehabilitative. Prophylactic knee braces (PKBs) are designed to protect the medial collateral ligament (MCL), by redirecting a lateral valgus force away from the joint itself to points more distal to the tibia and femur. Two general types of PKBs are the lateral and bilateral bar designs (**Fig. 6.15A**). Recent studies have concluded that, although individual PKBs may provide some increases in MCL failure loading, any knee ligament protection is modest (13,14).

Knee braces fall into three broad groups: prophylactic, functional, and rehabilitative

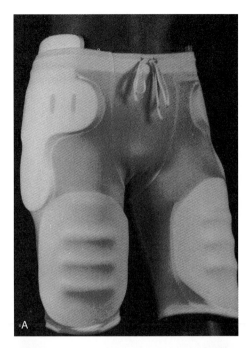

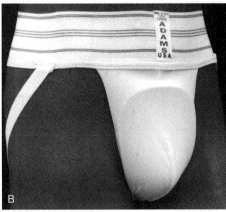

Figure 6.14. Girdle pads protect the gluteal and sacral area from high-velocity forces. Thigh pads can also be inserted to protect the quadriceps area (**A**). Protective cups placed inside an athletic supporter can reduce trauma to the male genital region (**B**).

Functional knee braces, commonly called derotation or anterior cruciate ligament (ACL) braces, control tibial translation and rotational stress relative to the femur, with a rigid, snug fit, and extension limitations **(Fig. 6.15B)** (15). There are two basic styles of derotation braces: hinge-post-strap and the hinge-post-shell (2). These braces may be prescribed by a physician for individuals with moderate ACL instability who participate in activities with low or moderate load potential, and following ACL ligament repair or reconstructive surgery. Range of motion blocks may be used to help control hyperflexion and hyperextension.

Functional knee braces, also called derotation or ACL braces, control tibial translation and rotational stress relative to the femur with a rigid, snug fit, and extension limitations

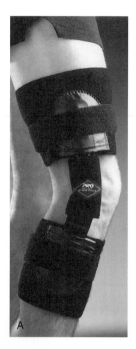

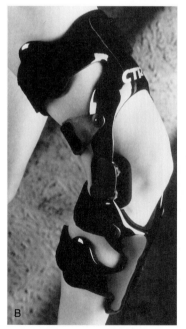

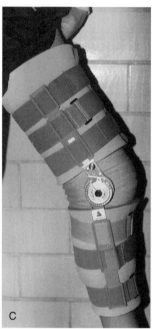

Figure 6.15. Knee braces come in three groups: prophylactic (**A**), functional (**B**), or rehabilitative (**C**).

Rehabilitative braces provide absolute immobilization at a selected angle following surgery, permit controlled range of motion through predetermined arcs, and provide protection from accidental loading in nonweight-bearing patients (**Fig. 6.15C**) (2). The braces are lighter in weight, adjustable for optimal fit, and can be easily removed and reapplied for wound inspection and rehabilitation. As the individual progresses in the rehabilitation program, the allowable range of motion is adjusted periodically by the clinician. Early motion prevents joint adhesions from forming, enhances proprioception, and increases synovial nutrient flow to promote healing of cartilage and collagen tissue.

Decisions to use any of the three major categories of knee braces should rest with the supervising physician or surgeon. Selection should be based on the projected objectives and needs of the sport participant relative to sport demands, cost effectiveness, durability, fit, and comfort (15).

Patellar braces are designed to dissipate force, maintain patellar alignment, and improve patellar tracking (2). A horseshoe-type pad sewn into an elastic or neoprene sleeve has been found to relieve pain and tension in recurring patellofemoral subluxation or dislocations **(Fig. 6.16A)** (16). These braces may also be helpful in relieving chronic patellar pain. An alternative brace for treating patella pain is a strap worn over the infrapatellar ligament **(Fig. 6.16B)**.

Lower Leg Protection

Pads for the anterior tibia area should involve a high-density padding covered by a molded shell. Velcro straps and stirrups help stabilize the pad inside the sock. Many styles can also incorporate

Newer rehabilitative braces are lighter in weight, adjustable for optimal fit, and can be easily removed and reapplied for wound inspection and rehabilitation

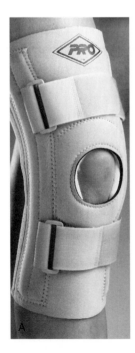
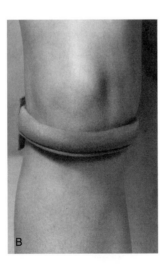

Figure 6.16. A. Patellofemoral braces can relieve chronic patella pain.
B. Patellar pain can also be reduced with an infrapatellar strap.

padding or plastic shells over the ankle malleoli, which is also subject to repeated contusions. Several commercial designs are available (**Fig. 6.17**).

Ankle and Foot Protection

Commercial ankle protectors used to stabilize the ankle joint post-injury include a lace-up brace, semirigid orthosis, or air bladder brace (**Fig. 6.18**). Lace-up braces have been shown to limit all ankle motions, whereas a semirigid orthosis and air bladder brace limit only inversion and eversion (17,18). In several studies, it was found that, after exercise, semirigid orthosis and air bladder devices provided the most inversion restraint, followed by the lace-up brace (19,20). Adhesive tape, when used to restrict inversion and eversion, lost maximal protection after 20 minutes or more of exercise (20,21). Semirigid and air bladder braces are more effective in reducing ankle injuries, are easier for the wearer to apply independently, do not produce some of the skin irritation problems associated with adhesive tape, provide better comfort and fit, do not adversely affect performance, and may be more cost effective (22–25).

Specific foot conditions, such as fallen arches, pronated feet, or medial tibial stress syndrome, can be padded and supported with innersoles, semirigid orthotics, and rigid orthotics (**Fig. 6.19A**). Research has found that a 6.5-mm thick polymetric foam rubber material is more effective in absorbing heel-strike impact than a viscoelastic polymetric shoe insert (26). Anti-shock heel

> Lace-up ankle braces limit all ankle motion, whereas a semirigid orthosis and an air bladder brace limit only inversion and eversion

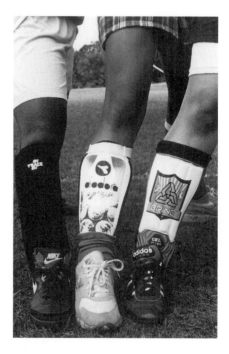

Figure 6.17. Shin guards.

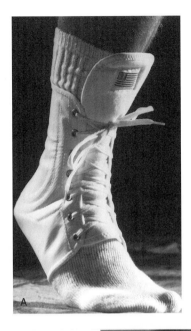

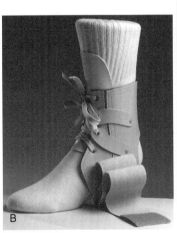

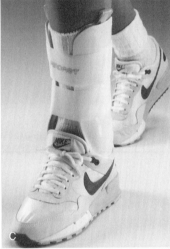

Figure 6.18. Ankle protectors can prevent ankle sprains, and include the lace-up brace (**A**), semirigid orthosis (**B**), and air bladder brace (**C**).

lifts may be used to relieve strain on the Achilles tendon and heel cups reduce tissue shearing and shock in the calcaneal region (**Fig. 6.19B**). Other commercially available pads may be used to protect the forefoot region, bunions, and toes, or adhesive felt (moleskin), felt, and foam can be cut to construct similar pads.

Selection and fit of shoes may also affect injuries to the lower extremity. Shoes should adequately cushion impact forces, support, and guide the foot during the stance and final pushoff phase of running. In sports requiring repeated heel impact, additional

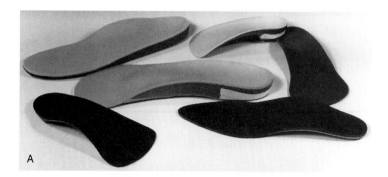

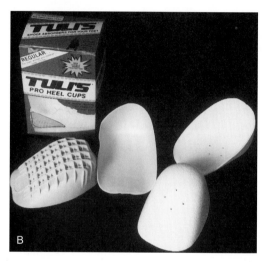

Figure 6.19. Semirigid orthotics provide more stability and support to the intrinsic structures of the foot (**A**); heel cups reduce tissue shearing and shock in the calcaneal region (**B**).

heel cushioning should be present. Length should be sufficient to allow all toes to be fully extended. Individuals with toe abnormalities or bunions may also require a wider toe box. **Field Strategy 6.4** lists several important points to remember when purchasing athletic shoes.

In field sports, shoes may have a flat-sole, long cleat, short cleat, or a multicleated design (**Fig. 6.20**). The cleats should be properly positioned under the major weight-bearing joints of the foot and should not be felt through the sole of the shoe. Research has shown that shoes with the longer irregular cleats placed at the peripheral margin of the sole, with a number of smaller pointed cleats positioned interiorly, produce significantly higher torsional resistance and are associated with a significantly higher anterior cruciate ligament injury rate, when compared to shoe models with flat cleats, screw-in cleats, or pivot disk models (27). When increased temperatures are a factor, such as when playing on turf, only the flat-soled basketball-style turf shoe had low-release coefficients at varying elevated temperatures (28). This may lead

Cleats should be positioned under the weight-bearing joints of the foot and should not be felt through the sole of the shoe

Field Strategy 6.4. Factors in the Selection and Fit of Athletic Shoes

Always fit shoes toward late afternoon or evening, preferably after a workout, and wear socks typically worn during sport participation

Fit shoes to the longest toe of the largest foot, leaving one thumb's width to the end of the toe box. Shoes should feel snug, but not too tight

The widest part of the shoe should coincide with the widest part of the foot. Eyelets should be at least 1 inch apart with normal lacing. Women with big or wider feet should consider purchasing boy's or men's shoes

The sole of the shoe should provide moderate support but should not be too rigid. The sole tread typically comes in a horizontal bar or waffle design. The horizontal bar design is commonly used on asphalt or concrete and the waffle tread is used on off-road terrain where traction is more important

The midsole is composed of ethylene vinyl acetate (EVA), polyurethane, or a combination of the two. EVA provides good cushioning, but will break down over time. Polyurethane has minimal compressibility and provides good durability and stability. A combination of the two materials is best

A thermoplastic heel counter maintains its shape and firmness even in adverse weather conditions. The running shoe should position the heel at least ½ inch above the outsole to minimize stretch on the Achilles tendon

While wearing the shoes, approximate athletic skills (walking, running, jumping, and changing directions)

Individuals with specific conditions need special shoes, such as:
Runners with normal feet—more forefoot and toe flexibility
Overpronation—greater control on the medial side
Achilles tendinitis—at least a 15-mm heel wedge
Court sports—added side-to-side stability
High, rigid arches—soft midsoles, curved lasts, and low or moderate hindfoot stability
Normal arches—firm midsole, semicurved lasts, and moderate hindfoot stability
Flexible, low arch—very firm midsole, straight last, and strong hindfoot stability

After purchasing the shoes, walk in the shoes for 2 to 3 days to allow them to adapt to the feet. Then begin running or practicing in the shoes for about 25 to 30% of the workout. To prevent blisters, gradually extend the length of time the shoes are worn

Avid runners should replace shoes every 3 months, recreational runners every 6 months

to a lower incidence of lower leg injuries. In individuals with arch problems, the shoe should include adequate forefoot, arch, and heel support. In all cases, individuals should select shoes based on the demands of the activity, not on the color, style, or price.

Did you determine that the baseball player could benefit from an external ankle supportive device? These devices are easy to apply, do not irritate the skin, provide better comfort and fit, and are more cost effective than adhesive tape. Use of any external support should be combined with a full rehabilitation program to strengthen muscles around the injured joint.

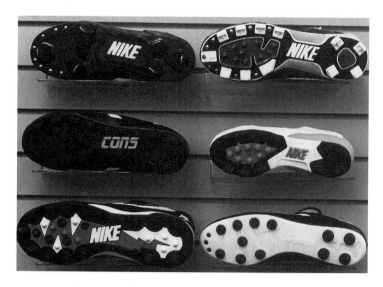

Figure 6.20. Shoes may have a flat-sole, long cleat, short cleat, or a multi-cleated design. Selection will depend on the surface and weather conditions.

SUMMARY

Protective equipment is only effective when it is properly fitted and maintained, periodically cleaned and disinfected, and utilized as it was intended. In athletic events involving impact and collisions, the sport participant must be protected from high-velocity–low-mass forces and low-velocity–high-mass forces. The design and selection of protective equipment is based on the optimal level of impact intensity afforded by the given thickness, density, resilience, and temperature of energy-absorbing material. Many sports, such as football and ice hockey, require full body protection. Many other sports require protection over specific body areas at risk for injury. It is imperative that the athletic trainer and coach be fully aware of the rules and standards governing the selection and fitting of protective equipment, to ensure safe participation in sport.

REFERENCES

1. Hodgson VR. Athletic equipment and injury prevention. In *Prevention of athletic injuries: the role of the sport medicine team*, edited by JO Mueller and AJ Ryan. Philadelphia: FA Davis, 1991.
2. Saliba E, Foreman S, and Abadie RT. Protective equipment considerations. In *Athletic injuries and rehabilitation*, edited by JE Zachazewski, DJ Magee, and WS Quillen. Philadelphia: WB Saunders, 1996.
3. LaPrade RF, Burnett QM, Zarzour R, and Moss R. 1995. The effect of the mandatory use of face masks on facial lacerations and head and neck injuries in ice hockey. Am J Spts Med 23(6):773–775.
4. Greenberg MS, and Springer PS. Diagnosis and management of oral injuries. In *Athletic injuries to the head, neck, and face*, edited by JS Torg. St. Louis: Mosby Year Book, 1991.

5. Morrow RM, Seals RR, Barnwell GM, Day EA, Moore RN, and Stephens MK. 1991. Report of a survey of oral injuries in male college and university athletes. Ath Train (JNATA) 26(4):338–342.

6. Wilkinson EE, and Powers JM. 1986. Properties of custom-made mouth-protector materials. Phys Sportsmed 14(6):77–84.

7. Pine D. 1991. Preventing sports-related eye injuries. Phys Sportsmed 19(2):129–134.

8. Gibbs R. 1984. A protective collar cervical radiculopathy. Phys Sportsmed 12(5):139.

9. Watkins RG, Dillin WH, and Maxwell J. Cervical spine injuries in football players. In *The spine in sports*, edited by SH Hochschuler. Philadelphia: Hanley & Belfus, 1990.

10. Haycock CE. 1987. How I manage breast problems in athletes. Phys Sportsmed 15(3):89–95.

11. Woodhouse ML, Heinen JRK, Shall L, and Bragg K. 1990. Selected isokinetic lifting parameters of adult male athletes utilizing lumbar/sacral supports. J Ortho Sports Phy Ther 11(10):467–473.

12. Aronen JG, and Chronister RD. 1992. Quadriceps contusions: hastening the return to play. Phys Sportsmed 20(7):130–136.

13. Salvaterra GF, Wang M, Morehouse CA, and Buckley WE. 1993. An in vitro biomechanical study of the static stabilizing effect of lateral prophylactic knee bracing on medial stability. Ath Train (JNATA) 28(20):113–119.

14. Brown TD, Hoeck JE, and Brand RA. Laboratory evaluation of prophylactic knee brace performance under dynamic valgus loading using a surrogate leg model. In *Clinics in Sports Medicine*, vol. 9, no. 4, edited by LE Paulos. Philadelphia: WB Saunders, 1990.

15. Zachazewski JE, and Geissler G. 1992. When to prescribe a knee brace. Phys Sportsmed 20(11):91–99.

16. Henry JH. Conservative treatment of patellofemoral subluxation. In *Clinics in sports medicine*, vol. 8, no. 2, edited by JH Henry. Philadelphia: WB Saunders, 1989.

17. Kimura I, Beninoato P, and Sitler M. 1992. Effect of sport ankle orthoses on range of motion and torque production during ankle motion. J Ath Train 27(2):150.

18. Gehlsen GM, Pearson D, and Bahamonde R. 1991. Ankle joint strength, total work, and ROM: comparison between prophylactic devices. Ath Train (JNATA) 26(1):62–65.

19. Carroll MJ, Rijke AM, and Perrin DH. 1993. Effect of the Swede-O ankle brace on subtalar joint displacement in subjects with unstable ankles. J Ath Train 28(2):154.

20. Martin N, and Harter RA. 1993. Comparison of inversion restraint provided by ankle prophylactic devices before and after exercise. Ath Train (JNATA) 28(4):324–329.

21. Mack KS, Douglas MS, Kum SKC, and Haskvits EM. 1993. Effects of Sport-stirrup and taping on ankle inversion before and after exercise. J Ath Train 28(2):167.

22. Sitler M, Ryan J, Wheeler B, McBride J, Arciero R, Anderson J, and Horodyski M. 1993. The clinical effectiveness of a semirigid ankle brace to reduce acute ankle injuries in basketball. J Ath Train 28(2):152–153.

23. Feuerback JW, and Grabiner MD. 1993. Effect of the Aircast on unilateral postural control: amplitude and frequency variables. J Ortho Sports Phys Ther 17(3):149–154.

24. Macpherson K, Sitler M, Kimura I, and Horodyski M. 1995. Effects of a semirigid and softshell prophylactic ankle stabilizer on selected performance tests among high school football players. JOSPT 21(3):147–152.

25. Pienkowski D, McMorrow M, Shapiro R, Caborn DNM, and Stayton J. 1995. The effect of ankle stabilizers on athletic performance. Am J Spts Med 23(6):757–762.

26. Shiba N, Kitaoka HB, Cahalan TD, and Chao EYS. 1995. Shock-absorbing effect of shoe insert materials commonly used in management of lower extremity disorders. Clin Orthop 310:130–135.
27. Lambson RB, Barnhill BS, and Higgins RW. 1996. Football cleat design and its effect on anterior cruciate ligament injuries: a three year prospective study. Am J Spts Med 24(2):155–159.
28. Torg JS, Stilwell G, and Rogers K. 1996. The effect of ambient temperature on the shoe-surface interface release coefficient. Am J Spts Med 24(1):79–82.

Chapter 7

Protective Taping and Wraps

After completing this chapter, you should be able to:

- Identify the types of prophylactic tape and wraps and their uses in sports-injury management

- Describe common principles used in the application of tape and wraps

- Apply common taping and wrapping techniques to specific joints or body regions to prevent injury or reduce the risk of reinjury

Key Terms:

Maceration	**Proprioceptors**
Prophylactic	**Spica**

Taping or wrapping a body part provides support and protection while allowing functional movement. Although both techniques may be used as a **prophylactic**, or preventative measure, taping and wrapping are used extensively during rehabilitation to reduce the risk of reinjury. Providing support to an injured body part may allow early return to activity, yet control undesirable movement that may impede the healing process (1–3).

In this chapter, you will learn about the principles of taping and wrapping body parts, the different types of tape and wraps available, their various uses, and common techniques of application. Although many specific skills will be illustrated, these are presented as a guide and should not be viewed as the only method of application. Each strapping must be customized for the particular athlete and condition.

Prophylactic
Preventative or protective

PRINCIPLES OF TAPING AND WRAPPING

? *A high school soccer player has been experiencing mild to moderate bilateral medial tibial pain during pre-season practice. You suspect that the pain may be due to an overload on the athlete's arches. How will you provide arch support to reduce strain on the supporting structures?*

Prior to any application of tape or a wrap, the injury must first be fully evaluated to determine the severity of injury. Injured anatomical structures must be identified and an appropriate therapeutic rehabilitation program should be developed to ensure safe return to activity (1,2). Too often, premature return to activity can lead to a chronic injury. Only those individuals who are in a supervised therapeutic exercise program should be braced or taped (4). The rehabilitation program, as discussed in Chapter 5, should focus on regaining full range of motion, proprioception and balance, strength, endurance, and power in the injured body part, while maintaining cardiovascular fitness. The individual should be able to complete all functional tests pain-free before being cleared for participation. At that time, the correct application technique can be selected and properly applied. A poorly applied strapping or wrap can lead to blisters or skin irritation, place stress on other body parts, and perhaps even increase the risk of injury to the region (**Fig. 7.1**).

Properly applied external support via taping or wrapping a joint can limit abnormal or excessive motion of an injured joint and the surrounding soft tissue structures. A **spica** is a common taping and wrapping technique whereby a figure-eight is applied around two body regions of differing sizes to limit motion. An example is a hip spica, commonly used with a groin strain (See **Figure 7.21**). This support is further enhanced through **proprioceptive** feedback. The body senses the external support and in-

> The use of tape, braces, or other supportive devices should not be a substitute for complete rehabilitation of the injury

Spica
Figure-eight pattern to limit motion around two body parts of differing sizes

Proprioceptors
Specialized deep sensory nerve cells in joints, ligaments, muscles, and tendons sensitive to stretch, tension, and pressure, which are responsible for position and movement

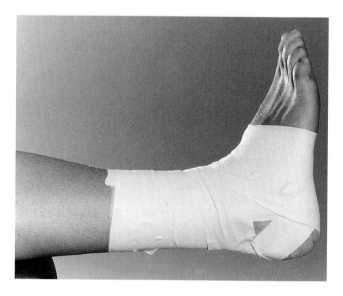

Figure 7.1. This ankle strapping has several "windows" and wrinkles that can lead to blisters or skin irritation. In addition, the tension in applying the individual strips is uneven and can place the individual at risk for further injury.

creases the athlete's conscious awareness of the injured area. As a result, the individual often avoids motions or situations that place the injured area at further risk for injury.

Uses of Tape and Wraps

Tape and wraps are prophylactic devices used to (a) provide immediate first aid, (b) limit excessive joint movement, (c) allow for pain-free functional movement, (d) support an injured body part, (e) secure protective pads, and (f) allow early resumption of activity (5). Several of these uses are illustrated in **Figure 7.2**. Although the use of taping and wraps may allow the individual to resume early activity, their use should never take the place of a comprehensive rehabilitation program designed to strengthen the area so that supplemental support is no longer necessary.

Types of Tape and Wraps

Many companies manufacture a variety of tape used in sports injury management. In a general sense, tape can be made of an elastic or nonelastic material. Elastic tape is often used to hold protective pads in place or around joints that require maximum movement while allowing muscles to contract without impeding circulation or neurologic function (3,6). The level of elasticity varies from brand to brand. The more elastic the tape, the easier the application. Elastic tape should be stretched to one-half to one-third of its elastic capability before application. If it is applied too tightly, it can restrict circulation and function of the body part, leading to increased pain or discomfort. The product comes in a variety of widths and must be selected according to the size of the injury site and desired effect **(Fig. 7.3)** (6).

> If tape is applied too tightly, it can restrict circulation and function of the body part, leading to increased pain or discomfort

Nonelastic tape provides support to joints by restricting excessive motions, and may be porous or nonporous. Porous tape allows heat and sweat to pass through the tape through minute openings. This action allows the skin to remain cool. Nonporous tape makes the application more occlusive, thus increasing the potential for damage to the underlying skin from friction and retained heat. Like elastic tape, nonelastic tape comes in a variety of widths, primarily ranging from ½ to 3 inches wide **(Fig. 7.3)** (6). Nonelastic tape may be bleached or unbleached. Bleached tape tends to be more aesthetically pleasing, but is more expensive and does not offer better support than unbleached tape. Many athletic training classes prefer unbleached tape, as it saves money while students learn strapping techniques. Nonelastic tape is more difficult to apply. The body's natural contours increase the potential for wrinkles and excessive pressure from friction on underlying tissues, which can lead to blisters or cuts under the tape. An effective wrinkle-free nonelastic strapping requires extensive practice and patience.

> Wrinkles and excessive pressure from friction over underlying tissues can lead to blisters or cuts under the tape

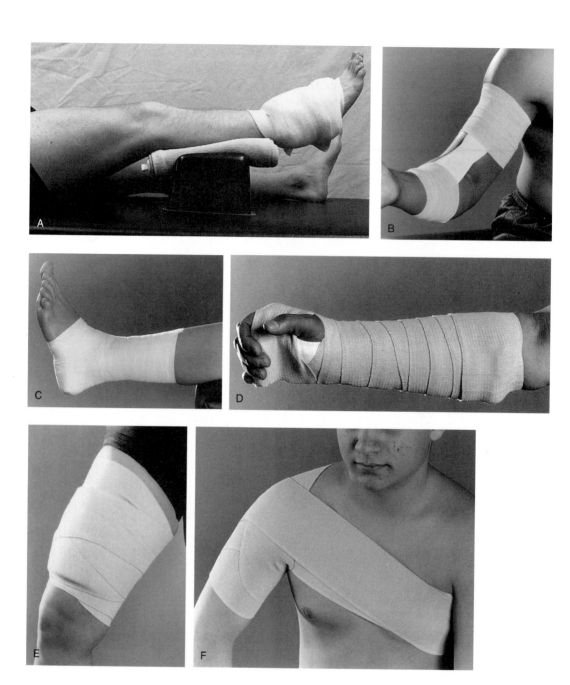

Figure 7.2. Tape and wraps are used to provide immediate first aid (**A**), limit excessive joint movement (**B**), allow for pain-free functional movement (**C**),support an injured body part (**D**), secure protective pads (**E**), and allow early return to activity (**F**).

There are two major types of wraps, elastic and nonelastic. Both are made of cloth; however, the elastic wrap contains fibers that allow it to be stretched. The elastic wrap, as mentioned earlier, is used during acute care to secure ice to the body part or may be used to hold protective pads in place. Nonelastic wraps are typically used only to limit joint motion and provide support. Although they are often used in lieu of tape, largely due to fiscal concerns, they are not as effective. Nonelastic wraps may be used in combination with nonelastic tape for additional support. Cloth wraps, for example, are often used at the ankle; however, they do not contour well to the sharp angles in the region, nor do they "give" with muscle contractions (See **Figure 7.13**).

Application of Tape

Prior to application, the body part should be washed, dried, and free of hair (5). Any minor open wounds, such as blisters or cuts, should be cleaned with normal saline and covered with a dry sterile dressing. Areas sensitive to friction, such as the Achilles tendon or dorsum of the foot, should be protected with a pad and lubricant (5). Petroleum jelly or a commercial skin lubricant may be applied to a nonsterile gauze pad or a commercially available heel and lace pad. Hair should be removed with an electric shaver or a disposable razor that should be discarded after use (5).

Occasionally, the athlete is required to stand on a table with the hip and knee placed in slight flexion. This can be accomplished by placing the athlete's heel on a 1.5- to 2-inch heel lift. Old tape cores wound with tape or a commercial taping block may be used.

> Prior to application, the body part should be clean, dry, and free of hair, and sensitive areas should be protected with a lubricated pad

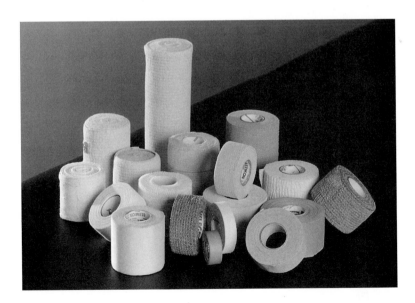

Figure 7.3. Tape and wraps comes in a variety of sizes and may be either elastic or nonelastic.

Tape rolls, while the appropriate height, will be compressed and become unusable.

When the skin has been appropriately prepared, a light layer of tape adherent is sprayed onto the skin surface and allowed to dry (5). This provides a somewhat sticky surface permitting the tape to adhere better to the skin. For individuals who are sensitive to tape, must be taped on a daily basis, or may be allergic to tape, a foam underwrap may be applied over the skin prior to tape application **(Fig. 7.4)** (5). It is critical that only one layer of underwrap be applied, as several layers may increase sweating under the tape, thus compromising the effectiveness of the strapping.

Proper positioning of the athletic trainer is as important as proper positioning of the athlete. To avoid unnecessary low back stress, use a table at an appropriate height to prevent having to bend over excessively at the waist (5). If it is necessary to reach above shoulder level, stand on a bench or have the athlete sit down. When several dozen athletes must be taped in a short amount of time, proper positioning is critical so as not to overtire the athletic trainer.

The athlete should be placed in a position of function to ensure the desired result. To avoid wrinkles in the tape, allow only a few inches of tape to be unrolled off the roll at one time (6). As the tape is guided around the contours of the body part, slight tension is applied. To tear the tape, the roll should be held in the dominant hand and pinched between the thumb and index finger of each hand **(Fig. 7.5)**. A quick push of the roll away from the body

> Proper positioning of the athletic trainer is as important as proper positioning of the athlete

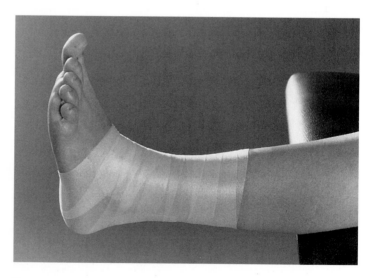

Figure 7.4. For individuals sensitive to tape or those who must be taped daily, a single layer of underwrap may be applied over the skin prior to tape application.

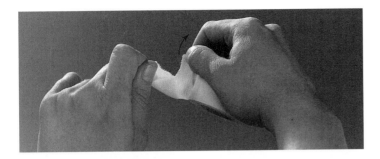

Figure 7.5. To tear tape, hold the roll in the dominant hand and pinch the thumb and index finger of each hand over the tear site. While holding the nondominant hand still, push the roll quickly away from the body.

while holding the nondominant hand still will result in the tape ends being evenly torn.

Each subsequent strip of tape should overlap the previous strip by one-half or one-third the width of the tape (6). Apply the tape snugly, but do not impair circulation. To check circulation, take a pulse distal to the strapping, feel for skin temperature, or blanch the nails and check capillary refill. Skin color and skin temperature should be the same as the uninjured body part above and below the strapping. After tape application, have the athlete check the body part for support and function.

Tape should be removed immediately after the practice or competition. Prolonged contact with the skin may cause the skin to breakdown and bacteria to build up (5). The tip of the tape cutters or scissors can be dipped in a skin lubricant to facilitate removing the tape from the skin. The scissors or tape cutter should lift the tape up and away from the skin and then advance along the body's natural contours **(Fig. 7.6)**. For example, with an injury to the lateral aspect of the ankle, start the tape cutters on the posteromedial aspect of the tape job (6,7). Slide the cutters distally around the posterior medial malleolus, extending through the arch toward the toes. In this manner, the tape cutter or scissors does not place any undue pressure on sensitive injured structures. Stabilize the skin and remove the tape in the direction of the natural hair growth (1). Tearing tape rapidly off the skin can lead to damaged skin, open wounds, and pain. After removal, the skin should be cleansed with tape remover, then washed with soap and water and dried thoroughly. Application of a skin moisturizer is suggested to prevent skin dryness and breakdown (5,6).

The skin should be inspected regularly for signs of irritation, blisters, or infection. Look for skin that is red, dry, hot, and tender (5). These signs indicate a possible allergic reaction to the tape or tape adherent. If the skin cannot be protected from irritation, it may be necessary to fit this individual with an appropriate brace rather than subject them to continued irritation. Refer to Chapter

The skin should be inspected regularly for signs of irritation, blisters, or infection

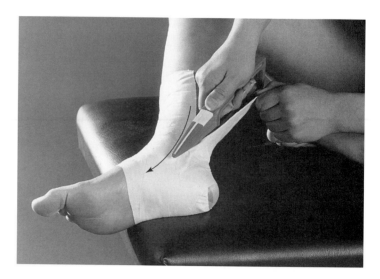

Figure 7.6. When cutting tape, lift the tape away from the skin and then advance the scissors or tape cutters along the body's natural contours, avoiding sensitive tissues.

6 for discussion on appropriate braces for the various body regions. **Field Strategy 7.1** summarizes application techniques for taping a body part.

Although tape is useful in the prevention, management, and rehabilitation of sports injuries, its effectiveness is limited unless the individual subscribes to a comprehensive rehabilitation program. For discussion on rehabilitation exercises for the various body parts, refer to the individual joint chapters.

Application of Wraps

Application of elastic wraps should begin with the body part in a position of maximum muscle contraction. This ensures that movement and circulation will not be impaired during activity. Begin distal to the injured area and move proximal to the injury. This prevents any edema formation from settling in the distal digits and provides support against gravitational forces. The wrap should be stretched from one-half to one-third of its total elastic capability prior to application. Stretching it more may cause constriction of the circulation, compression of superficial nerves, and impairment of function. Each turn of the wrap should be overlapped by at least one-half of the previous underlying strip. The end of the wrap may be secured with elastic tape for added support. **Field Strategy 7.2** summarizes application techniques for wrapping a body part.

The high school soccer player needed additional arch support. After developing a rehabilitation program to strength the intrinsic muscles of the foot and the muscles that support the

Field Strategy 7.1. Application Techniques for Taping a Body Part

Prior to Application

The body part should be clean, dry, and free of hair
Cover open wounds with a sterile dressing
Apply a lubricated pad over sensitive areas, such as the dorsum of the foot, Achilles tendon, or popliteal space
Spray a light layer of tape adherent onto the skin surface
For individuals sensitive or allergic to tape, or who must be taped on a daily basis, apply a single layer of foam underwrap

During Application

To limit low back stress from bending over, use a table at an appropriate height
Place the body part to be taped in a position of function to ensure the desired result
If the hip and knee must be slightly flexed, place the heel on a 1.5- to 2-inch heel lift
Should it be necessary to reach above the shoulder level, stand on a bench or have the athlete sit down
Allow only a few inches of tape to be unrolled off the roll at one time, to prevent wrinkles
Guide the tape around the contours of the body part while applying slight tension
Each strip of tape should overlap the previous strip by one-half to one-third the width of the tape
When completed, check circulation

After Athletic Participation

Remove the tape immediately to prevent skin breakdown
Dip the tip of the tape cutters or scissors in a skin lubricant, lift the tape up away from the skin, and cut along the body's natural contours
Always cut on the side opposite the injury site
Remove the tape in the direction of the natural hair growth
Cleanse the skin with tape remover and then soap and water. Dry thoroughly
Apply a skin moisturizer to prevent dry skin
Inspect the skin regularly for signs of irritation, blisters, or infection

medial longitudinal arch, you can apply an arch pad or an X-arch strapping to support the area.

COMMON TAPING AND WRAPPING TECHNIQUES

A football lineman separated his right shoulder at the acromioclavicular joint. How will you limit motion at the joint to allow some mobility of the shoulder joint, yet prevent excessive painful motion?

The following taping and wrapping techniques are provided as a guide to application. When strapping or bracing a particular body part, adapt the technique to the individual's needs.

Field Strategy 7.2. Application Techniques for Wrapping a Body Part

Cover open wounds with a sterile dressing and secure with tape

To limit low back stress from bending over, have the athlete sit down on a stool, use a table at an appropriate height, or ask the athlete to stand

Place the injured muscles in a shortened state, but have them maximally contracted

If the hip and knee must be slightly flexed, place the heel on a 1.5- to 2-inch heel lift

Begin distal to the injured area and move in a proximal direction lifting up against gravity

Stretch the wrap one-half to one-third of its total elastic capability prior to application

Overlap each turn of the wrap by at least one-half of the previous underlying strip

Secure the end of the wrap with elastic tape for added support

After participation, remove the wrap and wash it in a washing machine on a delicate cycle

If possible, hang the wrap to dry to prevent losing its elasticity

---

Taping and Wrapping Techniques for the Lower Extremity

Great Toe Taping

This strapping is used to limit motion at the great toe, primarily because of a joint sprain. To begin, place anchor strips on the great toe just proximal to the nail and at the midfoot (**Fig. 7.7**) (5). To prevent hyperextension of the toe, a strip of tape is applied from the distal anchor to the proximal anchor on the plantar surface of the foot (3). Additional supportive strips are applied until the base of the first metatarsal is covered. This procedure is completed by re-anchoring the strips at midfoot. For hyperflexion injuries, the supportive tape strips run on the dorsum of the toe and foot. Occasionally, the athlete may have both a hyperextension and hyperflexion injury. In this case, the two tapings may be combined to limit motion in both directions.

Arch Support: Technique 1

Arch support may be necessary for individuals with plantar fasciitis, high arches, or for those who run or jump excessively

Arch support may be necessary in individuals with plantar fasciitis, high arches, or in individuals who run or jump excessively. A simple arch support utilizes three to four circular strips of tape applied around the mid-foot region (**Fig. 7.8**) (6). The first strip is anchored on the dorsum of the foot and encircles the lateral border of the foot. As the strip moves across the plantar aspect, the strip is secured under the fifth metatarsal with one hand, while the other hand applies slight tension in an upward direction through the medial longitudinal arch. In this manner, tension is applied only through the arch area and will not constrict the blood

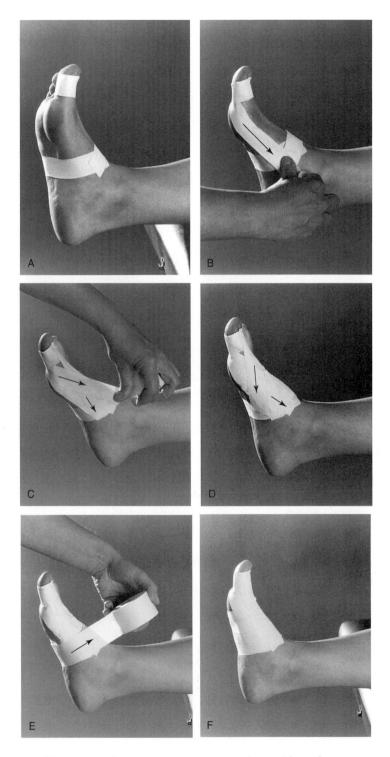

Figure 7.7. A–F. A great toe strapping may be used for turf toe.

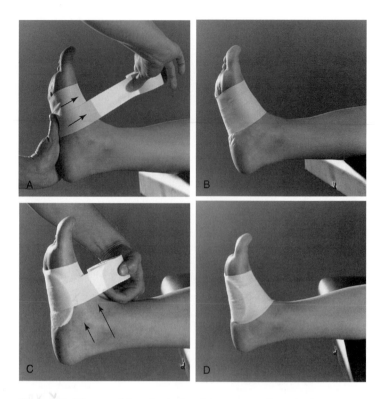

Figure 7.8. When applying circular bands to support the arch, do not constrict circulation to the toes. Rather, anchor the tape under the 5th metatarsal and lift only through the arch area (**A, B**). An arch pad may also be used under the circular straps for additional arch support (**C, D**).

vessels on the lateral aspect of the foot. The next strip overlaps the previous strip by one-half, until the entire arch is covered. By moving distal to proximal, the exposed edges of the tape will not roll when socks are placed on the foot (6). An arch pad may be added to this technique for further support.

Arch Support: Technique 2

If additional support is required, an alternative "X-arch" strapping may be applied (**Fig. 7.9**) (6). An anchor strip is placed at the level of the distal metatarsal heads. To avoid constricting circulation, this strip should not encircle the entire foot. Beginning at the base of the great toe, the tape is pulled along the medial aspect of the foot, around the heel, and angled across the arch to end at the starting point. The second strip begins at the base of the fifth metatarsal, moves along the lateral aspect of the foot, around the heel, and is angled across the arch, back to its point of origin. Alternating subsequent strips of tape follow the same pattern until the entire arch is covered. The tape job is then closed using the simple arch taping technique. An alternative closing technique is to use elastic tape, being careful not to constrict circulation.

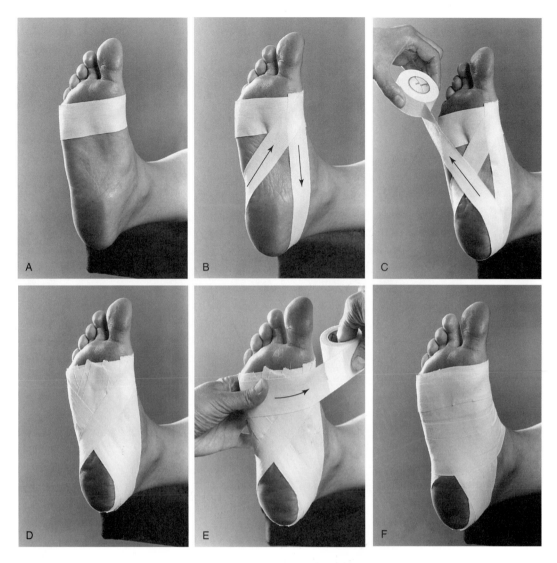

Figure 7.9. A–F. X-arch strappings provide additional arch support for individuals who do extensive running and jumping.

Open Basketweave Ankle Strapping

The open basketweave is used on an acute inversion or eversion ankle sprain to control swelling and limit motion (3,4). The athlete should sit on the table with the ankle flexed at 90°. Using nonelastic tape, apply one anchor 4 to 6 inches proximal to the ankle joint, and another anchor at the level of the metatarsal heads (3,6). Do not constrict circulation. These anchors help to secure the remaining strips of tape to the skin **(Fig. 7.10)**.

A "stirrup" strip of tape is applied, beginning from the medial aspect of the proximal anchor. The strip extends behind the medial malleolus, under the heel, behind the lateral malleolus, and is

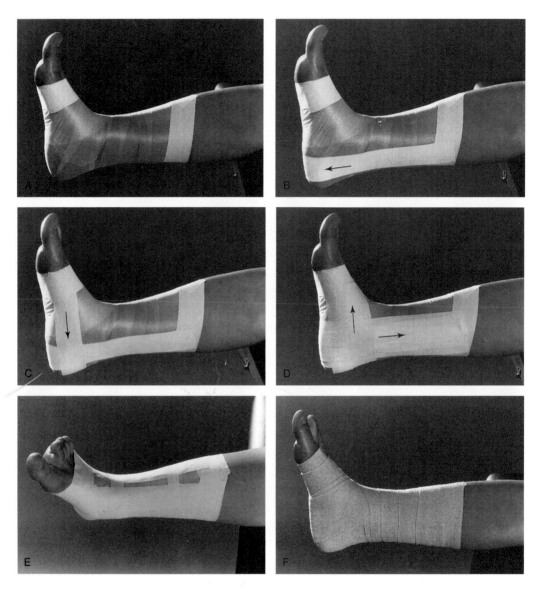

Figure 7.10. A–F. An open basketweave is used to control swelling and limit motion after an acute ankle sprain.

secured back to the proximal anchor. Next, a "horseshoe" strip of tape is applied, beginning on the medial aspect of the distal anchor. The horseshoe strip follows the base of the first metatarsal, travels behind the calcaneus, and continues to the base of the fifth metatarsal, ending on the distal anchor.

This process of alternating stirrups and horseshoes is continued, leaving approximately a ½- to 1-inch opening on the anterior aspect of the lower leg and foot (3). This opening allows for some swelling to occur, but limits gross effusion. The plantar aspect is then closed with semicircular strips of tape and the tape edges are then re-anchored. Two to three horizontal pieces of tape may then be applied to secure the anchors. If further stability is needed, heel locks may be applied (See closed basketweave).

An elastic wrap may then be applied over the tape for additional compression; however, it should be removed at night to avoid circulatory compromise (3–5). Ideally, the tape should be replaced daily when the individual is doing rehabilitative exercises. The strapping, however, may be left on for up to 2 days, as long as the skin under the tape is intact and circulation is normal. Ice may be applied directly over the tape, but avoid getting the tape wet (5). Tape that becomes wet from perspiration, ice treatments, or bathing should be removed to avoid skin **maceration**. To avoid getting the tape wet, the lower leg may be placed in a plastic bag during bathing. Any sign of skin maceration or breakdown warrants the immediate removal of the tape for further evaluation and treatment.

Maceration
Softening of tissues that may result in breaking, tearing, or wasting away

Closed Basketweave

The closed basketweave technique is used to provide external support to ankle ligaments during activity. Because most ankle sprains are caused by excessive inversion, this explanation will focus on providing support to the lateral ligaments. Adaptations can be made for eversion ankle sprains by reversing the pull of support.

The lower leg and foot should be clean, dry, and free of hair. Padding with a lubricant should be applied to the dorsum of the ankle and to the Achilles tendon area. The proximal anchor should be placed approximately 4 to 6 inches above the ankle joint, distal to the belly of the gastrocnemius. The distal anchor bisects the styloid process of the fifth metatarsal **(Fig. 7.11)** (6). Beginning on the medial aspect of the superior anchor, run a stirrup strip down behind the medial malleolus, under the heel, behind the lateral malleolus, and pull up on the lateral aspect, ending on the superior anchor.

Next, beginning on the medial aspect of the distal anchor, a horseshoe strip of tape is placed along the base of the first metatarsal, behind the heel, following the base of the fifth metatarsal, and ends on the lateral aspect of the distal anchor. The next stirrup overlaps the first by one-half to two-thirds of the previous stirrup. A second horseshoe is placed, working again from medial to lateral, overlapping one-half to two-thirds of the previous strip. This alternation occurs until there are at least three stirrups and three horseshoes in place. Alternating the directions of the tape will give the tape an appearance of a woven basket, hence the name. A figure-eight and heel locks are then applied. Finally, the strapping is closed from distal to proximal using horizontal strips, which

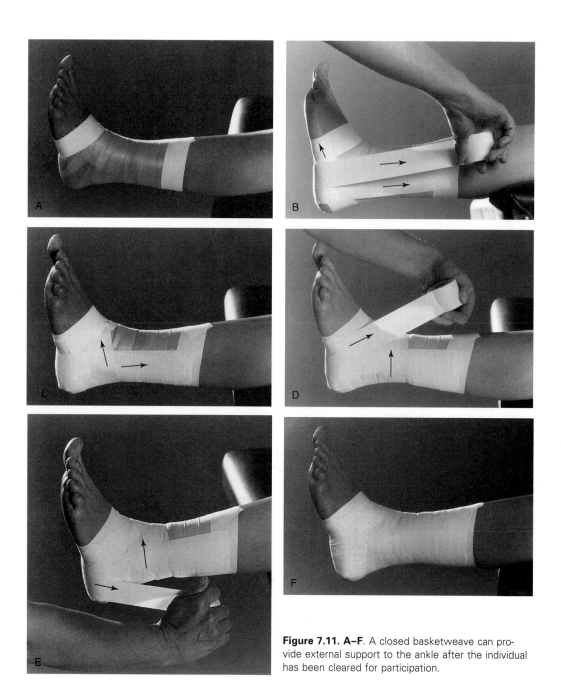

Figure 7.11. A–F. A closed basketweave can provide external support to the ankle after the individual has been cleared for participation.

The most common problem with tape application used to restrict motion is that it can be applied too tightly, leading to circulatory compromise and discomfort

overlap one-half to two-thirds of the previous strip. For additional support, a second figure-eight and heel locks may be applied (6).

The most common problem with applying tape that restricts motion is that it can be applied too tightly, so that it constricts circulation and causes discomfort. This is especially true with the distal anchor. To avoid this, place the distal anchor on the foot and do not apply any tension.

Game Strapping

This technique is fast and easy to apply, but provides only a moderate amount of support to the ankle. It is commonly used as both a preventive strapping and as a post-injury strapping for an individual who has completed the rehabilitation program. Athletes who require a more substantial amount of support can combine this taping with a brace or may wish to use the closed basketweave technique.

To begin, the foot is held at 90° of flexion. Anchors are applied to the foot, bisecting the styloid process of the fifth metatarsal. The second anchor is applied 4 to 6 inches above the ankle joint, just distal to the belly of the gastrocnemius. Three stirrups are placed, beginning on the medial aspect of the superior anchor **(Fig. 7.12)**. These run posterior to anterior, each overlapping one-half to two-thirds of the previous stirrup, completely covering the malleoli. Next, beginning on the medial malleolus, apply a figure-eight with heel locks in a continuous fashion. Use caution when crossing behind the Achilles tendon, as tight tape may cause skin irritation and blisters. A second figure-eight is then applied. Finally, the strapping is closed using successive circular strips around the foot, continuing proximal to distal.

Cloth Ankle Wrap

Cloth wrap is available in large rolls that can be cut into 72 inch lengths. When combined with the support offered by a minimal amount of nonelastic tape, cloth wraps provide adequate support for the ankle (6). Although not as supportive as nonelastic tape, they are washable, reusable, and a cost-effective alternative to a game strapping.

Although cloth ankle wraps are not as supportive as nonelastic tape, they are washable, reusable, and a cost-effective alternative to a game strapping

The cloth wrap is applied over a white athletic sock while the ankle is held at 90° (4,6). The sock should be snug and free of wrinkles (5). Place the wrap just distal to the medial malleolus and complete a figure-eight **(Fig. 7.13)**. Once completed, move directly into heel locks, pulling up on the lateral aspect of the ankle, and downward on the medial aspect of the ankle. Repeat the pattern until approximately 12 inches of the material is left. Then, secure this material in a circular fashion around the lower leg. Anchor the end of the material with nonelastic tape. Apply a figure-eight and heel locks over the cloth wrap with nonelastic tape to provide additional support (6).

Achilles Tendon Taping

Taping of the Achilles tendon limits excessive dorsiflexion, thus reducing tension on the tendon (6). Place the athlete in a prone position on the taping table with the lower leg extended over the table (6). Dorsiflex the foot and determine where the discomfort occurs. This indicates the point to which you allow motion, but restrict any further painful motion. The athlete holds the foot in

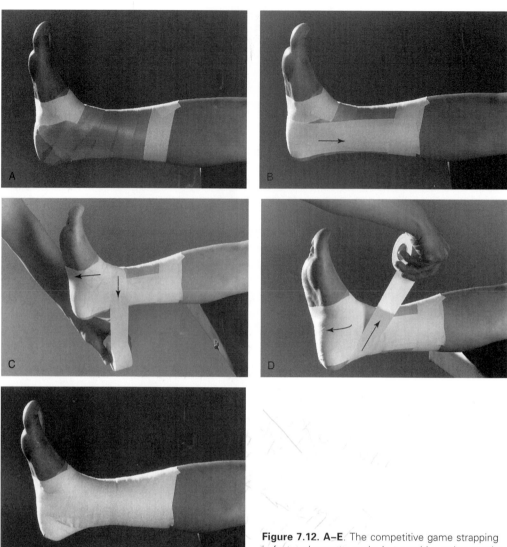

Figure 7.12. A–E. The competitive game strapping is fast and easy to apply, but provides only a moderate amount of support to the ankle.

a relaxed position (**Fig. 7.14**). Anchors, using nonelastic tape, are applied to the base of the metatarsals and 4 to 6 inches above the ankle joint, just distal to the belly of the gastrocnemius. A heel pad with lubricant is placed over the Achilles tendon. Using 2-inch elastic tape, three strips are applied in an "X" pattern from the distal to proximal anchor. The X is re-anchored distally and proximally with nonelastic tape. The athlete then moves to a seated position. Using elastic tape, a figure-eight and heel locks are then applied (3). Be careful not to apply added pressure over the irritated Achilles tendon area. Heel lifts may also be placed in the shoes to limit dorsiflexion; however, lifts should be placed in both shoes to prevent any undo stress on other body parts.

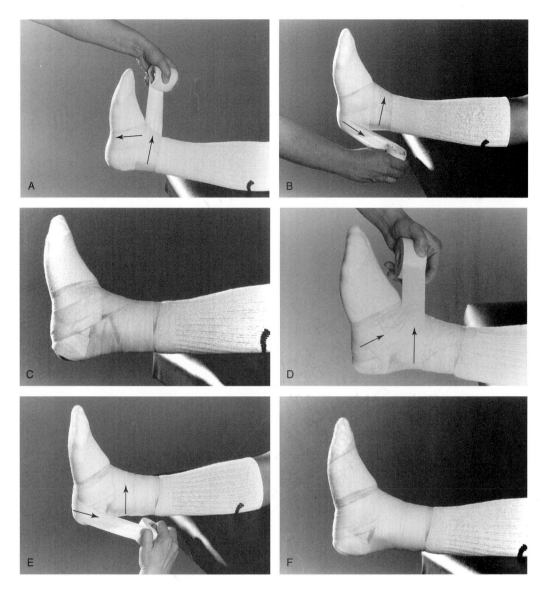

Figure 7.13. A–F. When combined with nonelastic tape, a cloth ankle wrap can provide adequate support to an ankle.

Shin Splints Taping

Shin splints is a generic term that refers to pain found on the anterior shin. Often, anterior shin pain is directly related to stress on the medial longitudinal arch; therefore, arch strappings may help alleviate symptoms. If the condition is related to tendinitis of the tibialis posterior muscle, strapping the ankle to limit eversion may provide some relief. Stress fractures and compartment syndromes will not benefit from strapping, and may actually be aggravated by compression from the tape. This strapping should not

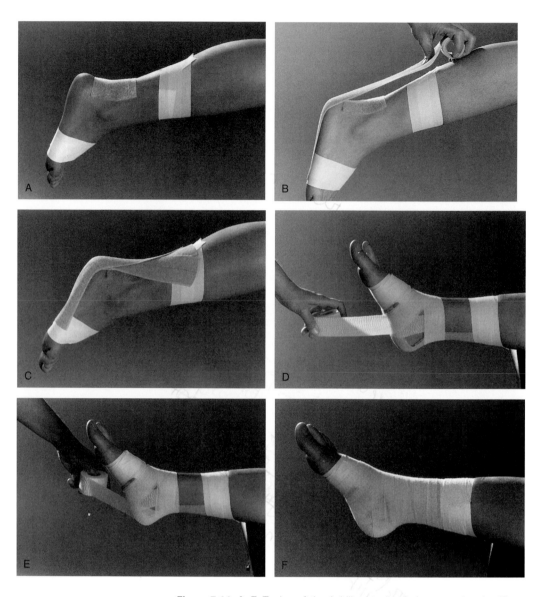

Figure 7.14. A–F. Taping of the Achilles tendon limits excessive dorsiflexion, thus reducing tension on the tendon. This strapping can also be combined with a heel lift placed in the shoe, to limit further stress on the tendon.

be applied until the actual source of pain has been identified by an experienced health-care provider.

Begin with the athlete standing on a table facing forward. A heel lift should be placed under the heel of the leg being taped to relax the muscles. Anchors are placed distally above the malleoli and proximally at the tibial tuberosity (6). Medial and lateral anchor strips are placed from distal to proximal, lifting up against gravity **(Fig. 7.15)**. These should follow the line of the malleoli.

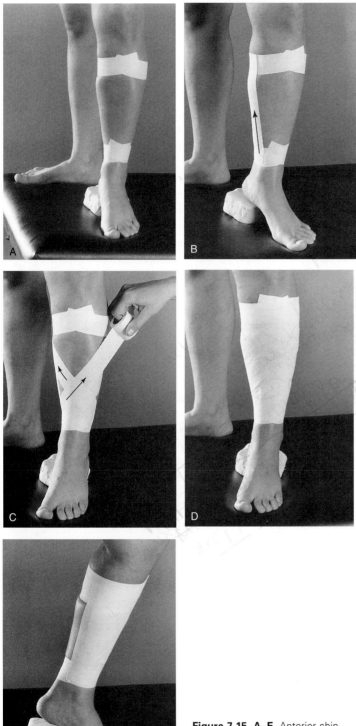

Figure 7.15. A–E. Anterior shin pain may originate from several different injuries. Therefore, this strapping should not be applied until the actual source of pain has been identified and treated.

Tape is applied in an alternating oblique direction, forming an X over the anterior shin, working distal to proximal until the entire anterior shin is covered. Medial and lateral anchors are then placed, followed by distal and proximal anchors.

Collateral Ligament Support for the Knee

The athlete should be standing on a table with the affected limb resting on a 1.5- to 2-inch heel lift (3). Taping is most effective when done directly to the skin or with the use of minimal underwrap after the area has been properly prepared. Elastic tape is commonly used because of the musculature involved (3). Apply the distal anchor 2 inches below the level of the tibial tuberosity and apply the proximal anchor at the midpoint of the quadriceps muscle group **(Fig. 7.16)**. Lateral and medial supportive strips are applied in an X fashion that outlines the medial and lateral collateral ligaments, but keeps the patella open (3). Successive interlocking Xs will give additional support to the collateral ligaments. The collateral taping may be further reinforced with nonelastic tape. Finally, the tape is closed off with successive circular strips, moving from the distal anchor to proximal anchor.

Rotary Knee Instability Taping

The athlete stands on the table with the heel elevated. Anchors are placed 2 to 3 inches below the tibial tuberosity and at the mid-quadriceps using elastic tape **(Fig. 7.17)**. A pad with lubricant is placed in the popliteal space. A piece of elastic tape is cut in the middle at both ends and torn to form an X. The divided ends are then placed around the patella and interlocked (6). Beginning at the superior anchor, a piece of elastic tape is angled down behind the knee, through the popliteal space, ending on the inferior anchor. In an opposite direction, a second piece of tape spirals down behind the knee, through the popliteal space, ending on the inferior anchor. Three to four spirals in each direction provide the necessary support (6). Once in place, the taping is closed with circular applied strips of tape. Additional support may be provided by using nonelastic tape to reinforce the spiral pattern. If the collateral ligaments also need support, the collateral taping technique may be applied under the rotary instability strapping.

Knee Hyperextension

This taping limits hyperextension of the knee and may be applied with elastic or nonelastic tape. With the athlete standing on a table with the heel elevated, the superior anchor is placed at mid-thigh, encircling the entire thigh, with a second anchor applied 2 to 3 inches below the tibial tuberosity **(Fig. 7.18)** (5). A gauze pad with lubricant is placed in the popliteal space, thus reducing the friction of the nerves and circulatory supply to the knee (6). From the inferior anchor, apply tape strips in a X pattern over

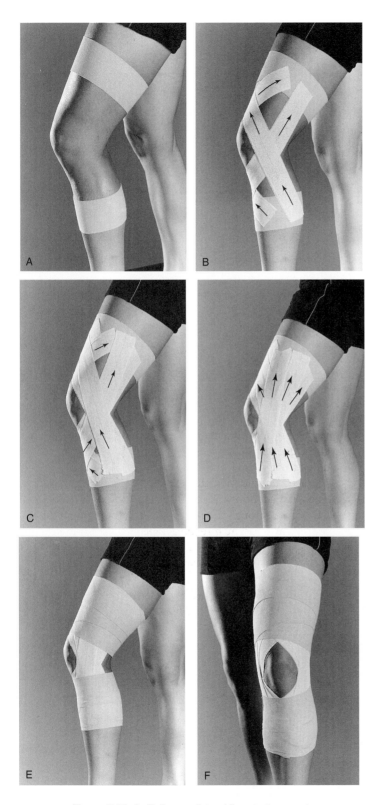

Figure 7.16. A–F. Knee collateral ligament support.

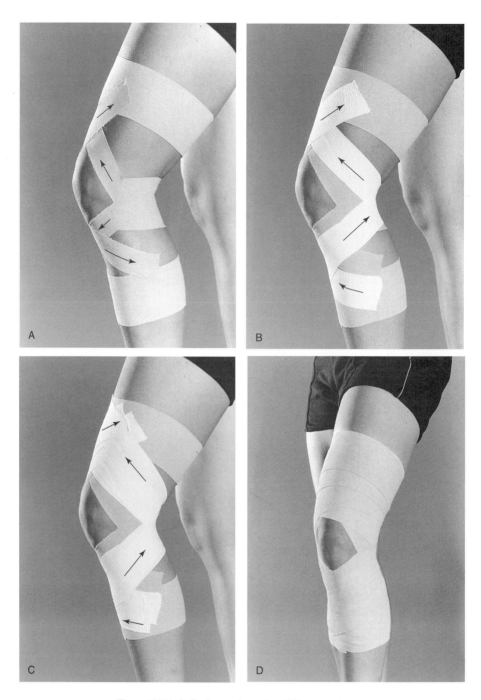

Figure 7.17. A–D. Rotary knee instability strapping.

the gauze in the popliteal space. The X pattern should begin wide and become narrower as the popliteal space is covered (6). The last strip will run perpendicular to the anchors. The strapping is completed by applying 2 to 3 anchors on the lower leg and 4 to 5 anchors on the thigh, each overlapping one-half to two-thirds

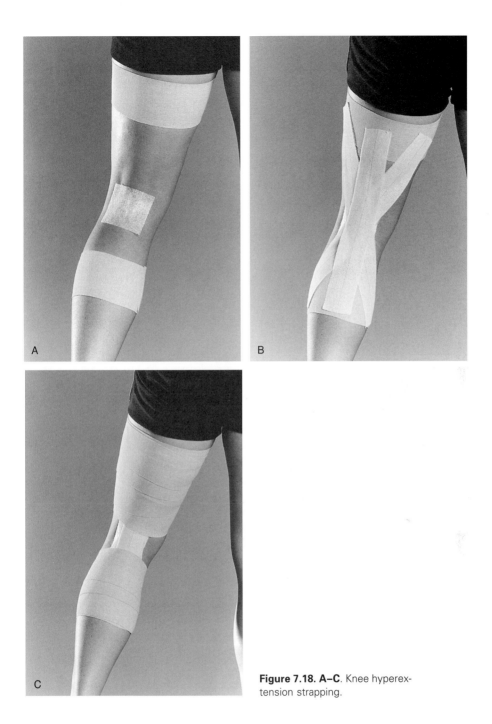

Figure 7.18. A–C. Knee hyperextension strapping.

of the previous strip. When completed, the taping should allow knee flexion and extension, but limit hyperextension.

Quadriceps and Hamstrings Wrap

A thigh strain may involve either the quadriceps or hamstrings muscle group. For the quadriceps muscles, the heel of the injured

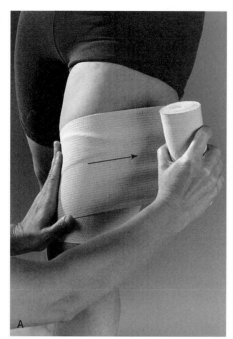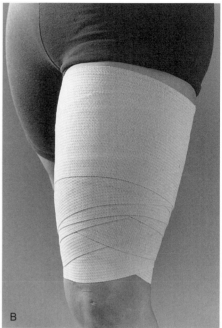

Figure 7.19. A, B. Quadriceps wrap.

leg should be elevated 2 to 3 inches on a taping block. With the thigh in a neutral position, begin on the anterior aspect of the mid-thigh distal to the painful site. Apply the wrap in an upward and lateral direction, encircling the thigh (**Fig. 7.19**). Elastic tape is then applied over the wrap to provide additional support.

With a hamstring strain, two techniques may be used. The first technique is used when the strain is to the distal portion of the muscle group and is applied in a manner similar to the quadriceps wrap. The tension of the wrap is applied in an upward and lateral direction, encircling the thigh. Elastic tape is then applied over the wrap to provide additional support. The second technique may be used when the injury occurs in the proximal portion of the muscle group. The wrap is placed on the posteromedial aspect of the thigh, and encircles the thigh several times, pulling from a medial to lateral direction. The wrap is then pulled up across the greater trochanter, continues around the lower abdomen, is brought around the opposite iliac crest over the waist and gluteals, then crosses the greater trochanter, ending back on the anterior thigh, to encircle the thigh again, moving in a medial to lateral direction (**Fig. 7.20**). The wrap is then reinforced with elastic tape, which repeats the same pattern.

Groin Wrap

Although groin strains may refer to damage to the hip flexors, hip adductors, or hip abductors, this explanation will focus on

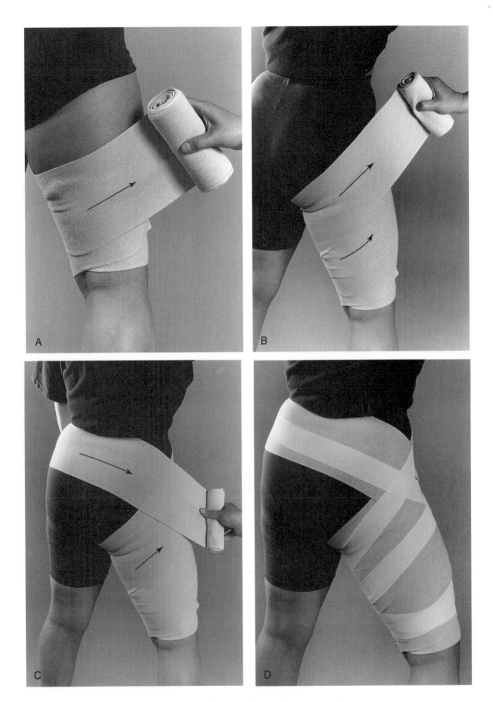

Figure 7.20. A–D. Although the hamstrings strain may be wrapped in a manner similar to the quadriceps wrap, the technique shown is used when the strain is located in the proximal portion of the muscle belly.

preventing stress on the hip adductors. When supporting the adductor muscles, the heel is elevated on a taping block, with the hip internally rotated. The wrap is then placed on the lateral aspect of the thigh, and encircles the thigh in a medial direction to further draw the thigh into internal rotation **(Fig. 7.21)** (5,6). The wrap continues around the thigh, crossing over the greater trochanter, continuing across the lower abdomen, covering the iliac crest, around the waist and gluteals, then crosses the greater trochanter, ending back on the thigh. The wrap is then reinforced with elastic tape, which repeats the same pattern.

Taping and Wrapping Techniques for the Upper Extremity

Acromioclavicular Taping

> The nipple should be protected with a gauze pad and lubricant to prevent chaffing

The nipple should be protected with a gauze pad and lubricant to prevent chaffing (5). The arm is placed in a relaxed position and supported at the elbow. Begin with an anchor of elastic tape that encircles the mid-biceps region. A second anchor is placed just below the spine of the scapula, extends over the shoulder through the midclavicular line, and ends just under the nipple. A third anchor is placed just under the nipple and runs horizontally around the trunk, connecting the two ends of the second anchor **(Fig. 7.22)** (6). Beginning on the biceps anchor, a strip of tape is pulled from the anchor up and over the acromion process, ending on the midclavicular anchor. A second strip, also originating on the biceps anchor, is pulled up and over the acromion process to anchor on the posterior back. These two strips form an X over the acromion process (5,6). A midclavicular strip is then applied, followed by another horizontal anchor. Each of the anchors should overlap one-half to two-thirds of the previous piece of tape. The pattern is then repeated, first crossing over the acromion process with the Xs, then the midclavicular anchor, and finally the horizontal anchor, until the acromion process is covered. The horizontal anchors should stop just below the axilla and should not impede arm motion. This taping may be reinforced by covering it with an elastic bandage wrapped as a shoulder spica (7).

Shoulder Spica Wrap

The athlete should hold the injured arm in internal rotation. Begin by encircling the arm in a posterior to anterior direction at the mid-biceps (5). Cross the anterior chest in the region of the pectoralis major **(Fig. 7.23)**. Wrapping in this direction maintains internal rotation of the glenohumeral joint and limits external rotation. The limitation of motion is determined by the amount of internal rotation the arm is placed in initially. The wrap is then brought under the opposite axilla, across the back, over the acromion process in an anterior direction. The wrap is then continued

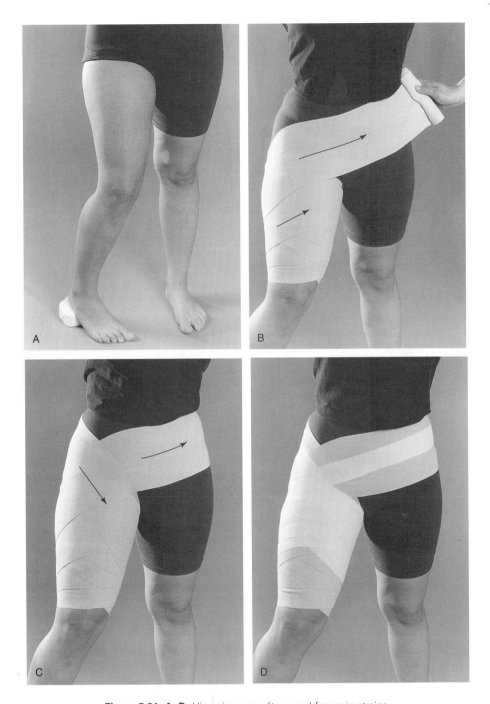

Figure 7.21. A–D. Hip spicas are often used for groin strains.

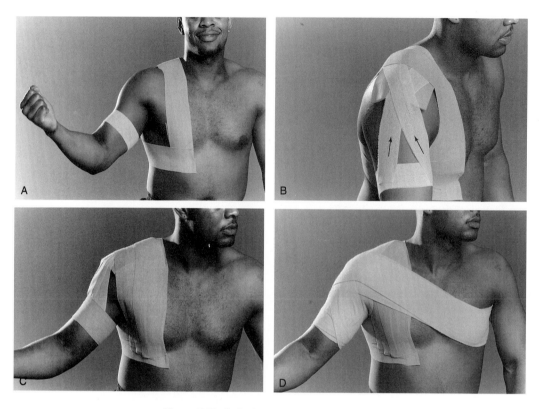

Figure 7.22. A–D. Acromioclavicular taping.

through the axilla, around the arm, and again across the anterior chest (6). The wrap is then secured with nonelastic tape.

Elbow Hyperextension

Flex the biceps brachii muscle and apply an anchor of either nonelastic tape or elastic tape just proximal to the muscle belly. The distance between the two anchors is approximated. Two pieces of tape approximately the same length are then torn from the roll. A checkrein is constructed by placing these two pieces of tape back to back then adding five to six additional pieces of tape over the template in an X fan shape **(Fig. 7.24)** (2,5,6).

The checkrein is then attached to the anchors by applying three to four additional anchors overlapping the previous anchor by one-half to two-thirds. A figure-eight with an elastic wrap may then be applied to further secure the taping and prevent slipping during competition. Check and monitor the radial pulse to determine if the tape is applied too tight.

Wrist: Technique 1

Hyperextension or hyperflexion of the wrist may damage the ligaments of the wrist. For a mild sprain, three or four circular strips

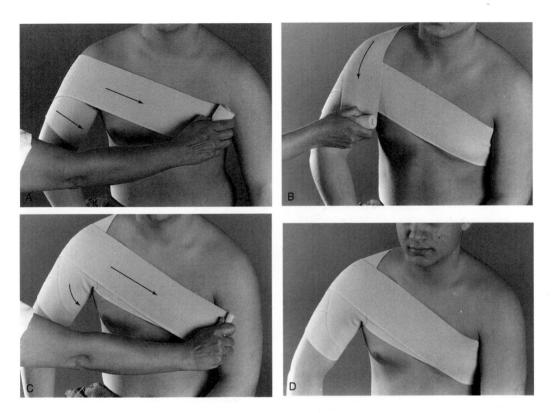

Figure 7.23. A–D. Shoulder spica.

of tape may be applied to the wrist, beginning distal to proximal. Overlap the previous strip by one-half to two-thirds of the width of the tape **(Fig. 7.25)** (2,5,6).

Wrist: Technique 2

If additional limitation of motion is needed, begin by placing an anchor strip around the wrist and at the heads of the metacarpals **(Fig. 7.26)**. To limit hyperextension, 3 to 4 strips of tape are placed in an X pattern over the palmar aspect of the hand (5,6). To limit hyperflexion, place the X pattern over the dorsum of the hand. Using either elastic or nonelastic tape, a figure-eight is then applied around the wrist and hand. The figure-eight should begin on the radial aspect of the proximal anchor, travel across the dorsum of the hand around the metacarpal heads, travel across the palm of the hand, and end on the ulnar side of the proximal anchor (5). As the tape is brought through the web space of the thumb and index finger, the tape is crimped to prevent irritation of the skin.

Thumb

Most thumb injuries occur when the thumb is hyperextended (1). Using nonelastic tape, apply an anchor on the wrist and another

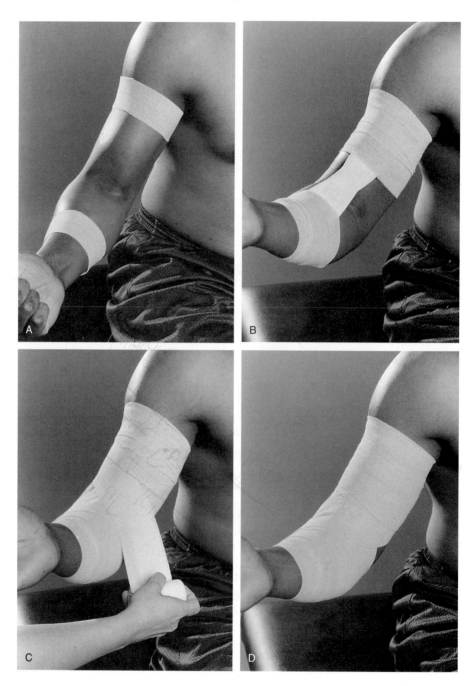

Figure 7.24. A–D. Elbow hyperextension.

on the metacarpophalangeal joint of the thumb (**Fig. 7.27**) (5). Next, apply a strip of tape beginning on the ulnar aspect of the proximal anchor and continue upward over the palmar aspect of the thenar eminence on the thumb. Cross over the metacarpophalangeal joint, encircling the thumb, and re-anchor the strip on the

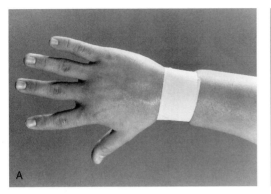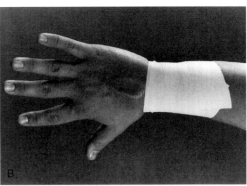

Figure 7.25. A, B. For a mild wrist sprain, three or four circular strips of tape may be applied to the wrist.

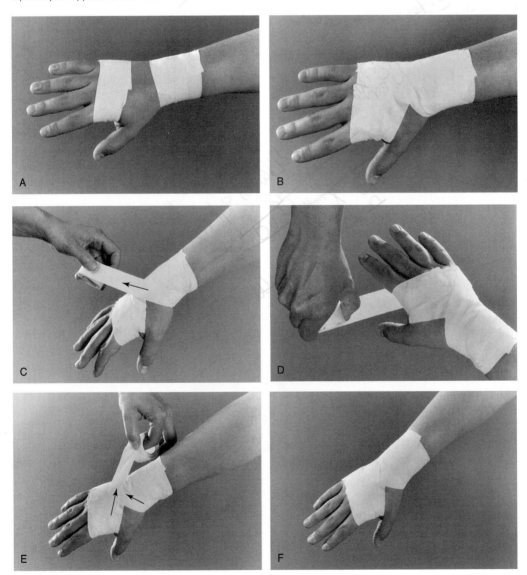

Figure 7.26. A–F. For a moderate wrist sprain, a more extensive strapping is necessary to limit painful motion.

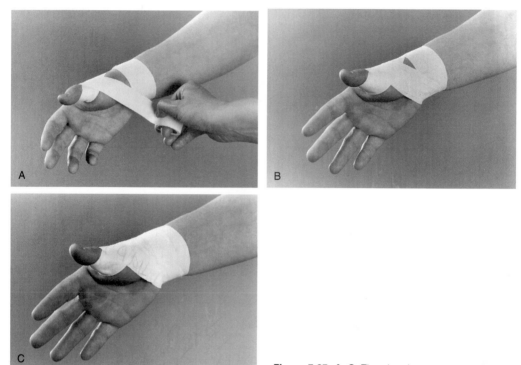

Figure 7.27. A–C. Thumb spica.

dorsal aspect of the anchor. This line of pull makes an X pattern. As the tape passes thru the web space of the thumb, adduct the thumb slightly. Do three to four Xs and finish the strapping with additional anchors (6).

Finger Taping Technique

The interphalangeal joints are often injured. "Buddy" taping for the fingers involves using an adjacent finger for support (5). Strips of narrow tape are applied around the proximal phalanx and distal

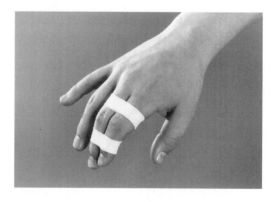

Figure 7.28. Buddy taping for the fingers.

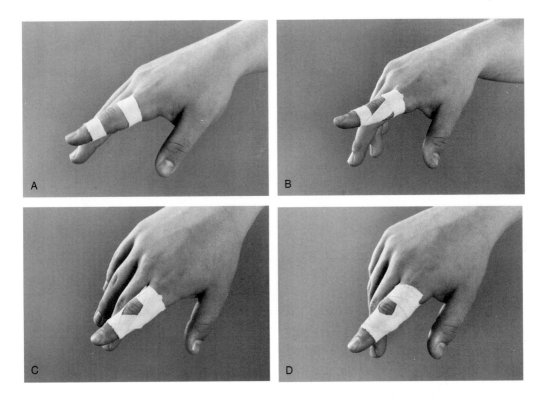

Figure 7.29. A–D. Added support for the collateral ligaments of the fingers can be provided by this strapping.

phalanx, leaving the joints uncovered to permit limited flexion and extension of the fingers **(Fig. 7.28)**.

If additional support for the medial and lateral collateral ligaments is needed, anchors can be placed just proximal and distal to the injured joint **(Fig. 7.29)**. Working from distal to proximal, apply two narrow strips of tape in an X pattern over the collateral ligaments, followed by a longitudinal strip to connect the two anchors. A figure-eight may be applied, using care not to impinge circulation. Capillary refill should be checked after taping, as the blood supply is very superficial and easily compressed.

The football lineman separated his right shoulder at the acromioclavicular joint. Did you determine that motion at this joint can be limited by applying restrictive strips of nonelastic tape in an X-like fashion over the joint and securing them to anchors around the biceps and midclavicular region? If so, you are correct. A shoulder spica elastic wrap can provide further support over the strapping.

SUMMARY

Taping and wrapping a body part provides support and protection while allowing functional movement. They may be used to provide immediate first aid, support an injured body part, or provide pain-free functional movement. Used in conjunction with a comprehensive rehabilitation program, tape or wraps can allow early resumption of activity without the threat of reinjury.

When using tape, the skin should be inspected regularly for signs of irritation, blisters, or infection. Look for skin that is red, dry, hot, and tender. These signs indicate a possible allergic reaction to the tape or tape adherent. If the skin cannot be protected from irritation, it may be necessary to fit this individual with an appropriate brace rather than subject them to continued irritation.

REFERENCES

1. Anderson MK, and Hall SJ. *Sports injury management*. Media, PA: Williams & Wilkins, 1995.
2. *Manual of athletic training*. Philadelphia: FA Davis, 1995.
3. Austine KA, Gwymn-Brelt KA, and Marshall SC. *Illustrated guide to taping techniques*. London: Mosby Year Book, 1994.
4. Mercier LR. *Practical orthopedics*. St. Louis: Mosby Year Book, 1995.
5. Kennedy R, and Berry D. *The sports therapy taping guide*. Ottawa, Ontario: Sports-medics, 1991.
6. Arnheim D. *Essentials of athletic training*. St. Louis: Mosby Year Book, 1995.
7. Starkey C, and Ryan JL. *Evaluation of orthopedic and athletic injuries*. Philadelphia: FA Davis, 1996.

Injuries to the Lower Extremity

Injuries to the Lower Extremity

Chapter 8: **Foot, Ankle, and Lower Leg**

Chapter 9: **The Knee**

Chapter 10: **Thigh, Hip, and Pelvis Injuries**

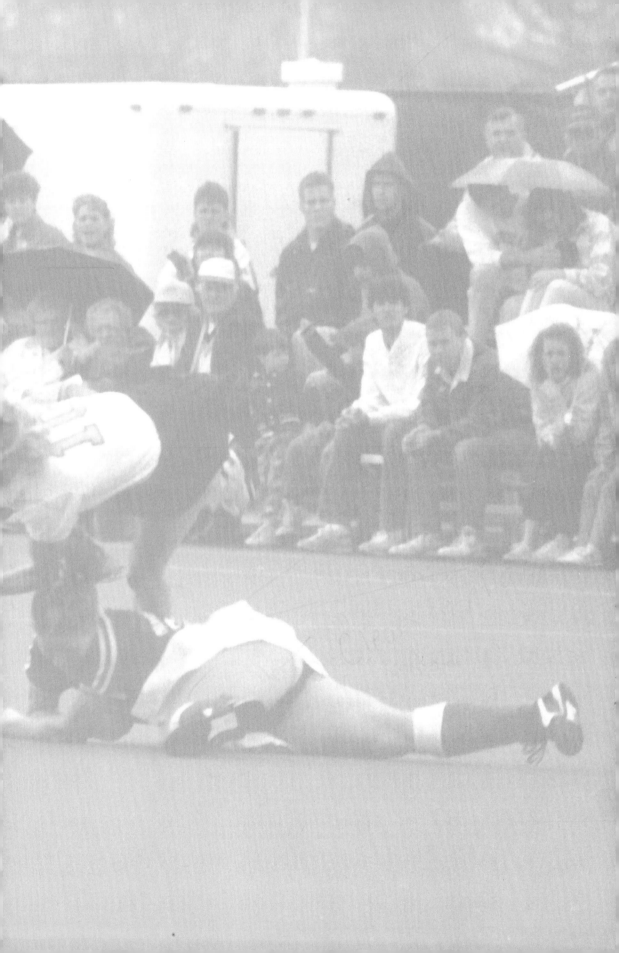

Ron O'Neil, BS, ATC

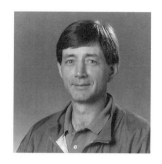

Although I started college studying to be an architect, I got interested in athletic training after an ankle injury occurred just prior to the baseball season. The two trainers who worked daily on my ankle took time to explain what they were doing and told me exactly what I needed to do to get ready for the season. When I showed an interest in the their work, they invited me to observe during the football season. It wasn't long before I knew that was what I wanted to do.

In my position as a professional football trainer, I work 12 months a year. A large part of the off-season in January through February involves supervising the rehabilitation of players who have been injured during the season or who have just had surgery. In late February, the medical staff travels to Indianapolis to evaluate the health status of over 350 college players. We see 110+ men a day as they complete a comprehensive physical examination. From that data, my staff and I call several colleges and universities to verify the athlete's health records. In April, we fly back to Indianapolis to re-evaluate those individuals who may not have had a complete exam in February due to an injury. All of this has to be done before the draft.

Starting in March, we have over 50 men training at the stadium. Our weight room is open from 6am to 6pm. Once training camp begins in mid-July, through the end of August, I work 18 to 20 hours every day of the week, and when the regular season starts in September, I work 12 to 14 hours every day. To say you have to be committed to this job is an understatement. There is very little down time, but I wouldn't give it up for the world.

It is so exciting to work with these elite athletes, especially when you realize that fewer than 0.5% of all men can play professional sports, and you're the one entrusted to keep these individuals healthy. It is really special, very gratifying. The players really appreciate what you do for them, not just taking care of the physical injury, but taking the time to talk to them, counsel them, and taking a sincere interest in their personal welfare. Our team physician and medical staff are totally committed to providing quality care to our players to increase their longevity, not only during the time they are with us, but more importantly, when they leave us. We want these individuals to have a healthy, long life, and we know that what we do every day for them will impact that goal.

Working on the professional level is hard work and there is a certain amount of stress to return these players to competition quickly. But you get to see a variety of injuries and can follow the player through the entire course of the rehabilitation. Because the medical staff is so extensive, we can have these players seen by a specialist almost immediately after injury. The team physician, Dr. Bert Zarins, is present at the stadium 2 days of the week and on game day. It is just a remarkably talented and complete medical staff.

For those of you thinking of working at the professional level, I recommend you develop a broad background in athletic training and personnel management. It's not enough just to know about prevention, treatment, rehabilitation, conditioning, weight training, and nutrition. You have to communicate this knowledge in daily interaction with your athletes. That means being physically fit, being a professional, and taking a sincere personal interest in your players. Working on the professional level is great, but you need to be willing to put in the long hours needed to provide total health care for your players. You need to volunteer at your area team locations to get your foot in the door, and you have to show initiative and commitment to your profession. Without commitment and dedication to the total health care of your athlete, you're in the wrong profession.

Ron O'Neil is the Head Athletic Trainer of the New England Patriots Professional Football Team in Foxboro, Massachusetts. As an athletic trainer for over two decades, Ron has distinguished himself as an educator and professional committed to providing comprehensive health care to his players.

Foot, Ankle, and Lower Leg

After completing this chapter, you should be able to:

- Locate the important bony and soft tissue structures of the foot, ankle, and lower leg

- Analyze the function of the plantar arches and their role in supporting and distributing body weight

- Describe motions of the foot and ankle and identify the muscles that produce them

- Identify basic principles in the prevention of injuries to the foot, ankle, and lower leg

- Recognize and manage specific injuries of the foot, ankle, and lower leg

- Demonstrate a basic assessment of the foot, ankle, and lower leg

- Demonstrate general rehabilitation exercises for the region

Key Terms:

Amenorrhea	Oligomenorrhea
Biparte	Paronychia
Claw toes	Pes planus
Compartment syndrome	Plantar fascia
Hallux	Pronation
Hammer toes	Sever's disease
Heel bruise	Shin bruise
Jones fracture	Snowball crepitation
Kinematics	Supination
Metatarsalgia	Tenosynovitis
Neuritis	Tinea pedis
Nonunion fracture	

Because of the essential roles played by the foot, ankle, and lower leg in all sport activities, injuries to this region are common. Sport participation often places both acute and chronic overloads on the lower extremity, leading to sprains, strains, and overuse injuries. Ankle injuries, in particular, comprise 20 to 25% of all injuries associated with running and jumping sports resulting in a loss of training time (1).

This chapter begins with an anatomical review, including the major muscle actions at the foot, ankle, and lower leg. Next, prevention of injuries will be followed by discussion on specific sports injuries and their management. Finally, a step-by-step basic injury assessment of the region will be presented, and examples of rehabilitative exercises will be provided.

ANATOMY REVIEW OF THE FOOT, ANKLE, AND LOWER LEG

? *A gymnast has pain on the plantar aspect of the midfoot during her floor routine. Although the pain is not too severe, it has worsened over the past week. What anatomical structures might be the source of pain?*

The foot, ankle, and lower leg provide support for the upright body, propel the body through space, absorb shock, and adapt for uneven terrain. In this section, discussion of the anatomical structures will begin with the bone and ligamentous structures, followed by the plantar arches, muscles, and, finally, the nerves and blood vessels of the region.

Bones of the Foot

The foot is made up of 26 bones, including 5 metatarsals and 14 phalanges **(Fig. 8.1)**. The toes function to smooth the weight shift to the opposite foot during walking and help maintain stability during weight bearing by pressing against the ground when necessary. The first digit is referred to as the **hallux**, or "great toe."

Hallux
The first, or great, toe

The tibia is the major weight-bearing bone of the lower leg. It articulates with the fibula at both proximal and distal ends **(Fig. 8.2)**. The fibula, which assists minimally with weight bearing, serves as a site for muscle attachments and contributes to stability at the ankle.

Ligaments of the Foot and Ankle

The joints of the foot include the metatarsophalangeal (MTP), proximal interphalangeal (PIP), and distal interphalangeal (DIP) joints. These joints, along with the tarsometatarsal and intertarsal joints, are bound together by several ligaments and enable the foot to adapt to uneven surfaces during gait.

The talocrural joint (ankle joint) is a uniaxial, modified hinge joint formed by the talus, the tibia, and the lateral malleolus of the fibula. Although the joint capsule is thin and especially weak anteriorly and posteriorly, the ankle is crossed by a number of strong ligaments that enhance its stability **(Fig. 8.3)**. The four separate bands of the medial collateral ligament, more commonly called the deltoid ligament, cross the ankle medially. Forces pro-

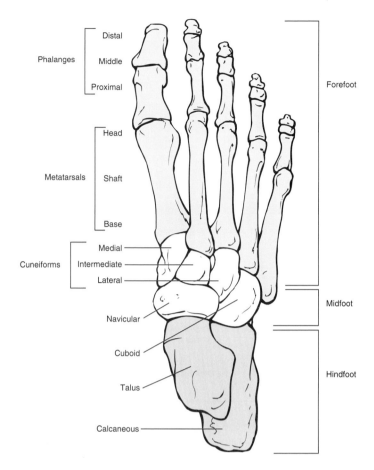

Figure 8.1. The bones of the foot are divided into three major regions—the forefoot, midfoot, and hindfoot.

ducing stress on the medial aspect of the ankle typically cause an avulsion fracture of the medial malleolus rather than a tear of the deltoid ligament. The lateral side of the ankle is crossed by three ligaments—the anterior and posterior talofibular and the calcaneofibular. The relative weakness of these lateral ligaments as compared to the deltoid ligament, coupled with less bony stability laterally than medially, contributes to a higher frequency of lateral ankle sprains.

As the name suggests, the subtalar joint lies beneath the talus and articulates with the sustentaculum tali on the superior calcaneus by four small talocalcaneal ligaments. This hinge joint has an axis aligned in an oblique direction.

The tibiofibular articulations are supported by the anterior and posterior tibiofibular ligaments, as well as by the crural interosseous tibiofibular ligament (**Fig. 8.2**). The tibia and fibula are also joined throughout most of their length by the interosseus membrane. This membrane is of such strength that strong lateral stresses will fracture the fibula rather than tear the membrane.

Lateral ankle sprains are more common because of less bony stability and ligamentous strength on the lateral aspect as compared to the medial aspect of the ankle

The tibiofibular interosseous ligament is so strong that excessive stress will fracture the fibula rather than rupture the ligament

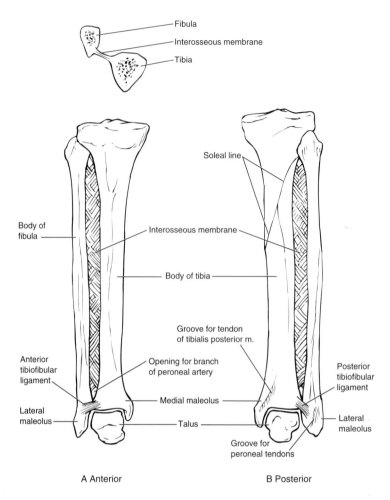

Figure 8.2. A,B. Little motion occurs at the proximal tibiofibular joint, but the distal tibiofibular joint forms the mortise for the talocrural joint. Note the interosseous membrane joining the full lengths of the tibia and fibula.

Plantar Arches

The bones and supporting ligamentous structures in the tarsal and metatarsal regions of the foot form interdependent longitudinal and transverse arches **(Fig. 8.4)**. They function to support and distribute body weight from the talus through the foot across changing weight-bearing conditions and over varying terrains.

The longitudinal arch runs from the anterior, inferior calcaneus to the metatarsal heads. Because the arch is higher medially than laterally, the medial side is usually the point of reference. The transverse arch runs across the anterior tarsals and the anterior metatarsals. The foundation of the arch is the medial cuneiform, with the apex of the arch formed by the second metatarsal. At the level of the metatarsal heads, the arch is reduced, with all metatarsals aligned parallel to the weight-bearing surface for the even distribution of body weight (2).

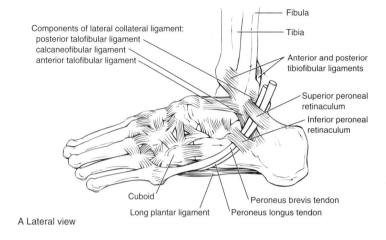

Components of lateral collateral ligament:
posterior talofibular ligament
calcaneofibular ligament
anterior talofibular ligament

Fibula
Tibia

Anterior and posterior
tibiofibular ligaments

Superior peroneal
retinaculum

Inferior peroneal
retinaculum

Cuboid
Long plantar ligament

Peroneus brevis tendon
Peroneus longus tendon

A Lateral view

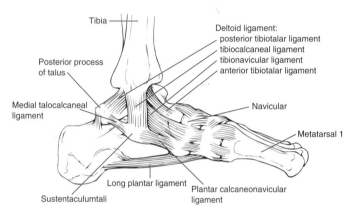

Tibia

Deltoid ligament:
posterior tibiotalar ligament
tibiocalcaneal ligament
tibionavicular ligament
anterior tibiotalar ligament

Posterior process
of talus

Navicular

Medial talocalcaneal
ligament

Metatarsal 1

Long plantar ligament
Sustentaculumtali

Plantar calcaneonavicular
ligament

B Medial view

Figure 8.3. A,B. Ligaments supporting the midfoot and hindfoot region.

The primary ligaments supporting the plantar arches are the spring (calcaneonavicular) ligament, long plantar ligament, plantar fascia (plantar aponeurosis), and the short plantar (plantar calcaneocuboid) ligament. When muscle tension is present, the muscles of the foot, particularly the tibialis posterior, also contribute support to the arches and joints as they cross them.

The **plantar fascia**, or plantar aponeurosis, is a thick interconnected band of fascia that covers the plantar surface of the foot, providing support for the longitudinal arch **(Fig. 8.5)**. It extends from the posterior medial calcaneus to the proximal phalanx of each toe. During the weight-bearing phase of the gait cycle, the plantar fascia functions like a spring to store mechanical energy that is then released to help the foot push off from the surface. The plantar fascia may be elongated by stretching the Achilles tendon, since both structures attach to the calcaneus.

Plantar fascia
Specialized band of fascia
that covers the plantar
surface of the foot and helps
support the longitudinal arch

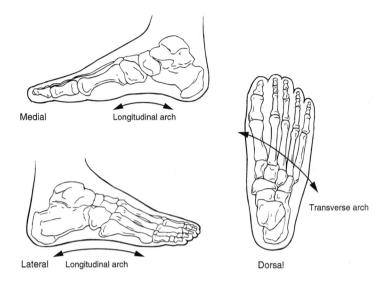

Figure 8.4. The arches of the foot.

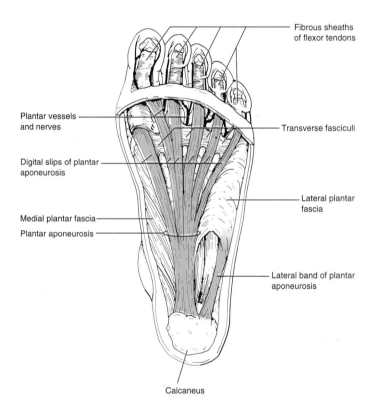

Figure 8.5. The plantar fascia stores mechanical energy each time the foot deforms during the weight-bearing phase of the gait cycle.

Muscles of the Lower Leg and Foot

Thick sheaths of fascia divide the muscles of the leg into four compartments—the anterior, deep and superficial posterior, and lateral compartments. The anterior compartment contains the tibialis anterior, extensor digitorum longus, extensor hallucis longus, and peroneus tertius (**Fig. 8.6**). These muscles can easily be remembered by using the mnemonic **T**om, **D**ick, and **H**arry too. Muscles in the deep posterior compartment can also be remembered by the Tom, Dick, and Harry mnemonic, and include the tibialis posterior, flexor digitorum longus, and flexor hallucis longus (**Fig. 8.7**). The superficial posterior compartment houses the gastrocnemius, soleus, and plantaris (**Fig. 8.8**). The lateral compartment contains the peroneus longus and peroneus brevis (**Fig. 8.9**).

The foot contains a number of both intrinsic and extrinsic muscles. The attachments and primary actions of the major extrinsic muscles of the foot, ankle, and leg are summarized in **Table 8.1**.

Nerves and Blood Supply of the Foot, Ankle, and Lower Leg

The sciatic nerve and its branches provide primary innervation for the foot, ankle, and leg (**Fig. 8.10**). Traveling down the posterior aspect of the leg from the lumbosacral spine, the sciatic nerve branches into smaller nerves just proximal to the popliteal fossa. The major branches are the tibial nerve that innervates the poste-

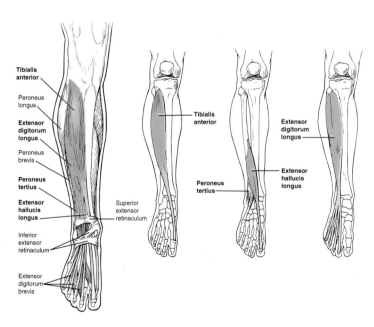

Figure 8.6. The anterior compartment of the leg contains the tibialis anterior, extensor digitorum longus, extensor hallucis longus, and peroneus tertius.

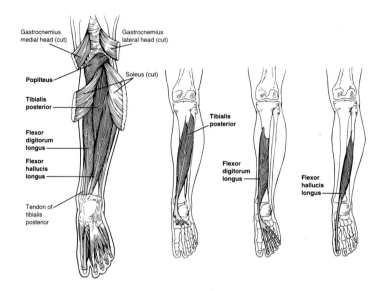

Figure 8.7. The muscles in the deep posterior compartment pass behind the medial malleolus to enter the foot. Using the **T**om, **D**ick, **and** **H**arry mnemonic, the structures pass anterior to posterior in this order: **t**ibialis posterior, flexor **d**igitorum longus, tibialis posterior **a**rtery, tibial **n**erve, and flexor **h**allucis longus.

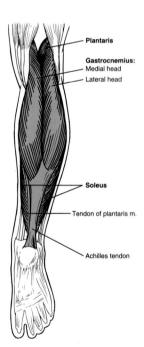

Figure 8.8. The superficial compartment is comprised of the gastrocnemius, soleus, and plantaris. They are collectively known as the triceps surae and attach to the calcaneus via the Achilles tendon.

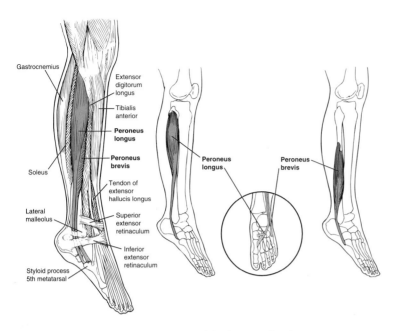

Figure 8.9. The lateral compartment of the leg contains the peroneus brevis and peroneus longus. Note that the peroneus tertius is an extension of the extensor digitorum longus and is in the anterior compartment.

rior aspect of the leg and the common peroneal nerve that spawns the deep and superficial peroneal nerves. Given the extensiveness of the sciatic nerve supply to the lower extremity, it is no surprise that impingement of the sciatic nerve by a herniated disc in the lumbosacral region often results in pain, numbness, and/or impaired function in the foot and ankle region.

The blood supply to the foot, ankle, and leg enters the lower extremity as the femoral artery **(Fig. 8.11)**. The femoral artery becomes the popliteal artery proximal and posterior to the knee, then branches into the anterior and posterior tibial arteries just distal to the knee. The anterior tibial artery becomes the dorsalis pedis artery to supply the dorsum of the foot. The posterior tibial artery gives off several branches that supply the posterior and lateral compartments and the plantar region of the foot.

Did you determine what structures may be causing the pain on the plantar aspect of the midfoot? If you determined the navicular, medial and middle cuneiforms, medial longitudinal arch and associated ligaments, or the tibialis posterior or toe flexors, you are correct.

The leg is innervated by the tibial nerve (posterior compartment), deep peroneal nerve (anterior compartment), and superficial peroneal nerve (lateral compartment)

MAJOR MUSCLE ACTIONS OF THE FOOT, ANKLE, AND LOWER LEG

Many styles of running shoes are designed to control pronation and supination of the foot. At what joint(s) do these motions occur?

Table 8.1. Major Muscles of the Foot and Leg

Muscle	Proximal Attachment	Distal Attachment	Primary Action(s)	Nerve Innervation
Anterior Compartment				
Tibialis anterior	Upper two-thirds lateral tibia & interosseus membrane	Medial surface of first cuneiform & first metatarsal	Dorsiflexion, inversion	Deep peroneal
Extensor digitorum longus	Upper three-fourths anterior fibula & interosseus membrane	Second and third phalanges of four lesser toes	Toe extension, dorsiflexion	Deep peroneal
Extensor hallucis longus	Middle anterior fibula & interosseus membrane	Dorsal surface of distal phalanx of great toe	Extension of great toe	Deep peroneal
Peroneus tertius	Distal third of anterior fibula & interosseus membrane	Dorsal surface styloid process, fifth metatarsal	Eversion, dorsiflexion	Deep peroneal
Lateral Compartment				
Peroneus longus	Proximal two-thirds lateral fibula	Plantar surface of first cuneiform & first metatarsal	Eversion, plantar flexion	Superficial peroneal
Peroneus brevis	Distal two-thirds fibula	Lateral side of styloid process, fifth metatarsal	Eversion, plantar flexion	Superficial peroneal
Posterior Deep Compartment				
Flexor digitorum longus	Posterior tibia	Distal phalanx of four lesser toes	Toe flexion, plantar flexion	Tibial
Flexor hallucis longus	Distal two-thirds posterior fibula	Distal phalanx of the great toe	Flexion of the great toe, plantar flexion	Tibial
Tibialis posterior	Upper two-thirds tibia, fibula & interosseus membrane	Cuboid, navicular, cuneiforms, & 2–4 metatarsals	Inversion, plantar flexion	Tibial
Posterior Superficial Compartment				
Gastrocnemius	Posterior medial & lateral condyles of the femur	Calcaneal tuberosity via Achilles tendon	Plantar flexion, knee flexion	Tibial
Soleus	Posterior proximal fibula and middle tibia	Calcaneal tuberosity via Achilles tendon	Plantar flexion	Tibial
Plantaris	Posterior femur above lateral condyle	Calcaneal tuberosity by Achilles tendon	Plantar flexion, knee flexion	Tibial

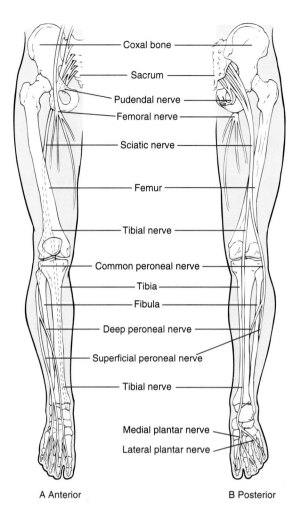

Labels on figure:
- Coxal bone
- Sacrum
- Pudendal nerve
- Femoral nerve
- Sciatic nerve
- Femur
- Tibial nerve
- Common peroneal nerve
- Tibia
- Fibula
- Deep peroneal nerve
- Superficial peroneal nerve
- Tibial nerve
- Medial plantar nerve
- Lateral plantar nerve

A Anterior   B Posterior

Figure 8.10. A, B. Motor function to the lower leg is supplied by the sciatic nerve (L4, L5, S1). Sensory innervation is supplied by the sciatic nerve and saphenous branch of the femoral nerve (L2, L3, L4).

Kinematics is the study of spatial and temporal aspects of motion that translate to movement form or technique. Evaluation of the kinematics of a particular movement can provide information about timing and sequencing of the movement, which can then yield important clues for injury prevention. This section describes the kinematics of the foot, ankle, and lower leg, and identifies muscles responsible for specific movements.

Kinematics
Study of the spatial and temporal aspects of movement

Toe Flexion and Extension

A number of muscles contribute to flexion of the second through fifth toes. These include the flexor digitorum longus, flexor digitorum brevis, quadratus plantae, lumbricals, and interossei. The flexor hallucis longus and brevis produce flexion of the hallux. Conversely, the extensor hallucis longus, extensor digitorum longus, and extensor digitorum brevis are responsible for extension and hyperextension of the toes.

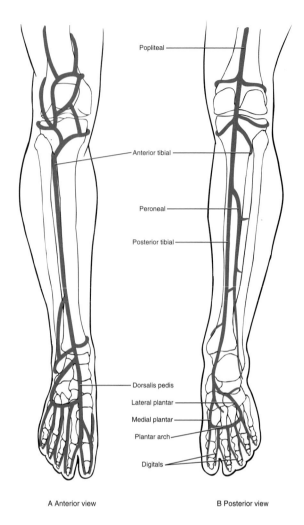

Popliteal

Anterior tibial

Peroneal

Posterior tibial

Dorsalis pedis

Lateral plantar

Medial plantar

Plantar arch

Digitals

A Anterior view

B Posterior view

Figure 8.11. A,B. The blood supply to the leg, ankle, and foot region. The dorsalis pedis artery is easily palpated in the midfoot region between the second and third tendons of the extensor digitorum longus.

Dorsiflexion and Plantar Flexion

Flexion and extension at the ankle are termed dorsiflexion and plantar flexion, respectively **(Fig. 8.12)**. The medial and lateral malleoli serve as pulleys to channel the tendons of the leg muscles either posterior or anterior to the axis of rotation, thereby enabling their contributions to either dorsiflexion or plantar flexion. Muscles with tendons passing anterior to the malleoli, such as tibialis anterior, extensor digitorum longus, and peroneus tertius, are dorsiflexors. Those with tendinous attachments running posterior to the malleoli, such as the soleus, gastrocnemius, and plantaris, contribute to plantar flexion.

Muscles with tendons that pass anterior to the malleoli are dorsiflexors, and tendons that pass posterior are plantar flexors

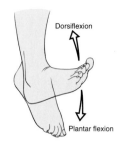

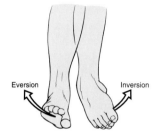

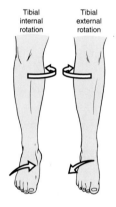

Figure 8.12. Motions of the leg and ankle. Supination of the subtalar joint results in external rotation of the tibia. Pronation is linked with internal rotation of the tibia.

Inversion and Eversion

Rotations of the foot in the medial and lateral directions are termed inversion and eversion, respectively **(Fig. 8.12)**. These movements occur primarily at the subtalar joint, with secondary contributions from gliding movements at the intertarsal and tarsometatarsal joints. The tibialis posterior and tibialis anterior are the major inverters. Peroneus longus and peroneus brevis, with tendons passing behind the lateral malleolus, are primarily responsible for eversion, with assistance provided by the peroneus tertius.

Pronation and Supination

The lower extremity moves through a cyclical sequence of movements during gait. Among these, the action at the subtalar joint during weight bearing has the most significant implications for lower extremity injury potential. During heel contact with the support surface, the hindfoot is typically somewhat inverted. As

Supination

At the foot, combined motions of calcaneal inversion, foot adduction, and plantar flexion

Pronation

At the foot, combined motions of calcaneal eversion, foot abduction, and dorsiflexion

Pes planus

Flat feet

Excessive pronation can result in increased stress within the plantar fascia and Achilles tendon

the foot rolls forward and the forefoot initially contacts the ground, the foot is plantar flexed. This combination of calcaneal inversion, foot adduction, and plantar flexion, all at the subtalar joint, is known as **supination**. During weight bearing at midstance, there is a tendency for calcaneal eversion and foot abduction to occur, as the foot moves into dorsiflexion. These movements are known collectively as **pronation**. Supination of the subtalar joint also results in external rotation of the tibia, with pronation linked to internal tibial rotation (**Fig. 8.12**).

Although a normal amount of pronation is useful in reducing the peak forces sustained during impact, studies have indicated a link between excessive pronation and running-related injuries of the lower extremity (3,4). Normal walking gait typically involves about 6 to 8° of pronation, although individuals with **pes planus** (flat feet) may undergo as much as 10 to 12° of pronation (5). Because pronation also causes a compensatory inward rotation of the tibia, excessive pronation can result in increased stress within the plantar fascia and Achilles tendon.

Pronation and supination occur at the subtalar joint. Combined action of all the major joints of the foot, however, are required for smooth, coordinated locomotion.

PREVENTION OF INJURIES

What exercises should be included in a preseason program to reduce the risk of injury to the foot, ankle, and lower leg region?

Several steps can be taken to reduce the incidence and severity of injury in the foot, ankle, and lower leg. Chapter 6 discussed protective equipment and provided guidelines for proper shoe selection (See **Field Strategy 6.4**). Chapter 7 reviewed common taping and bracing techniques for the region. In addition to external protection, a flexibility and strengthening program should be initiated prior to any sport participation. A tight Achilles tendon has been shown to increase the risk of plantar fasciitis, Achilles tendinitis, and lateral ankle sprains. To build strength in the foot, for example, pick up marbles or dice with the toes and place them in a container close to the foot. Place a tennis ball between the soles of the feet and roll the ball back and forth from the heel to the forefoot. To increase strength in the lower leg muscles, secure elastic tubing around a table leg, place leg in elastic loop, and move the leg through the range of motion. Bilateral toe raises and heel raises may also be used. **Field Strategy 8.1** demonstrates several exercises used to prevent injuries to the foot, ankle, and lower leg.

Strengthening exercises for muscles of the foot and lower leg should be included in a regular preventative program and should be supplemented by an extensive flexibility program. Where appropriate, protective equipment or taping and bracing can be used to support and protect the region.

Field Strategy 8.1. Exercises to Prevent Injury to the Lower Leg

Foot Intrinsic Muscle Exercises

  Plantar fascia stretch. Place a towel around the toes and slowly over-extend them. To stretch the Achilles tendon, combine with dorsiflexion of the ankle

  Towel crunches. Place a towel between the plantar surfaces of the toes and feet. Push the toes and feet together, crunching the towel between the toes

  Toe curls. With the foot resting on a towel, slowly curl the toes under, bunching the towel beneath the foot. Variation: use two feet. Place a book or small weight on the towel for added resistance

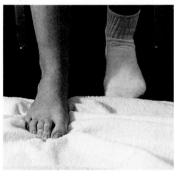

  Picking up objects. Pick up small objects, such as marbles or dice, with the toes and place in a nearby container, or use therapeutic putty to work the toe flexors

  Unilateral balance activities. Stand on uneven surfaces with the eyes first open, then closed

  BAPS board. Seated position: roll the board slowly clockwise then counterclockwise 20 times

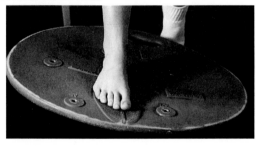

Ankle/Lower Leg Muscle Exercises

  Ankle alphabet. Using the ankle and foot only, trace the letters of the alphabet from A to Z; 3 times with capital letters and 3 times with lowercase.

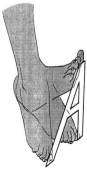

Field Strategy 8.1. Exercises to Prevent Injury to the Lower Leg (continued)

Triceps surae stretch. Keeping the back leg straight and heel on the floor, lean against a wall until tension is felt in the calf muscles (**A**). To isolate the soleus, bend both knees (**B**)

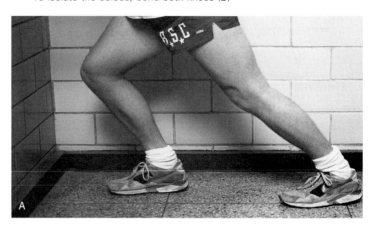

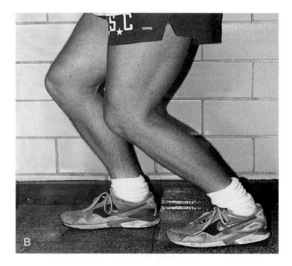

Field Strategy 8.1. Exercises to Prevent Injury to the Lower Leg (continued)

Plantar fascia and triceps surae stretch. Standing with the ball of the foot on a stair step, allow body weight to drop the heels below the step until tension is felt in the arch and calf muscles. Combine with toe raises. Variation: use a tilt board. In both exercises, point the toes outward, straight ahead, and inward to stretch the various fibers of the Achilles tendon

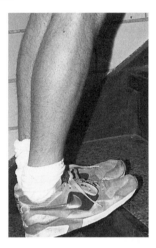

Theraband or surgical tubing exercises. Secure the Theraband or tubing around a table leg and do resisted dorsiflexion, plantar flexion, inversion, and eversion.

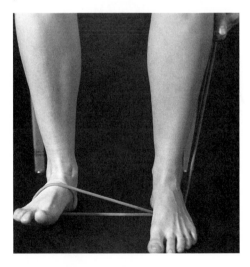

Unilateral balance exercises. Balance on the opposite leg while doing Theraband exercises in all directions.

BAPS board. Standing position: Balance on the involved foot and repeat the process. Additional challenges, such as using no support, or dribbling with a basketball while balancing, can be added.

During practice, a basketball player sensed that a hot spot was developing on the back of the heel from the constant friction between the heel and shoe. What steps can you take to prevent a blister from forming?

Many individuals are at risk for toe and foot problems because of a leg length discrepancy, postural deviation, muscle imbalance, or a malalignment syndrome (pes cavus, pes planus, pes equinus, hammer or claw toes) **(Figs. 8.13 and 8.14)**. Although many of these conditions are minor and may even be asymptomatic, each condition can become painful and disabling.

Turf Toe

Turf toe is caused by jamming the great toe into the end of the shoe, or hyperextending the MTP joint of the great toe. It is related to artificial turf, lightweight shoes that are too flexible, and positions that require forced hyperextension of the toes, as in football linebackers and offensive lineman. The individual will have pain, tenderness, and swelling at the MTP joint of the great toe. The push-off phase of running is particularly painful, as is passive extension of the great toe. Initial treatment involves ice therapy, NSAIDs, rest, and protection from excessive motion. Taping to limit motion at the MTP joint, a metatarsal pad to lower

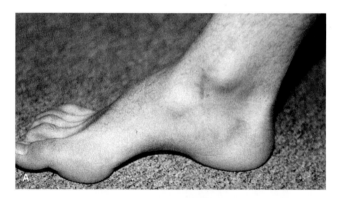

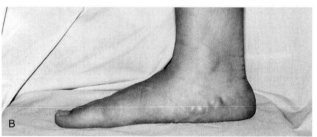

Figure 8.13. Common foot deformities. (**A**) Pes cavus. (**B**) Pes planus.

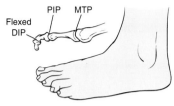

A Hammer toe

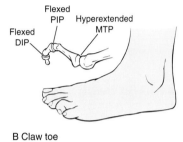

B Claw toe

Figure 8.14. Toe deformities. (**A**) A hammer toe is a flexion deformity of the DIP joint. (**B**) A claw toe involves hyperextension of the MTP joint and hyperflexion of the DIP and PIP joints.

stress on the first metatarsal, or use of a stiff-soled shoe may be helpful. Running is not permitted until the individual is asymptomatic (6).

Hammer and Claw Toes

Although often congenital, hammer and claw toes can occur because of improperly fitted shoes, muscle contractures, or malalignment of bony structures. **Hammer toes** are a flexion deformity of the DIP joint. **Claw toes** involve hyperextension of the MTP joint and hyperflexion of the DIP and PIP joints (**Fig. 8.14**). Both can lead to painful callus formation on the dorsum of the toe or under the metatarsal head, particularly the second toe. A metatarsal pad may assist in controlling symptoms, but surgical resection of the head of the proximal phalanx is often necessary to treat the condition.

Ingrown Toenail

Improper cutting of the toenails, improper shoe size, or constant sliding of the foot inside the shoe can traumatize the nail, causing its edge to grow into the lateral nail fold and surrounding skin. The nail margin reddens and becomes inflamed and painful. If a fungal/bacteria infection is present, the condition is called **paronychia**. Two methods to treat this condition are discussed in **Field Strategy 8.2**.

Blisters and Calluses

Blisters and calluses are caused by excessive localized pressure or friction between the foot and improperly fitted shoes or from constant sliding of the foot inside a shoe. Shearing forces cause

Hammer toes
A flexion deformity of the DIP joint of the toes

Claw toes
A toe deformity characterized by hyperextension of the metatarsophalangeal (MTP) joint and hyperflexion of the interphalangeal (IP) joints

Improper cutting of the toe nail, improper shoe size, or constant sliding of the foot inside the shoe can lead to ingrown toenails

Paronychia
A fungal/bacterial infection in the folds of skin surrounding a fingernail or toenail

Blisters, calluses, and corns are caused by excessive localized pressure against the foot and toes from improperly fitted shoes, constant sliding of the foot inside a shoe, or with certain toe conditions

Field Strategy 8.2. Prevention and Management of an Ingrown Toenail

Prevention

Cut toenails straight across to prevent the edges from growing under the skin on the side of the nail

Allow the toenail to be long enough to extend beyond the underlying skin, but short enough so as not to push into the shoe toe box

Wear properly fitted shoes and socks

Management—Method 1

Soak the involved toe in hot water (108° to 116°) until the nail bed is soft (usually 10 to 15 minutes)

Lift the edge of the nail and place a small piece of cotton under the nail to elevate the nail out of the skinfold (**A**)

Apply antiseptic to the area and cover with a sterile dressing

Repeat the procedure daily; keep the area clean and dry

If a purulent infection is present, refer to a physician for antibiotics and drainage of the infection

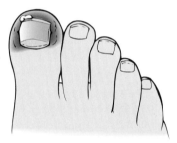

A

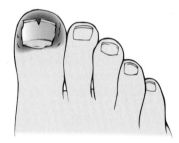

B

Management—Method 2

Soak the toe as above and cut a V in the center of the nail (**B**)

As the nail grows, its edges will pull toward the center, drawing the nail edges from under the skin

Apply an antiseptic, cover with a sterile dressing, and keep the area clean and dry

If a purulent infection is present, refer to a physician for antibiotics and drainage of the infection

skin irritation and fluid accumulation to separate the skin layers. Often the fluid is clear; however, blood may be mixed with the fluid. The blister should not be opened unless absolutely necessary, as this opens an avenue for infection. Ice application may cause the fluid to resorb on its own. If the blister is large and painful, special steps should be taken to drain the blister and prevent further friction and fluid formation. **Field Strategy 8.3** explains the management of blisters.

Calluses on the plantar aspect of the foot are treated with a felt or commercial metatarsal pad secured proximal to the head. Regular debridement with a callus file or emery board can help keep calluses to a minimum. If you feel an edge on the callus, it is too thick and needs to be reduced. A large callus can become detached from the underlying skin layer, tearing small capillaries, leading to a blood blister under the callus. Do not drain the blood, as it opens an avenue for infection. Soak the foot in ice water, apply a compression pad over the area, and elevate the foot whenever possible, to assist in reabsorption of the blood and fluid. If drainage is necessary, refer to a physician.

> Regular debridement with a callus board or callus shaver can keep calluses to a minimum

 ### Field Strategy 8.3. Prevention and Management of Blisters

Prevention

Wear properly fitted shoes and one pair of sweat socks
Break the shoes in gradually during practice
Lubricants, such as petroleum jelly, can be applied to susceptible areas
Toes glides, a Teflon-coated paper, can be worn under the socks to relieve friction in the toes and ball of the foot
Wear heel and lace pads under an ankle strapping to prevent rubbing and chafing

Management

If a hot spot arises, apply cryotherapy (ice massage, ice bags, or ice immersion) to reduce local heat caused by the friction. Pad the area to protect it
If fluid-filled, apply latex gloves and cleanse the area with soap and water or an iodine-providine solution. Lance the blister with a sterile number 11 scalpel, scissors, or a large needle. The optimal place for drainage is the most inferior junction between the intact skin and blister. Do not remove the skin overlying the blister, as this helps to prevent infection
Drain the fluid with a sterile gauze pad. Place an antibiotic cream under the fold of skin and cover with a sterile dressing or 2nd skin. This can be secured with a thin strip of moleskin or several strips of adhesive tape. A doughnut pad may create additional friction because of the added bulk, and should not be used
Recheck the area daily for signs of infection (redness or pus). After 3 to 4 days, trim the dead skin, apply an antibiotic ointment, and cover the area with a sterile dressing
If a blood blister is present, follow the same procedure.

Morton's Neuroma

Morton's neuroma is characterized by pain on the plantar side of the foot, primarily in the second and third metatarsal space, that often radiates into the respective toes (**Fig. 8.15**). Occasionally it is preceded by **metatarsalgia**. The plantar nerves become compressed between the metatarsal heads due to tight-fitting shoes or a pronated foot. This leads to a painful irritation of the nerves, or **neuritis**. Conservative management involves a wider toe box and a lower heel, metatarsal pads, and NSAIDs, but local corticosteroid injections or a surgical incision may be necessary to remedy the situation (6).

Bunions (Hallux Valgus)

Bunions are typically found on the medial aspect of the MTP joint of the great toe, but when they occur on the lateral aspect of the fifth toe they are called bunionettes. Pronation of the foot, arthritis, and generalized ligamentous laxity can lead to an inflammation of the bursa overlying the medial side of the first metatarsal head as it is constantly rubbed against the inside of the shoe. As the condition worsens, the great toe may shift laterally and overlap the second toe, leading to a rigid nonfunctional hallux valgus deformity (**Fig. 8.16**). This condition is exacerbated by high heels and pointed shoe toe boxes, factors that account for women having this condition more often than men. Once the deformity has occurred, little can be done. Although strapping the great toe as closely to proper anatomical position as possible and wearing wider shoes can provide some relief, surgical correction is indicated in severe cases.

Bursitis (Pump Bump, Runner's Bump)

External pressure from a constrictive heel cup, excessive pronation, or a poorly supported and poorly padded heel counter in the shoe can lead to swelling, erythema (redness of the skin), and irritation of bursa associated with the Achilles tendon. The retrocalcaneal bursa is located between the anterior Achilles ten-

Metatarsalgia
A condition involving general discomfort around the metatarsal's heads

Neuritis
Inflammation or irritation of a nerve commonly found between the third and fourth metatarsal heads

Bunions typically occur on the medial aspect of the MTP joint of the great toe, but when they occur on the lateral aspect of the fifth toe they are called bunionettes

When bursitis is suspected, pain can be palpated in the soft tissue just anterior to the Achilles tendon

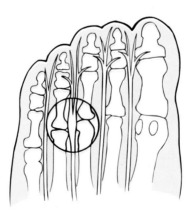

Figure 8.15. Plantar's neuroma (Morton's neuroma) is caused by pinching the interdigital nerve between the metatarsal heads. While weight bearing in shoes, the individual will have an agonizing pain on the lateral side of the foot, but will be relieved when going barefoot.

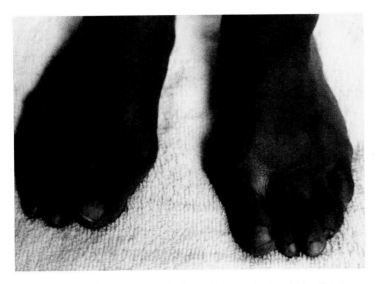

Figure 8.16. Bunions are generally formed by constantly rubbing the medial aspect of the MTP joint of the great toe against the inside of the shoe. The toe then shifts laterally, forming the hallux valgus deformity.

don insertion and calcaneus **(Fig. 8.17)**. Pain is elicited when you reach around the Achilles tendon to palpate the soft tissue just anterior to the tendon. Active plantar flexion during push-off compresses the bursa between the tendon and bone, leading to increased irritation and pain. Treatment involves ice therapy, NSAIDs, gentle stretching exercises for the Achilles tendon, shoe modification, or a heel lift to relieve external pressure on the bursa. Occasionally, an inflamed bursa can lead to a dramatic large mass referred to as a "pump bump," and is commonly seen in figure skaters and runners (runner's bump). This bump may be related to an underlying bony spur caused by frequent microtrauma or microavulsions surrounding the distal attachment of the Achilles tendon.

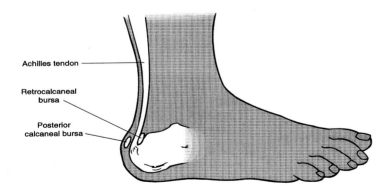

Figure 8.17. The retrocalcaneal bursa is commonly inflamed when it is pinched between the Achilles tendon and calcaneus during plantar flexion.

Field Strategy 8.4. Prevention and Management of Athlete's Foot

Prevention

Shower after every practice and competition

Always dry the feet thoroughly after every shower, especially between the toes

Apply absorbant powder, such as Desenex and Tinactin, to the shoes, socks, and feet, especially between toes

Change socks daily and allow wet shoes to dry thoroughly before wearing them

Wear nonocclusive street shoes

Clean and disinfect the floors in the shower room, dressing room, and training room daily

Management

Apply topical antifungal agents, such as Micatin, Tinactin, Lotrimin, and Halotex, twice daily for 1 month

In resistant infections, oral griseofulvin can be used for 4 to 8 weeks

Follow proper foot hygiene as listed above

Athlete's Foot

Tinea pedis

A fungal infection including small vesicles, itching, and scaling between the toes

Athlete's foot, or **tinea pedis**, is a common fungal infection that can spread during casual handling of contaminated socks or can be picked up by another player on the floor or shower stall. It is, however, based on individual susceptibility and may not affect certain people. The condition is characterized by extreme itching, burning, and irritation on the sole of the foot and between the toes. Scratching leads to scaling, peeling, and cracking fissures in the skin, particularly between the toes. **Field Strategy 8.4** summarizes the prevention and management of athlete's foot.

Did you determine what steps might be taken to prevent the hot spot from becoming a blister? You might immerse the heel in ice water to cool the hot spot, apply a lubricant to the area to facilitate sliding inside the shoe, or you may recommend that the player wear another pair of shoes that fit more comfortably, until the other shoes are broken in.

CONTUSIONS

A softball player was hit on the shin by a line drive. What should be done immediately to control inflammation? Are there any complications that may arise from the injury?

Contusions of the foot and leg frequently result from direct trauma, such as dropping a weight on the foot, being stepped on, being kicked, or being hit by a speeding ball or implement. Although many of the injuries are minor and easily treated with immediate ice therapy, compression, elevation, and rest, a few injuries can result in complications.

Foot Contusions

Most contusions to the foot can be treated with ice, compression, and elevation. When pain and edema have subsided, the area can be padded to safely return the individual to participation. A contusion to the hindfoot, called a "**heel bruise**," can be more serious. Elastic adipose tissue lies between the thick skin and plantar aspect of the calcaneus. It is constantly subjected to extreme stresses in running, jumping, and changing directions. Excessive body weight, age, poorly cushioned or worn-out running shoes, increases in training, and hard, uneven training surfaces can also complicate this condition. Ice treatments to minimize pain and inflammation should be followed by regular use of a heel cup or doughnut pad. Despite excellent care, the condition may persist for months.

Heel bruise
Contusion to the subcutaneous fat pad located over the inferior aspect of the calcaneus

Lower Leg Contusions

Contusions to the gastrocnemius result in immediate pain, weakness, and partial loss of motion. Hemorrhage and muscle spasm quickly lead to a tender, firm mass that is easily palpable. While applying ice, keep the muscle on static stretch to decrease muscle spasm. If the condition does not improve in 2 to 3 days, refer the individual to a physician.

Contusions to the gastrocnemius result in immediate pain, weakness, and partial loss of motion

The shin is particularly vulnerable to direct blows that irritate the periosteal tissue around the tibia. This contusion, called a **shin bruise**, can be prevented by wearing appropriate shin guards to protect this highly vulnerable area. Although painful, the condition can be managed with ice, compression, elevation, and rest. A doughnut pad over the area and additional shin protection can allow the individual to participate.

Shin bruise
A contusion to the tibia, sometimes referred to as tibial periostitis

Acute Compartment Syndrome

A direct blow to the anterolateral aspect of the leg can lead to a crushing injury, fracture, or circulatory occlusion. The rapid accumulation of hemorrhage and edema can lead to circulatory and tissue dysfunction within 30 minutes of onset and may become a medical emergency. Signs and symptoms include increasing pain and swelling over the anterior compartment that does not cease with rest. A firm mass, tight skin (because it has been stretched to its limits from the edema), loss of sensation between the great toe and second toe on the dorsum of the foot, and diminished pulse at the dorsalis pedis are all late and dangerous signs. Immediate action is necessary, because irreversible damage can occur within 12 to 24 hours. Immediate care involves ice and total rest. Compression is not recommended because the compartment is already unduly compressed, and additional external compression will only hasten the deterioration. Furthermore, the limb must not be elevated, as this decreases arterial pressure and further compromises capillary filling. Referral to a physician for immediate care is absolutely necessary.

If you suspect an acute compartment syndrome, immediate action is necessary, since irreversible damage can occur within 12 to 24 hours

The softball player was struck on the anterior leg. After applying standard acute care, did you determine that the individual should be watched for a possible anterior compartment syndrome? If so, you are correct.

FOOT AND ANKLE SPRAINS

After going up for a rebound, a basketball player stepped on the foot of an opponent and rolled off the side of the foot, inverting the ankle. Although the player iced the ankle during the night, the ankle appeared swollen and discolored the next morning and ached while walking. What may have been overlooked in the initial ankle evaluation?

Sprains to the foot and ankle region constitute about 25% of all injuries that occur in running and jumping sports, with 75% of these injuries occurring as ankle sprains (7). Uneven terrain, stepping in a hole, landing on another player's foot and sliding off the side, or muscle strength imbalance are all contributing factors to sprains in this vulnerable area.

Toe and Foot Sprains/Dislocations

Sprains and dislocations of the toes may occur by tripping or stubbing the toe. Pain, dysfunction, immediate swelling, and, if dislocated, gross deformity are clearly evidence of a sprain or dislocation. Radiographs should be taken to determine a possible fracture, but closed reduction and strapping to the next toe for 10 to 14 days is usually sufficient to remedy the problem.

Midfoot sprains are more frequent in activities in which the foot is unsupported, such as in gymnastics or dance, where slippers are typically worn, or in track athletes, who wear running flats. Pain and swelling is deep on the medial aspect of the foot and weight bearing may be very painful. Depending on the location and severity of pain, adequate strapping, arch supports, and limited weight bearing is warranted during the acute stage. If the condition does not improve, refer the individual to a physician. Reconditioning exercises should include range of motion and strengthening for the intrinsic muscles of the foot.

> Midfoot sprains are more frequently seen in activities in which the foot is unsupported

Lateral Ankle Sprains

Acute inversion ankle sprains commonly occur when stress is applied to the ankle during plantar flexion and inversion, injuring the anterior talofibular ligament. If the strain continues, the medial malleolus acts as a fulcrum to further invert and stretch or rupture the calcaneofibular ligament (**Fig. 8.18**). The peroneal tendons can absorb some strain to prevent this ligament from being injured; however, if the peroneal muscles are weak, they are unable to stabilize the joint. With severe injuries, the posterior talofibular ligament is also involved.

> If the peroneal muscles are weak, they cannot help stabilize the joint, leading to tearing of the calcaneofibular ligament

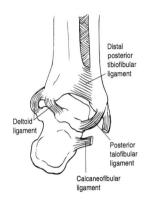

Distal
posterior
tibiofibular
ligament

Deltoid
ligament

Posterior
talofibular
ligament

Calcaneofibular
ligament

Figure 8.18. During inversion, the medial malleolus acts like a fulcrum to further invert the talus, leading to stretching or tearing of the calcaneofibular ligament.

The individual will usually report a cracking or tearing sound at the time of injury. Swelling and ecchymosis will be rapid and diffuse. Point tenderness will be localized over the anterior talofibular ligament and may extend over the calcaneofibular ligament. After assessment for possible fracture and ligamentous damage, initial treatment should consist of ice therapy, compression (with or without a horseshoe pad), elevation, and restricted activity. If the individual is unable to bear weight, crutches should be used. **Field Strategy 8.5** summarizes management of lateral ankle sprains. If chronic pain persists during the rehabilitation process, the individual should be referred to a physician. The pain may indicate lateral ankle instability, a previously undetected trauma, an impingement disorder, congenital abnormality, or a tumor (8).

Medial Ankle Sprains

Eversion ankle sprains are less common than inversion ankle sprains because of the strong deltoid ligament and bony structure of the ankle joint. In mild to moderate injuries, the individual may report pain at the ankle when it was initially everted, but as the ankle returns to its normal anatomical position, pain subsides. The individual continues to play, only to have the pain slowly intensify. Swelling may not be as evident as in a lateral sprain. Point tenderness can be elicited over the deltoid ligament and the anterior and posterior joint line. If standard acute care does not reduce the symptoms, referral to a physician is warranted to determine the presence of more extensive ligamentous disruption or fracture.

After seeing the swollen ankle the next day, did you reassess the ankle for possible fracture? If fracture tests are negative, continue ice therapy, apply a horseshoe pad or open basketweave strapping, and elastic wrap for compression, and fit the individual with crutches. If pain persists, refer the individual to a physician.

Field Strategy 8.5. Management of a Lateral Ankle Sprain

	Signs and Symptoms	Treatment
First degree	Pain and swelling on anterolateral aspect of lateral malleolus Point tenderness over anterior talofibular ligament No laxity with stress tests	Immediate ice therapy with wet-wrap compression and elevation 15 to 20 minutes; repeat every hour until swelling is controlled Apply horseshoe pad or open basketweave with tape and/or elastic wrap to protect area, but instruct individual to remove elastic wrap during sleeping If limping, fit with crutches Reassess in the morning and start rehabilitation
Second degree	Tearing or popping sensation felt on lateral aspect Pain and swelling on anterolateral and inferior aspect of lateral malleolus Painful palpation over anterior talofibular and calcaneofibular ligaments. May also be tender over posterior talofibular, deltoid ligament, and anterior capsule area Positive anterior drawer and talar tilt test	Treatment as above If fracture is suspected, refer to physician
Third degree	Tearing or popping sensation felt on lateral aspect Diffuse swelling over entire lateral aspect with or without anterior swelling Can be very painful or absent of pain right after injury Positive anterior drawer and talar tilt test	Suspect possible fracture Immobilize and apply ice Fit with crutches and refer to physician (A short walking cast may need to be applied)

ACUTE STRAINS OF THE FOOT AND LOWER LEG

A middle-aged tennis player was playing on a cool day when the individual felt a sudden, painful tearing sensation in the calf, leading to immediate disability. What factors have contributed to this injury and how you will manage this acute condition?

Direct blows or chronic overuse frequently strain the muscles of the foot and lower leg. **Tenosynovitis** is a condition caused by friction and subsequent irritation between the tendon and its surrounding sheath. The muscles and tendons that run across the dorsum of the foot may be injured as a result of shoe laces being tied too tight or having the feet repeatedly stepped on. Pain and localized edema may be present. During assessment, the involved

Tenosynovitis
Inflammation of a tendon sheath

tendon(s) will have pain on passive stretching and active and resisted motion. Palpation during active motion may reveal a sound similar to that heard when crunching a snowball together, hence the sound is called "**snowball**" crepitation. Treatment involves ice therapy, NSAIDs, and strapping to limit active motion of the musculotendinous unit. Range of motion and strengthening exercises should be started once acute pain has subsided.

Snowball crepitation
Sound similar to that heard while crunching snow into a snowball; indicative of tenosynovitis

Muscle Cramps

Although the specific nature of cramping is unknown, it is commonly attributed to dehydration, electrolyte imbalance, or prolonged muscle fatigue. For some, acute spasms may waken them in the night following a day of strenuous exercise. Acute cramps are best treated with ice, pressure, and slow stretch of the muscle as it begins to relax. Prevention involves an adequate water intake during strenuous activity and a regular stretching program for the gastrocnemius-soleus complex. When participation may extend over 2 hours in hot weather, water intake with a weak electrolyte solution should be increased during and after strenuous activity.

Muscles cramps are associated with dehydration, electrolyte imbalance, or prolonged muscle fatigue

Lower Leg Tendon Strains

Lower leg tendon strains may be acute or chronic. If acute, the individual may experience a tearing sensation, followed by an inability to walk without intense pain. Swelling and tenderness is typically localized over the involved tendon and may lead to acute tendinitis and tenosynovitis. If the tendon ruptures, a painful pop can be felt. Point tenderness, swelling, and muscle weakness will be present. In chronic conditions, symptoms progressively get worse, until the pain becomes overwhelming. Treatment will depend on the severity of injury, and may include ice therapy, NSAIDs, restricted activity, support with tape, or a heel pad on both feet to relieve tension on posterior muscles. In chronic cases involving a partial tear of a tendon, painful, palpable nodular scar tissue may build up in the tendon sheath, requiring surgical debridement.

Achilles Tendon Rupture

Rupture of the Achilles tendon is probably the most severe acute muscular problem in the lower leg. Nearly 75% of these injuries are seen in muscular male athletes between the ages of 30 to 40 who participate in intermittent athletic activities (9). The usual mechanism is a push-off of the forefoot while the knee is extending, a common move in many propulsive activities. Because of the poor blood supply, most ruptures occur 1 to 2 inches proximal to the distal attachment of the tendon on the calcaneus **(Fig. 8.19)**. The individual experiences sharp pain and hears or feels a characteristic "pop" sensation in the tendon area. A common sensation is that of being struck in the back of the leg (9). Other symptoms

Achilles tendon ruptures are commonly seen in muscular male athletes between the ages of 30 to 40 years old who participate intermittently in athletic activities

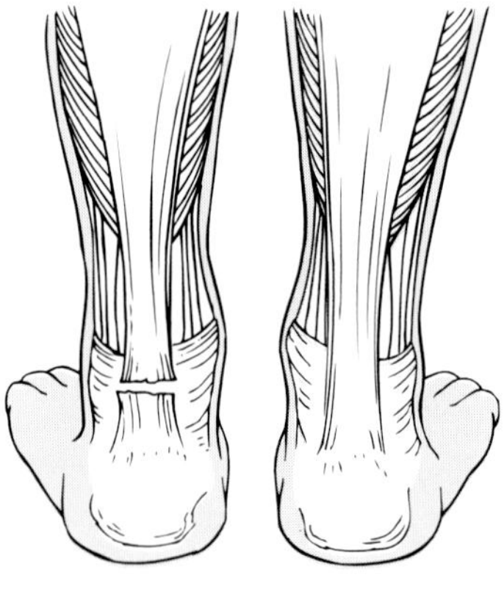

Figure 8.19. The Achilles tendon is often ruptured 1 to 2 inches proximal to its distal attachment. The individual will hear and feel a characteristic "pop" sensation of being kicked in the tendon.

include a visible defect in the tendon, inability to stand on tiptoes or even balance on the affected leg, swelling and bruising around the malleoli, and excessive passive dorsiflexion. A compression wrap should be applied from the toes to the knee and the individual should be referred immediately to a physician.

💡 *Did you determine that the middle-aged tennis player probably strained the gastrocnemius muscle? Age, physical condition, and cool climate may have contributed to this injury. What suggestions might you make to prevent the injury from recurring?*

OVERUSE CONDITIONS

❓ *During pre-season track, a novice distance runner is complaining about pain along the distal medial tibial border at the beginning of the workout. As activity progresses, the pain diminishes only to recur hours after activity has ended. What factors may have initiated this condition? How will you manage this injury?*

The leg is subjected to a number of overuse conditions. Repetitive overloading of tendinous structures leads to inflammation that overwhelms the tissue's ability to repair itself. Other factors, such as faulty biomechanics, poor cushioning or stiff-soled shoes, or excessive downhill running, all contribute to inflammation of the tendons. Many individuals complain of vague leg pain caused by activity, but will have no history of a specific injury that caused the pain.

> A common complaint with overuse injuries is pain brought on by activity

Plantar Fasciitis

Excessive tightness of the Achilles tendon, excessive or prolonged pronation, or obesity can overload the plantar fascia origin on the calcaneus during weight-bearing activities. Predisposing factors include training errors, overuse, hyperpronation, poor strength and/or flexibility of the triceps surae and Achilles tendon, degenerative changes, and systemic disorders (10). The individual will complain of pain upon arising in the morning that diminishes within 5 to 10 minutes, but builds throughout the day. Point tenderness is elicited over the medial calcaneus and increases with forefoot dorsiflexion and toe extension. Treatment may involve relative rest, ice massage, ultrasound, NSAIDs, stretching exercises for the Achilles tendon and toe flexors, intrinsic muscle strengthening, and use of a heel lift, doughnut pad, or figure-eight strapping for support. Circular strips of tape around the foot, however, are contraindicated, because they may overstretch the fascia and prolong recovery. Athletes with hyperpronation may also benefit from rigid, semirigid, or flexible orthoses, or an antipronatory shoe (straight last with good hindfoot control). Running shoes should be flexible at the ball of the foot, but not in the middle of the arch (10). **Field Strategy 8.6** explains the management of plantar fasciitis.

With plantar fasciitis, pain is elicited over the medial tubercle of the calcaneus and increases with forefoot dorsiflexion and toe extension

Achilles Tendinitis

Achilles tendinitis is the most common form of tendinitis seen in athletes. Risk factors include vascular insufficiency, a tight heel cord, Achilles contractures, hyperpronation, repetitive heel running, a recent change in shoes or running surface, a sudden increase in distance or intensity during a workout session, or excessive hill climbing (6,9). Pain is present during and after activity and increases with passive dorsiflexion and resisted plantar flexion.

 ## Field Strategy 8.6. Management of Plantar Fasciitis

Signs and Symptoms

Pain in the foot upon arising in the morning, particularly in the proximal medial longitudinal arch
Point tenderness can be elicited just over and distal to the medial calcaneal tubercle
Passive extension of the great toe and dorsiflexion of the ankle will increase pain and discomfort
Pain increases with weight bearing
Initial pain is relieved with activity, but returns with rest
As condition worsens, pain will be present during and after activity

Treatment

Stop running. Use ice massage 3 times/day for 10 to 12 minutes
NSAIDs for about 3 weeks
Insert a shock-absorbing heel pad or soft plantar arch orthotic that controls excessive pronation
Figure-eight strapping may help during activity

Rehabilitation

Heel cord stretching 3 times/day in three positions: toes straight ahead, toes in, and toes out
Initiate gentle isometric contractions for intrinsic muscles of the foot and progress to active range of motion within pain-free ranges (toe curls, marble pick-up, towel crunches, and towel curls to fatigue)
Maintain cardiovascular fitness with nonweight-bearing activities

---

Point tenderness can be elicited on the tendon and diffuse or localized swelling can be seen. Occasionally, fine crepitation can be palpated in the middle of the tendon during movement, indicating friction between the tendon and its sheath.

Acute treatment involves decreasing inflammation with a cold whirlpool bath, ice massage, or contrast bath, NSAIDs, 3/8 inch heel lifts, and decreasing activity by at least 50%. An intensive stretching and strengthening exercise program must also be developed for the gastrocnemius and soleus muscles. Once inflammation has decreased, low-impact activities, such as a stationary bike, rowing, stair climbing, or exercise with surgical tubing, can begin. High-impact exercises should be avoided until all symptoms are resolved and low-impact activity is tolerated (9). In moderate to severe cases, nonactivity may be necessary for 3 weeks and the individual may be required to wear corrective orthotics.

Medial Tibial Stress Syndrome (MTSS)

> In MTSS, pain initially is present at the start of activity, but diminishes as activity progresses only to recur hours after activity has ceased

Medial tibial stress syndrome encompasses any pain along the posteromedial tibial border, usually in the distal third, not associated with a stress fracture or compartment syndrome (11). Contributing factors include excessive pronation, prolonged pronation, and recent changes in running distance, speed, form, stretching, footwear, or running surface. Pain is initially present at the start of activity, but as activity progresses, pain diminishes, only to recur hours after activity has ceased. In later stages, pain will be present before, during, and after activity, and may restrict performance. Pain is aggravated by active plantar flexion and inversion of the ankle, indicating strain of the tibialis posterior muscle.

Cryotherapy, NSAIDs, and activity modification, such as non-impact or low-impact activities, relieve initial acute symptoms. Pain-free stretching of the heel cord and deep posterior musculature will improve joint mobility and increase muscle and tendon strength and coordination. **Field Strategy 8.7** summarizes management of medial tibial stress syndrome.

Exercise-induced Compartment Syndrome

> **Compartment syndrome**
> Condition in which increased intramuscular pressure impedes blood flow and function of tissues within that compartment

A **compartment syndrome** exists when increased intracompartmental pressure during exercise impedes blood flow and function of the tissues within that compartment. Although the condition may be either acute or chronic, chronic compartment syndrome is more common, and frequently involves the anterior and deep posterior compartments of the lower leg. Virtually any injury (fracture, strain, contusion, or overuse condition) associated with bleeding or edema formation within the compartment can lead to a compartment syndrome (12).

Chronic lower leg pain usually arises at a specific point in the training session, depending on speed and terrain, and does not seem to worsen over time. Pain, often described as a deep cramping sensation and feeling of fullness in the midthird of the leg, is

Field Strategy 8.7. Management of Medial Tibial Stress Syndrome

Signs and Symptoms

Initial pain begins at start of activity, then ceases, but recurs hours after activity stops

In late stages, pain is present before, during, and after activity

In experienced runners, condition is usually secondary to mechanical abnormalities

Pain is along posterior medial border of tibia in a 3- to 6-cm area, usually in distal third

Pain is aggravated by active plantar flexion and inversion of ankle (posterior tibialis muscle)

Treatment

Rest, ice, compression, elevation, and NSAIDs

If condition does not improve in 2 to 3 days, refer to physician for a possible bone scan to rule out a stress fracture

Evaluate and correct any foot anomaly

Increase flexibility in the heel cord and tibialis posterior

Increase strength in the deep posterior muscles

Change running surface and possibly shoes

---

relieved by rest, usually within 20 minutes of exercise, only to recur on returning to exercise. About 50% to 70% of individuals will have bilateral involvement, with one side being somewhat worse (13). In a chronic anterior compartment syndrome, dorsiflexion is limited and weak. If swelling becomes excessive within the fascial compartment, pressure on the deep neurovascular structures leads to numbness and tingling in the foot and toes. Conservative treatment involves cryotherapy, NSAIDs, and activity modification. Intrinsic factors, such as muscle imbalance, flexibility, and limb alignments (especially hindfoot pronation), are addressed with strengthening and stretching exercises and orthoses; however, these efforts may not be effective (13). If no improvement is seen, refer the individual to a physician.

Did you determine the runner may have medial tibial stress syndrome? If so, you are correct. This individual may be putting in too much mileage before the bones and muscles can adapt to the increased load. As part of the assessment, check foot alignment, gait, and shoes for problems that may have contributed to the condition. Watch this individual for any signs that may indicate the development of a possible stress fracture or compartment syndrome.

FRACTURES

A volleyball player is complaining of pain in the forefoot region. When you encircle the region and compress the metatarsals together, the individual winces in pain, but says it only hurts "a little." What should you suspect?

> Pain often arises at a specific point in the training session and does not seem to worsen over time, but is relieved by rest within 20 minutes of exercise, only to recur upon resumption of activity

Sever's disease
A traction-type injury, or osteochondrosis, of the calcaneal apophysis, seen in young adolescents

Amenorrhea
Absence or abnormal cessation of menstruation

Oligomenorrhea
Menstruation involving scant blood loss

Bipartite
Having two parts

Fractures in the foot and lower leg region seldom result from a single traumatic episode. Often, repetitive microtraumas lead to apophyseal or stress fractures, or tensile forces associated with severe ankle sprains lead to avulsion fractures.

In adolescents aged 10 to 15, a special condition called **Sever's disease**, or calcaneal apophysitis, occurs on the calcaneus where the Achilles tendon attaches. Being kicked in the region or landing off-balance may also lead to this condition. The individual will complain of posterior heel pain during activity. Palpable heel pain occurs just below the Achilles tendon attachment. The condition usually resolves itself with closure of the apophysis. Until then, rest, NSAIDs, heel lifts, or strapping the foot in slight plantar flexion to relieve some strain on the Achilles tendon will usually relieve symptoms.

Stress fractures are often seen in running and jumping, particularly after a significant increase in the training regimen or changing to a less resilient surface, or in individuals who wear shoes that no longer provide adequate padding or support for the foot. Women with **amenorrhea** and **oligomenorrhea** have a higher incidence of stress fractures of the foot and leg during sport activity (14). The neck of the second metatarsal is the most common site for a stress fracture, but they may occur in any bone. Metatarsal stress fractures produce pain on weight bearing and will have swelling and point tenderness over the fracture site. Encircling the forefoot with your hand and squeezing the fingers together will produce added discomfort. Stress fractures to the calcaneus produce significant pain on heel strike, as does squeezing the calcaneus.

The two sesamoid bones of the great toe are often fractured as a result of constant weight bearing on a hyperextended great toe, or because of prolonged pronation during running. Pain and swelling are present on the ball of the foot and the individual will be unable to roll through the foot to stand on the toes. Radiographs may be inconclusive, because it is common for sesamoid bones to be **bipartite**.

Stress fractures to the tibia and fibula occur as a result of repetitive stress to the leg, leading to muscle fatigue. Symptoms begin with mild discomfort during running, but decrease or stop after activity and when nonweight bearing. Localized pain over the fracture site can be elicited with percussion or vibration. Bone scans usually reveal the presence of a fracture long before it becomes evident on radiographs (**Fig. 8.20**). Early treatment involves ice therapy, NSAIDs, activity modification, and correcting any factors that may have contributed to the condition. Most stress fractures heal in 4 to 6 weeks, but can take as long as 12 weeks. The individual should be asymptomatic before returning to participation.

Avulsion fractures can occur at the site of any ligamentous or tendinous attachment, due to excessive tensile forces. In eversion, the deltoid ligament may avulse a portion of the distal medial

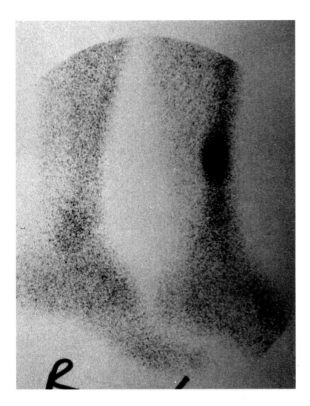

Figure 8.20. Bone scans detect stress fractures long before the fractures become apparent on x-rays.

malleolus rather than tear the ligament. Inversion ankle sprains may cause the peroneus brevis tendon to avulse the base of the fifth metatarsal, called a **Jones fracture**. Healing may be delayed or may result in a **nonunion fracture**. Unless there is wide displacement, a short leg cast and weight bearing, as tolerated, is employed.

Displaced and undisplaced fractures result from direct compression in acute trauma (e.g., falling from a height or being stepped on) or from combined compression and shearing forces, such as during a severe twisting action. Signs of fracture include pain, swelling, ecchymosis, deformity, grating or crepitus, guarding, or exposed bone ends. Assessment and recognition is confirmed through the use of palpation, percussion, compression, and distraction (see **Fig. 3.16**). For specific techniques used to determine a possible fracture in the foot and lower leg, refer to **Field Strategy 8.10**.

Because of the proximity of major blood vessels and nerves, many fractures necessitate immediate immobilization and referral to the nearest trauma center. The neurovascular integrity should be assessed before and after immobilization by taking a distal pulse at the posterior tibial artery, dorsalis pedis artery, or blanching the toe nails to determine capillary refill. Stroke the pulp of your

Jones fracture
A transverse stress fracture of the proximal shaft of the fifth metatarsal

Nonunion fracture
A fracture in which healing is delayed or fails to unite at all

finger across the top of the distal metatarsal heads and ask the individual if they can feel your finger. Repeat with the finger nail. Nondisplaced fractures are treated conservatively with cast immobilization for 4 to 6 weeks, followed by a functional brace until completely healed. Displaced fractures involving joint stability require surgical intervention with open reduction and internal fixation. Healing after surgery usually takes 2 to 3 months or longer, followed by an extensive rehabilitation program.

Did you determine the volleyball player had a possible stress fracture of the metatarsal due to repetitive overloading of the region? If so, you are correct. This individual should be referred to a physician for assessment and treatment.

ASSESSMENT OF THE FOOT, ANKLE, AND LOWER LEG

An basketball player is complaining about vague pain on the dorsum of the foot during activity. Can you limit the assessment to only the foot or should you assess the entire lower leg? How will you proceed?

Although pain, discomfort, or weakness may occur at a specific site, the lower extremities work as a unit to provide a foundation of support for the upright body, propulsion through space, absorption of shock, and adaptation to varying terrains. As such, assessment must include the entire lower extremity, to evaluate how the body segments work together to provide motion. Always enter the assessment with an open mind, because pain may be referred to the foot, ankle, and lower leg from conditions in the lumbar spine, sacrum, hip, or knee. Keep this in mind as you progress through the assessment.

HISTORY

What information do you need from the individual complaining of vague pain on the dorsum of the foot? How will you phrase the questions to identify the main components of the primary complaint?

Many conditions in the foot, ankle, and lower leg are related to family history, congenital deformities, poor technique, and recent changes in training programs, surfaces, or foot attire. In addition to general questions discussed in Chapter 4, specific questions related to the foot, ankle, and lower leg are listed in **Field Strategy 8.8**.

You have learned from the basketball player that dorsal foot pain started at the start of pre-season and intensified during the practice session. Today, the pain was so intense the individual had to stop and remove the shoe because the laces were irritating the top of the foot. Nothing like this has ever happened before, nor does the athlete recall any member of the family having a similar experience.

Field Strategy 8.8. Developing a History of the Injury

Current Injury Status

1. How did the injury occur (mechanism)?
2. Ask about the pain location, severity, onset (sudden or gradual), and type (sharp, aching, burning, radiating). Did you hear any sounds during the incident, such as a snap, pop, or crack?
3. Was there any swelling, discoloration, muscle spasms, or numbness with the injury?
4. What actions or motions replicate the pain? Does it wake you up at night? Do you stand, sit, or walk on uneven surfaces for long periods? Have you recently increased your training frequency, intensity, or duration?
5. What types of surfaces give you the most problem? What shoes do you wear when the pain sets in? (Check the heel height, wear pattern on bottom, and internal arch and heel padding)
6. Are there certain activities you cannot perform because of the pain or weakness? How old are you? Which foot is dominant?

Past Injury Status

1. Have you ever injured your leg or ankle before? When? How did that occur? What was done for injury?
2. Have you had any medical problems recently? (Look for problems that may refer pain to the area from the lumbar spine, hip, or knee.) Are you on any medication? Do you have any musculoskeletal problems elsewhere in the body? (Changes in gait or technique may transfer abnormal forces to structures in the involved limb)

OBSERVATION AND INSPECTION

Think for a minute or two about what specific factors you want to observe in this individual. Would it help to look at the athlete's general posture and gait? What specific conditions might contribute to pain in the foot?

Both lower legs should be clearly visible to denote symmetry, any congenital deformity, swelling, discoloration, hypertrophy, muscle atrophy, or previous surgical incisions. The individual should wear running shorts to allow full view of the lower extremity. Ask them to bring along the shoes they normally wear when pain is present. Inspect the sole, heel box, toe box, and general condition of the shoes for unusual wear, thus indicating a biomechanical abnormality.

In an ambulatory patient, begin observations by completing a general postural exam. At the foot, note the presence, or lack, of an arch on weight bearing and nonweight bearing. Ask the person to walk several steps. Note any abnormalities in gait, favoring one limb, heel–toe floor contact, and heel alignment. Specific areas to focus on in the lower extremity are summarized in **Field Strategy 8.9**. Inspect the injury site for obvious deformities, discoloration, and edema. Remember to compare the affected limb with the unaffected limb.

Field Strategy 8.9. Postural Assessment of the Lower Extremity

Anterior View

The iliac crests should be level and both thighs should look the same

Check for hypertrophy or atrophy. The patellas should be at the same height and face straight forward

The legs should be straight. The knees may be genu valgus (knock kneed) or genu varus (bow legged)

The medial and lateral malleoli should be level as compared to the opposite foot. Is there swelling in the ankle joint?

Both feet should be angled equally. Tibial torsion may result in the foot pointing medially ("pigeon toes"), or pointing slightly lateral. Both feet should have visible equal arches. Note any pes cavus (high arch), or pes planus (flatfoot). Are the feet splayed (widening of the forefoot)? Are the toes straight and parallel? Do the nails appear normal?

Check the skin for normal contours, discolored lesions, exostosis or other bumps, corns, calluses, and scars indicating a previous injury or surgery. Note any signs of circulatory impairment or varicose veins

Posterior View

The gluteal folds and knee folds should be level. The hamstrings and calf muscles should have equal bulk

The Achilles tendons should go straight down to the calcaneus. If they appear to angle out, excessive pronation may be present. The heels should appear to be straight, with equal shape and position

The lateral malleoli should extend slightly more distal than the medial malleoli

Side View

The knees should be slightly flexed (0 to 5°)

The lateral malleolus should be slightly posterior to the center of the knee

Nonweight Bearing View

Check for abnormal calluses, plantar warts, arches, and scars on the plantar side of the foot

---

The individual has bilateral low arches and the calcaneus appears to evert slightly; however, gait appears normal. The dorsa of both feet are red and swollen.

PALPATIONS

With pain centered on the dorsum of each foot, think for a minute where you should begin to palpate the various structures. During palpations, what factors are you looking for?

Bilateral palpations can determine temperature, swelling, point tenderness, crepitus, deformity, muscle spasm, and cutaneous sensation. Vascular pulses can be taken at the posterior tibial artery behind the medial malleolus and at the dorsalis pedis artery on the dorsum of the foot. Proceed proximal to distal, but palpate the most painful areas last. Allow the individual to sit on a table so you can perform bilateral palpations.

Bony Palpations

1. Tibia and medial malleolus
2. Fibula and lateral malleolus
3. Tarsal bones (talus, navicular, calcaneus, cuboid, and cunei-forms)
4. Metatarsals
5. Phalanges

Soft Tissue Palpations

1. Muscles of the anterior compartment
2. Dorsalis pedis pulse
3. Deltoid ligament
4. Posterior tibial artery
5. Muscles of the posterior compartment, Achilles tendon, and retrocalcaneal bursa
6. Muscles of the lateral compartment
7. Anterior and posterior talofibular ligaments and calcaneofibular ligament
8. Plantar fascia

If a fracture is suspected, perform percussion, compression, vibration, and distraction prior to any movement of the limb or any weight bearing. **Field Strategy 8.10** lists several techniques used to determine a possible fracture in the region. If a fracture is suspected, check sensation and circulation distal to the fracture site. Immobilize the area and refer to a physician for follow-up care.

 You found increased pain and warmth on palpation of the toe extensor tendons on the dorsum of the foot. Localized swelling and a slight increase in skin temperature are also present in the region.

Field Strategy 8.10. Determining a Possible Fracture in the Foot and Lower Leg

Percussion or tapping on the head of the fibula or tibial shaft can detect a possible fracture of the malleolus

Strike the bottom of the heel with the palm to drive the talus into the mortise. Increased pain may indicate an osteochondral fracture, malleolar fracture, or increased mortise spread

Compress the tibia and fibula together just inferior to the knee. This causes the distal malleoli to distract. Increased distal pain may indicate a fracture at the ankle

Encircle the midfoot with the hand and slowly squeeze the metatarsal heads. Increased pain may indicate a tarsal or metatarsal fracture

Place a vibrating tuning fork near the suspected fracture site. Increased localized pain is a positive sign

Tap the ends of the toes and compress the toes and metatarsals along the long axis of the bone. Follow this with distraction along the long axis. If a fracture is present, percussion and compression should increase pain, but distraction should decrease pain

> **?** *Pain and swelling are localized over the dorsum of the foot, with pain increasing with palpation of the toe extensor tendons. What special tests can be performed to determine if the injury is muscular, bony, or ligamentous?*

Special tests should be performed in a comfortable position, with the individual lying on a table with the feet hanging over the end, or with the individual sitting. Bilateral comparison is used to assess normal level of function.

Joint Range of Motion

Active movements are best performed with the individual sitting on a table with the leg flexed over the end of the table. Stabilize the thigh and knee. Actions causing pain should be performed last to prevent any painful symptoms from overflowing into the next movement. Perform the following motions:

1. Dorsiflexion and plantar flexion of the ankle
2. Pronation (eversion) and supination (inversion) of the ankle
3. Toe extension and toe flexion
4. Toe abduction and adduction

Resisted Manual Muscle Testing

Stabilize the thigh and repeat each active motion with resistance throughout the full range of motion. As always, painful motions should be delayed until last. **Figure 8.21** demonstrates what motions should be tested, including:

1. Ankle dorsiflexion
2. Ankle plantar flexion
3. Ankle pronation (eversion)
4. Ankle supination (inversion)
5. Toe extension
6. Toe flexion

Neurologic Assessment

Neurologic integrity is tested with resisted manual muscle testing (already completed), reflex testing, and cutaneous sensation. Always compare results bilaterally to determine what is normal for the individual.

Reflexes in the lower leg region include the patella (L_3, L_4) and Achilles tendon (S_1). Test each reflex by striking the tendon with the flat end of the reflex hammer, using a crisp wrist-flexion action **(Fig. 8.22)**. A normal patella reflex exhibits a slight jerking motion in extension and a normal Achilles tendon reflex elicits slight plantar flexion.

In testing cutaneous sensation, run a sharp and dull object over the skin, i.e., blunt tip of taping scissors vs. flat edge of taping scissors. With their eyes closed or looking away, ask the individual

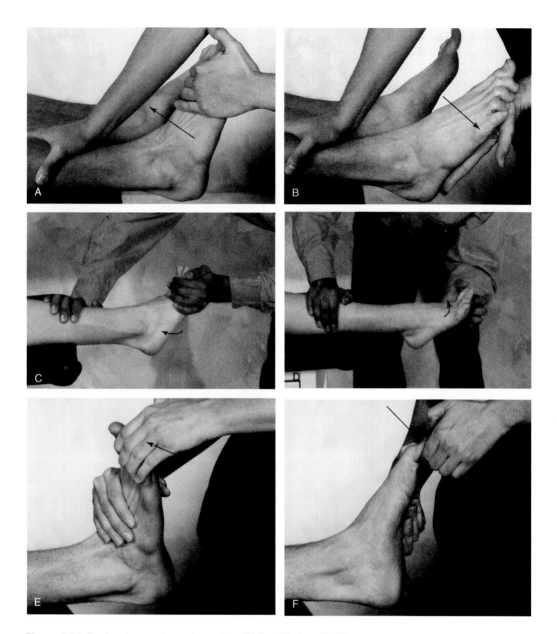

Figure 8.21. Resisted manual muscle testing. (**A**) Dorsiflexion. (**B**) Plantar flexion. (**C**) Pronation. (**D**) Supination. (**E**) Toe extension. (**F**) Toe flexion. Arrows indicate the direction the athlete moves the body part against the applied resistance.

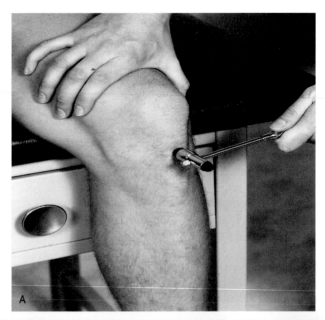

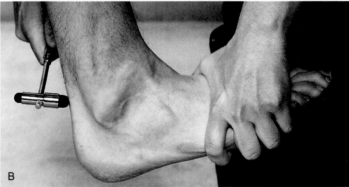

Figure 8.22. Reflex testing. (**A**) The patellar reflex. (**B**) The Achilles reflex.

if they can distinguish sharp and dull. Any variations, such as tingling or numbness, from the uninjured leg should be documented, and the individual should be referred to a physician for more extensive evaluation.

Stress and Functional Tests

From information gathered during the history, observation, inspection, and palpation, determine which tests most effectively assess the condition. Only those tests deemed relevant should be used.

Thompson's Test for Achilles Tendon Rupture

With the individual prone on a table, squeeze the calf muscles. A normal response will elicit slight plantar flexion. Always compare bilaterally, as some plantar flexion may occur if other posterior muscles are intact. A positive test, indicating a rupture of the Achilles tendon, is indicated by the absence of plantar flexion (**Fig. 8.23**).

Anterior Drawer Test

This test can assess collateral ligament integrity of the ankle. Place the individual supine and extend the foot beyond the table. Stabilize the tibia and fibula in one hand and cup the individual's heel in the other hand. To isolate the anterior talofibular ligament and anterolateral capsule, apply a straight anterior movement with slight plantar flexion and inversion (**Fig. 8.24A**). If the talus shifts forward, the test is positive, indicating anterolateral instability.

Talar Tilt

The calcaneofibular ligament and deltoid ligaments are tested in the same position described for the anterior drawer test. Maintain the calcaneus in normal anatomic position (90° flexion). The talus is then slowly rocked between inversion and eversion (**Fig. 8.24B**). Inversion tests the calcaneofibular ligament; eversion tests the deltoid ligament.

Functional Tests

Functional tests should be performed pain-free without a limp or antalgic gait before clearing any individual for re-entry into competition. These may include any or all of the following:

1. Squatting with both heels maintained on the floor
2. Going up on the toes at least 20 times with no pain
3. Walking on the toes for 20 to 30 feet
4. Balancing on one foot at a time
5. Running straight ahead, stopping, and running backwards

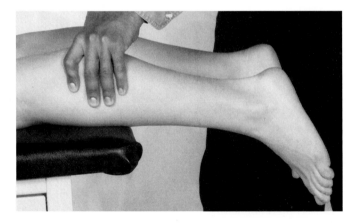

Figure 8.23. To perform the Thompson test, do passive compression of the calf muscles. This should produce slight plantar flexion at the ankle. If no plantar flexion occurs, suspect a possible rupture of the gastrocnemius-soleus complex or the Achilles tendon.

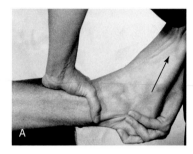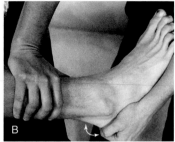

Figure 8.24. Stress tests for the ankle collateral ligaments. (**A**) Anterior drawer test. (**B**) Talar tilt test. Arrows indicate the direction the clinician moves the body part to determine possible joint laxity.

6. Running figure-eights with large circles slowly decreasing in size
7. Running at an angle sideways and making V-cuts
8. Jumping rope for at least 1 minute
9. Jumping straight up and going to a 90° squat

💡 *Increased pain occurred on toe extension of the middle three toes and on dorsiflexion. While palpating the tendons you felt slight snowball crepitation during resisted motion. All other tests were negative. If you determined that the basketball player had tenosynovitis of the toe extensors, you are correct. Irritation of these tendons probably occurred because of the increased compression from the tight shoe laces. How will you manage this injury?*

REHABILITATION

❓ *A soccer player is recovering from a mild second degree inversion ankle sprain. After controlling acute swelling and inflammation, what exercises should be included in the rehabilitation program?*

Rehabilitation exercises for the foot, ankle, and lower leg can be initiated during the acute inflammatory phase as long as the condition is not further irritated. For example, while icing an ankle, the gastrocnemius and soleus can be passively stretched or strengthening exercises for the foot intrinsic muscles can begin. Pain and swelling will dictate the amount of exercise tolerated and may necessitate restricted weight bearing. The rehabilitation program should restore motion and proprioception, maintain cardiovascular fitness, and improve muscular strength, endurance, and power, predominantly through closed-chain exercises. **Field Strategy 8.1** introduced several nonweight-bearing range-of-motion and strengthening exercises. Maintenance of cardiovascular fitness can begin immediately after injury, with use of an upper body ergometer (UBE), or hydrotherapeutic exercise. Running in

The rehabilitation program should restore motion and proprioception, maintain cardiovascular fitness, and improve muscular strength, endurance, and power, predominantly through closed-chain exercises

Field Strategy 8.11. Rehabilitation Exercises for the Lower Leg

Phase one. Control edema formation. Minimize inversion and eversion motion to allow for healing. Dorsiflexion and plantar flexion can be performed within the limits of pain, and may be combined with ice therapy and elevation. Use those exercises listed in Field Strategy 8.1, as tolerated
 Plantar fascia stretch
 Towel crunches
 Toe curls
 Picking up objects
 BAPS board in seated position
 Triceps surae stretch, nonweight bearing
 Pool therapy or upper body ergometer (UBE) exercises for
  cardiovascular fitness
Phase two. As pain and tenderness subside, initiate inversion and eversion range-of-motion and strengthening exercises as tolerated
Include:
 Shin curls
 Ankle alphabet
 Triceps surae stretch, standing position
 Toe raises
 Theraband or tubing exercises in dorsiflexion, plantar flexion,
  inversion, and eversion
 Unilateral balance—BAPS board activities with support
 Pool therapy, UBE, and stationary bike (if tolerated) for cardiovascular
  fitness
Phase three
 Toe raises with weights
 Multiaxial ankle machine
 Squats and lunges
 Balance exercises with challenges, such as dribbling while balancing
  on one leg, doing Theraband exercises while balancing on one leg,
  or balancing on an uneven surface
 If able to walk without a limp, do straight ahead jogging
Phase four. Use external support for the ankle as needed
 Isokinetic exercises to work functional speeds
 Multiangle plyometrics, including single- and double-limb jumping;
  front to front, side to side, and diagonals
 Side-to-side running
 Running backwards
 Jumping for height and distance (long jump)
 Slide board
 Gradual return to sport activity with protection

deep water and performing sport-specific exercises can provide mild resistance in a nonweight-bearing medium. **Field Strategy 8.11** lists several rehabilitation exercises that may be incorporated in a complete program for the lower leg.

If indicated, the individual should be assessed for biomechanical anomalies so that appropriate orthoses can be fabricated to correct any malalignment. With ankle injuries, it may be necessary to provide external support. When cleared for full participation, a proper maintenance program of stretching and strengthening exercises should be provided to the individual.

 Initiate early strengthening exercises for the intrinsic muscles of the foot and maintain plantar flexion and dorsiflexion at the ankle. If the condition is irritated, adjustments must be made in the intensity of exercise. As the condition improves, surgical tubing exercises and closed-chain exercises can be added. A UBE or aquatic exercises can maintain cardiovascular fitness until the condition allows for light jogging and more intense weight-bearing activities.

SUMMARY

The foot, ankle, and lower leg are highly susceptible to injury during sports participation. In addition, congenital abnormalities, muscle imbalance or dysfunction, and postural deviations can predispose an individual to many chronic injuries. Because of this, a

---

Field Strategy 8.12. Foot, Ankle, and Lower Leg Evaluation

History

Primary complaint and mechanism of injury
Onset of symptoms, including pain and discomfort
Disability and functional impairments from the injury
Previous injuries to the area, and family history

Observation and Inspection

Observe general posture and gait
Inspect:

Muscle symmetry	Hypertrophy or atrophy
Swelling	Congenital deformity
Discoloration	Surgical incisions or scars

Palpation

Bony structures, to determine possible fracture
Soft tissue structures, to determine:

Temperature	Crepitus
Swelling	Muscle spasm
Point tenderness	Cutaneous sensation
Deformity	Vascular pulses

Special Tests

Active range of motion
Resisted manual muscle testing
Neurologic testing
Stress and functional tests
   Thompson's test for Achilles tendon rupture
   Anterior drawer test
   Talar tilt
   Functional tests

systematic, thorough assessment must be completed for all lower leg injuries and is summarized in **Field Strategy 8.12**.

Throughout the assessment, remember that pain may be referred from the lumbar spine, hip, or knee. If a significant finding is assessed, immediately refer the individual to a physician for further evaluation. Conditions that warrant immediate referral include: obvious deformity suggesting a dislocation or fracture; significant loss of motion or muscle weakness; excessive joint swelling; possible epiphyseal or apophyseal injuries; abnormal or absent reflexes; abnormal cutaneous sensation; absent or weak pulse; gross joint instability; or any unexplained pain. The final rule of thumb is always "When in doubt, refer!"

Should you decide to refer the individual to a physician, immobilize the limb in a comfortable position using an appropriate brace, splint, or strapping. Apply ice with compression to limit swelling and, if necessary, fit the individual with crutches. Transport the individual appropriately.

Functional tests should be performed pain-free without a limp or antalgic gait before clearing any individual for re-entry into competition. In addition, the individual should have bilaterally equal range of motion, strength, proprioception, and a high cardiovascular fitness level. If seen by a physician, permission to return to competition should be documented in writing from the supervising physician. When necessary, protective equipment or braces should be used to prevent reinjury.

REFERENCES

1. Johnson RE, and Rust RJ. 1985. Sports related injury: an anatomic approach, part 2. Minn Med 68(11):829–831.
2. Norkin CC, and Levangie PK. *Joint structure and function: a comprehensive analysis*. Philadelphia: FA Davis, 1992.
3. Frederick EC. 1986. Kinematically mediated effects of sport shoe design: a review. J Sport Sci 4(3):169–184.
4. Nigg BM, and Bahlsen HA. 1988. Influence of heel flare and midsole construction on pronation, supination and impact forces for heel-toe running. Int J Sport Biomech, 4(3):205–219.
5. Renstrom P, and Johnson RJ. 1985. Overuse injuries in sports: a review. Sports Med 2(5):316–333.
6. Jones DC, and Singer KM. Soft-tissue conditions of the ankle and foot. In *The lower extremity & spine*, edited by JA Nicholas and EB Hershmann. St. Louis: Mosby Year Book, 1995.
7. Baumhauer JF, Alosa DB, Renström PAFH, Trevino S, and Beynnon B. 1995. A prospective study of ankle injury risk factors. Am J Sports Med 23(5):564–570.
8. Grana WA. 1995. Chronic pain after ankle sprain: consider the differential diagnosis. Phys Sportsmed 23(5):67–79.
9. Myerson MS, and Biddinger K. 1995. Achilles tendon disorders: practical management strategies. Phys Sportsmed 23(12):47–54.
10. Batt ME, and Tanji JL. 1995. Management options for plantar fasciitis. Phys Sportsmed 23(6):77–86.
11. Fick DS, Albright JP, and Murray BP. 1992. Relieving painful 'shin splints.' Phys Sportsmed 20(12):105–113.

12. Allen MJ. 1990. Compartment syndromes of the lower limb. J R Coll Surg Edinb 35(6 Suppl):S33–36.
13. Edwards P, and Myerson MS. 1996. Exertional compartment syndrome of the leg: steps for expedient return to activity. Phys Sportsmed 24(4):31–46.
14. Warren MP, Brooks-Gunn J, Hamilton LH, Warren LF, and Hamilton WG. 1986. Scoliosis and fractures in young ballet dancers: relation to delayed menarche and secondary amenorrhea, N Eng J Med 314(21):1348–1353.

Chapter 9

The Knee

After completing this chapter, you should be able to:

- Locate the important bony and soft tissue structures of the knee region

- Describe the motions of the knee and identify the muscles that produce them

- Identify basic principles in the prevention of knee injuries

- Recognize and manage specific injuries at the knee

- Demonstrate a basic assessment of the knee and patellofemoral joint

- Demonstrate general rehabilitation exercises for the region

Key Terms:

Chondral fracture	**Osteochondral fracture**
Chondromalacia patellae	**Osteochondritis dissecans**
Collateral ligaments	**Patellofemoral stress syndrome**
Cruciate ligaments	**Patellofemoral joint**
Extensor mechanism	**Q-angle**
Hemarthrosis	**Screwing home mechanism**
Larsen-Johansson disease	**Tibiofemoral joint**
Menisci	**Valgus laxity**
Osgood-Schlatter disease	**Varus laxity**

The knee is a large, complex joint frequently injured during sport participation. During walking and running, the knee moves through a considerable range of motion while bearing loads equivalent to three to four times body weight. The knee is also positioned between the two longest bones in the body, the femur and tibia, creating the potential for large, injurious torques at the joint. These factors, coupled with minimal bony stability, make the knee susceptible to injury, particularly during participation in field and/or contact sports.

This chapter begins with a review of the anatomy of the knee and major muscle actions at the knee. General principles to prevent injuries will then be followed by discussion of common injuries to the knee complex. Finally, a step-by-step injury assessment of the region is presented and examples of rehabilitative exercises will be provided.

> ❓ *A basketball player is complaining of pain on the proximal anterior tibia where the patellar tendon attaches. Pain is very noticeable during jumping drills and when sprinting. What structures might be inflamed in this region?*

The knee is a large synovial joint including three articulations within the joint capsule. The weight-bearing joints are the two condylar articulations of the tibiofemoral joint, with the third articulation being the patellofemoral joint. The soft tissue connections of the proximal tibiofibular joint also exert a minor influence on knee motion (1).

Tibiofemoral Joint

The distal femur and proximal tibia articulate to form two side-by-side condyloid joints known collectively as the **tibiofemoral joint, (Fig. 9.1)**. These joints function together primarily as a modified hinge joint because of the restricting ligaments, with some lateral and rotational motions allowed. Because the medial and lateral condyles of the femur differ somewhat in size, shape, and orientation, the tibia rotates laterally on the femur during the last few degrees of extension to produce "locking" of the knee. This phenomenon is known as the **"screwing-home" mechanism**.

Tibiofemoral joint
Dual condyloid joints between the tibial and femoral condyles that function primarily as a modified hinge joint

Screwing-home mechanism
Rotation of the tibia on the femur during extension that produces an anatomic "locking" of the knee

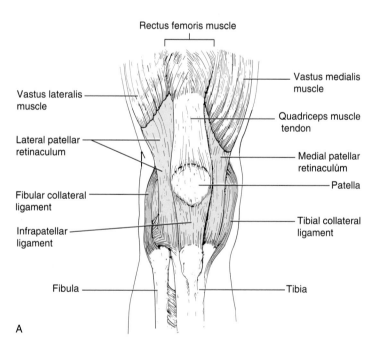

A

Figure 9.1. The knee. **A.** Ligaments of the knee (anterior view). **B.** Ligaments of the knee (posterior view—superficial and deep structures). **C.** Bursae of the knee. **D.** Superior surface of tibia with menisci and associated structures.

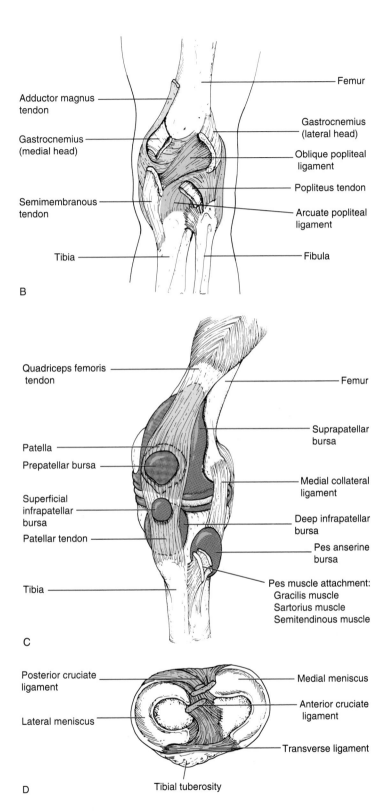

B

Adductor magnus tendon

Gastrocnemius (medial head)

Semimembranous tendon

Tibia

Femur

Gastrocnemius (lateral head)

Oblique popliteal ligament

Popliteus tendon

Arcuate popliteal ligament

Fibula

Quadriceps femoris tendon

Patella

Prepatellar bursa

Superficial infrapatellar bursa

Patellar tendon

Tibia

C

Femur

Suprapatellar bursa

Medial collateral ligament

Deep infrapatellar bursa

Pes anserine bursa

Pes muscle attachment:
Gracilis muscle
Sartorius muscle
Semitendinous muscle

Posterior cruciate ligament

Lateral meniscus

D

Tibial tuberosity

Medial meniscus

Anterior cruciate ligament

Transverse ligament

Figure 9.1. (continued)

Menisci

Menisci
Fibrocartilagenous discs
within the knee that reduce
joint stress

The **menisci** are discs of fibrocartilage firmly attached to the superior plateaus of the tibia by the coronary ligaments and joint capsule (**Fig. 9.1**) (2). The menisci are thicker along the lateral margin and thinner on the medial margin, serving to deepen the concavities of the tibial plateaus. The medial meniscus is injured much more frequently than the lateral meniscus. This is partly due to the medial meniscus being more securely attached to the tibia and, therefore, less mobile.

Joint Capsule and Bursae

The joint capsule at the knee is large and lax, encompassing both the tibiofemoral and patellofemoral joints (**Fig. 9.1**). Anteriorly, it extends about two-and-one-half centimeters above the patella to attach along the edges of the superior patellar surface. The deep bursa formed by this capsule above the patella, the suprapatellar bursa, is the largest bursa in the body. It lies between the femur and quadriceps femoris tendon and functions to reduce friction between the two structures. Posteriorly, the subpopliteal bursa lies between the lateral condyle of the femur and popliteal muscle, and the semimembranosus bursa lies between the medial head of the gastrocnemius and semimembranosus tendons.

The largest bursa of the
body is the suprapatellar,
located between the femur
and quadriceps femoris
muscle tendon

During flexion and extension, the synovial fluid moves throughout the bursal recesses to lubricate the articular surfaces (2). In extension, the gastrocnemius and subpopliteal bursae are compressed, driving the synovial fluid anteriorly. In flexion, the suprapatellar bursa is compressed, forcing fluid posteriorly (2). When the knee joint is in a semi-flexed position, the synovial fluid is under the least amount of pressure. This position provides relief of pain caused by swelling in the joint capsule and surrounding bursae.

During motion at the knee,
the synovial fluid moves
throughout the synovial
cavity to lubricate the
articular surfaces

Three other key bursae associated with the knee, but not contained in the joint capsule, are the prepatellar, superficial infrapatellar, and deep infrapatellar bursae. The prepatellar bursa is located between the skin and anterior surface of the patella, allowing free movement of the skin over the patella during flexion and extension. The superficial infrapatellar bursa is located between the skin and patellar tendon. Inflammation of this bursa due to excessive kneeling is sometimes referred to as "housemaid's knee." The deep infrapatellar bursa, located between the tibial tuberosity and the patellar tendon, serves to reduce friction between the ligament and the bony tuberosity.

Ligaments of the Knee

Cruciate ligaments
Major ligaments that
criss-cross the knee in the
anteroposterior direction

Because the shallow articular surfaces of the tibiofemoral joint contribute little to knee stability, the stabilizing role of the ligaments crossing the knee is of great significance. Two major ligaments of the knee are the anterior and posterior **cruciate**

ligaments (Fig. 9.1). The name *cruciate* is derived from the fact that these ligaments cross each other, with *anterior* and *posterior* referring to their respective tibial attachments. These ligaments restrict the anterior and posterior sliding of the femur on the tibial plateaus during knee flexion and extension, and also serve to limit knee hyperextension. The anterior cruciate is considered to be the weaker of the two ligaments, and is frequently subject to deceleration injuries.

The medial and lateral **collateral ligaments** are referred to, respectively, as the tibial and fibular collateral ligaments after their distal attachments. The medial collateral ligament connects the medial epicondyle of the femur to the medial tibia. The distal attachment is just below the pes anserinus, the common attachment of the semitendinosus, semimembranosus, and gracilis to the tibia, thereby positioning the ligament to resist medially directed shear (valgus) and rotational forces acting on the knee. The lateral collateral ligament connects the lateral epicondyle of the femur to the head of the fibula, contributing to lateral stability of the knee.

Patellofemoral Joint

The patella is a triangular-shaped bone commonly known as the kneecap. It articulates with the patellofemoral groove between the femoral condyles to form the **patellofemoral joint (Fig. 9.1).**

The **Q-angle** is the angle formed between the line of resultant force produced by the quadriceps muscles and the line of the patellar tendon **(Fig. 9.2).** The normal Q-angle ranges from approximately 13° in males to approximately 18° in females, when the knee is extended. A Q-angle less than 13° or greater than 18° is considered abnormal and can predispose the sport participant to patellar injuries or degeneration (3).

In the sagittal plane, the patella serves to increase the angle of pull of the patellar tendon on the tibia, thereby improving the mechanical advantage of the quadriceps muscles for producing knee extension. The patella also provides some protection for the anterior aspect of the knee.

Muscles Crossing the Knee

The muscles of the knee develop tension to produce motion at the knee and also contribute to the knee's stability. The attachments and primary actions of the muscles crossing the knee are summarized in **Table 9.1.**

Nerves and Blood Supply of the Knee

The tibial nerve is the largest and most medial branch of the sciatic nerve. It innervates all of the muscles in the hamstring group, except the short head of the biceps femoris, and then continues to supply all of the remaining posterior muscles in the

The cruciate ligaments restrict the sliding of the femur on the tibial plateaus and limit hyperextension

Collateral ligaments
Major ligaments that cross the medial and lateral aspects of the knee

The medial collateral ligament resists medially directed rotational forces and the lateral collateral ligament resists laterally directed forces

Patellofemoral joint
Gliding joint between the patella and the patellar groove of the femur

Q-angle
Angle between the line of quadriceps force and the patellar tendon

A Q-angle less than 13° and greater than 18° can predispose the athlete to patellar injuries

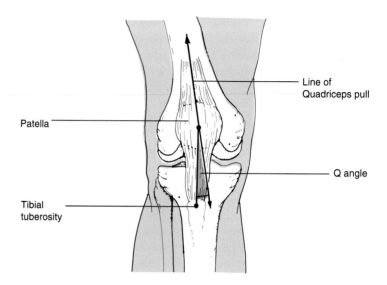

Line of
Quadriceps pull

Patella

Q angle

Tibial
tuberosity

Figure 9.2. The Q-angle is formed between the line of quadriceps pull and the imaginary line connecting the center of the patella to the center of the tibial tuberosity.

Table 9.1. Muscles Acting on the Knee

Muscle	Proximal Attachment	Distal Attachment	Primary Action(s)	Nerve Innervation
Rectus femoris	Anterior inferior iliac spine (AIIS)	Patella	Extension	Femoral
Vastus lateralis	Greater trochanter and lateral linea aspera	Patella	Extension	Femoral
Vastus intermedius	Anterior femur	Patella	Extension	Femoral
Vastus medialis	Medial linea aspera	Patella	Extension	Femoral
Semitendinosus	Ischial tuberosity	Proximal, medial tibia at pes	Knee flexion and medial rotation	Sciatic
Semimembranosus	Ischial tuberosity	Proximal, medial tibia	Knee flexion and medial rotation	Sciatic
Biceps femoris	*Long head:* ischial tuberosity. *Short head:* lateral linea aspera	Fibular head and lateral condyle of tibia	Knee flexion and external rotation	Sciatic
Sartorius	Anterior superior iliac spine (ASIS)	Proximal medial tibia at pes	Knee flexion and medial rotation	Femoral
Gracilis	Symphysis pubis and the pubic arch	Proximal medial tibia at pes	Knee flexion and medial rotation	Obturator
Popliteus	Lateral condyle of the femur	Posterior, medial tibia	Medial rotation, knee flexion	Tibial
Gastrocnemius	Posterior medial and lateral femoral condyles	Calcaneus, via the Achilles tendon	Knee flexion	Tibial
Plantaris	Posterior femur above lateral condyle	Calcaneus	Knee flexion	Tibial

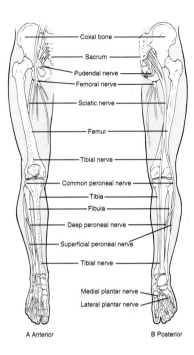

Coxal bone

Sacrum

Pudendal nerve

Femoral nerve

Sciatic nerve

Femur

Tibial nerve

Common peroneal nerve

Tibia

Fibula

Deep peroneal nerve

Superficial peroneal nerve

Tibial nerve

Medial plantar nerve

Lateral plantar nerve

A Anterior

B Posterior

Figure 9.3. A, B. The innervation of the knee.

lower leg **(Fig. 9.3)**. The common peroneal nerve is the lateral branch of the sciatic nerve. It innervates the short head of the biceps femoris, then passes through the popliteal fossa, winds around the head of the fibula, and divides into the superficial and

The tibial nerve innervates all muscles in the hamstring group except the short head of the biceps femoris

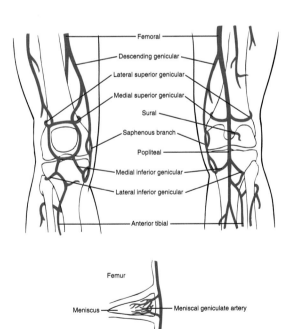

Femoral

Descending genicular

Lateral superior genicular

Medial superior genicular

Sural

Saphenous branch

Popliteal

Medial inferior genicular

Lateral inferior genicular

Anterior tibial

Femur

Meniscus

Meniscal geniculate artery

Tibia

Figure 9.4. Collateral circulation around the knee.

deep peroneal nerves, with an articular branch to the knee. The femoral nerve courses down the anterior aspect of the thigh to supply the quadriceps group and the sartorius.

Just proximal to the knee, the main branch of the femoral artery becomes the popliteal artery. The popliteal artery then courses through the popliteal fossa and branches to form the medial and lateral superior genicular, the middle genicular, and the medial and lateral inferior genicular arteries to supply the knee (**Fig. 9.4**).

The genicular arteries are branches of the popliteal artery that supply the knee with nourishment

💡 *The structure most likely to be irritated on the proximal anterior aspect of the tibia is the tibial tubercle where the patellar tendon attaches. This irritation may be due to the repeated tension of the tendon pulling on its distal attachment during running and jumping activities. The deep infrapatellar bursa and patellar tendon itself may also be irritated.*

MAJOR MUSCLE ACTIONS OF THE KNEE

❓ *Why does the rotational capability of the knee vary throughout the range of flexion/extension? What anatomical features are responsible for this phenomenon?*

The knee functions primarily as a hinge joint. The different shapes of the femoral condyles, however, serve to complicate joint function.

Flexion and Extension

The primary motions permitted at the tibiofemoral joint are flexion and extension (**Fig. 9.5**). In full extension, the joint is anatomically "locked." This occurs because the articulating surface of the medial condyle of the femur is longer than that of the lateral condyle in this position, rendering motion almost completely impossible (2). For flexion to be initiated from a position of full extension, the knee must first be "unlocked." The popliteus acts as a locksmith by laterally rotating the femur with respect to the tibia, thereby freeing the joint for motion.

Once the knee is unlocked from full extension, bony contact is diminished and motion in the transverse and frontal planes becomes freer. As the knee moves into flexion, the femur slides anteriorly on the tibia and, during extension, the reverse occurs, with the femur sliding posteriorly on the tibia.

Rotation and Passive Abduction and Adduction

Rotation of the tibia is maximal at about 90° of knee flexion

Rotational capability of the tibia with respect to the femur is maximal at approximately 90° of knee flexion. A few degrees of passive abduction and adduction are also permitted when the joint is positioned in the vicinity of 30° of flexion (4).

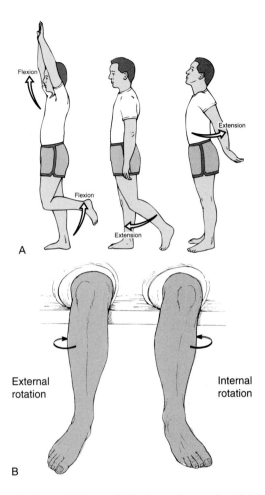

Figure 9.5. Motions at the knee. **A.** Flexion and extension of the knee. **B.** Supination of the subtalar joint results in external rotation of the tibia. Pronation is linked with internal rotation of the tibia.

External rotation

Internal rotation

Patellofemoral Joint Motion

During flexion/extension movements, the patella glides superiorly and inferiorly against the distal end of the femur in a primarily vertical direction with an excursion of as much as 8 cm (1). The patella also undergoes medial and lateral displacement as the tibia is rotated laterally and medially, respectively.

Tracking of the patella against the femur is dependent on the direction of the net force produced by the attached quadriceps. The vastus lateralis tends to pull the patella laterally in the direction of the muscle's action line, parallel to the femoral shaft. The iliotibial band and lateral extensor retinaculum also exert a lateral force on the patella. Although there is considerable debate as to the role of the vastus medialis oblique (VMO), it seems to oppose the lateral pull of the vastus lateralis, thereby keeping the patella centered in the patellofemoral groove. If the magnitude of the force produced by the vastus lateralis exceeds that produced by the VMO, the patella is pulled laterally out of its groove during tracking. Mistracking the patella during knee movement can lead to pain and dysfunction.

Rotational capabilities at the knee varies throughout the range of motion, depending on where the femoral condyles are in relation to the tibia. Rotation is maximal at about 90° of knee flexion.

PREVENTION OF INJURIES

What exercises should be included in a pre-season conditioning program to reduce the risk of injury at the knee? Does gender affect the potential for knee or patellofemoral injuries?

The potential for injuries at the knee is enormous. A well-rounded physical conditioning program is the key to injury prevention. Because many of the muscles that move the knee have their proximal attachments in the hip and thigh region, exercises for the knee can also prevent hip injuries.

Exercises should include the elements of flexibility, muscular strength, endurance, and power, as well as speed, agility, balance, and cardiovascular fitness. Focus on the quadriceps, hamstrings, gastrocnemius, iliotibial tract, and adductors, since many of these muscles contribute to knee stability. Specific preventive exercises are listed in **Field Strategy 9.1**.

In Chapter 6, shoe design was discussed. In football, a cleated shoe with a higher number of shorter, more broad cleats can prevent the foot from becoming fixed to the ground. The length of the cleats still allows for good traction on running and cutting maneuvers. Other athletes, particularly those who participate on artificial turf surfaces, prefer the multi-cleated soccer style shoe.

Flexibility, muscular strength, endurance, and power exercises should be included in a preventive conditioning program. In addition, agility, speed, balance, and a high cardiovascular fitness level can prevent injury. Women, because of their wider hips and larger Q-angle, may be at risk for knee or patellofemoral injuries.

CONTUSIONS AND BURSITIS

A wrestler has had a sore knee for several days. The joint is now warm, swollen, and aching. Visual inspection does not show an outline of the patella. Is the swelling intra-articular or extra-articular? Should this individual be referred to a physician? Why?

Contusions resulting from compressive forces (i.e., a kick, getting hit with a ball, or falling on the knee) are common injuries at the knee. General signs and symptoms include localized tenderness, pain, swelling, and ecchymosis.

If swelling is extensive, other injuries may be obscured. For example, being kicked on the proximal tibia or fibula may appear as a contusion, when, in fact, the impact may have caused an

Field Strategy 9.1. Exercises to Prevent Injury at the Knee

1. Hamstrings stretch, seated position
   Place the leg to be stretched straight out, with the opposite foot tucked toward the groin. Reach toward the toes until a stretch is felt

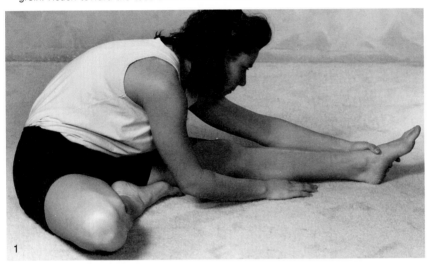

2. Quadriceps stretch, prone position
   Push the heel toward the buttocks, then raise the knee off the floor until tension is felt

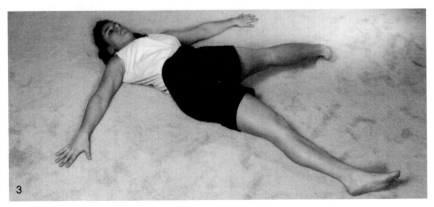

3. Iliotibial band stretch, supine position
   With the trunk stabilized, adduct the leg to be stretched over the other leg and allow gravity to passively stretch the iliotibial band

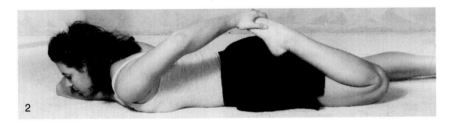

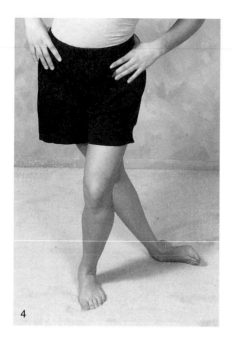

4

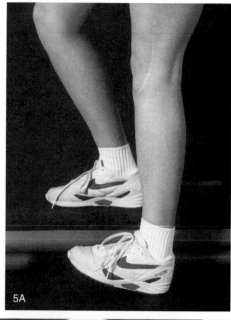

5A

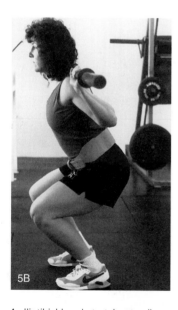

5B

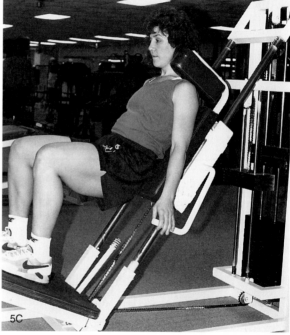

5C

4. Iliotibial band stretch, standing position
   Cross the limb to be stretched behind the other, extending and adducting the hip as far as possible
5. Closed-chain exercises
   a. Step ups, step downs, and lateral step ups
   b. Squats (never below 85 to 90°)
   c. Leg press

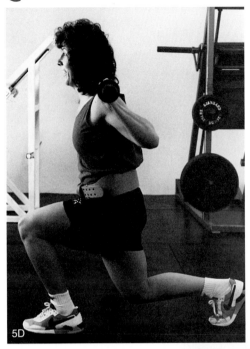

d. Lunges
6. Open-chain exercises
   a. Knee extension (quadriceps)
   b. Knee flexion (hamstrings)

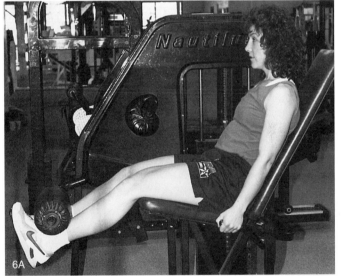

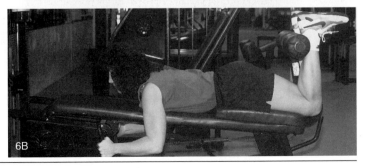

avulsion fracture of one of the collateral ligaments, or an epiphyseal injury in an adolescent. Extreme point tenderness and positive findings on fracture tests should indicate a more serious injury is present and referral to a physician is indicated.

Bursitis may be caused by direct trauma, infections, or metabolic disorders. The most commonly injured bursa is the prepatellar bursa, because of its location on the anterior surface of the patella. Swelling may occur immediately or over a 24-hour period, obscuring the visible outline of the patella (**Fig. 9.6**). Direct pressure over the bursa and passive flexion of the knee will lead to considerable pain. In contrast to the prepatellar bursa, inflammations of the deep infrapatellar bursa and pes anserinus bursa (**Fig. 9.1**) are usually caused by overuse and subsequent friction when local tendons are compressed against the underlying bone.

Treatment consists of cryotherapy, a compressive wrap, nonsteroidal anti-inflammatory medication (NSAIDs), avoiding activities that irritate the condition, or total rest until acute symptoms subside. A protective foam, or donut-shaped pad may protect the area from further insult. If signs of infection become apparent, or the joint appears grossly distended and warm to the touch, refer the individual to a physician.

Did you determine that the wrestler probably had prepatellar bursitis? If so, you are correct. Because the inflammation is anterior to the patella, it is considered to be extra-articular. After initial acute care, refer this individual to a physician, because the warm, swollen, painful knee may need to be aspirated and cultured to rule out an infected bursa.

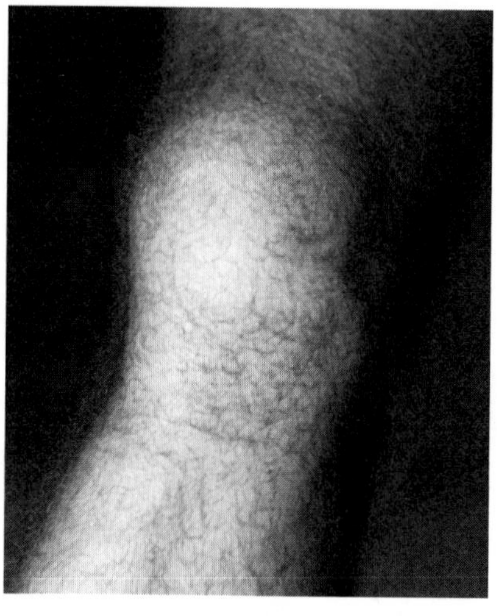

> Acute traumatic bursitis leads to a grossly distended, warm bursa sac filled with bloody effusion

Figure 9.6. The prepatellar bursa is commonly injured by compression from a direct blow or during a fall on a flexed knee.

LIGAMENTOUS INJURIES

> **?** A basketball player decelerated, set the left foot, then force-fully pushed off the left leg to perform a right-handed lay-up shot. The player felt a sudden popping sensation, intense pain, and then the knee collapsed. There is extreme pain on the anteromedial joint line. What structure(s) may have been injured? What is your course of action?

Knee joint stability depends primarily on a static system of support from its ligaments and capsular structures, rather than from the surrounding muscles. Bones and menisci provide some additional stability via their shape and inherent stability when two adjoining structures are in a close-packed position. Knowing the knee position at the moment of impact, and the direction the tibia displaces or rotates after impact, will denote what structures are damaged. At this level of understanding, ligamentous injuries will be described based on unidirectional or straight laxity.

Knee stability is dependent on static support from its ligaments and capsular structures

Unidirectional Instabilities

In straight medial laxity, or **valgus laxity**, lateral forces cause tension on the medial aspect of the knee, potentially damaging the medial (tibial) collateral ligament (MCL), posterior oblique ligament, and posteromedial capsular ligaments (**Fig. 9.7**). Pain and swelling are localized on the medial joint line.

Straight lateral laxity, or **varus laxity**, results from medial forces that produce tension on the lateral aspect of the knee, damaging the lateral (fibular) collateral ligament (LCL), lateral capsular ligaments, and joint structures (**Fig. 9.8**). Swelling and pain are limited to the lateral knee; however, if pain is detected on the head of the fibula, an avulsion fracture should be suspected.

With straight anterior laxity, the anterior cruciate ligament (ACL) is damaged. Isolated anterior laxity is rare. Instead, an anteromedial or anterolateral laxity usually occurs. Recent research has shown that women involved in intercollegiate soccer and basketball have significantly higher ACL injury rates than their male counterparts (5). This may be due to extrinsic factors, such as body movement, muscular strength, shoe-surface interface, and skill level, or to intrinsic factors, such as joint laxity, limb alignment, notch dimensions, and size of the ligament (5). Children's ligaments are generally stronger than their growth plates and bones. Therefore, ACL injuries in children typically involve an avulsion fracture of the tibial eminence. This injury typically occurs when the child's knee hyperextends and twists (6). Damage to the adult ACL may arise from a cutting or turning maneuver, landing in an off-balance position after a jump, or during sudden deceleration (**Fig. 9.9**). Pain may be described as being located deep in the knee or on either side of the patellar tendon. Joint effusion is typically mixed with blood and may not

Valgus laxity
An opening on the medial side of a joint caused by the distal segment moving laterally

Varus laxity
An opening on the lateral side of a joint caused by the distal segment moving medially

Damage to the anterior cruciate ligament commonly occurs during a cutting maneuver, sudden deceleration, or landing in an off-balance position after a jump

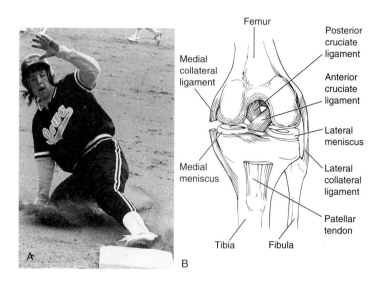

Figure 9.7. A, B. When a valgus force is applied to the knee, the tibial collateral ligament and medial capsular ligaments are damaged, leading to valgus laxity.

become evident until 24 hours postinjury, even if standard acute care is followed.

In straight posterior laxity, the tibia is displaced posteriorly, damaging the posterior cruciate ligament (PCL). Hyperextension is the most common mechanism, although the ligament can also be damaged when the knee is flexed and the upper tibia is driven posteriorly, such as when a hockey player collides with the boards

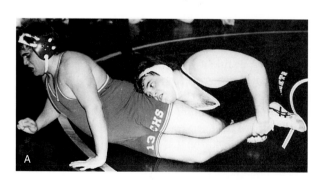

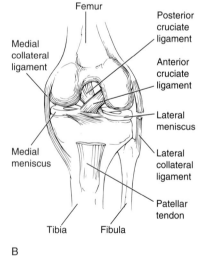

Figure 9.8. A, B. In wrestling, the opponent is often between the athlete's legs and is able to deliver an isolated varus force damaging the fibular collateral ligament, leading to varus laxity.

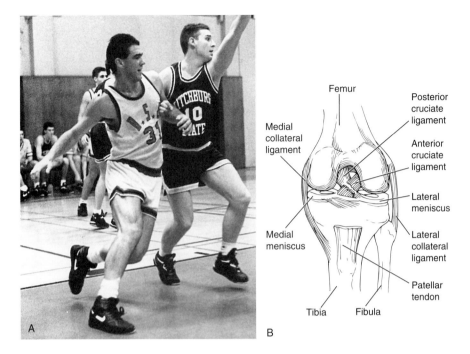

Femur

Posterior cruciate ligament

Medial collateral ligament

Anterior cruciate ligament

Lateral meniscus

Medial meniscus

Lateral collateral ligament

Patellar tendon

Tibia   Fibula

Figure 9.9. A, B. The anterior cruciate ligament can be damaged during deceleration, when changing directions.

(**Fig. 9.10**). Intense pain and a sense of stretching are felt in the posterior aspect of the knee. Effusion and **hemarthrosis** occur rapidly and knee extension is limited due to the effusion and stretching of the posterior capsule and gastrocnemius. **Table 9.2** explains the signs and symptoms seen in the various stages of ligament failure.

Hemarthrosis
Blood in a joint or its cavity

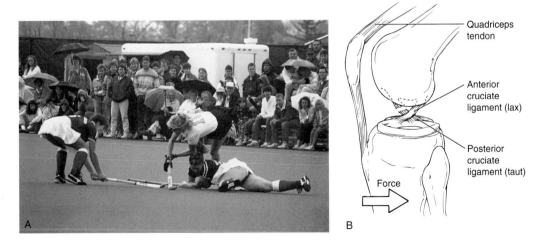

Quadriceps tendon

Anterior cruciate ligament (lax)

Posterior cruciate ligament (taut)

Force

Figure 9.10. A, B. The posterior cruciate ligament can be damaged during hyperextension of the knee or when the knee is flexed and the tibia is driven posterior.

Table 9.2. Signs and Symptoms of Ligament Failure

First-Degree (Mild) Sprain with Minimal Ligament Failure
(Less than 5 mm Distraction)

Less than one-third of the fibers are torn
Mild pain and swelling is localized over the injury site
Joint range of motion and muscular strength will be normal
No joint laxity is apparent during stress test

Second-Degree (Moderate) Sprain with Partial Ligament Failure
(5 to 10 mm Distraction)

One-third to two-thirds of the ligament has been torn
Localized swelling and joint effusion limits range of motion
Pain is usually sharp and may be transient or lasting
Individual may complain of instability and is unable to walk with the heel
  on the ground
Active knee extension is limited
Visible moderate joint laxity during the stress tests

Third-Degree (Severe) Sprain with Complete Ligament Failure
(Over 10 mm Distraction)

Over two-thirds of the ligament is torn or ruptured
Swelling is diffuse, severely limiting range of motion
Pain is initially sharp and often disappears within a minute
Individual can feel the knee giving way
Significant visible joint laxity during the stress tests

Management of Ligament Injuries

Injuries involving minimal ligament failure are managed conservatively with ice application, compression, elevation, and protected rest until acute symptoms subside. A compression wrap, consisting of an inverted horseshoe around the patella secured by an elastic wrap, can be used with a knee immobilizer to reduce swelling. Modalities and NSAIDs can also reduce pain and edema.

In a moderate injury with partial ligament failure, ice, compression, elevation, and protected rest should be continued for 24 to 72 hours. Crutches are used until the individual can walk without a limp. Progression to partial weight bearing with heel-to-toe gait can begin as tolerated. Range-of-motion exercises should include assisted knee flexion and knee extension. Isometric exercises of the quadriceps and straight leg raises in all directions can progress to resisted exercises throughout the full range of motion. Closed kinetic chain exercises, such as one-third knee bends, seated leg presses, and use of surgical tubing with hamstring curls, forward and backward walking, or side-to-side sliding may be used in the early stages of the rehabilitation program (7). In ligament injuries in which complete ligament failure has occurred, or when more than one major ligament is involved, referral to an orthopedist is warranted for possible surgical repair. **Field Strategy 9.2** lists management and rehabilitation of a mild ligament injury.

Field Strategy 9.2. Management of a Ligamentous Injury

Phase 1 (PRICE)

Ice, elevation, compression wrap, and rest with a knee immobilizer to
    reduce swelling. Use crutches if needed
Range-of-motion exercises within pain-free limits
    Heel slides
    Prone knee flexion assisted with the opposite leg
    Passive knee extension in a supine or seated position
Strengthening exercises
    Bent leg raises in all directions
    Multiangle isometric exercises for the quadriceps, hamstrings, and hip
        adductors
Cardiovascular fitness may include UBE and unilateral leg cycling

Phase 2

Range-of-motion exercises continued to regain full ROM
Unilateral balance activities (standing on one foot with the eyes closed or
    BAPS board)
Strengthening exercises
    Do slow, controlled, closed-chain exercises (two-legged squats to 60°,
        step ups, step downs, and lateral step ups)
    Calf raises (seated position) progressing to standing position when pain
        free
    Straight leg raises in all directions with tubing added as tolerated
Cardiovascular fitness continues with UBE or hydrotherapy

Phase 3

Maintain range of motion and flexibility in the lower extremity
Strengthening
    Hip leg press and squats
    Toe raises with weights
    Lunges
Open- and closed-chain exercises for major muscle groups
Cardiovascular fitness
    Bilateral minimal tension cycling if 110 to 115° of knee flexion is
        present. Avoid full knee extension
    Pool running, swimming with a flutter kick, jogging in place on a
        trampoline, and power walking

Phase 4

Balance and proprioception. Continue exercises from above and add slide
    board
Functional activities
    Running drills (circles, figure-eights, cross-over steps); jumping with
        double limb/single limb, progressing from standing in place, front to
        back, to diagonals
    Multidirectional high-speed balance drills are added after the individual
        can run 2 to 3 miles
    Jumping, bounding, and skipping (plyometrics)

The basketball player reported a popping sensation and buckling of the knee after deceleration. Did you suspect a possible anterior cruciate injury? If so, you are correct. Because anterior cruciate injuries seldom occur as an isolated injury, this individual should be referred to a physician for further assessment.

MENISCAL INJURIES

A softball catcher is complaining of mild swelling and posteromedial joint line tenderness. Although the pain has been persistent over the past several weeks, it now hurts to remain in a prolonged squatting position. What may be occurring?

Menisci become more stiff and less resilient with age, and are injured in manners similar to ligamentous structures. In addition to compression and tensile forces, shearing forces caused when the femur rotates on a fixed tibia trap the posterior horns of both menisci, leading to some tearing. Tears may be described as longitudinal, bucket-handle, horizontal, or parrot-beak **(Fig. 9.11)**. Peak incidence of injuries has been found to occur in men between the ages of 21 and 40, and in girls and women between the ages of 11 and 20, and again between 61 and 70 (8). Medial meniscus damage is more common than lateral meniscus damage.

Meniscal injuries are difficult to assess because of the limited sensory nerve supply. The individual may experience a popping, grinding, or clicking sensation that can lead to the knee buckling or giving way, causing the individual to stumble or fall. In addition, the individual will have difficulty doing a deep squat or doing a duck walk.

Mild cases of pain and swelling can be managed with standard acute care—ice, compression, elevation, protected rest, and crutches as needed. If joint effusion is extensive, aspiration of the fluid by a physician may be necessary. Occasionally, the meniscal tear may lodge in the knee joint, causing the knee to lock in place. When the knee cannot be spontaneously reduced, surgical intervention is necessary.

In the softball catcher, did you suspect a possible chronic meniscal tear aggravated when the knee is fully flexed? If so, you are correct. This individual should be referred to a physician.

> **Menisci become more stiff and less resilient with age**

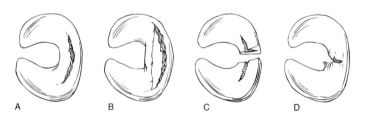

Figure 9.11. Mensical tears. **A.** Longitudinal. **B.** Bucket-handle. **C.** Horizontal. **D.** Parrot-beak.

PATELLA AND RELATED INJURIES

❓ *A female rower is complaining of a deep, aching pain in the knee during activity. Slight joint effusion is present. Palpable pain is elicited over the lateral patellar border. Intense pain is felt when the patella is pushed downward into the patellofemoral groove. What factors may contribute to this condition? What long-term management should be considered after acute symptoms have subsided?*

The patellofemoral joint is the region most commonly associated with anterior knee pain. The quadriceps mechanism, more accurately called the **extensor mechanism**, places the femur and patella in specific positions to provide stability and function at the knee **(Fig. 9.12)**. The VMO is the dynamic medial stabilizer that resists lateral displacement of the patella. Atrophy of this muscle is nearly always evident in patellofemoral dysfunction. Patellar tracking disorders and instability within the joint, along with overweight, direct trauma, and repetitive motions, all contribute to a variety of injuries.

Patellofemoral Stress Syndrome

Patellofemoral stress syndrome occurs when either the VMO is weak or the lateral retinaculum that holds the patella firmly to the femoral condyle is excessively tight. In either case, the end result is lateral excursion of the patella. The condition is found more commonly in women because of their higher Q-angle. Pain often results when a tense lateral retinaculum passes over the trochlear groove. The individual may report a dull, aching pain in the center of the knee. Point tenderness can be located over the lateral edge of the patella, with intense pain and crepitus

Extensor mechanism
Complex interaction of muscles, ligaments, and tendons that stabilize and provide motion at the patellofemoral joint

The VMO is the dynamic medial stabilizer that resists lateral displacement of the patella

Patellofemoral stress syndrome
Condition whereby the lateral retinaculum is tight or the vastus medialis oblique (VMO) is weak, leading to lateral excursion and pressure on the lateral facet of the patella, causing a painful condition

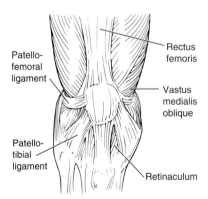

Figure 9.12. The extensor mechanism is composed of dynamic and static stabilizers. Working together, they combine rolling and gliding motions to place the femur and patella in specific positions to effect the deceleration mechanism of the patellofemoral articulation, to provide stability and function at the knee. Oblique condensations of the retinacula produce the patellofemoral ligament and medial and lateral patellotibial ligaments.

elicited when the patella is manually compressed into the patello-femoral groove.

Treatment involves standard acute care and NSAIDs. A patellar taping technique may be applied to correct patellar position and tracking during knee motion; however, recent studies suggest no beneficial effects are gained by adding a patellar taping program in the conservative treatment of patellofemoral pain (9). Other patellofemoral support devices, such as those demonstrated in Chapter 6, may be used to prevent lateral displacement of the patella. Rehabilitation exercises should include isometric hip adduction, isometric quadriceps contractions in the 60 to 90° arc of motion, straight leg raises in hip flexion and adduction, resisted terminal knee extension, knee flexion in 30 to 70°, and lateral steps up from 1 to 8 inches, to allow eccentric and concentric movements (10,11). Closed-chain exercises allow for better patellar tracking than open-chain exercises during full knee extension and through 20° of knee flexion. Open-chain strengthening appears to be more appropriate after 30° of knee flexion (12). Exercises, however, that load the patellofemoral joint, such as deep-knee bends, should be avoided.

> Exercises that load the patellofemoral joint, such as deep knee bends, should be avoided

Chondromalacia Patellae

Chondromalacia patellae is a true degenerative change in the articular cartilage of the patella. This condition occurs when compressive forces exceed the normal range or when alterations in patellar excursion produce abnormal shear forces that damage the articular surface. It is generally described in four stages **(Fig. 9.13)**:

> **Chrondromalacia patellae**
> Degenerative condition in the articular cartilage of the patella caused by abnormal compression or shearing forces

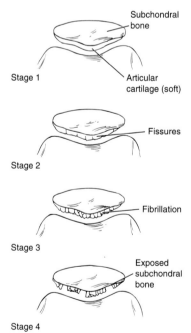

Figure 9.13. Four stages of chondromalacia patellae. Stage 1 involves softening or blistering of the cartilage. Stage 2 reveals fissures in the cartilage. Stage 3 is reached when fibrillation of the cartilage occurs, causing a "crabmeat" appearance. Stage 4 reveals cartilage defects with subchondral bone exposed.

Stage 1. Articular cartilage shows only softening or blistering

Stage 2. Fissures appear in the cartilage

Stage 3. Fibrillation of the cartilage occurs, causing a "crab-meat" appearance

Stage 4. Full cartilage defects are present and subchondral bone is exposed

Asymptomatic chondromalacia does not require treatment. If symptomatic, standard acute care protocol and mild NSAIDs, medial quadriceps strengthening, and a hamstrings flexibility program may be implemented. Exercises such as crouches or deep-knee bends should be avoided, since these positions may aggravate the condition. A knee sleeve with a patellar cutout may be helpful for many individuals.

> Exercises, such as crouches or deep knee bends, should be avoided, since these positions may aggravate the condition

Acute Patellar Subluxation and Dislocation

A subluxation or dislocation of the patella commonly occurs during deceleration with a cutting maneuver. During this action, the patella moves laterally and may tear the medial muscular and retinaculum attachments from the medial aspect of the patella, leading to an audible pop and violent collapse of the knee. In addition to soft tissue damage, the lateral femoral condyle and medial patellar bone may be bruised (13). The patella can remain dislocated or can spontaneously reduce, leaving a painful, swollen, tender knee. The individual will resist any attempt to displace the patella laterally (positive patellar apprehension test). Immediate treatment involves ice, elevation, immobilization, and immediate referral to a physician.

> Dislocation of the patella commonly occurs during deceleration with a cutting maneuver

Patellar Tendinitis (Jumper's Knee)

The patellar tendon frequently becomes inflamed and tender from repetitive or eccentric knee extension activities, such as in running and jumping, hence the name "Jumper's Knee." Pain is concentrated on the infrapatellar tendon, but can also occur at the insertion of the infrapatellar tendon into the tibial tuberosity **(Fig. 9.14)**. Increased pain occurs while ascending and descending stairs, after prolonged sitting, and during resisted knee extension.

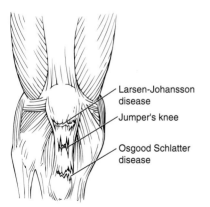

Larsen-Johansson disease

Jumper's knee

Osgood Schlatter disease

Figure 9.14. Patellar conditions may involve Larsen-Johansson disease, patellar tendinitis, or Osgood-Schlatter disease. The pain location will typically define which problem is present.

Immediate treatment involves ice, compression, elevation, relative rest, and NSAIDs. Aquatic therapy is very useful in early stages to reduce gravitational forces. Eccentric quadriceps strengthening and a stretching program for the quadriceps, hamstrings, plantar flexors, hip flexors, and extensors will assist in absorbing some of the strain. **Field Strategy 9.3** summarizes the management and suggested exercises for patellar tendinitis.

Osgood-Schlatter Disease

Osgood-Schlatter disease is a traction-type injury to the tibial apophysis where the infrapatellar tendon attaches onto the tibial tuberosity, and is more common in boys ages 10 to 15. Pain and swelling are present with activity and are relieved with rest. Point tenderness can be elicited directly over the tuberosity, but range of motion is usually not affected. In cases of long duration, the tibial tuberosity may appear enlarged and prominent. Treatment is symptomatic. In most cases, activity is not restricted unless pain is disabling. The condition will rectify itself with closure of the apophysis. A similar condition, **Larsen-Johansson disease**, occurs at the inferior pole of the patella. Treatment is similar to Osgood-Schlatter disease.

Osgood-Schlatter disease
Inflammation or partial avulsion of the tibial apophysis due to traction forces

Larsen-Johansson disease
Inflammation or partial avulsion of the apex of the patella due to traction forces

---

 Field Strategy 9.3. Management of Patellar Tendinitis

Signs and Symptoms

Initially, pain occurs on the inferior pole of the patella or on the tibial tuberosity

Pain is present at the start of activity, subsides with warm up, then reappears after activity, and is particularly bothersome while ascending and descending stairs

Pain occurs on passive knee flexion beyond 120° and during resisted knee extension

Management

Follow PRICE protocol and avoid activities that cause pain
Focus on flexibility for the Achilles tendon, quadriceps, and hamstrings
Strengthening exercises
    Straight-leg raises in all directions
    Short-arc knee extension exercises
    One-quarter knee squats
    Eccentric loading for the quadriceps and dorsiflexors, such as drop squats (e.g., landing from a jump). Later, plyometrics may be used (single-leg hop, double-leg hop, single-leg vertical jump, and bounding)
Cardiovascular exercises may include UBE, swimming, stationary bike with minimal tension, or slide board
A patellofemoral knee sleeve may help during activity

Extensor Tendon Rupture

Extensor tendon ruptures occur as a result of a powerful muscle contraction or in conjunction with severe knee ligamentous disruption. The rupture may be partial or total. A partial rupture will produce pain and muscle weakness in knee extension. If a total rupture occurs distal to the patella, assessment will reveal a high riding patella and an inability to do knee extension. If the rupture is superior to the patella and the extensor retinaculum is still intact, knee extension is still possible, although it will be weak and painful. Treatment will depend on the location and displacement of any bony fragment. In partial ruptures involving a shredded tendon, wiring may be necessary through the patella to relieve tension on the healing tendon. In total ruptures, surgical repair is necessary.

The repetitive motions performed by the female rower, coupled with an increased Q-angle, can lead to stress on the patellofemoral region. The VMO should be strengthened with eccentric and concentric closed-chain exercises.

ILIOTIBIAL BAND FRICTION SYNDROME

A female runner is complaining of pain on the lateral side of her left knee just about at the joint line. The pain in more noticeable when she runs on the local city streets facing traffic and when going up and down stairs. How will you handle this situation?

The iliotibial band continues the line of pull from the tensor fascia latae and gluteus maximus muscle to Gerdy's tubercle on the lateral proximal tibia. The band drops posteriorly behind the lateral femoral epicondyle with knee flexion, then snaps forward over the epicondyle during extension (**Fig. 9.15**). Excessive com-

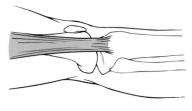

A Extension

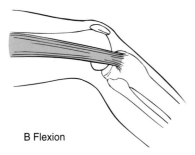

B Flexion

Figure 9.15. A, B. The iliotibial band drops posteriorly behind the lateral femoral epicondyle during knee flexion, then snaps forward over the epicondyle during extension. Malalignment problems or constant irritation can inflame the iliotibial band or lead to bursitis.

Runners, particularly women, who constantly run on the same side of the street are at risk for iliotibial band friction syndrome

pression and friction forces over the greater trochanter and lateral femoral condyle can be caused by a large Q-angle, genu valgus, excessive foot pronation, or constantly running on the same side of the street. Most streets are crowned for water run off, therefore, one leg is always lower than the other, placing considerable strain on lateral joint structures.

Initially, pain is present only while running, particularly uphill and downhill. As the condition progresses, pain is evident in climbing stairs and during walking. Point tenderness is localized over the lateral femoral condyle. A positive Ober's test can confirm the condition (see Assessment). **Field Strategy 9.4** lists signs and symptoms and management of iliotibial band friction syndrome (8).

 Because the runner is female, the increased Q-angle, coupled with the extensive knee flexion and extension required during running, particularly on crowned streets, can contribute to additional strain of the iliotibial band as it passes over the lateral femoral condyle. After controlling inflammation, an extensive flexibility program for the iliotibial band should be initiated.

FRACTURES

A basketball player has had a progressively persistent pain on the proximal tibia since the start of the basketball season, and now reports that it hurts just to walk. There is mild swelling

---

✂ Field Strategy 9.4. Management of Iliotibial Band Friction Syndrome

Signs and Symptoms

Initially, pain does not restrict distance or speed, but, as the condition worsens, distance and speed are limited

Pain is especially noticeable during weight-bearing flexion and extension, such as walking down stairs, and can be palpated over the lateral femoral epicondyle with the leg flexed at 30°

Eventually pain is continuous during daily activities and may produce a creaking sound during knee flexion and extension

Positive Ober's test

Management

Follow PRICE protocol until acute symptoms subside

Increase flexibility in the hip abductors, hip flexors, and lateral thigh muscles

Begin with nonweight-bearing strengthening exercises, such as leg lifts, isometric exercises for knee flexion and knee extension, hip abduction, and hip adduction

Progress to closed-chain strengthening of the hip and thigh muscles

Running or training should be modified to prevent the onset of pain. Hill running should be avoided until asymptomatic

Maintain cardiovascular fitness with swimming

Ice massage before and after running may be helpful

Foot orthodics may correct some structural problems

present on the anteromedial aspect of the proximal tibia just below the joint line, but no other obvious signs. What might be happening to this player?

Traumatic fractures around the knee area are rare in sports, unless you include high-velocity sports such as motorcycling and auto racing. These fractures are usually associated with multiple trauma. Other fractures, however, can occur.

Avulsion fractures may be caused by compressive forces from direct trauma or excessive tensile forces. The individual will have localized pain and tenderness over the bony site and a fragment may be palpated. If a musculotendinous unit is involved, muscle function will be limited.

The tibial tuberosity is a common site for apophyseal fractures in boys and may occur as a result of Osgood-Schlatter disease, which has already been discussed. These injuries are commonly seen in jumping activities like basketball, long jump, and high jump, or in hurdling. The individual will have pain, swelling, and tenderness directly over the tuberosity. When a small fragment of the tuberosity avulses, knee extension will be painful and weak.

Fractures to the proximal tibial epiphysis and distal femoral epiphysis are more serious because of possible arterial damage to the growth plate of each bone. The mechanism of injury is often a varus or valgus stress applied on a fixed weight-bearing foot. These fractures may require internal fixation and can result in an angular or leg length discrepancy.

Stress fractures result from repetitive overload of the bone due to sudden changes in training intensity, duration, frequency, running surface, or poorly worn shoes (14). The individual will complain of localized pain, before and after activity, that is relieved with rest and nonweight bearing. As the condition progresses, pain becomes more persistent. Early bone scans are highly recommended. Treatment involves rest, crutches, or casting.

A **chondral fracture** is a fracture involving the articular cartilage at a joint. An **osteochondral fracture** involves the articular cartilage and underlying bone. These fractures occur when compression from a direct blow to the knee causes shearing or forceful rotation.

Osteochondritis dissecans occurs when a fragment of bone adjacent to the articular surface of a joint is deprived of its blood supply, leading to avascular necrosis. Although found in several joints, it is typically associated with the knee, particularly in males ages 10 to 20 **(Fig. 9.16)**. The most frequent symptom is an aching, diffuse pain and/or swelling with activity. If the bony fragment has displaced and is free floating within the joint, the knee may momentarily lock. A positive diagnosis is made with a radiograph.

A patella fracture will produce diffuse extra-articular swelling on and about the knee. A defect may be palpated and a straight-leg raise will be impossible to perform. Apply ice, elevate, and splint the region with a knee immobilizer.

Chondral fracture
Fracture involving the articular cartilage at a joint

Osteochondral fracture
Fracture involving the articular cartilage and underlying bone

Osteochondritis dissecans
Localized area of avascular necrosis resulting from complete or incomplete separation of joint cartilage and subchondral bone

A straight-leg raise will be impossible to perform with a patella fracture

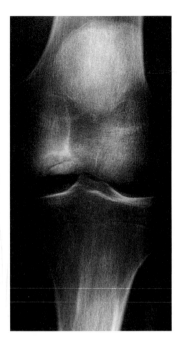

Figure 9.16. Osteochondritis dissecans occurs when a fragment of bone adjacent to the articular surface of a joint is deprived of its blood supply, leading to avascular necrosis. In this patient, a portion of the medial condyle of the femur is damaged.

Distal femoral fractures result from axial loading or rotational forces with added valgus or varus stress, and tend to angulate and displace posteriorly. The adductor muscles contract to rotate and shorten the femoral shaft, giving a characteristic posture (**Fig. 9.17**). Femoral fractures can be life-threatening if the neurovascular structures are damaged by bony fragments leading to

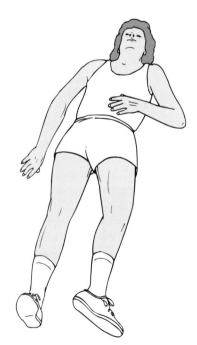

Figure 9.17. In a fractured femur the adductor muscles contract, leading to internal rotation of the femur, external rotation of the tibia, and a shortened appearance of the leg.

excessive blood loss and shock. Summon EMS to properly immobilize the limb in a traction splint and transport the individual to the nearest medical center.

The basketball player may have a stress fracture of the medial tibial plateau. This may be due to repetitive overuse on a hard surface, or lack of adequate support in the shoes to absorb and disperse force. This individual should be referred to a physician for assessment.

ASSESSMENT OF THE KNEE

A high school football player is complaining of anterior knee pain during running and in ascending and descending stairs. Knowing that the knee is a complex joint, can you limit the assessment to only the knee region? Why not?

The lower extremity works as a unit to provide motion. Several biomechanical problems of the foot directly impact strain on the knee. In addition, the knee plays a major role in supporting the body during dynamic and static activities. Furthermore, referred pain from the hip and lumbar spine may also be involved. As such, assessment of the knee complex must encompass an overview of the entire lower extremity.

HISTORY

What information should be gathered from the football player complaining of anterior knee pain during running and in going up and down stairs? What questions can identify the main components of the primary complaint?

Many conditions at the knee are related to family history, age, congenital deformities, mechanical dysfunction, and recent changes in training programs, surfaces, or foot attire. In addition to general questions covered in Chapter 4, specific questions related to the knee can be seen in **Field Strategy 9.5**.

The player reported that pain came on gradually and hurts during running and blocking drills when he attempts to maintain position against an oncoming opponent. It is particularly bothersome while descending stairs or after sitting for a prolonged period of time. He rested for 2 days, iced, and took over-the-counter anti-inflammatory medication, but pain returned when activity resumed. Family history or past related medical history does not appear to be a factor.

OBSERVATION AND INSPECTION

What position(s) do you want to observe this individual in? Should you do a posture and gait analysis? Why? What specific congenital anomalies might contribute to pain at the knee?

Both legs should be clearly visible to denote symmetry, any congenital deformity, swelling, discoloration, hypertrophy, muscle atrophy, or previous surgical incisions. The individual should wear

Field Strategy 9.5. Developing a History of the Injury

Current Injury Status

1. How did the injury occur? What position was the leg in and from what direction did the force originate? Was the foot fixed when impact occurred?
2. Ask about the pain location, severity, onset (sudden or gradual), and type (sharp, aching, burning, radiating). Did you hear any sounds during the incident, such as a snap, pop, or crack? (Snaps or pops may indicate ligament rupture or osteochondral fracture.)
3. Was there any swelling, discoloration, muscle spasms, or numbness with the injury? Did the joint lock or catch? Can you bear weight on the leg?
4. Does it hurt to walk, run, twist, or change directions? Have you recently increased your training frequency, intensity, or duration? Do you wear any equipment or braces that may be aggravating the condition? What type of shoes do you wear when the pain sets in? (Check the height of the heel, wear pattern on bottom, internal arch, and heel padding.)
5. Are there certain activities you cannot perform because of the pain or weakness? How old are you? Which leg is dominant?

Past Injury Status

1. Have you ever injured your knee before? When? How did that occur? What was done for injury?
2. Have you had any medical problems recently? (Look for referred pain from the lumbar spine, hip, or knee.) Are you on any medication? Do you have any other musculoskeletal problems that may have altered your gait?

running shorts to allow full view of the entire lower extremity. Ask the individual to bring the shoes they normally wear when pain is present. Inspect the sole, heel box, and general condition of the shoe for unusual wear, indicating a biomechanical abnormality that may be affecting the knee.

In an ambulatory patient, observe overall body symmetry and gait (refer to **Field Strategy 8.9**). Ask the individual to do a deep knee squat, and to step up and down on a low stool or cement block. Note any abnormalities in gait, favoring one limb, unusual swelling, or discoloration. With the individual sitting on a table, place the injured knee on a folded towel or pillow at 30° flexion to relieve any strain on the joint structures. Inspect the injury site for obvious deformities, discoloration, swelling or scars that might indicate previous surgery, and note the general condition of the skin. Compare the affected limb with the unaffected limb.

The individual appears to walk with a slight antalgic gait. Stepping up and down on a low stool was painful and limited. A deep-knee bend caused considerable anterior knee pain. Slight redness and swelling is noticeable around the patellar tendon.

PALPATIONS

? *With pain centered on the anterior knee region, where should you begin to palpate the various structures? During palpation, what factors are you looking for?*

Bilateral palpations can determine temperature, swelling, point tenderness, crepitus, deformity, muscle spasm, and cutaneous sensation. Vascular pulses can be taken at the popliteal artery in the posterior knee, or at the ankle (see Chapter 8). Proceed proximal to distal, leaving the most painful area to last.

Palpation of bony structures, and compression, distraction, percussion, and vibration, may detect a possible fracture. For example, compression at the distal tibia and fibula causes distraction at the proximal tibiofibular joint. Percussion or tapping on the malleoli and epicondyles of the femur, or use of a tuning fork, may produce positive fracture signs. If you suspect a fracture, immobilize the joint in a knee immobilizer, or summon EMS if a traction splint is necessary. Assess circulatory and neural integrity distal to the fracture site, and take vital signs.

Bony Palpations

1. Patella
2. Medial and lateral femoral condyles and epicondyles
3. Joint line, medial and lateral tibial plateaus, tibial tuberosity, and head of the fibula

Soft Tissue Palpations

1. Quadriceps muscles and adductor muscles
2. Patellar tendon and medial and lateral collateral ligaments
3. Posterior joint capsule, popliteus, hamstring muscles, and gastrocnemius

Palpation for Swelling

At the knee, it is of major importance to palpate for joint effusion, to determine whether swelling is intra-articular or extra-articular. One such test, the patella tap ("ballotable patella") test, is performed with the leg slightly relaxed. The patella is pushed downward into the patellofemoral groove (**Fig. 9.18**). If swelling is intra-articular, the fluid under the patella will cause it to rebound, making the outline of the floating patella clearly visible. This indicates a serious internal joint injury. If the swelling is extra-articular, a click or definite stopping point will be felt when the patella strikes the patellofemoral groove. The outline of the patella will usually be obscured by swelling, typically from a ruptured bursa.

Q *Pain increased on palpation of the superior half of the patellar tendon. Slight swelling and an increase in temperature is also present.*

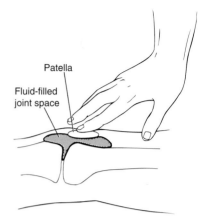

Patella

Fluid-filled
joint space

Figure 9.18. To perform the patella tap ("ballotable patella") test, the leg should be relaxed. Gently push the patella downward into the groove. If joint effusion is present, the patella will rebound and float back up.

SPECIAL TESTS

> *Pain and swelling are present on the superior half of the patellar tendon. What special tests will determine if the injury is a contusion, bursitis, or tendinitis?*

Perform special tests in a comfortable position, preferably supine. Pain and muscle spasm can restrict motion, giving an inaccurate result. Do not force the limb through any sudden motions. It may be necessary to place a rolled towel under the knee to relieve strain on the joint structures.

Joint Range of Motion

Active movements are best with the individual sitting on a table, with the leg flexed over the end of the table. Stabilize the thigh and, as always, perform the most painful movements last to prevent painful symptoms from overflowing into the next movement. Perform the following motions:

1. Knee flexion and extension
2. Medial and lateral rotation of the tibia on the femur with the knee flexed at 90°

Resisted Manual Muscle Testing

Stabilize the hip and provide resistance throughout the full range of motion in a seated position for all motions except knee flexion, which is done in the prone position. As the quadriceps extend the knee, observe any abnormal tibial movement or excessive pain from patellar compression. **Figure 9.19** demonstrates motions that should be tested:

1. Knee extension
2. Ankle plantar flexion
3. Ankle dorsiflexion
4. Knee flexion

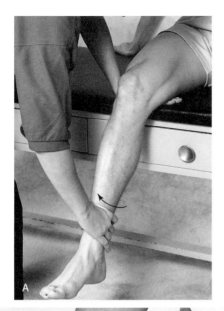

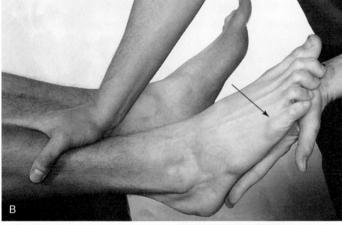

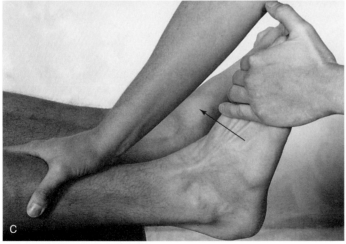

Figure 9.19. Resisted manual muscle testing. **A.** Knee extension. **B.** Ankle plantar flexion. **C.** Ankle dorsiflexion. **D.** Knee flexion. Arrows indicate the direction the athlete moves the body part against the applied resistance.

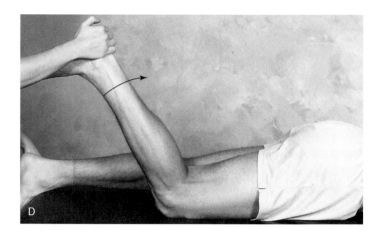

Figure 9.19. (continued)

Neurologic Assessment

Neurologic integrity is assessed with manual muscle testing (already completed), reflex testing, and cutaneous sensation. Always compare results bilaterally to determine what is normal for the individual.

Reflexes in the lower extremity include the patella (L_3, L_4) and Achilles tendon reflex (S_1), and were demonstrated in Chapter 8 (see **Fig. 8.22**). In testing cutaneous sensation, run a sharp and dull object over the skin, i.e., blunt tip of taping scissors vs. flat edge of taping scissors. With their eyes closed or looking away, ask the individual if they can distinguish sharp and dull. Any variations in sensation, such as numbness or tingling, should be documented and the individual referred to a physician for more extensive evaluation.

Stress and Functional Tests

From information gathered during the history, observation, inspection, and palpation, determine which tests most effectively assess the condition. Perform only those tests you believe to be absolutely necessary.

Valgus Stress Test

With the individual supine and leg extended, place the heel of one hand on the lateral joint line. The other hand should stabilize the distal lower leg. Apply a lateral or valgus stress at the joint line, with the lower leg fully extended, and again at 30° flexion (**Fig. 9.20A**). If positive (i.e., the tibia abducts), primary damage is to the medial collateral ligament and posteromedial joint structures.

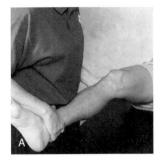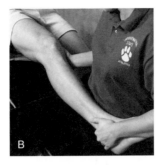

Figure 9.20. A. Valgus stress test. Flex the knee at 30° and apply a gentle valgus stress at the knee joint while moving the lower leg laterally. Repeat the test with the knee fully extended. **B.** Varus stress test. Flex the knee at 30° and apply a gently varus stress at the knee joint while moving the lower leg medially. Repeat the test with the knee fully extended.

Varus Stress Test

The knee is placed in a position similar to the valgus test; however, a medial or varus stress is applied at the knee joint **(Fig. 9.20B)**. Laxity in full extension indicates major instability. When testing at 20 to 30° of flexion, the true test for one-plane lateral instability, a positive test indicates damage to the lateral collateral ligament.

Anterior and Posterior Drawer Test

The anterior cruciate ligament and posterior cruciate ligament can be assessed with the drawer test. Have the patient seated while reclining against the room wall. Flex the knee at approximately 90° and stabilize the foot by placing it under your thigh to prevent any tibial rotation. An alternative position is to have the patient seated at the edge of the table with the foot stabilized between your legs. Place both thumbs on either side of the patella tendon, extending the fingers into the popliteal fossa. Apply alternating anterior and posterior displacement force on the proximal tibia **(Fig. 9.21A)**. Stability can be visualized from a lateral view or palpated with the thumb at the joint line. The test is positive for an anterior cruciate injury if the tibia shifts abnormally anterior, and positive for an posterior cruciate injury if the tibia shifts abnormally posterior.

Gravity Drawer Test (Posterior "Sag" Sign)

A one-plane posterior instability can also be tested by flexing the hip and knee at 90°. In this position the tibia sags back on the femur if the posterior cruciate ligament is torn **(Fig. 9.21B)**. It is important to note the sag, since it may produce a false-positive Drawer test if the sag goes unnoticed.

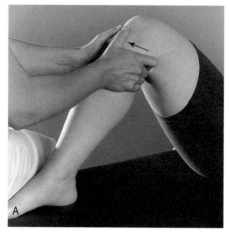
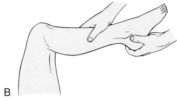

Figure 9.21. A. Drawer test. Flex the knee at approximately 90° and stabilize the foot. Place both thumbs on either side of the patella tendon and apply an anterior and posterior displacement force on the proximal tibia. **B.** The posterior "sag" test. Flex both hip and knees. Look from the side and compare the anterior contours of both legs. If one leg sags back and the prominence of the tibial tuberosity is lost, the posterior cruciate may be damaged.

Meniscal Test

At this level of experience, meniscal injuries are difficult to assess; suspicion is your best tool. Ask the individual to show the maneuver that last reproduced the symptoms. Can they do a deep knee squat? Can they bear weight on the affected limb and cross the opposite foot in front of and behind that limb (cross-over test)? You are attempting to trap the torn meniscus in the joint, producing pain and an audible click.

Patella Compression or Grind Test

Place a rolled towel under the knee, flexing it at about 20°. Compress the patella into the patellofemoral groove **(Fig. 9.22A)**. The test is positive if pain is felt or a grinding sound is heard. You can also place the web of your hand just proximal to the patella **(Fig. 9.22B)**. Ask the individual to contract the quadriceps while you gently push downward. If the individual has pain, the test is positive for chondromalacia patellae. This test can elicit pain in any individual if the pressure is significant, so caution is warranted.

Patella Apprehension Test

With the knee in a relaxed position, push the patella laterally **(Fig. 9.23)**. If the individual voluntarily or involuntarily shows apprehension, it is a positive test for subluxating patella.

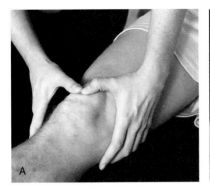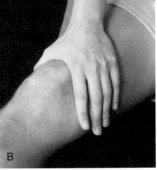

A

B

Figure 9.22. A. Pain on compression of the patella into the groove indicates pathology to the patella articular cartilage. **B.** An alterative method is to apply slight compression just proximal to the superior pole of the patella and ask the individual to contract the quadriceps. The test is positive for chondromalacia patella if the individual has pain or is unable to hold the contraction.

Ober's Test for Iliotibial Tract Contracture

The individual lies on their side with the lower leg slightly flexed at the hip and knee for stability. Stabilize the pelvis with one hand, to prevent the pelvis from shifting posteriorly during the test. Passively abduct and slightly extend the hip so the iliotibial

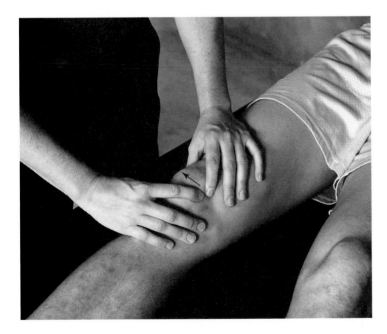

Figure 9.23. To perform the patella apprehension test, gently displace the patella laterally. The test is a positive sign for subluxating patella if the individual shows apprehension.

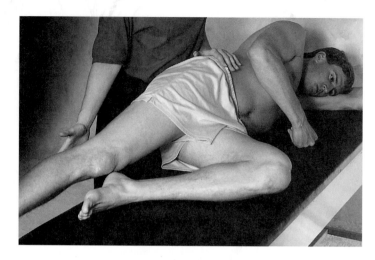

Figure 9.24. To perform Ober's test, passively abduct and slightly extend the hip. Slowly lower the extended leg. If the iliotibial band is tight, the leg will remain in the abducted position.

tract passes over the greater trochanter (**Fig. 9.24**). Although the original Ober's test called for the knee to be flexed at 90°, the iliotibial tract has a greater stretch if the knee is extended. Slowly lower the upper leg. If the iliotibial band is tight, the leg will remain in the abducted position.

Functional Tests

Functional tests should be performed pain-free without a limp or antalgic gait before clearing the individual for return to participation. Examples of functional tests include forward running, crossover stepping, running figure-8s or V-cuts, side-step running, and karioca running. When appropriate, functional braces or protective supportive devices should be used to prevent reinjury.

💡 *During special tests you found increased pain and weakness during active and resisted knee extension. Passive knee flexion at the extremes of motion led to pain in the anterior knee region, but extension was not painful. Neurologic assessment was normal, and other stress tests were negative. Did you determine the individual may have patellar tendinitis? If so, you are correct. How will you manage this condition?*

REHABILITATION

❓ *What major components must be included in a knee rehabilitation program? What criteria determine when an individual can return to sport participation?*

Rehabilitation attempts to minimize edema and the effects of limited activity by initiating early mobilization and controlled movement, to allow healing tissues to be stressed gradually and progressively until normal joint function is restored. Sample exer-

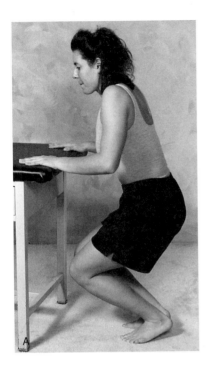
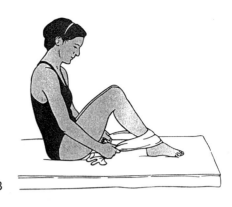
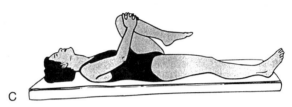

Figure 9.25. Range-of-motion exercises. **A.** Half squat. **B.** Assisted heel slide. **C.** Assisted knee flexion.

cise programs for specific injuries were listed in several Field Strategies, therefore, discussion here will be very general.

Range-of-motion exercises can begin on the first day of injury. Continuous passive motion (CPM) machines are primarily used post-surgically at the knee or after knee manipulation (See **Fig. 5.17**). When a CPM machine is not needed, range-of-motion exercises, such as the wall slide, heel slide, assisted knee flexion and extension, half squats, or PNF stretching exercises can be performed (**Fig. 9.25**).

Proprioception can be regained early through shifting one's weight while on crutches, straight leg raises, bilateral mini squats, or use of a BAPS board with support. As balance improves, unassisted use of the BAPS board, running in place on a mini-tramp, or use of a slide board may be incorporated, along with other closed-chain exercises.

Strengthening exercises should focus on the quadriceps musculature, particularly the vastus medialis and VMO. These muscles aid in the stabilization of the patella superiorly and medially. Isometric contractions, called quad sets, are performed at, or near, 0°, 45°, 60°, and 90° flexion. Isometric hip adduction exercises are also used to recruit the VMO, and can be performed by squeezing a rolled towel between the knees in a seated position.

Closed-chain exercises may include terminal knee extension

> Because of their importance in patellar stabilization, strengthening exercises should focus on the vastus medialis and vastus medialis oblique (VMO)

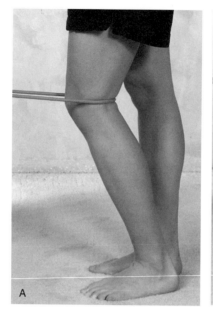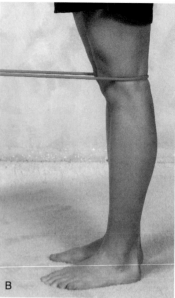

Figure 9.26. Closed-chain terminal extension. **A.** Starting position. **B.** Ending position.

(**Fig. 9.26**), step ups, step downs, lateral step ups, mini squats from 0° to 40°, leg presses on a machine from 0° to 60°, or use of a stepping machine (9). Several of these exercises were illustrated in **Field Strategy 9.1**. Exercises can be made progressively more difficult by using surgical tubing, increasing the resistance and speed of movement, or changing the individual's visual feedback, such as looking at the ceiling, looking at the floor, or closing the eyes (15).

Plyometric jumping in the later stages of rehabilitation can use small boxes and directional changes to improve power and proprioceptive function. Because of the increased eccentric contraction and the associated muscle microtrauma that results from the power maneuvers, these exercises should only be performed two or three times weekly.

Maintenance of cardiovascular fitness can begin immediately with use of an upper body ergometer (UBE) or hydrotherapeutic exercise. When range of motion is adequate, a stationary bicycle may be used. The seat should be adjusted so that the knee is flexed 15° to 30°. The individual should be instructed to pedal with the ball of the foot, using toe clips, and pull through the bottom of the stroke. A low to moderate workload is recommended to reduce patellofemoral compressive forces. Other exercises, such as walking, light jogging, and functional activities can progress as tolerated.

The rehabilitation program should restore motion and proprioception, maintain cardiovascular fitness, and improve muscular strength, endurance, and power. The individual can return to sport participation after completing all functional tests pain free and must be cleared by the supervising physician. These tests might include timed sprints, shuttle runs, agility runs, karioca runs, hop or vertical jump tests.

SUMMARY

The knee is highly susceptible to stress during sport activities, particularly in running and jumping that involve deceleration and rotation. Congenital abnormalities, muscle imbalance, muscle dysfunction, and postural deviations can also lead to injury. During the assessment, remember that referred pain may originate in the lumbar spine, hip, or ankle. **Field Strategy 9.6** lists the steps in assessing a knee.

Refer the individual to a physician if any of the following condi-

---

 Field Strategy 9.6. Knee Evaluation

History

Primary complaint and mechanism of injury
Onset of symptoms, including pain and discomfort
Changes in training/equipment/shoes
Disability and functional impairments from the injury
Previous injuries to the area and family history

Observation and Inspection

Observe general posture and gait
Inspect:
    Muscle symmetry   Hypertrophy or muscle atrophy
    Swelling   Congenital deformity
    Discoloration   Surgical incisions or scars

Palpation

Bony structures to determine possible fracture
Soft tissue structures to determine:
    Temperature   Crepitus
    Swelling   Muscle spasm
    Point tenderness   Cutaneous sensation
    Deformity   Vascular pulses
Patella tap test for joint swelling

Special Tests

Active range of motion
Resisted manual muscle testing
Neurologic testing
Stress and functional tests
    Valgus and varus stress tests
    Drawer test and posterior "sag" test
    Meniscal test (deep knee bends, cross-over test)
    Patella compression test
    Patella apprehension test
    Ober's test
    Functional tests

tions are suspected: obvious deformity suggesting a dislocation or fracture; significant loss of motion or locking of the knee; excessive joint swelling; gross joint instability; sounds, such as popping, snapping, clicking, or giving way of the knee; possible epiphyseal injuries; abnormal or absent reflexes; abnormal cutaneous sensations; absent or weak pulse; muscle weakness; or any unexplained or chronic pain. Any knee injury that disrupts an individual's play or performance should be diagnosed by a physician.

If the individual is referred to a physician, remove the person from activity and splint the limb in a knee immobilizer or other appropriate splint. If necessary, fit the individual for crutches if they are unable to walk without a limp or pain. Apply cryotherapy to control swelling and transport the individual in an appropriate manner. The individual should not return to activity until they can perform all functional tests pain-free and receive a medical clearance to participate.

REFERENCES

1. Soderberg GL. *Kinesiology: Application to pathological motion*. Baltimore: Williams & Wilkins, 1986.
2. Beaupré A, et al. 1986. Knee menisci: correlation between microstructure and biomechanics. Clin Orthop & Rel Res 208:72–75.
3. McGee DJ. *Orthopedic physical assessment*. Philadelphia: WB Saunders, 1987.
4. Jenkins DB. *Hollinshead's functional anatomy of the limbs and back*. Philadelphia: WB Saunders, 1991.
5. Arendt E, and Dick R. 1995. Knee injury patterns among men and women in collegiate basketball and soccer: NCAA data and review of literature. Am J Sports Med 23(6):694–701.
6. Lastihenos M, and Nicholas SJ. 1996. Managing ACL injuries in children: are kids' injuries different? Phys Sportsmed 24(4):59–70.
7. Bynym EB, Barrack RL, and Alexander AH. 1995. Open versus closed chain kinetic exercises after anterior cruciate ligament reconstruction: a prospective randomized study. Am J Sports Med 23(4):401–406.
8. Cooper DE, Arnoczky SP, and Warren RF. Arthroscopic meniscal repair. In *Clinics in sports medicine*, edited by KM Singer. vol. 9, no. 3. Philadelphia: WB Saunders, 1990.
9. Kowall MG, Kolk G, Nuber GW, Cassisi JE, and Stern SH. 1996. Patellar taping the treatment of patellofemoral pain: a prospective randomized study. Am J Sports Med 24(1):61–71.
10. Westfall DC, and Worrell TW. 1992. Anterior knee pain syndrome: role of the vastus medialis oblique. J Spt Rehab 1(4):317–325.
11. Spiker JC, and Massie DL. 1992. Comprehensive management of patellofemoral pain. J Spt Rehab 1(3):258–263.
12. Doucette SA, and Child DD. 1996. The effect of open and closed chain exercise and knee joint position on patellar tracking in lateral patellar compression syndrome. JOSPT 23(2):104–110.
13. Sallay PI, Poggi J, Speer KP, and Garrett WE. 1996. Acute dislocation of the patella: a correlative pathoanatomic study. Am J Sports Med 24(1):52–60.
14. Brown DE. Ankle and leg injuries. In *The team physician's handbook*, edited by MB Mellion, WM Walsh, and GL Shelton. Philadelphia: Hanley & Belfus, Inc, 1990.
15. Harrelson GL. Knee rehabilitation. In *Physical rehabilitation of the injured athlete*, edited by JR Andrews and GL Harrelson. Philadelphia: WB Saunders, 1991.

Thigh, Hip, and Pelvis Injuries

After completing this chapter, you should be able to:

- Locate the important bony and soft tissue structures of the thigh, hip, and pelvis

- Describe the motions of the hip and identify the muscles that produce them

- Identify measures that can prevent injury to the region

- Recognize specific injuries at the thigh, hip, and pelvis

- Demonstrate a basic assessment of the hip region

- Demonstrate general rehabilitation exercises for the region

Key Terms:

Hip pointer	**Osteitis pubis**
Hypovolemic shock	**Pulmonary embolism**
Innominate bones	**Sacral plexus**
Legg-Calvé-Perthes disease	**Snapping hip syndrome**
Lumbar plexus	**Thrombophlebitis**
Myositis ossificans	

Although the thigh, hip, and pelvis have a sturdy anatomical composition and are seldom injured in sport participation, the soft tissues of the thigh are frequently injured. Compressive forces can lead to contusions and strains, but usually are not serious unless they are mismanaged. Daily activities, such as sitting, walking, or climbing stairs, rarely involve stretching of the hamstrings. As a result, this inflexibility, and a strength imbalance between the hamstrings and the more frequently exercised quadriceps, place the sport participant at a higher risk for strain of the hamstrings.

This chapter begins with a review of the anatomy and major muscle actions of the thigh, hip, and pelvis. Next, preventative measures will be discussed, followed by information on basic injuries to the region. A step-by-step basic injury assessment process is then presented, followed by examples of rehabilitation exercises for the region.

ANATOMY OF THE THIGH, HIP, AND PELVIS

? *Although the hip has a larger range of motion than the knee and ankle joints, injuries to the hip are less common. Why is this true?*

The thigh, hip, and pelvis have an extremely stable bony structure that is further reinforced by a number of large, strong ligaments and muscles. This region is anatomically well-suited for withstanding the large forces to which it is subjected during daily activities.

Bony Structure of the Thigh, Hip, and Pelvis

The femur of the thigh is a major weight-bearing bone and is the longest, largest, and strongest bone in the body (**Fig. 10.1**). Its weakest component is the femoral neck, which is smaller in diameter than the rest of the bone, and weak internally because it is primarily composed of cancellous bone. The femur angles medially downward from the hip during the support phase of walking and running, enabling single leg support beneath the body's center of gravity. Because women have a wider pelvis, this angulation tends to be more pronounced in women.

The hip joint is the articulation between the concave acetabulum of the pelvis and the head of the femur. The acetabulum functions as a classic ball and socket joint. The acetabulum angles obliquely in an inferior, anterior, and lateral direction. Because the socket is deep, it provides considerable bony stability to the joint.

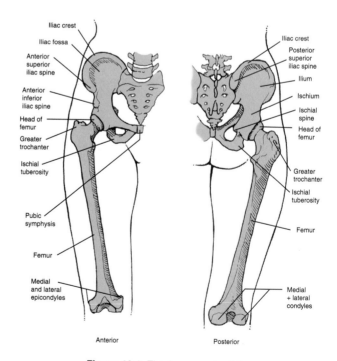

Figure 10.1. The femur and pelvis.

The pelvis, or pelvic girdle, consists of a protective bony ring formed by four fused bones—the two **innominate bones**, the sacrum, and coccyx (**Fig. 10.1**). The innominate bones articulate with each other anteriorly at the symphysis pubis, and with the sacrum posteriorly at the sacroiliac joints. Each innominate bone consists of three fused bones—the ilium, ischium, and pubis. Among these, the ilium forms the major portion of the innominate bone, including the prominent iliac crests. The anterior superior iliac spine (ASIS) is a readily palpable landmark. The posterior superior iliac spine (PSIS) is typically marked by an indentation in the soft tissues just lateral to the sacrum. The pelvis protects the enclosed inner organs, transmits loads between the trunk and lower extremity, and provides a site for a number of major muscle attachments.

Innominate bones
Without a name; used to describe anatomic structures

The pelvic girdle consists of the sacrum, coccyx, and two innominate bones, which are a combination of the fused ilium, ischium, and pubis

Hip Joint

The joint capsule of the hip is large and loose. It completely surrounds the joint. Because the capsular fibers attaching to the femoral neck are arranged in a circular fashion, they are known as the zona orbicularis. The zona orbicularis is an important contributor to hip stability.

The interior of the capsule is covered by a synovial membrane and several bursae are present. The iliopsoas bursa is positioned between the iliopsoas and the articular capsule, serving to reduce the friction between these structures. The deep trochanteric bursa provides a cushion between the greater trochanter of the femur and the gluteus maximus at its attachment to the iliotibial tract.

Several large, strong ligaments support the hip (**Fig. 10.2**). On the anterior aspect, the extremely strong Y-shaped iliofemoral ligament and the pubofemoral ligament limit hip hyperextension. The ischiofemoral ligament reinforces the hip posteriorly. Tension in these major ligaments acts to twist the head of the femur into

The pelvis protects the abdominal organs, transmits loads between the trunk and lower extremity, and provides a site for muscle attachments

The most prominent bursae at the hip joint are the iliopsoas bursa and deep trochanteric bursa

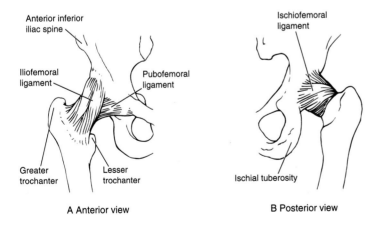

Figure 10.2. The ligaments of the hip.

Anterior inferior iliac spine

Iliofemoral ligament

Pubofemoral ligament

Greater trochanter

Lesser trochanter

A Anterior view

Ischiofemoral ligament

Ischial tuberosity

B Posterior view

The iliofemoral and pubofemoral ligaments, located on the anterior aspect of the hip, severely limit hip hyperextension

Lumbar plexus
Interconnected roots of the first four lumbar spinal nerves

The sciatic nerve is the largest and longest nerve in the body and innervates the hamstrings and adductor magnus

Sacral plexus
Interconnected roots of the L_4 to S_4 spinal nerves

The femoral arteries provide the major blood supply to the lower extremity, with the lateral and medial circumflex arteries providing blood supply to the hip joint

the acetabulum upon hip extension, as when a person rises from a seated position.

A number of large, strong muscles cross the hip, enhancing its stability. The muscles of the hip are summarized in **Table 10.1** and the actions of the major muscles are discussed later in the chapter.

Nerves and Blood Vessels of the Thigh, Hip, and Pelvis

The major nerve supply to the thigh, hip, and pelvis arises from the lumbar and sacral plexi. The **lumbar plexus** is formed from the first four lumbar spinal nerves **(Fig. 10.3)**. It spawns the femoral nerve that supplies the muscles and skin of the anterior thigh. Another branch, the obturator nerve, provides innervation to the hip adductor muscles.

The lower spinal nerves, including L_4 through S_4, form the **sacral plexus**, which spawns the largest and longest single nerve in the body, the sciatic nerve **(Fig. 10.3)**. The sciatic nerve innervates the hamstrings and adductor magnus. The tibial and common peroneal nerves that branch from the sciatic nerve in the posterior thigh region are discussed in Chapters 8 and 9.

The external iliac arteries become the femoral arteries at the level of the thighs, providing the major blood supply to the lower extremity **(Fig. 10.4)**. The femoral artery gives off several branches in the thigh region, including the deep femoral artery, which serves the posterior and lateral thigh muscles, and the lateral and medial femoral circumflex arteries, which supply the region of the femoral head.

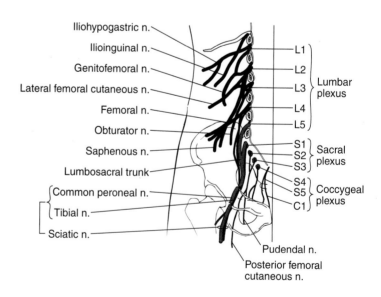

Figure 10.3. The lumbar and sacral plexus.

Table 10.1. Muscles of the Hip

Muscle	Proximal Attachment	Distal Attachment	Primary Action(s)	Nerve Innervation
Rectus femoris	Anterior inferior iliac spine (AIIS)	Patella	Hip flexion & knee extension	Femoral
Iliopsoas			Hip flexion	L_1 & Femoral
Iliacus	Iliac fossa and adjacent sacrum	Lesser trochanter		
Psoas major	12th thoracic and lumbar vertebrae and lumbar discs	Lesser trochanter		
Sartorius	Anterior superior iliac spine (ASIS)	Upper medial tibia	Assists with flexion, abduction, and lateral rotation	Femoral
Pectineus	Pectineal crest of pubic ramus	Medial proximal femur	Flexion and adduction	Femoral
Tensor fascia lata	Anterior crest of the ilium & ASIS	Iliotibial band	Assists with flexion, abduction and medial rotation	Superior gluteal
Gluteus maximus	Posterior ilium, iliac crest, sacrum, and coccyx	Gluteal tuberosity of the femur and iliotibial band	Hip extension & lateral rotation	Inferior gluteal
Gluteus medius	Between posterior and anterior gluteal lines on the posterior ilium	Superior, lateral greater trochanter	Abduction	Superior gluteal
Gluteus minimus	Between anterior and inferior gluteal lines on posterior ilium	Anterior surface of the greater trochanter	Medial rotation	Superior gluteal
Gracilis	Anterior, inferior symphysis pubis	Medial, proximal tibia	Adduction	Obturator
Adductor magnus	Inferior ramus of pubis and ischium	Entire linea aspera	Adduction	Obturator
Adductor longus	Anterior pubis	Middle linea aspera	Adduction	Obturator
Adductor brevis	Inferior ramus of the pubis	Upper lineal aspera	Adduction	Obturator
Semitendinosus	Medial ischial tuberosity	Proximal, medial tibia	Hip extension & knee flexion	Tibial
Semimembranosus	Lateral ischial tuberosity	Proximal, medial tibia	Hip extension & knee flexion	Tibial
Biceps femoris				
Long head	Lateral ischial tuberosity	Head of fibula & condyle of tibia	Hip extension & knee flexion	Tibial
Short head	Lateral linea aspera		Knee flexion	Common peroneal
Lateral rotators	Sacrum, ilium, and ischium	Posterior greater trochanter	Lateral rotation	L_5 to S_2

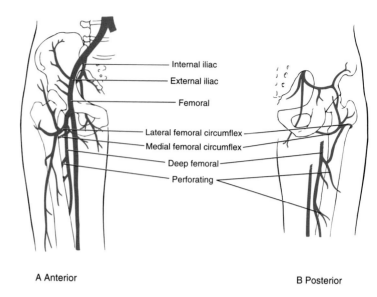

Internal iliac	
External iliac	
Femoral	
Lateral femoral circumflex	
Medial femoral circumflex	
Deep femoral	
Perforating	

A Anterior   B Posterior

Figure 10.4. The arterial supply to the hip region.

The hip is the most stable joint in the body. Not only does it have a substantial amount of bony stability, but it is reinforced by several large, strong ligaments and muscles. As such, the hip joint is seldom injured.

MAJOR MUSCLE ACTIONS OF THE HIP

Which muscles that move the hip also contribute to motion of the knee? What is the functional significance of these two-joint muscles?

Since the hip is a ball and socket joint, the femur can move in all planes of motion (**Fig. 10.5**). However, the massive muscles crossing the hip tend to limit range of motion, particularly in the posterior direction.

Flexion

The major hip flexors are the iliacus and psoas major, referred to jointly as the iliopsoas because of their common attachment at the femur (**Fig. 10.6**). Four other muscles cross the anterior aspect of the hip that also contribute to hip flexion. These include the pectineus, rectus femoris, sartorius, and tensor fascia latae. Because the rectus femoris is a two-joint muscle active during both hip flexion and knee extension, it functions more effectively as a hip flexor when the knee is in flexion, as when a person kicks a ball. The sartorius is also a two-joint muscle. Crossing from the ASIS to the medial surface of the proximal tibia just below the tuberosity, the sartorius is the longest muscle in the body.

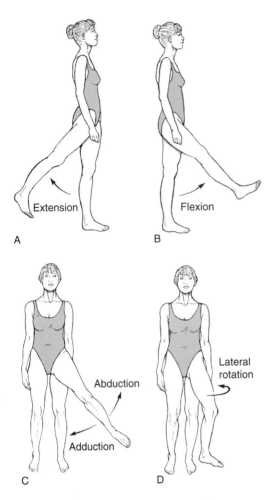

Figure 10.5. A–D. Motions at the hip.

Extension

The hip extensors are the gluteus maximus and the three hamstrings—the biceps femoris, semitendinosus, and semimembranosus (**Fig. 10.6**). The gluteus maximus is usually active only when
the hip is in flexion, as during stair climbing or cycling, or when
extension at the hip is resisted. The nickname "hamstrings" derives
from the prominent tendons of the three muscles, which are
readily palpable on the posterior aspect of the knee. The hamstrings cross both the hip and knee, contributing to hip extension
and knee flexion.

> The hamstrings contribute
> to both hip extension and
> knee flexion

Abduction

The gluteus medius is the major abductor at the hip, with assistance from the gluteus minimus. The hip abductors are active in

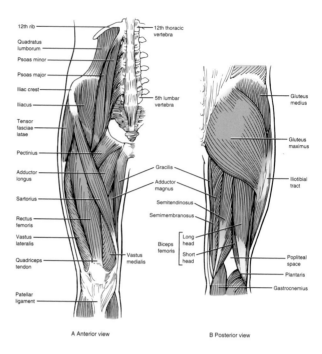

Figure 10.6. The superficial muscles of the hip and thigh.

stabilizing the pelvis during single leg support of the body and during the support phase of walking and running. For example, when body weight is supported by the right foot during walking, the right hip abductors contract isometrically and eccentrically to prevent the left side of the pelvis from being pulled downward by the weight of the swinging left leg. This allows the left leg to move freely through the swing phase without scuffing the toes. If the hip abductors are too weak to perform this function, then lateral pelvic tilt occurs with every step during gait.

Adduction

The hip adductors include the adductor longus, adductor brevis, and adductor magnus (**Fig. 10.6**). These muscles are active during the swing phase of gait to bring the foot beneath the body's center of gravity for placement during the support phase. The relatively weak gracilis also assists with hip adduction. The hip adductors also contribute to flexion and internal rotation at the hip, especially when the femur is externally rotated.

The hip adductors also contribute to flexion and internal rotation at the hip

Medial and Lateral Rotation of the Femur

Although several muscles contribute to lateral rotation of the femur, there are six muscles that function solely as lateral rotators. These are the piriformis, gemellus superior, gemellus inferior, obturator internus, obturator externus, and quadratus femoris

346 Section 3 Injuries to the Lower Extremity

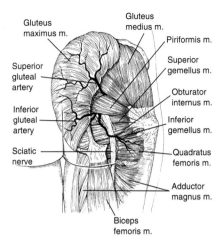

Gluteus maximus m.
Gluteus medius m.
Piriformis m.
Superior gluteal artery
Superior gemellus m.
Obturator internus m.
Inferior gluteal artery
Inferior gemellus m.
Sciatic nerve
Quadratus femoris m.
Adductor magnus m.
Biceps femoris m.

Figure 10.7. The deep muscles of the posterior hip. Note that the sciatic nerve passes inferior to the piriformis muscle to enter the posterior thigh.

(**Fig. 10.7**). Lateral rotation of the femur of the swinging leg occurs during gait to accommodate the lateral rotation of the pelvis.

The major medial rotator of the femur is the gluteus minimus, with assistance from the tensor fascia latae, gluteus medius, and the four adductor muscles. The medial rotators are weak in comparison to the lateral rotators, with the estimated strength of the medial rotators only approximately a third of the lateral rotators (1).

When a muscle crosses two joints, the positions of both joints affect the amount of stretch or tension present in the muscle. Both joint positions, therefore, affect the extent to which a muscle can be stretched during a warm-up exercise and the amount of force the muscle can produce upon contraction. This principle will have significance during injury assessment.

PREVENTION OF INJURIES

Muscles of the thigh, hip, and pelvis are used extensively in nearly every physical activity. What exercises will strengthen the muscles in this region to prevent injury?

The hip joint is well-protected within the pelvic girdle and is seldom injured. Many collision and contact sports require special hip and buttock protection to pad the iliac crests, sacrum and coccyx, and genital region. In addition, the male genital region can be further protected by a protective cup worn inside an athletic supporter. Inflammation of the hip joint and stress fractures to the femoral neck or pubis can be prevented by proper heel cushioning to absorb and disperse ground shock during running. Many of these commercial pads were illustrated in Chapter 6.

Field Strategy 10.1. Exercises to Prevent Injury at the Thigh, Hip, and Pelvis

Field Strategy 9.1 demonstrated stretching exercises for the hamstrings, quadriceps, and iliotibial band, and strengthening exercises for the muscles that cross the knee joint. In addition, the following may be performed:

A. **Hip flexor stretch (lunge)**. Extend the leg to be stretched behind you. Bend the contralateral knee in front of you as you move the hips forward. While keeping the back straight, flex the forward knee

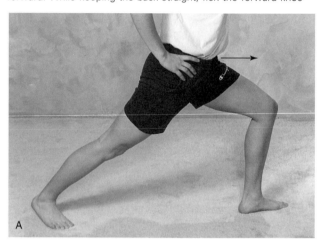

B. **Lateral rotator stretch, seated position**. Cross one leg over the thigh and place the elbow on the outside of the knee. Gently stretch the buttock muscles by pushing the flexed knee across the body while keeping the pelvis on the floor

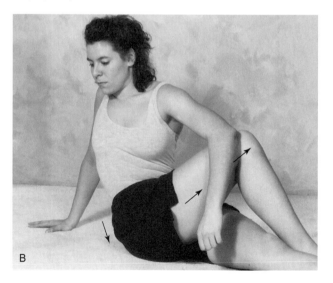

Field Strategy 10.1. Exercises to Prevent Injury at the Thigh, Hip, and Pelvis (continued)

C. **Adductor stretch, standing position**. Place the leg to be stretched out to the side, on a chair, or on a table. Slowly flex the contralateral knee. Keep the hips in a neutral or extended position

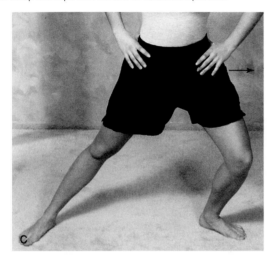

D. **Theraband or tubing exercises**. Secure Theraband or surgical tubing to a table. Perform hip flexion, extension, abduction, adduction, and medial and lateral rotation in a single plane or in multidirectional patterns

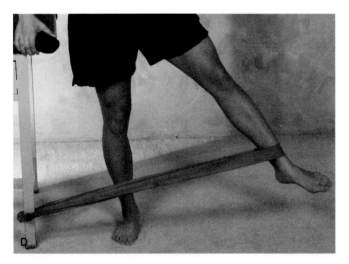

E. **Full squats**. A weight belt should be worn during this exercise with heavy weights. Place the feet a shoulder-width apart. Keep the back straight by keeping the chest out and the head up at all times. Flex the knees and hips to no greater than 90°. Begin the upward motion by extending the hips first.

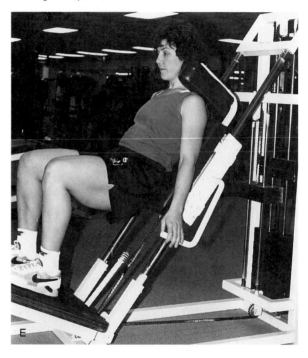

F. **Hip extension**. With the trunk stabilized and the back flat, extend the hip while keeping the knee flexed. Alternate legs

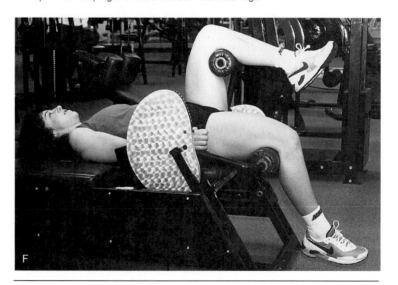

Many flexibility and strengthening exercises of the quadriceps, hamstrings, and tensor fascia latae were illustrated in Chapter 9. **Field Strategy 10.1** illustrates some additional exercises for the hip flexors, extensors, adductors, abductors, and medial and lateral rotators.

Muscles that move the hip must be flexible enough to prevent muscular strains. In addition, strengthening exercises for the hip should be incorporated into a year-round physical conditioning program.

CONTUSIONS

A pitcher was struck on the anterior thigh from a line drive, leading to immediate pain and loss of function. After assessing the injury, you determined the player should move to the dugout to ice the region to control acute swelling. What position should the leg be placed in to limit the amount of edema formation?

Contusions may occur anywhere in the hip region, but are typically seen in the quadriceps muscle group, often referred to as a charley horse, or on the crest of the ilium, called a hip pointer. Football and hockey have special athletic girdles to allow hip and thigh pads to be slipped conveniently into slots, thus protecting the area. These girdles can also be worn in other sports to protect this vulnerable area.

Contusions to the quadriceps muscle group are often referred to as a charley horse; to the iliac crest, hip pointers

Quadriceps Contusion

The most common site for a quadriceps contusion is the anterolateral thigh and it almost always damages muscle tissue. Immediately after impact, pain and swelling may be extensive. In a moderate contusion, the individual can flex the knee only between 45 and 90° and will walk with a noticeable limp. If severe, the individual will be unable to bear weight or fully flex the knee. Within 24 hours, there may be a palpable firm hematoma, resulting in an inability to contract the quadriceps or do a straight-leg raise (2). Treatment involves ice application and a compressive wrap for the first 24 hours, applied with the knee in maximal flexion **(Fig. 10.8)**. This position preserves the needed flexion and limits intramuscular bleeding and spasm. **Field Strategy 10.2** further explains the care of a quadriceps contusion.

Myositis Ossificans

Myositis ossificans is an abnormal ossification involving bone deposition within muscle tissue and may stem from a single traumatic blow, or several repeated blows to the quadriceps **(Fig. 10.9)**. Common sites involve the anterior and lateral thigh. Examination reveals a warm, firm, swollen thigh nearly 2 to 4 cm larger than the unaffected thigh. A palpable mass may limit passive knee flexion to 20 to 30 degrees. Active quadriceps contractions

Myositis ossificans
Accumulation of mineral deposits in muscle tissue

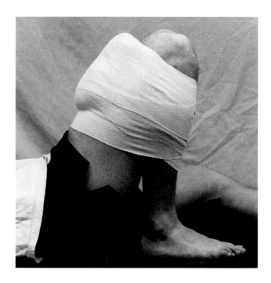

Figure 10.8. Ice a quadriceps contusion with the knee in maximal flexion to place the muscles on stretch.

 Field Strategy 10.2. Management of a Quadriceps Contusion

Acute Phase (first 24 to 48 hours)

Apply ice packs and compression with knee flexed at 120°
Crutches with non- or partial weight bearing
Pain-free passive stretching and gentle, active range-of-motion exercises
Anti-inflammatory medication after 24 hours

Subacute Phase (2 to 5 days)

Continue NSAIDs, cryotherapy, and passive stretching exercises
Active range-of-motion and pain-free resisted PNF strengthening exercises
Swimming with gentle kicking exercises
Partial weight bearing continued until 90° flexion is attained

Full Weight Bearing

Continue active range-of-motion exercises and initiate progressive
    resistance exercises
Cycling or light jogging as tolerated
Radiograph at 3 weeks to rule out myositis ossificans

Final Phase

Range of motion within 10° of unaffected leg
Bilateral equal strength and endurance
Work on jumping, running, starts, stops, and changing directions
If progress is slow, consider a bone scan
Return to participation after passing all functional tests pain-free
Consider protective padding to prevent reinjury

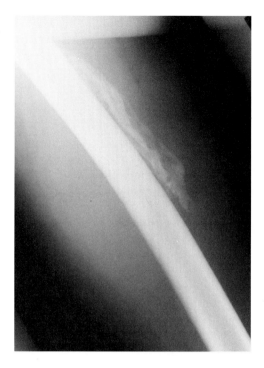

Figure 10.9. With myositis ossificans, full resorption of the calcification may not occur, leaving a visible cortical-type bony lesion.

and straight-leg raises may be impossible. Refer this individual to a physician. If the mass fails to reabsorb completely within 6 to 12 months and activity is limited by pain, weakness, and loss of motion, surgery is indicated. Excision before the mass matures may result in reformation, sometimes larger than the original mass.

Hip Pointers

Hip pointers are contusions to an unprotected iliac crest. Because so many trunk and abdominal muscles attach to the crest, any movement of the trunk will be painful, including coughing, laughing, and even breathing. Immediate pain and spasm will prevent the individual from rotating the trunk or laterally flexing the trunk toward the injured side. In severe injury, the individual may be unable to walk or bear weight, even with crutches, because of the intense pain caused by muscular tension pulling on the injury site. Ice, compression, non-steroidal anti-inflammatory drugs (NSAIDs), and total inactivity should be initiated during the first 2 to 3 days following injury. Because the mechanism may also lead to a fracture to the iliac crest, refer the individual to a physician for follow-up radiographs. Gradual return to activity with a dense foam donut pad fitted into a custom-formed plastic shell can be used to protect the area from further injury.

Hip pointer
Contusions caused by direct compression to an unprotected iliac crest that crushes soft tissue and, sometimes, the bone itself

💡 *The knee should be maximally flexed during any ice treatment to reduce intramuscular bleeding, spasm, and edema. Check range of motion after the ice treatment and the next day to determine if injury to the muscle is involved.*

BURSITIS

❓ *A 47-year-old woman is complaining of pain over the greater trochanter while running and, occasionally, the pain is accompanied by a snapping sensation. What structure(s) are located in this area that might be irritated during repetitive running motions?*

The trochanteric bursa can be compressed between the greater trochanter and iliotibial tract during the running motion and this is more common in runners, particularly women because of the wider pelvis and larger Q-angle. Because streets are crowned to allow for run off, the condition usually affects the down leg, referring to the leg closest to the gutter. A burning or deep, aching feeling is felt just posterior to the greater trochanter and can be aggravated by contraction of the hip abductors against resistance **(Fig. 10.10)**. The iliopsoas bursa can be irritated when the iliopsoas muscle repeatedly compresses the bursa against either the joint capsule of the hip or the lesser trochanter of the femur. Pain can be elicited with passive rotary motions at the hip, or with resisted hip flexion. Treatment involves cryotherapy, protected rest, NSAIDs, and a stretching program for the involved muscle(s). Different shoes, orthoses, or altering the running technique may correct the problem and avoid recurrence. If the condition does not rapidly improve, a bone scan may be necessary to rule out possible femoral neck stress fractures.

Chronic bursitis can lead to **snapping hip syndrome** and is particularly prominent in dancers. The condition is characterized by a snapping sensation either heard or felt during certain distinct motions at the hip. The condition is usually handled with anti-inflammatories and a stretching program. If associated with pain

Snapping hip syndrome
A snapping sensation either heard or felt during motion at the hip

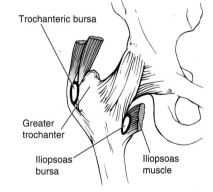

Figure 10.10. Bursitis at the hip may involve the trochanteric bursa or iliopsoas bursa.

Trochanteric bursa

Greater trochanter

Iliopsoas bursa

Iliopsoas muscle

or a sense of hip joint instability, however, the individual should be referred to a physician.

The runner probably has trochanteric bursitis. This individual should stretch the iliotibial tract and alter the direction she runs to avoid having the same leg as the down leg when running in the street.

SPRAINS AND DISLOCATIONS

A football player was tackled by an opponent when his hip and knee were flexed at 90°. The individual is now lying on the ground in great pain with the hip slightly flexed and internally rotated in a fixed position. Any attempt to move the leg leads to intense pain. What injury should you suspect? Should EMS be summoned to take care of this injury?

Hip joint sprains are rare because of the multitude of movements allowed at the ball and socket joint, and the level of protection provided by layers of muscles. Injury can occur in violent twisting actions or in catastrophic trauma when the knee is driven into a stationary object, such as in an automobile accident when the knee is driven into the dashboard. Symptoms of a mild or moderate hip sprain mimic those of synovitis, or stress fractures about the hip, and involve pain on hip rotation. Treatment is symptomatic and may include cryotherapy, NSAIDS, rest, and protected weight bearing on crutches until walking is pain-free.

Severe hip sprains and dislocations result in immediate intense pain and an inability to walk or even move the hip. The hip remains in a characteristic flexed and internally rotated position, indicating a posterior, superior dislocation (**Fig. 10.11**). With this injury,

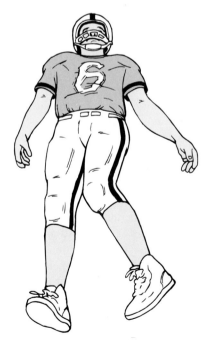

Hip sprains and dislocations occur in violent twisting actions or in catastrophic trauma, such as when a flexed knee is driven into a stationary object

Figure 10.11. Most hip dislocations drive the head of the femur posterior and superior, leaving the leg in a characteristic flexed and internally rotated position.

initiate the emergency plan and summon EMS. Because the sciatic nerve may be damaged, assess nerve function. Run your fingers down both legs and ask the individual where you are touching the leg and what it feels like. Do they have full or partial sensation? Monitor vital signs and treat for shock. It is imperative not to move the individual until the ambulance arrives, because of a possible fracture to the acetabulum or head of the femur.

💡 *Because of the fixed position of the leg and the intense pain, a possible hip dislocation may be present. EMS should be summoned immediately to immobilize the leg and transport the individual to the nearest hospital for further care.*

STRAINS

❓ *A lacrosse player is complaining of a tightness and pulling sensation in the anterior groin region. It is uncomfortable when running straight ahead and backwards, but is very painful when running side-to-side. What muscle group may be injured? What is your course of action?*

Muscular strains to the hip and thigh muscles are frequently seen not only in sport, but in many occupations involving repetitive motions. Strains range from mild to severe, with the severity of symptoms paralleling the amount of disruption to the fibers. **Table 10.2** summarizes the signs and symptoms of muscular strains in the hip and thigh region.

A strain of the quadriceps is less common than strains to the hamstrings, and may be caused by an explosive knee extension and hip flexion movement, or by compressive forces from a helmet or knee, leading to a massive contusion. The individual may report a snapping or tearing sensation during an explosive jumping, kicking, or running motion, followed by immediate pain, loss of function, and, if severe, an inability to bear weight. Assessment will reveal tenderness, swelling, a palpable defect if continuity is disrupted, pain on passive knee flexion, particularly past 90°, and pain and weakness during resisted hip flexion.

The hamstrings are the most frequently strained muscles in the body and these may be caused by a rapid contraction or a violent stretch. Recent research has also linked injury to the biceps femoris muscle, in particular, to anterior translation instability at the knee (3). A hamstrings strain has a reputation of being both chronic and recurring, largely due to a failure to adequately restrengthen the hamstrings after injury, setting up a muscle imbalance with the quadriceps. In mild strains, the individual will complain of tightness and tension in the muscle. Moderate strains will produce an accompanying tearing sensation, leading to immediate pain and weakness in knee flexion. In more severe cases, a sharp pain will be present in the posterior thigh and may occur during mid-stride. The individual will limp and be unable to fully extend the knee. Pain and muscle weakness is elicited during active knee flexion. Although total rupture of the ischial origin is rare, it often

A snapping or tearing sensation during an explosive jumping, kicking, or running movement, followed by immediate anterior pain and muscle weakness, signifies a quadriceps strain

Many individuals fail to restrengthen the hamstrings after injury, thereby setting up a muscle imbalance with the quadriceps

In a hamstring strain, the individual will limp and be unable to fully extended the knee

Table 10.2. Muscular Strains and Associated Signs

History

Quadriceps. A snapping or tearing sensation at AIIS or at mid-thigh during an explosive kicking, jumping, or running movement

Hamstrings. History of poor posture, inflexibility, and muscle imbalance. May occur mid-stride with sharp pain in the posterior thigh

Adductors. Running straight ahead and backward does not cause discomfort, but sliding sidways does

Gluteals. History of muscle overload or repetitive muscular contractions, such as in weightlifting or rowing in crew

Piriformis. History of prolonged sitting, overuse, or a recent increase in activity. A dull ache in the midbuttock region worsens at night and may be accompanied by weakness and numbness extending down the back of the leg

Observation

Mild strain. No noticeable limp, but mild swelling is present

Moderate to severe strains. A noticeable limp and moderate swelling is present

Palpation

Mild strain. Mild point tenderness over the injury site

Moderate strain. Moderate pain over the injury site. A possible defect may be palpated if continuity of the muscle is disrupted. A warm tender mass indicates swelling

Severe strain. Severe pain and a defect in muscle continuity is palpable. A warm painful mass indicates severe swelling

Special Tests for Muscles

Pain with passive stretching and active muscle contraction of the involved muscle. Severity is gauged by the amount of limited motion. For example:

Quadriceps. Passive knee flexion will cause pain, but resisted knee extension will lead to more discomfort

Hamstrings. Pain will occur on passive hip flexion with the knee extended and on active knee flexion

Adductors. Pain will occur on passive hip abduction, external hip rotation, and on active hip adduction

Gluteals. Pain will occur on passive hip flexion and on active hip abduction (gluteus medius and gluteus minimus) or hip extension (gluteus maximus)

Piriformis. Pain will occur on passive hip flexion, adduction, and internal rotation, and on resisted external rotation

results from a sudden forceful flexion of the hip joint when the knee is extended and the hamstring muscles powerfully contract. These severe injuries are treated promptly with surgery (4).

Adductor strains are common in activities that require quick changes of direction and explosive propulsion and acceleration. The individual will often experience a previous "twinge" or "pull" of the groin muscles and is unable to walk because of the intense, sharp pain (5). As the condition worsens, increased pain, stiffness,

With an adductor (groin) strain, running straight ahead and backward may be tolerable, but any side-to-side movement causes intense pain

and weakness in hip adduction and flexion become apparent. Running straight ahead or backwards may be tolerable, but any side-to-side movement will lead to more discomfort and pain. Increased pain will be present during passive stretching with the hip extended, abducted, and externally rotated, and with resisted hip adduction.

The gluteal muscles are rarely injured because of their size and strength, except in activities that require muscle overload, such as in power weightlifting or rowing in crew. Symptoms will be the same as in other muscular strains. Passive stretching and resisted hip extension or abduction will cause discomfort.

The sciatic nerve passes through the sciatic notch beneath the piriformis muscle to travel into the posterior thigh (**Fig. 10.8**). In about 10 to 15% of the population, however, the nerve passes through or above the muscle, subjecting the nerve to compression from trauma, hemorrhage, or spasm of the piriformis muscle (2). Resulting symptoms may mimic a herniated lumbar disk problem, with nerve root impingement. The individual may complain of a dull ache in the midbuttock region, pain that worsens at night, difficulty walking up stairs or an incline, and weakness or numbness down the back of the leg. Low back pain is not unusual. Assessment will reveal point tenderness in the midbuttock region and weakness on hip abduction and external rotation. Pain can be elicited with the individual supine and the hip flexed, adducted and internally rotated, as this stretches the piriformis muscle.

If the piriformis muscle is involved, the individual may have a dull ache in the midbuttock region, pain that worsens at night, difficulty climbing stairs, and numbness down the posterior leg

Treatment for muscle strains involves immediate ice, compression, elevation, protected rest, and NSAIDs. Whenever possible, muscles should be iced in a stretched position and crutches used if the individual walks with a limp. In severe strains, a compression wrap may be indicated from the toe to groin to prevent venous thrombosis and/or distal edema (6). After the acute phase, pain-free gentle stretching and isometric contractions can begin. Active stretching, progressive resistance exercises, swimming, cycling, mild jogging, and stair climbing can begin when the region is pain-free and range of motion is within 10° of the uninvolved limb. Rapid stops, starts, and changing directions are not allowed until the individual can achieve full pain-free motion. The individual should not be returned to sport participation until normal muscle strength and power are achieved. In cases where pain persists, referral to a physician is necessary to rule out nontraumatic diagnostic possibilities, such as an avulsion fracture, osteitis pubis, myositis ossificans, hip joint disease, nerve entrapment, hernia-related conditions, urologic disorders, or gynecologic problems (7).

In severe strains, a compression wrap should be applied from the toe to groin to prevent venous thrombosis and/or distal edema

Did you determine the lacrosse player strained the adductors? If so, you are correct. This individual should incorporate a stretching program and strengthen the muscles to prevent reoccurrence. During participation, a hip spica may help to reduce the discomfort.

? *An adolescent basketball player has been complaining of chronic groin pain that is so uncomfortable, he now limps from the pain. After a week of rest and regular ice therapy, the condition does not seem to be improving. What condition might you suspect? Should this individual be seen by a physician?*

Vascular disorders should be suspected in any lower extremity injury caused by a high-velocity–low-mass projectile, and in an injury where no physical findings support the continued discomfort. If an acute circulatory problem exists, the lower leg and foot may appear pale, cyanotic, be cool to the touch, or have diminished or total loss of sensitivity. Immobilization of the limb and transportation to the nearest trauma center is a priority to restore proper circulation to the involved extremity.

Legg-Calvé-Perthes disease, or avascular necrosis of the proximal femoral epiphysis, is a noninflammatory, self-limiting disorder of the hip seen in young children, especially males, ages 3 to 8 **(Fig. 10.12)** (6). The most common complaint is a gradual onset of a limp and mild hip or knee pain of several months' duration. The pain is most often referred to the groin region, but up to 15% of patients report knee pain as the primary symptom (8). The pain may be aggravated by physical activity and will lead to a decreased range of motion at the hip. If pain persists for

> Vascular disorders should be suspected in injuries caused by compression, or in an injury in which no physical findings support the continued discomfort

Legg-Calvé-Perthes disease
Avascular necrosis of the proximal femoral epiphysis seen especially in young males ages 3 to 8

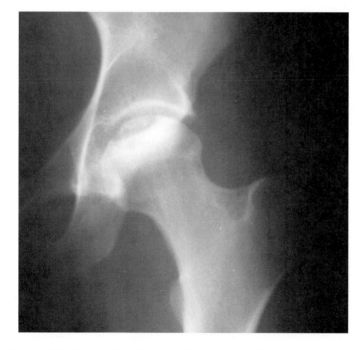

Figure 10.12. In Legg-Calvé-Perthes disease, destruction occurs to the articular cartilage, sometimes called osteochondrosis. In mild cases, no restriction in activity is indicated.

more than a week after initial acute care, or if the individual continues to limp after activity, immediate referral to a physician is needed to rule out other nontraumatic causes of the pain. Possibilities may include slipped capital femoral epiphysis, septic arthritis, transient synovitis, juvenile rheumatoid arthritis, or a bone tumor (9).

Thrombophlebitis
Acute inflammation of a vein

A direct blow may also lead to **thrombophlebitis** or inflammation of a vein. An aching or burning pain and superficial tenderness will be present and may be associated with varicose veins (10). If deep veins are affected, the condition may not become apparent until a pulmonary embolism occurs. A **pulmonary embolism** results when a blood clot travels through the circulatory system to lodge in a blood vessel in the lungs. Chronic swelling and edema in the involved extremity is the most reliable sign. Refer this individual to a physician.

Pulmonary embolism
A blood clot that travels through the circulatory system and lodges in the lungs

💡 *In an adolescent, any groin pain that is not relieved by ice therapy and rest after a few days should be suspected of having a more serious underlying condition, such as Legg-Calvé-Perthes disease, and should be immediately referred to a physician.*

HIP FRACTURES

❓ *An individual has been running 2 to 3 miles a day and doing 20 minutes of aerobics every other day to get in shape for soccer. In the past 3 weeks, however, she has increased her mileage to 5 miles a day and aerobics twice a day. An aching pain has developed in the anterior groin area over the last week that is not relieved with ice or rest. What might this individual be developing? Should she be referred to a physician?*

Individuals who perform rapid, sudden acceleration and deceleration moves are at risk for avulsion fractures to the ASIS with the sartorius being displaced, anterior inferior iliac spine (AIIS) with the rectus femoris being displaced, ischial tuberosity with the hamstrings being displaced, and the lesser trochanter with the iliopsoas being displaced (**Fig. 10.13**). The individual will

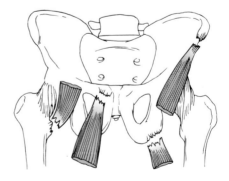

Figure 10.13. Several major muscles attach to the pelvis, but can be avulsed from their bony attachment during muscular action. Can you name the muscles illustrated here?

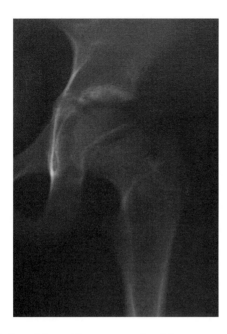

Figure 10.14. An epiphyseal fracture seen in adolescents ages 12 to 15 occurs through the growth plate at the femoral head. With this fracture, the patient will be unable to internally rotate the femur.

complain of sudden acute localized pain that may radiate down the muscle. Examination will reveal severe pain, swelling, and discoloration directly over the tendinous attachment on the bony landmark. In a complete displaced avulsion fracture, a gap may be palpated between the tendon's attachment and bone. Pain increases with passive stretching of the involved muscle and during active and resisted motion. Depending of the fracture site, immobilization from an elastic compression spica wrap may limit motion and decrease pain. After fitting the individual with crutches, refer the individual to a physician for radiograph examination.

An epiphyseal fracture seen in adolescent boys ages 8 to 15 occurs across the capital femoral epiphysis, the growth plate at the femoral head (**Fig. 10.14**). The condition is seen in obese or rapidly growing slender boys and is often congenital. As the proximal femoral growth plate deteriorates, the individual begins to develop a painful limp with groin pain. Pain may also be referred to the anterior thigh or knee region. The individual will be unable to internally rotate the femur or stand on one leg. In nearly all cases, surgery is indicated.

Stress fractures to the pubis, femoral neck, and proximal third of the femur are seen in individuals who do extensive jogging or aerobic dance activities, to the point at which muscle fatigue occurs (11). An aching pain is localized in the anterior groin or thigh region during weight-bearing activity, but is relieved with rest. Night pain is a frequent complaint. Bone scans are frequently

> In a complete displaced avulsion fracture, a gap may be palpated between the tendon's attachment and bone

> With an injury to the proximal femoral epiphysis, the individual will be unable to internally rotate the femur or stand on one leg

> Stress fractures to the hip region are often seen in individuals who do extensive jogging or aerobic activities to the point of muscle fatigue

Osteitis pubis
Stress fracture to the pubic symphysis caused by repeated overload of the adductor muscles or repetitive stress activities

used for early diagnosis to prevent delayed treatment. Swimming can maintain cardiovascular fitness; however, the whip kick and scissors kick should be avoided. **Osteitis pubis** is an inflammatory process involving continued stress on the symphysis pubis from repeated overload of the adductor muscles or from repetitive running activities. The most common complaint is a gradual onset of pain in the adductor musculature, which is aggravated by kicking, running, and pivoting on one leg. Pain over the symphysis pubis and lower abdominal muscles will increase with sit-ups and abdominal muscle strengthening exercises (12). Treatment is symptomatic with ice, protected rest, and NSAIDs, until the condition is resolved; however, prolonged rest is usually required to alleviate symptoms. Hydrotherapy exercises, such as running, "cycling," stretching, and strengthening the hip abductors and adductors while in the water may help in the rehabilitation of the condition. Use of a stationary bike and light jogging may be added as tolerated (13).

Major fractures to the pelvis seldom occur in sport participation except in activities such as equestrian sports, hockey, rugby, skiing, or football. This crushing injury produces severe pain, total loss of function, and in many cases, severe loss of blood leading to **hypovolemic shock**. A possible pelvic fracture can be determined with slight compression to the sides of the ilium and the ASIS. Fractures to the acetabulum can be detected by gently placing upward pressure on the femur against the acetabulum (see **Figures 10.15 and 10.16**). If a fracture is suspected, summon EMS. Cover the individual with a blanket to maintain body temperature. Monitor vital signs frequently and watch for signs of internal hemorrhage and shock.

Major pelvic fractures produce severe pain, total loss of function, and severe loss of blood that can lead to hypovolemic shock and subsequent death

Hypovolemic shock
Shock caused by excessive loss of whole blood or plasma

Fractures to the femoral shaft can be very serious because of potential damage to the neurovascular structures from bony fragments. Signs and symptoms of a fracture include a shortened limb deformity, severe angulation with the thigh externally rotated, swelling into the soft tissues, severe pain, and total loss of function. Distal neurovascular function should be assessed immediately and monitored frequently. Palpate a pulse at the posterior tibial artery and dorsalis pedis artery. Look for pale skin at the foot and feel for cool skin temperature. Stroke the dorsum and plantar aspect of both feet and ask the individual if it feels the same on the involved leg as it feels on the uninvolved leg. Summon EMS immediately. The leg should be totally immobilized and the individual transported immediately to the nearest trauma center. **Table 10.3** summarizes signs and symptoms of the various fractures seen in the pelvis and thigh region.

Signs and symptoms of a femoral fracture are a shortened limb deformity, severe angulation, with the thigh externally rotated, severe pain and swelling, and total loss of function

A stress fracture may be developing in the pelvis or femoral neck due to the rapid excessive increase in the daily workout. This individual should be referred to a physician for radiographs or a bone scan.

Table 10.3. Fractures and Associated Signs

Fracture	Common Sites	History	Observation	Palpation	Signs & Symptoms
Avulsion & apophyseal	ASIS, AIIS, ischial tuberosity, lesser trochanter	Violent or explosive muscular contraction against fixed resistance or by direct trauma	Possible swelling at site	Severe pain & tenderness directly over bony landmark	Increased pain with active motion of involved muscle
Epiphyseal	Capital femoral epiphysis	May occur in conjunction with hip dislocation or subluxation. May describe pain in groin, medial thigh, or knee	Joint may appear normal	May not provide significant findings	Unable to internally rotate the thigh
Stress	Pubis, femoral neck, proximal third of femur	Repeated muscle overload or excessive increased activity level, especially in females. Pain is worse before and after activity, but relieved with rest	Joint may appear normal	May have point tenderness over the fracture site	Possible limp as fracture progresses
Pelvic girdle	Wing of ilium or acetabulum	Severe crushing or compression injury	May show signs of shock	Severe pain directly over fracture site. + pelvic gapping test. + compression test along long axis of femur	Total loss of function. May show signs of shock
Femoral	Shaft of femur or femoral neck	Severe shearing, torsion, or direct compressive force	Deformity and severe angulation with thigh externally rotated; shortened limb; swelling into soft tissues	Severe pain and crepitation at fracture site; + compression test along long axis of femur	Total loss of function. May show signs of shock. May have vascular damage leading to pale, cold, pulseless foot

ASSESSMENT OF THE THIGH, HIP, AND PELVIS

? *A basketball player has come into the training room complaining of pain in the hamstrings in the left leg during running and jumping motions. Can you assume the injury is only muscle related? Why not?*

The lower extremity works as a unit to transmit loads from the upper body to the ground, and also absorbs and dissipates ground force throughout the various structures. When excessive stress and load exceed the tissues yield point, injury occurs. The hip is also a common site for referred pain from visceral, low back, and knee conditions. As such, evaluations must be inclusive, particularly with adolescents complaining of groin pain. In the absence of trauma to the hip, or when improvement is not seen in 2 to 5 days, always refer the individual to a physician to rule out serious underlying conditions.

HISTORY

? *What information should be gathered from the individual complaining of pain during running and jumping activities. What questions can identify the four main components of the primary complaint?*

Many hip injuries may be related to family history, age, congenital deformity, improper biomechanical execution of skills, and recent changes in training programs, surfaces, or foot attire

Many hip conditions may be related to family history, age, congenital deformity, improper biomechanical execution of skills, or recent changes in training programs, surfaces, or foot attire. Gather information on the mechanism of injury, associated symptoms, the progression of those symptoms, any functional disabilities related to the injury, and medical history. In addition to general questions discussed in Chapter 4, specific questions related to the thigh, hip, and pelvis region can be seen in **Field Strategy 10.3**.

? *The 17-year-old basketball player has been plagued with chronic hamstring pain since preseason. Pain increases throughout practice and is very painful when the left leg is used to pushoff, when changing directions quickly, or when jumping up for a rebound. A few days of rest with ice treatments did help, but pain returned when participation was reinitiated. Nothing in the family history or past related medical history seems to be a factor.*

OBSERVATION AND INSPECTION

? *Would a posture and gait analysis be indicated with this individual? Why? What specific postural factors might contribute to pain in the hip and pelvic region?*

During examination, the individual should wear running shorts to allow full view of the lower extremity. However, this may not be possible in an acute injury on the field, such as in football or hockey, when protective equipment or the uniform may obstruct the view. In these cases, determination of the condition may rest

Field Strategy 10.3. Developing a History of the Injury

Current Injury Status

1. How did the injury occur? What position was the leg in and from what direction did the force originate? Was the foot fixed when impact occurred?
2. Ask about the pain location, severity, onset (sudden or gradual), and type (sharp, aching, burning, radiating). Did you hear any sounds, such as a snap, pop, or crack? (Snapping may indicate bursitis; tearing may indicate a muscle strain.) Does it hurt when you walk, run, twist, or change directions?
3. Was there any swelling, discoloration, muscle spasms, or numbness with the injury? Can you bear weight on the leg? What have you done for the condition?
4. Have you recently increased your training frequency, intensity, or duration? What type of shoes do you wear? (Check the heel height, wear pattern, arch, and heel padding.)
5. Are there certain activities you cannot perform because of the pain or weakness? How old are you? Which leg is dominant?

Past Injury Status

1. Have you ever injured your hip or low back before? When? How did that occur? What was done for the injury?
2. Have you had any medical problems recently? (Look for referred pain from the abdominal viscera or lumbar spine.) Are you on any medication? Do you have any musculoskeletal problems that may have altered your gait?

---

more heavily on palpation and special tests. With individuals who are non-ambulatory, complete all observations, inspection, and palpations for possible fractures and dislocations prior to moving the individual.

Observe for symmetry in the region. Note any visible congenital deformity, discoloration, hypertrophy, muscle atrophy, or previous surgical incisions. If time permits, a general posture and gait analysis can be completed (see **Field Strategy 8.9**). Note any abnormalities in gait. Ask the person if any actions cause pain or discomfort. In adolescent boys who limp, ask when the limp started. Does the pain or limp come and go? What activities make it worse, better? You are investigating the possibility of a congenital defect in the femoral head with these questions and observations. Inspect the specific injury site for obvious deformities, discoloration, edema, scars that might indicate previous surgery, and note the general condition of the skin. Always do bilateral comparison.

> *You observed no postural anomalies; however, the individual's pain increased when standing up from a seated position, and a slight limp was noticed during walking. No visible discoloration or swelling is present in the posterior thigh region.*

> Observe for symmetry, visible congenital deformity, discoloration, hypertrophy, muscle atrophy, or previous surgical incisions

PALPATIONS

? *With pain centered on the posterior thigh region, think for a minute where you will begin to palpate the various structures. Should you start in the posterior thigh or begin away from the painful area?*

Bilateral palpations can determine temperature, swelling, point tenderness, crepitus, deformity, muscle spasm, and cutaneous sensation. Vascular pulses can be taken at the femoral artery in the groin, popliteal artery in the posterior knee, and posterior tibial artery and dorsalis pedis artery in the foot (**Figs. 8.11** and **9.4**). Proceed proximal to distal, but leave the most painful area to last. Have the individual nonweight bearing, preferably on a table. When the individual is face down or prone on the table, always place a pillow under the hip and abdominal area to reduce strain on the low back region.

Pain during palpation of bony structures, along with compression, distraction, percussion, and vibration on a specific bony landmark, indicate a possible fracture. For example, to determine a possible fracture to the acetabulum, femoral head and neck, or femoral shaft, slowly apply a compressive force through the longitudinal axis of the femur (**Fig. 10.15**). A possible pelvic fracture can be determined with the pelvic gapping test. With the individual supine, apply a cross-arm pressure down and outward to the ASIS with your thumbs (**Fig. 10.16**). Bilateral compression of the iliac crests may also be performed. Sharp pain along the pelvic ring indicates a possible pelvic fracture. Unilateral gluteal or posterior leg pain may indicate a sprain to the anterior sacroiliac ligaments. If you suspect a fracture, immediately assess circulatory and neural integrity distal to the fracture site, summon EMS, take vital signs, and treat for shock.

> Vascular pulses may be taken at the femoral artery (groin), popliteal artery (posterior knee), or at the posterior tibial artery and dorsalis pedis artery (foot)

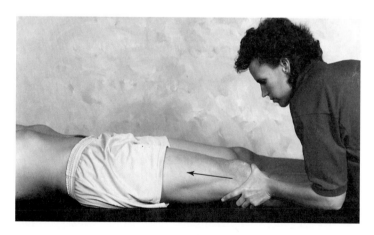

Figure 10.15. Increased pain with gentle compression along the long axis of the femur (indicated by the arrow) helps to determine a possible fracture of the femur or acetabulum.

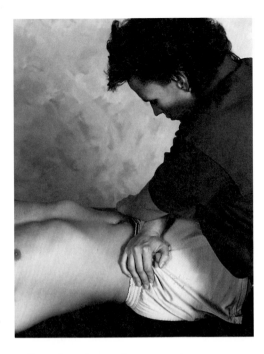

Figure 10.16. To perform the gapping test, apply a cross-arm pressure down and outward to the ASIS with your thumbs. Increased pain indicates a possible pelvic fracture.

Bony Palpations

1. Iliac crest, anterior and posterior superior iliac spines
2. Greater trochanter and ischial tuberosity

Soft Tissue Palpations

1. Quadriceps muscles
2. Inguinal ligament and femoral triangle
3. Hip abductors and adductors
4. Hip extensors and hamstring muscles

Painful palpation in the proximal posterior thigh was predominantly centered over the ischial tuberosity. The area was warm to the touch and slightly swollen. No other painful or warm sites were palpable.

SPECIAL TESTS

Pain and discomfort are centered around the ischial tuberosity. What special tests can be performed to determine if the injury is muscular, capsular, or neurovascular?

Always perform any special tests in a comfortable position and begin with gentle stress. Pain and muscle spasm may prevent an accurate assessment of the extent of weakness or instability, but do not force the limb through any sudden motions, nor cause any undue pain. Proceed cautiously through the examination.

Joint Range of Motion

Active movements can be performed in a seated or prone position with the most painful movements done last. The following movements should be assessed with a hip injury:

1. Hip flexion with the knee flexed
2. Knee extension
3. Lateral and medial hip rotation
4. Hip abduction and adduction
5. Hip extension and knee flexion

Resisted Manual Muscle Testing

Stabilize the hip during manual muscle testing to prevent any muscle substitution. Begin with the muscle on stretch and apply resistance throughout the full range of motion. Note any muscle weakness when compared to the uninvolved limb. As always, painful motions should be completed last. **Figure 10.17** demonstrates motions that should be tested:

1. Hip flexion	5. Hip abduction
2. Knee extension	6. Hip adduction
3. Lateral rotation of the hip	7. Hip extension
4. Medial rotation of the hip	8. Knee flexion

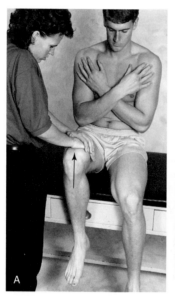 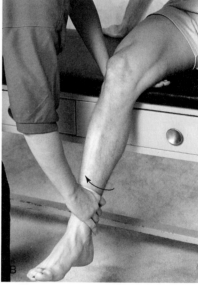

Figure 10.17. Resisted manual muscle testing. **A.** Hip flexion. **B.** Knee extension. **C.** Hip lateral rotation. **D.** Hip medial rotation. **E.** Hip abduction. **F.** Hip adduction. **G.** Hip extension. **H.** Knee flexion. Arrows indicate the direction the athlete moves the body segment against applied resistance.

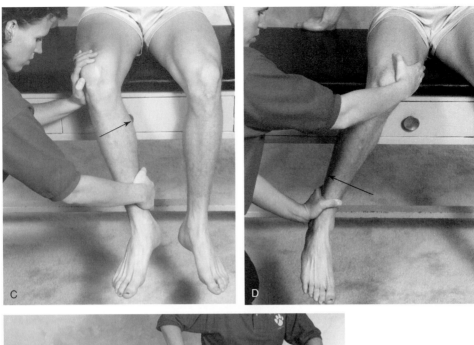

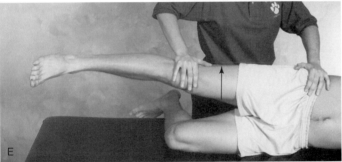

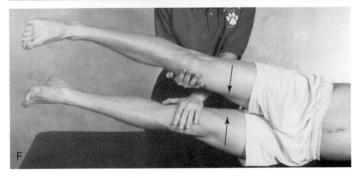

Figure 10.17. (continued)

Neurologic Assessment

Neurologic integrity is generally assessed with manual muscle testing (already completed), reflex testing, and cutaneous sensation. Although there are no specific reflexes in the pelvic or hip

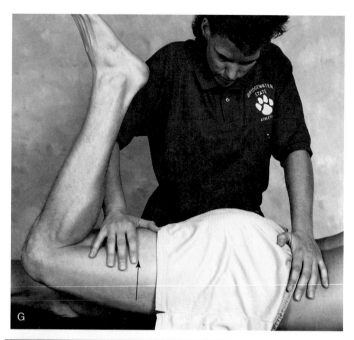

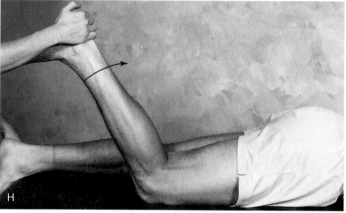

Figure 10.17. (continued)

area, the patella and Achilles tendon reflexes may be assessed (see **Figure 8.22**). In testing cutaneous sensation, run a sharp and dull object over the skin, such as the blunt tip of taping scissors vs. flat edge of taping scissors. With their eyes closed or looking away, ask the individual if they can distinguish sharp and dull and pinpoint the area being tested. Any variations in sensation, such as numbness or tingling, should be documented, and the individual referred to a physician for more extensive evaluation.

Stress and Functional Tests

Always be alert to possible congenital defects and epiphyseal injuries when dealing with adolescents. As you progress through the

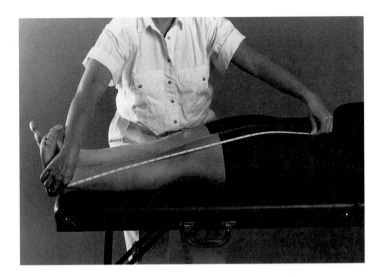

Figure 10.18. To measure leg length, make sure the pelvis is square, level, and balanced. Measure from the ASIS to the lateral malleolus of each ankle.

assessment process, perform only those tests you believe to be absolutely necessary.

Leg Length Measurement

To measure true leg length, place the individual in a supine position with the pelvis square, level, and balanced. The legs should be parallel to each other, with the heels approximately 6 to 8 inches apart. Measure between the distal edge of the ASIS to the distal aspect of the lateral malleolus of each ankle **(Fig. 10.18)**. A difference of 1.0 to 1.5 cm is considered normal. Functional discrepancies as a result of lateral pelvic tilt and flexion or adduction deformities are measured from the umbilicus to the medial malleolus of each ankle.

Thomas Test for Hip Flexion Contractures

In a supine position, observe any noticeable lumbar lordosis. If contractures are present, you may be able to slip your hand under the low back. Ask the individual to flex the uninvolved leg to the chest and hold it in that position. This should flatten the lumbar region. If the test is negative, the straight leg will remain in contact with the table. If the test is positive, however, the straight leg (involved leg) will rise off the table **(Fig. 10.19)**. Both legs are tested and compared.

Kendall Test for Rectus Femoris Contracture

In a supine position, with both knees flexed over the edge of the table, the individual flexes and holds the unaffected knee to the

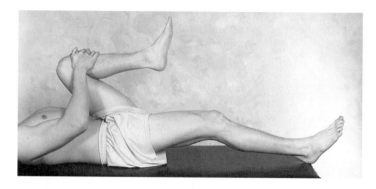

Figure 10.19. To perform a Thomas test, ask the individual to flex and hold the uninvolved leg to the chest. A positive test occurs when the extended leg rises off the table, indicating hip flexion contractures.

chest. The other knee should remain flexed at 90°. If the knee slightly extends, a contracture in the rectus femoris may be present on that leg **(Fig. 10.20)**. If the hip abducts during the test, it may be due to iliotibial band tightness and an Ober's test should be performed bilaterally (see **Figure 9.24**).

Hamstrings Contracture Test

In a seated position on a table, flex the hip, bringing one leg against the chest to stabilize the pelvic region. Ask the individual to touch the toes of the extended leg **(Fig. 10.21)**. If they are unable to do so, it indicates tight hamstrings on the extended leg. Test both legs and compare.

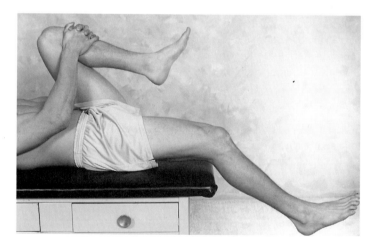

Figure 10.20. The Kendall test is similar to the Thomas test, except the individual lies supine with both knees flexed over the edge of the table. The uninvolved leg is flexed and held to the chest. A positive test occurs when the remaining leg passively extends.

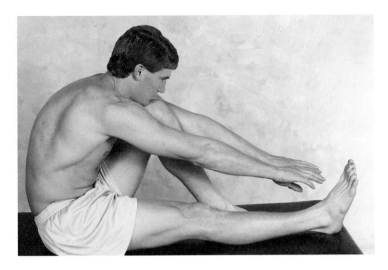

Figure 10.21. To test for possible hamstring contractures, have the individual flex one hip against the chest to stabilize the pelvic region. The test is positive if the individual cannot touch the toes of the extended leg.

Straight Leg Raising (Lasègue's) Test

Although this test is typically used to stretch the dura mater of the spinal cord to assess possible intervertebral disc lesions, it is also used to rule out tight hamstrings. In a supine position, passively flex the individual's hip while keeping the knee extended, until the individual complains of tightness or pain **(Fig. 10.22)**. Slowly lower the leg until the pain or tightness disappears. Then, dorsiflex the foot, have the individual flex the neck, or do both actions simultaneously. Pain that increases with dorsiflexion and neck flexion, or both, indicates stretching of the dura mater of the spinal cord. Pain that does not increase with dorsiflexion or neck flexion usually indicates tight hamstrings.

Functional Tests

Functional tests should be performed before clearing any individual for re-entry into sports participation. The individual should be able to perform activities pain-free with no limp or antalgic gait. Examples of functional activities include walking, going up and down stairs, jogging, squatting, jumping, running straight ahead, running sideways, and changing directions while running. Whenever possible, protective equipment or padding should be used to prevent reinjury.

You have completed assessing the basketball player. You found pain and weakness on active and resistive hip extension and knee flexion. Cutaneous sensation and stress tests were normal. Did you determine the individual had a hamstrings strain? If so, you are correct.

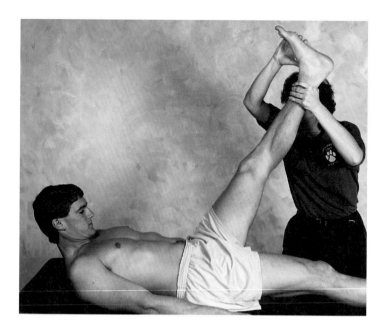

Figure 10.22. Passively flex the individual's hip while keeping the knee extended until pain or tension is felt in the hamstrings. Slowly lower the leg until the pain or tension disappears. Then, dorsiflex the foot, have the individual flex the neck, or do both simultaneously. If pain does not increase with dorsiflexion of the ankle or flexion of the neck, it indicates tight hamstrings.

REHABILITATION

? *The basketball player is doing ice therapy to control inflammation and pain. What range-of-motion exercises and strengthening exercises should be included in the rehabilitation program?*

Rehabilitation for the hip area should include flexibility and strengthening exercises for the hip flexors, extensors, abductors, adductors, medial and lateral rotators, and the quadriceps and hamstrings. Many of the stretching exercises were demonstrated in **Field Strategy 9.1**, **Fig. 9.25**, and **Field Strategy 10.1**. These exercises can be active or passive, and should include PNF stretching techniques.

Proprioception and balance in the early stages of exercise may include shifting one's weight while on crutches, doing straight-leg raises while weight bearing on one leg, performing bilateral minisquats, full squats, lunges, and using the BAPS board, slide board, or minitramp. Each of these exercises can be further supplemented with ankle weights, surgical tubing, hand-held weights, or a weighted bar. Movement patterns can work in a single plane or in multidirectional patterns. A variety of commercial machines or free weight exercises are also available to strengthen the individual muscle groups.

Cardiovascular fitness exercises can include early use of an upper body ergometer (UBE), or hydrotherapeutic exercise. Running in water and performing sport-specific exercises in deeper water can allow the individual to maintain sport-specific functional skills in a nonweight-bearing position. When range of motion is adequate, a stationary bike should be used, beginning with a light to moderate load and increasing the load as tolerated. Light jogging can begin with one-quarter speed, and progress to half speed, three-quarter speed, and full sprints. Plyometric exercises, including jumping, skipping, and bounding, can be combined with running, side-to-side running, or cutting and changing directions. Timed sprints, shuttle runs, karioca runs, hops or vertical jump tests may be used to measure return to full activity. At that time, the individual should have bilaterally equal range of motion, balance, muscular strength, endurance, and power, and an appropriate level of cardiovascular fitness for their specific sport.

The basketball player should focus on flexibility of the hamstrings in addition to general range-of-motion exercises for the entire hip region. Furthermore, muscular strength, endurance, and power in the hamstrings should be at least 60 to 70% of the quadriceps, and proprioception, balance, and cardiovascular fitness should be at or better than the pre-injury level.

SUMMARY

The thigh and pelvic region are highly susceptible to compression forces from direct trauma and tensile forces from explosive muscular contractions. These forces lead to a high incidence of contusions and muscular strains. Although a tremendous amount of stress is placed on the hip and pelvic joints during running and jumping activities, joint injuries are rare. Muscle imbalance and dysfunction, congenital abnormalities, or postural deviations can, however, predispose an individual to injury. **Field Strategy 10.4** lists the steps in assessing the thigh, hip, and pelvic region.

During the assessment, remember that the individual may be experiencing referred pain from the abdominal, lumbar, or knee region. Furthermore, in an adolescent, congenital defects and epiphyseal and apophyseal injuries are common. Refer the individual to a physician if any of the following conditions are suspected: obvious deformity, suggesting a dislocation or fracture; significant loss of motion or a palpable defect in a muscle; severe joint disability, evident by a noticeable limp; excessive soft tissue swelling; possible epiphyseal and apophyseal injuries; any groin pain that does not improve within 5 to 7 days; any abnormal or absent reflexes; abnormal cutaneous sensations; absent or weak pulse; or weakness in a myotome.

If the individual is referred to a physician, remove the player from any activity and immobilize the limb in a comfortable position, or fit the individual for crutches if they are unable to walk without pain or a limp. Apply ice to control inflammation and

Field Strategy 10.4. Hip Evaluation

History

Primary complaint and mechanism of injury
Onset of symptoms, including pain and discomfort
Disability and functional impairments from the injury
Previous injuries to the area and family history

Observation and Inspection

Observe general posture and gait
Inspect:

Muscle symmetry	Hypertrophy or muscle atrophy
Swelling	Visible congenital deformity
Discoloration	Surgical incisions or scars

Palpation

Bony structures, to determine possible fracture
Soft tissue structures, to determine:

Temperature	Deformity
Swelling	Muscle spasm
Point tenderness	Cutaneous sensation
Crepitus	Vascular pulses

Special Tests

Joint range of motion
Resisted manual muscle testing
Neurologic testing
Stress and functional tests
  Leg length measurement
  Contracture tests
    Thomas test
    Kendall rectus femoris test
    Hamstrings test
  Straight leg raising
  Functional tests

swelling, and transport the individual in an appropriate manner. Prior to return to activity, the individual should have a medical clearance from the supervising physician and should have passed all functional tests pain-free without a limp or antalgic gait.

REFERENCES

1. Johnston RC. 1973. Mechanical considerations of the hip joint. Arch Surg 107:411–417.
2. Reid DC. *Sports injury assessment and rehabilitation*. New York: Churchill Livingstone, 1992.
3. Terry GC, and LaPrade RF. 1996. The biceps femoris muscle complex at the knee: its anatomy and injury patterns associated with acute anterolateral-anteromedial rotatory instability. Am J Sports Med 24(1):2–8.
4. Orava S, and Kujala UM. 1995. Rupture of the ischial origin of the hamstring muscles. Am J Sports Med 23(6):702–705.
5. Hasselman CT, Best RM, and Garrett WE. 1995. When groin pain signals an adductor strain. Phys Sportsmed 23(7):53–60.

6. Esposito PW. Pelvis, hip and thigh injuries. In *The team physician's handbook*, edited by MB Mellion, WM Walsh, and GL Shelton. Philadelphia: Hanley & Belfus, 1990.

7. Swain R, and Snodgrass S. 1995. Managing groin pain: even when the cause is not obvious. Phys Sportsmed 23(11):55–66.

8. Paletta GA, and Andrish JT. Injuries about the hip and pelvis in the young athlete. In *Clinics in sports medicine*, edited by LJ Micheli, vol. 14, no. 3. Philadelphia: WB Saunders, 1995.

9. Gerberg LF, and Micheli LJ. 1996. Nontraumatic hip pain in active children: a critical differential. Phys Sportsmed 24(1):69–74.

10. Price SA, and Wilson LM. *Pathophysiology: clinical concepts of disease processes*. St. Louis: Mosby Year Book, 1992.

11. Fullerton LR, and Snowdy HA. 1988. Femoral neck stress fractures. Am J Sports Med 16(4):365–377.

12. Holt MA, Keene JS, Graf BK, and Helwig DC. 1995. Treatment of osteitis pubis in athletes: results of corticosteroid injections. Am J Sports Med 23(6):601–606.

13. Sing R, Cordes R, and Siberski D. 1995. Osteitis pubis in the active patient. Phys Sportsmed 23(12):67–73.

Injuries to the Upper Extremity

Chapter 11: **Shoulder Injuries**

Chapter 12: **Upper Arm, Elbow, and Forearm Injuries**

Chapter 13: **Wrist and Hand Injuries**

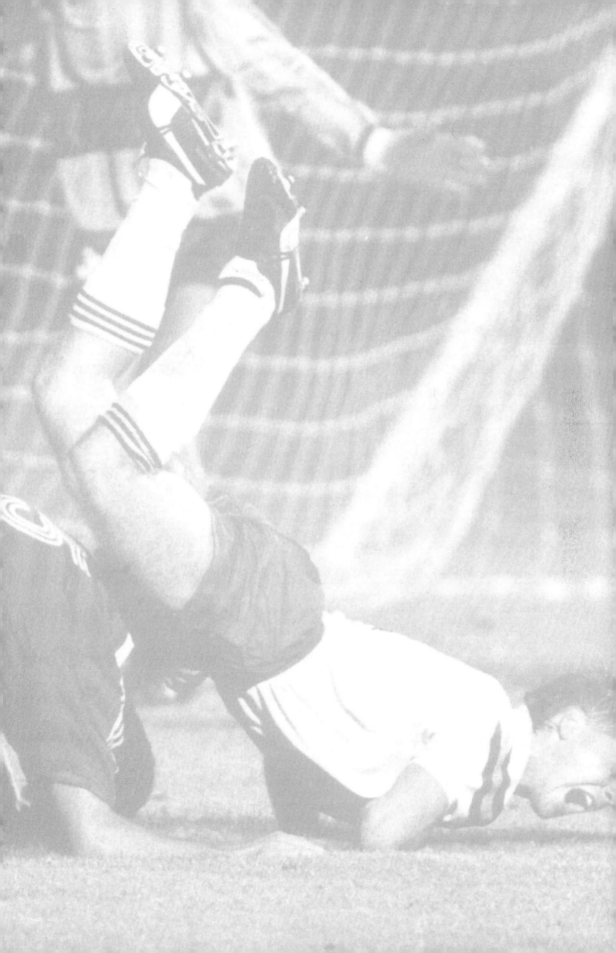

Yoshitaka Ando, BS, LATC

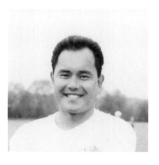

I came to the United States from Japan to play American football and learn to speak fluent English. During a high school game, I got injured and was taken care of by a student athletic trainer who was finishing his degree at Northeastern University. In talking with him and my guidance counselor, I decided to pursue a career in athletic training at Bridgewater State College.

Yoshitaka Ando is a full-time athletic trainer at Lincoln-Sudbury Regional High School in Sudbury, Massachusetts. As a regional high school trainer, he provides health care coverage to over 600 high school athletes throughout the year.

As a high school athletic trainer, I order, fit, clean, and inspect all protective equipment, develop pre-season conditioning programs for the sports, and provide on-site medical coverage for the high school athletes. A team physician and physical therapist work directly with me to provide a very comprehensive health care program for the athletes. In addition to the daily management of the training room, I also provide a fair amount of counseling to athletes on weight control, nutrition, substance abuse, and other health issues.

Our school has around 1000 students, 600 of which participate on athletic teams. Many of these individuals are three-season athletes. We have 15 competitive sports, with nearly all sports fielding three separate teams. In our league, six of the eight high schools have NATA-certified athletic trainers, so we know our athletes are getting good health-care coverage. Communication among the athletic trainers is excellent. After an away event, I always get a call from the on-site athletic trainer to let me know if anything happened to my athletes, and I return the courtesy to my other colleagues.

Working at this school is really a delight. The parents, superintendent, athletic director, and coaches really appreciate the service I provide them. My budget is adequate, and if I really need something that the school can't provide, the booster's club is right there to help. The athletes also see this tremendous support and appreciate what I do for them. Many go on to play at the college level, and continually return during home games just to say hi.

One thing about working with so many teams is that you need to be in multiple places at the same time. We know that's impossible, but our on-site communication is excellent. Although my athletic director doesn't expect to see me before noon, I come in early in the morning to update my files on the computer, clean the coolers and water bottles, and make my phone calls to the physicians and other league athletic trainers. I work six days a week and, during the winter, the days can be very long, but I wouldn't trade it for anything.

If you would like to work at the high school level, I would suggest doing a clinical rotation there to find out what it's all about. Your taping skills have to be excellent, due to the incredible volume of people you have to tape and get out on the field ready for practice. You also have to remember that you are working with minors, children under 18, so you can't take anything for granted. All injury assessments must be thorough and complete, and you have to develop a good follow-up system to recheck injuries and develop easy rehabilitation programs that the students can do on their own. Developing a good working relationship with the parents is also a must. They can be your best ally or your worst nightmare. You have to make yourself visible and demonstrate your professional style by always placing the health of the athletes in the forefront. Each day is a new challenge, especially when you realize you are there to safeguard these young athletes. You know it's worth that extra effort, and I wouldn't trade it for the world.

Shoulder Injuries

After completing this chapter, you should be able to:

- Locate the important bony and soft tissue structures of the shoulder

- Describe the major motions at the shoulder and identify the muscles that produce them

- Explain general principles and exercises used to prevent injuries to the shoulder

- Recognize and manage specific injuries in the shoulder region

- Demonstrate a basic assessment of the shoulder region

- Demonstrate general rehabilitation exercises for the shoulder complex

Key Terms:

Bankart lesion	**Impingement syndrome**
Brachial plexus	**Little league shoulder**
Dead arm syndrome	**Rotator cuff**
Glenoid labrum	**Scapulohumeral rhythm**

The loose structure of the shoulder complex enables extreme mobility, but provides little stability. As a result, the shoulder is much more prone to injury than the hip. The shoulder is involved in 8 to 13% of all sport-related injuries, with reports indicating complaints of shoulder pain in over 50 to 80% of competitive swimmers (1,2). Shoulder injuries are a major concern in activities involving an overhead motion, such as in baseball, swimming, tennis, volleyball, and weightlifting. These activities place significant demands on the shoulder and other joints of the upper extremity, leading to many acute and chronic conditions. Common injuries include bursitis, sprains, rotator cuff and impingement injuries, and bicipital tendinitis. Dislocations of the shoulder articulations are not uncommon, particularly in contact sports such as wrestling or football.

This chapter begins with a general anatomy review of the shoulder region, including major muscle actions in the region. Discussion on prevention of injuries is followed by an overview of common injuries to the shoulder complex. Injury management for specific injuries and the assessment process are then followed by examples of rehabilitation exercises.

? *A swimmer is complaining of throbbing pain on the anterior aspect of the right shoulder during the crawl stroke. The pain intensifies following practice sessions. What anatomical structure(s) might be the source of this pain?*

The shoulder region encompasses five separate articulations—the sternoclavicular (SC) joint, acromioclavicular (AC) joint, coracoclavicular joint, glenohumeral joint, and the scapulothoracic joint. The articulation referred to specifically as the shoulder joint is the glenohumeral joint, whereas the other articulations are joints of the shoulder girdle. The SC and AC joints enhance motion of the clavicle and scapula that position the glenohumeral joint to provide a greater range of motion for the humerus.

> The glenohumeral joint is the major joint of the shoulder

Sternoclavicular Joint

As the name suggests, the SC joint consists of the articulation of the superior sternum, or manubrium, with the proximal clavicle **(Fig. 11.1)**. The SC joint is a synovial joint surrounded by a joint capsule thickened anteriorly and posteriorly by four ligaments, including the interclavicular, costoclavicular, and anterior and posterior sternoclavicular ligaments. The SC joint is a ball and socket joint that enables rotation of the clavicle with respect to the sternum. The joint allows motion of the distal clavicle in superior, inferior, anterior, and posterior directions, along with some forward and backward rotation of the clavicle. Thus, rotation occurs at the SC joint during motions such as shrugging the shoulders, reaching above the head, and in most throwing-like activities.

> The sternoclavicular (SC) joint enables rotation of the clavicle with respect to the sternum during motions such as shrugging the shoulders or reaching above the head

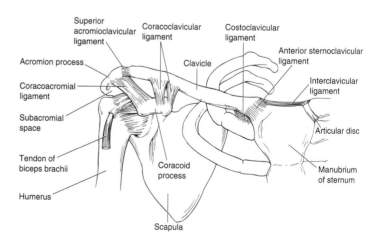

Figure 11.1. The bony and ligamentous structure of the shoulder girdle.

Acromioclavicular Joint

The AC joint consists of the articulation of the acromion process of the scapula with the distal end of the clavicle (**Fig. 11.1**). This is an irregular diarthrodial joint, with limited motion permitted in all three planes. The joint is enclosed by a capsule and is reinforced by the strong superior and inferior acromioclavicular ligaments. The coracoacromial ligament also attaches to the inferior lip of the AC joint to serve as a buffer between the rotator cuff muscles and the bony acromion process. The coracoclavicular ligament resists independent upward movement of the clavicle, downward movement of the scapula, and anteroposterior movement of the clavicle or scapula.

Coracoclavicular Joint

The coracoclavicular joint is a syndesmosis formed by the binding together of the coracoid process of the scapula and the inferior surface of the clavicle by the coracoclavicular ligament (**Fig. 11.1**). Very little movement is permitted at this joint.

Glenohumeral Joint

The glenohumeral joint is the articulation between the glenoid fossa of the scapula and the head of the humerus. Although the joint enables a greater total range of motion than any other joint in the human body, it is lacking in bony stability (**Fig. 11.2**). This is partially because the hemisphere-shaped head of the humerus has three to four times the amount of surface area of the shallow glenoid fossa. Because the glenoid fossa is also less curved than the humeral head, the humerus not only rotates, but moves linearly across the surface of the glenoid fossa when humeral motion occurs.

The glenoid fossa is somewhat deepened around its perimeter by the **glenoid labrum**, a narrow rim of fibrocartilage around the edge of the fossa (**Fig. 11.2**). The glenohumeral joint capsule is joined by the superior, middle, and inferior glenohumeral ligaments on the anterior side, and the coracohumeral ligament on the

> The head of the humerus not only rotates, but can move linearly across the surface of the glenoid fossa during arm movements

Glenoid labrum
Soft tissue lip around the periphery of the glenoid fossa that widens and deepens the socket to add stability to the joint

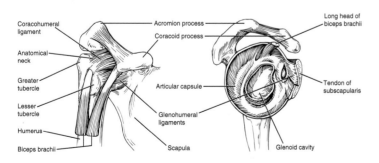

Figure 11.2. The glenohumeral joint.

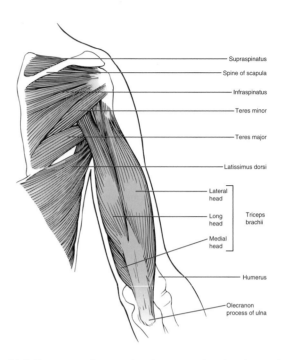

Figure 11.3. Deep posterior muscles that move the glenohumeral joint.

superior side. Although joint displacements can occur in anterior, posterior, and inferior directions, the strong coracohumeral ligament protects against superior dislocations.

The tendons of four muscles, including the supraspinatus, infraspinatus, teres minor, and subscapularis, also join the joint capsule (**Figs. 11.3 and 11.4**). These muscles are referred to as the SITS muscles, after the first letter of each muscle's name. They are also known as the **rotator cuff** muscles, because they all act to rotate the humerus, and their tendons merge to form a collagenous cuff around the joint. Tension in the rotator cuff muscles helps to hold the head of the humerus against the glenoid fossa, further contributing to joint stability.

Scapulothoracic Joint

Because muscles attaching to the scapula permit its motion with respect to the trunk or thorax, this region is sometimes described as the scapulothoracic joint. Muscles attaching to the scapula include the levator scapula, rhomboids, serratus anterior, pectoralis minor, subclavius, deltoid, subscapularis, supraspinatus, infraspinatus, teres major, teres minor, coracobrachialis, the short head of the biceps brachii, long head of the triceps brachii, and the trapezius (**Figs. 11.3 through 11.6**).

The scapular muscles perform two functions. The first is stabilization of the shoulder region. For example, when a barbell is lifted from the floor, the levator scapula, trapezius, and rhomboids

Rotator cuff
The SITS (supraspinatus, infraspinatus, teres minor, and subscapularis) muscles that hold the head of the humerus in the glenoid fossa and produce humeral rotation

The scapular muscles stabilize and/or position the scapula to facilitate movement at the glenohumeral joint

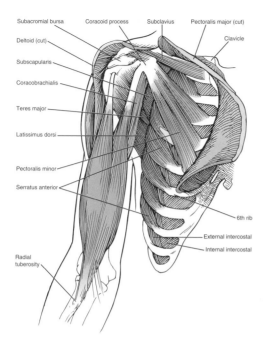

Figure 11.4. Deep anterior muscles that move the glenohumeral joint.

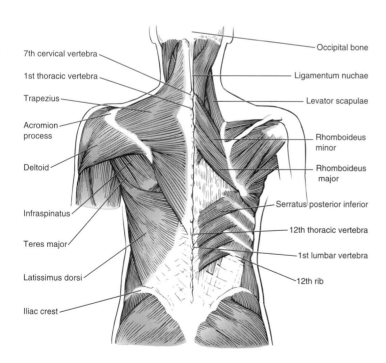

Figure 11.5. Superficial posterior muscles of the back.

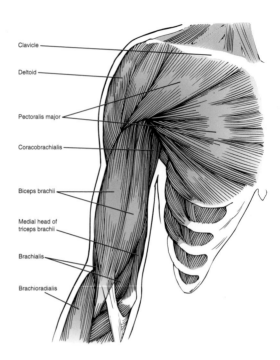

Clavicle

Deltoid

Pectoralis major

Coracobrachialis

Biceps brachii

Medial head of
triceps brachii

Brachialis

Brachioradialis

Figure 11.6. Superficial anterior muscles of the shoulder.

develop tension to support the scapula and, in turn, the entire shoulder, through the AC joint. The second function is to facilitate movements of the upper extremity through appropriate positioning of the glenohumeral joint. During an overhand throw, for example, the rhomboids contract to move the entire shoulder posteriorly, as the arm and hand move backward during the preparatory phase. As the arm and hand then move forward to execute the throw, tension in the rhomboids is released to permit forward movement of the shoulder, enabling medial rotation of the humerus.

Muscles of the Shoulder

A large number of muscles cross the glenohumeral joint, as shown in **Table 11.1**. Identifying actions of these muscles is complicated by the fact that, due to the large range of motion at the shoulder, the action produced by contraction of a given muscle may change with the orientation of the humerus.

Bursae

The shoulder is surrounded by several bursae, including the subcoracoid, subscapularis, and, most importantly, the subacromial. The subacromial bursa lies in the subacromial space, where it is surrounded by the acromion process of the scapula and the

Table 11.1. Muscles of the Shoulder

Muscle	Proximal Attachment	Distal Attachment	Primary Action(s)	Nerve Innervation
Deltoid	Outer third of the clavicle, top of the acromion, and scapula spine	Deltoid tuberosity of the humerus		Axillary
Anterior			Flexion, horizontal adduction	
Middle			Abduction, horizontal abduction	
Posterior			Extension, horizontal abduction	
Pectoralis major		Lateral aspect of the humerus just below the head		
Clavicular	Medial two-thirds of the clavicle		Flexion, horizontal adduction	Lateral pectoral
Sternal	Anterior sternum and cartilage of first six ribs		Extension, adduction, horizontal adduction	Medial pectoral
Supraspinatus	Supraspinous fossa	Greater tubercle of the humerus	Abduction	Suprascapular
Coracobrachialis	Coracoid process of the scapula	Medial anterior humerus	Horizontal adduction	Musculocutaneous
Latissimus dorsi	Lower six thoracic, all lumbar vertebrae, posterior sacrum, iliac crest, lower three ribs	Anterior humerus	Extension, adduction	Thoracodorsal
Teres major	Lower, lateral, dorsal scapula	Anterior humerus	Extension, adduction, medial rotation	Subscapular
Teres minor	Posterior, lateral border of scapula	Greater tubercle and adjacent shaft of humerus	Lateral rotation, horizontal abduction	Axillary
Subscapularis	Entire anterior surface of scapula	Lesser tubercle of the humerus	Inward rotation	Subscapular
Biceps brachii		Tuberosity of the radius		Musculocutaneous
Long head	Upper rim of the glenoid fossa		Assists with abduction	
Short head	Coracoid process of the scapula		Assists with flexion, adduction, inward rotation, and horizontal adduction	
Triceps brachii	Just inferior to the glenoid fossa	Olecranon process of the ulna	Assists with extension and adduction	Radial
Long head				

coracoacromial ligament above and the glenohumeral joint below (**Fig. 11.4**). The bursa cushions the rotator cuff muscles, particularly the supraspinatus, from the overlying bony acromion. This bursa may become irritated when repeatedly compressed during overhead arm action.

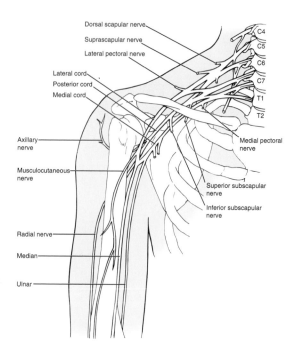

Dorsal scapular nerve

Suprascapular nerve

Lateral pectoral nerve

Lateral cord

Posterior cord

Medial cord

C4
C5
C6
C7
T1
T2

Axillary nerve

Musculocutaneous nerve

Radial nerve

Median

Ulnar

Medial pectoral nerve

Superior subscapular nerve

Inferior subscapular nerve

Figure 11.7. The brachial plexus and nerve supply to the shoulder region.

Nerves and Blood Vessels of the Shoulder

Brachial plexus
Large mass of interwoven spinal nerves (C$_5$ to T$_1$) that innervate the upper extremity

Innervation of the upper extremity arises from the **brachial plexus**, a complex web of neural pathways branching primarily from the lower four cervical (C$_5$ to C$_8$) and the first thoracic (T$_1$) spinal nerves (**Fig. 11.7**). A network of branches from these nerves extends from the neck anteriorly and laterally, passing between the clavicle and first rib. Injuries to the clavicle in this region can damage the brachial plexus. Major nerves arising from the brachial plexus that supply the shoulder region are the axillary, musculocutaneous, dorsal scapular, subscapular, suprascapular, and pectoral nerves. The nerve–muscle associations are presented in **Table 11.1**.

The subclavian artery passes beneath the clavicle to become the axillary artery, providing the major blood supply to the shoulder (**Fig. 11.8**). Branches of the axillary artery include the thoracoacromial trunk, lateral thoracic artery, subscapular artery, and thoracodorsal artery, as well as the anterior and posterior humeral circumflex arteries that supply the head of the humerus.

Forceful overhead arm movement seen in many swimming strokes can, when performed repetitively, irritate the subacromial bursa, coracoacromial ligament, or supraspinatus tendon, leading to pain and inflammation.

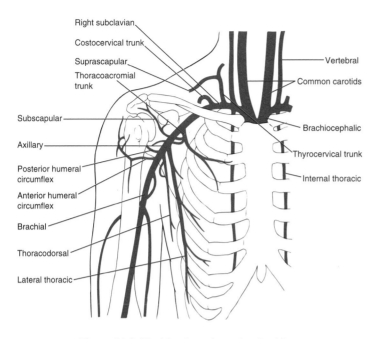

Right subclavian

Costocervical trunk

Suprascapular

Thoracoacromial
trunk

Subscapular

Axillary

Posterior humeral
circumflex

Anterior humeral
circumflex

Brachial

Thoracodorsal

Lateral thoracic

Vertebral

Common carotids

Brachiocephalic

Thyrocervical trunk

Internal thoracic

Figure 11.8. The blood supply to the shoulder.

MAJOR MUSCLE ACTIONS OF THE SHOULDER COMPLEX

 Why would an injury to the SC joint impair an individual's ability to throw a ball?

The shoulder is the most freely moveable joint in the body, with motion capability in all three planes (**Fig. 11.9**). Sagittal plane movements of the humerus at the shoulder include flexion, or elevation of the arm in an anterior direction; extension, or return of the arm from a position of flexion to the side of the body; and hyperextension, or elevation of the arm in a posterior direction. Frontal plane movements consist of abduction, or elevation of the arm in a lateral direction, and adduction, or return of the arm from a position of abduction to the side of the body. Transverse plane movements of the horizontally extended arm are termed horizontal adduction, when the arm is moved medially, and horizontal abduction, when the arm is moved laterally. The humerus can also rotate medially and laterally.

Throwing

Throwing and related motions produce a variety of both acute and chronic injuries to the shoulder. Throwing styles vary from individual to individual, even across overarm, sidearm, and underarm styles of the throw. To further complicate matters, some sport skills, casually referred to as throwing, actually involve more of a pushing motion than a throwing motion. An example is putting the shot.

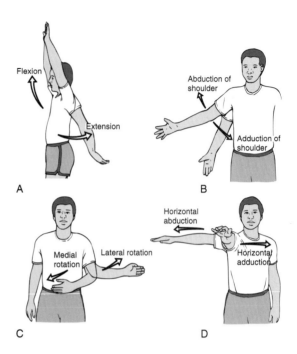

Figure 11.9. Movements at the glenohumeral joint. **A.** Flexion and extension. **B.** Abduction and adduction. **C.** Medial (internal) and lateral (external) rotation. **D.** Horizontal abduction and adduction. Combined motions are called circumduction.

Nevertheless, overarm throwing can be divided into three phases **(Fig. 11.10)**. Although skillful throwing involves the coordinated action of the entire body, this description focuses on the shoulder girdle and glenohumeral joint. In the preparatory or cocking phase, the arm and hand are drawn behind the body, through horizontal abduction, hyperextension, and maximal external rotation of the humerus. Eccentric loading of the horizontal adductors and internal rotators of the shoulder is very high during this action. To facilitate the cocking motion, the rhomboids contract to pull the scapula and the glenohumeral joint posteriorly, while the serratus anterior provides additional scapular stabilization. As the shoulder proceeds into horizontal abduction and external rotation, the humeral head tends to sublux, first posteriorly and then anteriorly, against the anterior capsule; consequently, tendinitis of the anterior muscle tendons is quite common (3). Just prior to maximal shoulder external rotation, elbow extension begins. This is immediately followed by the onset of shoulder internal rotation.

During the acceleration or delivery phase, the ball is brought forward and released. Humeral horizontal adduction, elbow extension, and rapid internal rotation of the humerus is coupled with relaxation of the rhomboids to enable anterior movement of the

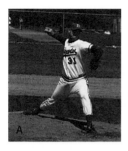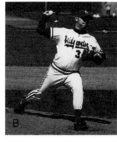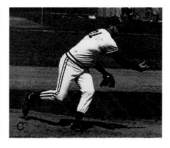

Figure 11.10. The overarm throwing motion includes three primary phases: (**A**) preparatory or cocking phase, (**B**) acceleration or delivery phase, and (**C**) deceleration or follow-through phase.

glenohumeral joint. This action, however, can lead to shoulder grinding (3). At ball release, the elbow is almost fully extended and positioned slightly anterior to the trunk. Because throwing can involve a whip-like action of the arm, large stresses can be placed on the tendons, ligaments, and epiphyses of the throwing arm during delivery.

Arm deceleration occurs after ball release, until maximal shoulder internal rotation occurs, and consists primarily of a snap-like flexion of the wrist and pronation of the forearm. Large eccentric loads at the elbow and shoulder decelerate the arm. The infraspinatus, supraspinatus, teres major and minor, latissimus dorsi, and posterior deltoid play major roles in resisting shoulder distraction and anterior subluxation forces. If the rotator cuff muscles are weak, fatigued, or injured, the humeral head will distract and translate in an anterior direction, leading to stress on the posterior capsule (3). Injuries common to the specific phases of throwing can be seen in **Table 11.2**.

Coordination of Shoulder Movements

The extensive range of motion afforded by the shoulder is partially due to the loose structure of the glenohumeral joint, and partially due to the proximity of the other shoulder articulations and the movement capabilities they provide. Movement at the shoulder typically involves some rotation at all three shoulder joints. For example, as the arm is elevated past 30° of abduction or the first 45 to 60° of flexion, the scapula also rotates, contributing approximately one-third of the total rotational movement of the humerus (5). This important coordination of scapular and humeral movements, known as **scapulohumeral rhythm**, enables a much greater range of motion at the shoulder than if the scapula were fixed **(Fig. 11.11)**. Also contributing to the first 90° of humeral elevation is the elevation of the clavicle through approximately 35 to 45° of motion at the SC joint (6). The AC joint contributes to overall movement capability as well, with rotation occurring during

Movement at the shoulder typically involves some rotation at all three shoulder joints

Scapulohumeral rhythm
Coordinated rotational movement of the scapula that accompanies abduction and adduction of the humerus

Table 11.2. Common Injuries Sustained During the Throwing Motion

Cocking Phase

Anterior glenohumeral instability or subluxation
Anterior inferior glenoid labral tears
AC joint pathology
Subacromial bursitis

Acceleration Phase

Anterior subluxation
Rotator cuff tendinitis/partial tears
Subacromial bursitis
Proximal humeral apophysitis
Glenoid labral pathology

Deceleration and Follow-through Phase

Rotator cuff tendinitis/partial tears
Biceps tendinitis/rupture
Posterior glenohumeral subluxation
Posterior capsulitis
AC joint pathology

the first 30° of humeral elevation, and then again as the arm is moved past 135° (7).

Glenohumeral Flexion

The muscles that cross the glenohumeral joint anteriorly are positioned to contribute to flexion (**Figs. 11.4 and 11.6**). The anterior deltoid and the clavicular pectoralis major are the primary shoulder

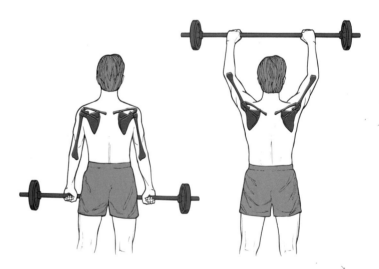

Figure 11.11. The coordinated movement of the scapula needed to facilitate motion of the humerus is known as scapulohumeral rhythm.

flexors, with assistance provided by the coracobrachialis and short head of the biceps brachii. Since the biceps also crosses the elbow joint, it is capable of exerting more force at the shoulder when the elbow is in full extension.

Glenohumeral Extension

When extension is unresisted, the action is caused by gravity. Eccentric contraction of the flexor muscles serves as a controlling or braking mechanism. When resistance to extension is offered, the posterior glenohumeral muscles act, including the sternocostal pectoralis, latissimus dorsi, and teres major, with assistance provided by the posterior deltoid and long head of the triceps brachii (**Figs. 11.3 and 11.5**).

Glenohumeral Abduction

The muscles superior to the glenohumeral joint produce abduction and include the middle deltoid and supraspinatus (**Fig. 11.3**). During the contribution of the middle deltoid, from approximately 90° through 180° of abduction, the infraspinatus, subscapularis, and teres minor produce inferiorly directed force to neutralize the superiorly directed dislocating force produced by the middle deltoid. This action serves an important function in preventing impingement of the supraspinatus and subacromial bursa.

Because the glenohumeral joint is lacking in stability, the development of tension in one shoulder group must often be accompanied by the development of tension in an antagonist (opposing) muscle group to prevent impingement of the structures

Glenohumeral Adduction

As with extension, adduction in the absence of resistance results from gravitational force, with the abductors controlling the speed of motion. When resistance is present, adduction is accomplished through the action of the muscles positioned on the inferior side of the glenohumeral joint, including the latissimus dorsi, teres major, and sternocostal pectoralis (**Fig. 11.5**).

Lateral and Medial Rotation of the Humerus

Lateral rotators of the humerus lie on the posterior aspect of the humerus, including the infraspinatus and teres minor, with assistance provided by the posterior deltoid. Muscles on the anterior side of the humerus contribute to medial rotation. These include the subscapularis and teres major, with assistance from the pectoralis major, anterior deltoid, latissimus dorsi, and the short head of the biceps (**Fig. 11.3**).

Although the glenohumeral joint provides most of the range of motion needed to throw a ball, a forceful movement of the upper extremity requires the coordinated contribution of motion from all of the joints in the shoulder complex. Consequently, an injury to one joint can affect the ability of the other joints to work effectively.

? *The glenohumeral joint provides a wide range of motion, yet has little bony stability. As a result, injuries are common to the region. What protection is available to prevent injury to this highly mobile region?*

Acute and chronic injuries to the shoulder complex are common in sport participation. Many contact and collision sports, such as football, lacrosse, and ice hockey, require shoulder pads to protect exposed bony protuberances. **Field Strategy 6.3** outlined guidelines in fitting football shoulder pads. Several other commercial pads and braces used to protect the region were also illustrated in the chapter.

Lack of flexibility can predispose an individual to joint sprains and muscular strains. Warm-up exercises should focus on general joint flexibility and may be performed alone or with a partner, utilizing proprioceptive neuromuscular facilitation (PNF) stretching techniques. Individuals using the throwing motion in their sport should increase range of motion in external rotation, as it has been shown to increase the velocity of the throwing arm and decrease shearing forces on the glenohumeral joint (8). Several flexibility exercises for the shoulder complex are demonstrated in **Field Strategy 11.1**.

Strengthening programs should focus on muscles acting on both the glenohumeral and scapulothoracic region. Strength in the infraspinatus, teres minor, and posterior shoulder musculature is necessary to (a) begin the cocking phase of throwing, (b) fix the shoulder girdle during the acceleration phase, and (c) provide adequate muscle tension through eccentric contractions for smooth deceleration through the follow-through phase (8). In many chronic shoulder problems, particularly among throwers, a weakened supraspinatus is present. Concentric and eccentric contractions, with light resistance in the first 30° of abduction, can strengthen this muscle. To strengthen the scapular stabilizers, do push-ups or move the arm through a resisted diagonal pattern of external rotation and horizontal abduction. Other strengthening exercises are demonstrated in **Field Strategy 11.2**.

In addition to proper throwing techniques, participants in contact and collision sports should be taught the shoulder roll method of falling, rather than falling on an outstretched arm. This technique reduces direct compression of the articular joints and disperses the force over a wider area.

💡 *Flexibility at the glenohumeral joint is necessary to provide adequate range of motion to perform throwing-like activities. In addition, adequate strength in the glenohumeral and scapulothoracic muscles allows for a synchronized throwing action that can reduce stress on the glenohumeral joint and reduce the incidence of many shoulder injuries.*

Field Strategy 11.1. Flexibility Exercises for the Shoulder Region

A. Posterior capsular stretch. Horizontally adduct the arm across the chest while the opposite hand assists the stretch
B. Inferior capsular stretch. Hold the involved arm over the head with the elbow flexed. Use the opposite hand to assist in the stretching. Add a side stretch

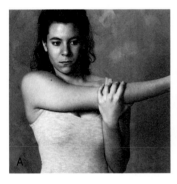
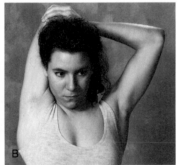

C. Anterior and posterior capsular stretch. Hold onto both sides of a doorway with your hands behind you. Let the arms straighten as you lean forward. Repeat with your hands in front of you as you lean backward
D. Medial and lateral rotators. Using a towel, bat, or racquet, pull the arm to be stretched into medial rotation. Repeat in lateral rotation

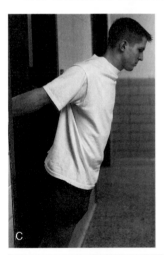
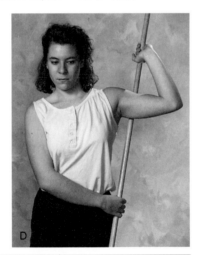

A. Shoulder shrugs. Elevate the shoulders toward the ears and hold. Pull
the shoulders back, pinch the shoulder blades together, and hold. Relax
and repeat

B. Scapular abduction (protraction). Thrust the weight directly upward, lifting
the posterior shoulder from the table. Relax and repeat

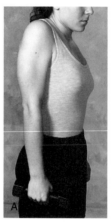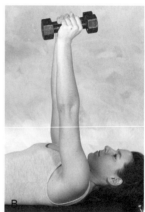

C. Scapular adduction (retraction). Do bent-over rowing while flexing the
elbows. At the end of the motion, pinch the shoulder blades together
and hold

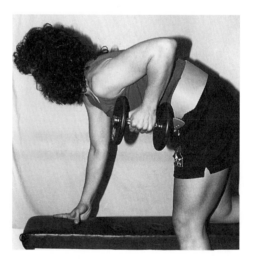

D. Bench press or incline press. Use a weight belt and spotter. Place the
hands, shoulder-width apart and push the barbell directly above the
shoulder joint

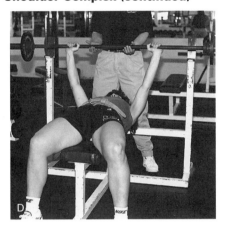

E. Bent arm lateral flies, supine position. With the elbows slightly flexed, bring the dumbbells directly over the shoulders. Lower the dumbbells until they are parallel to the floor, then repeat. In the prone position, the exercise strengthens the trapzius (trap flies)

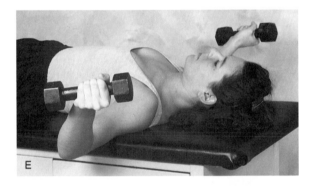

F. Lat pull-downs. In a seated position, grasp the handle and pull the bar behind the head. An alternative method is to pull the bar in front of the body
G. Surgical tubing. With the tubing secured, work in diagonal patterns

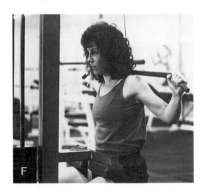

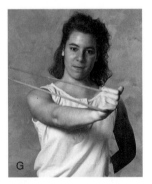

> An opposing player tackled the quarterback onto the hard turf. The quarterback landed sideways on his dominant shoulder and the arm was forced slightly anterior. Pain is centered on the superior shoulder region and you can feel a slight deformity between the acromion process and the clavicle. What structure(s) may be involved in this injury? How will you manage this condition?

Ligamentous injuries to the SC joint, AC joint, and glenohumeral joint can result from compression, tension, and shearing forces occurring in a single episode or from repetitive overload (**Fig. 11.12**). A common method of injury is a fall or direct hit on the lateral aspect of the acromion. The force is first transmitted to the site of impact, then to the AC joint, the clavicle, and, finally, to the SC joint. Failure can occur at any one of these sites (9). Acute sprains are commonly seen in hockey, rugby, football, soccer, and equestrian sports.

Sternoclavicular Joint Sprain

The SC joint is the main axis of rotation for movements of the clavicle and scapula. Nearly all injuries result from compression from a direct blow, as when a supine athlete is landed on by another participant, or more commonly, by indirect forces transmitted from a blow to the shoulder (10). The disruption typically drives the proximal clavicle superior, medial, and anterior causing anterior displacement.

First degree injuries are characterized by point tenderness and mild pain over the SC joint, with no visible deformity. Second degree injuries cause bruising, swelling, and significant pain, and the individual will be unable to horizontally adduct the arm without considerable pain. The athlete may hold the arm forward and close to the body, supporting it across the chest (10). Third degree sprains involve a prominent displacement of the sternal end of the clavicle and may involve a fracture. Pain is severe when the shoulders are brought together by a lateral force (10). **Field Strategy 11.3** summarizes the management of anterior sternoclavicular sprains.

Posterior displacement, although rare, is more serious because of possible injury to the esophagus, trachea, and subclavian artery. The individual will have a palpable depression, is unable to do shoulder protraction, and may have difficulty swallowing and breathing. Posterior dislocations can become life-threatening and EMS should be summoned.

Acromioclavicular Joint Sprain

The AC joint is weak and easily injured by a direct blow, a fall on the point of the shoulder (called a shoulder pointer), and, occasionally, from a force transmitted up the long axis of the

> Indirect forces can drive the proximal clavicle superior, medial, and forward, causing an anterior displacement

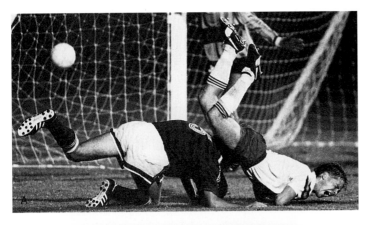

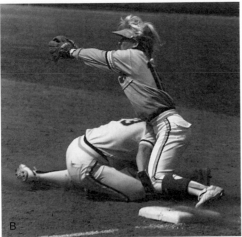

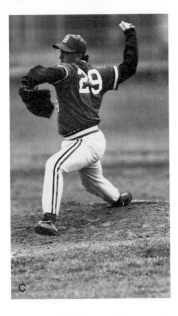

Figure 11.12. Injuries to the shoulder complex may be caused by (**A**) indirect forces, (**B**) direct forces, or (**C**) through repetitive overuse forces.

humerus during a fall on an outstretched arm. As with other joint sprains, symptoms parallel the amount of damage done to the supporting ligaments. In a first degree injury, minimal swelling and pain is present. In a second degree injury, the AC ligaments are torn, but the coracoclavicular ligament is only mildly sprained, but still intact. The clavicle rides above the level of the acromion and a minor step or gap is present at the joint line (**Fig. 11.13**). Pain increases when the distal clavicle is depressed or moved in an anteroposterior direction, and during passive horizontal adduction. In a third degree injury, there is a complete tear of the coracoclavicular and AC ligaments, resulting in obvious swelling and bruising, and a step deformity will be present.

First and second degree injuries are treated with ice and range-of-motion exercises as tolerated. Immobilization is necessary only if pain is present. The individual may return to certain activities earlier than others, but the area should be padded to protect it from further insult. Most third degree injuries are treated conservatively, with 90 to 100% having satisfactory results (9). After initial immobilization and acute care, gentle range-of-motion exercises can begin at 2 weeks, progressing to strengthening exercises. Return to sports, however, may take as long as 10 to 12 weeks (9). **Field Strategy 11.4** summarizes management of acromioclavicular sprains.

> With an AC joint sprain, pain increases with movement of the clavicle and passive horizontal adduction of the arm

 Field Strategy 11.3. Management of a Sternoclavicular Sprain

Signs and Symptoms	Mild—First Degree	Moderate—Second Degree	Severe—Third Degree
Deformity	None	Slight prominence of medial end of the clavicle	Gross prominence of medial end of the clavicle
Swelling	Slight	Moderate	Severe
Palpable pain	Mild	Moderate	Severe
Movement	Usually unlimited, but may have discomfort with movement	Unable to abduct the arm or horizontally adduct the arm across the chest without noticeable pain	Limited as in second degree, but pain will be more severe
Treatment	Ice, rest, immobilize with sling and swathe	Ice, rest, immobilize with figure-8 or clavicular strap with sling for 3 to 4 weeks. Start ROM exercises in 7 to 10 days, with strengthening exercises in 3 to 4 weeks	Figure-8 immobilizer with scapulas retracted. Refer to physician

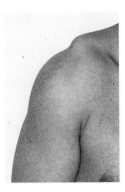

Figure 11.13. With an acromioclavicular separation, the distal clavicle is elevated, presenting what is called a step deformity.

Glenohumeral Joint Sprain

Damage to the glenohumeral joint can occur when the arm is forcefully abducted (i.e., when making an arm tackle in football), or abducted and externally rotated. In nearly all cases (95%), the anterior capsule is stretched or torn, leading to the humeral head

 Field Strategy 11.4. Management of an Acromioclavicular Sprain

Signs and Symptoms	Mild—First Degree	Moderate—Second Degree	Severe—Third Degree
Deformity	None, ligaments are still intact	Slight elevation of lateral clavicle; AC ligaments are disrupted, but coracoclavicular is still intact	Prominent elevation of clavicle; AC ligaments and coracoclavicular ligaments are disrupted
Swelling	Slight	Moderate	Severe
Palpable pain	Mild over joint line	Moderate with downward pressure on distal clavicle; palpable gap or minor step present; snapping may be felt on horizontal adduction	Severe on palpation and downward displacement of acromion process; definite step deformity present
Movement	Usually unlimited, but may have some discomfort on abduction over 90°	Unable to abduct the arm or horizontally adduct the arm across the chest without noticeable pain	Limited as in second degree, but pain will be more severe
Stability	No instability	Some instability	Demonstrable instability
Treatment	Ice, NSAIDs, and return to activity as tolerated, with protection	Ice, NSAIDs, immobilize with sling 1 to 4 weeks if pain is present. Return to activity with protection	Ice, immobilize, and refer to physician

slipping out of the glenoid fossa in an anterior-inferior direction (**Fig. 11.14**). A direct blow or forceful movement that pushes the humerus posteriorly can also result in damage to the joint capsule.

In a first degree injury, the anterior shoulder is particularly painful to palpation and movement, especially when the mechanism of injury is reproduced. A second degree sprain will produce some joint laxity. Pain, swelling, and bruising are usually severe and range of motion, particularly abduction, is limited. Treatment involves cryotherapy, rest, nonsteroidal anti-inflammatory drugs (NSAIDs), and immobilization with a sling during the initial 12 to 24 hours. Early emphasis is placed on pain-free range-of-motion exercises, elastic band strengthening, and PNF exercises. Exercises to regain full external rotation and abduction should be delayed at least 3 weeks to allow adequate time for capsular healing (6). A more extensive resistance program can start as tolerated.

> The individual will complain of pain during passive arm movement, especially when the mechanism of injury is reproduced

Glenohumeral Dislocations

Anterior dislocations are commonly due to excessive indirect forces that push the arm into abduction, external rotation, and extension. The ligaments are significantly damaged, causing the head of the humerus to lodge under the anterior-inferior portion of the glenoid fossa adjacent to the coracoid process. The labrum may be also be damaged or avulsed from the anterior lip of the glenoid as the humerus slides forward (**Bankart lesion**).

There is intense pain with the initial dislocation, although recurrent dislocations may be less painful. Tingling and numbness may

Bankart lesion
Avulsion or damage to the anterior lip of the glenoid as the humerus slides forward in an anterior dislocation

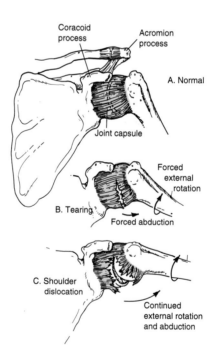

Figure 11.14. Glenohumeral sprains. **A.** Normal abduction, with some stretching of the fibers. **B.** Forced external rotation and abduction, with minimal tears to the joint capsule, leading to a moderate or second degree sprain. **C.** Continuation of the forced movement causes a third degree sprain or shoulder dislocation.

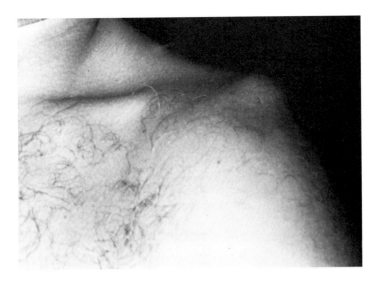

Figure 11.15. In a typical anterior dislocation, the head of the humerus is forced out of the glenoid fossa and comes to rest adjacent to the coracoid process. As a result, the acromion process becomes very prominent, the deltoid musculature appears flat, and the athlete may hold the arm away from the side.

extend down the arm into the hand. With a first-time dislocation, the injured arm is often held in slight abduction (20 to 30°) and external rotation, and is stabilized against the body by the opposite hand. Visually, a sharp contour on the affected shoulder, with a prominent acromion process, can be seen when compared to the smooth deltoid outline on the unaffected shoulder (**Fig. 11.15**). The individual will not allow the arm to be brought across the chest. Assessment of both the axillary nerve and artery is imperative, since both structures can be damaged in a dislocation. A pulse may be taken on the medial proximal humerus over the brachial artery, and the axillary nerve can be assessed by stroking the skin on the upper lateral arm. Ask the individual if it feels the same on both arms.

In a first-time dislocation, the injured arm is held in slight abduction and external rotation, and may be stabilized against the body with the opposite hand

Management of a first-time dislocation requires immediate reduction by a physician, because many are associated with a fracture. Treat the injury as a fracture and immobilize the arm in a comfortable position. To prevent unnecessary movement of the humerus, place a rolled towel or thin pillow between the thoracic wall and humerus prior to applying a sling. Ice is then applied to control hemorrhage and muscle spasm as the individual is transported to the nearest medical facility.

Occasionally, a posterior dislocation occurs from a fall on, or blow to, the anterior surface of the shoulder, driving the head of the humerus posterior. If dislocated, the arm will be carried tightly against the chest and across the front of the trunk in rigid adduction and internal rotation. The anterior shoulder will appear flat, the coracoid process is prominent, and a corresponding bulge may be

In a posterior dislocation, the arm will be splinted tightly against the chest and trunk in rigid adduction and internal rotation. Any attempt to move the arm will produce severe pain

seen posteriorly, if not masked by a heavy deltoid musculature (4). Any attempt to move the arm into external rotation and abduction produces severe pain. Treatment is the same as with an acute anterior dislocation, with immobilization in a sling and immediate transportation to a physician.

Recurrent Subluxations and Dislocations

In recurrent anterior subluxations or dislocations, the mechanism of injury is the same as acute dislocations. As the number of occurrences increases, however, the forces needed to produce the injury decrease, as does the associated muscle spasm, pain, and swelling. The individual is aware of the shoulder displacing because the arm will give the sensation of "going dead," referred to as the **dead arm syndrome**. Often it is reduced by the individual or with the help of a teammate.

Dead arm syndrome
Common sensation felt with a recurrent anterior shoulder dislocation

Recurrent posterior subluxations are common in activities, such as the follow-through phase of throwing or a racquet swing, ascent phase of push-ups or bench pressing, linebacker recoil, certain swimming strokes, or during crew sweep strokes. Pain is the major complaint with crepitation and/or clicking when the arm shifts into the appropriate position. After reduction by a physician, conservative treatment involves rest and immobilization, restoring shoulder motion, and strengthening the rotator cuff muscles. If persistent instability occurs, surgery may be indicated.

Recurrent posterior subluxations are common in activities such as the follow-through phase of throwing, ascent phase of push-ups or bench pressing, linebacker recoil, or during crew sweep strokes

💡 *During the tackle, the quarterback landed on the lateral shoulder and probably sprained the acromioclavicular ligament. This would account for the pain on the superior shoulder and the slight step deformity between the acromion process and clavicle.*

OVERUSE INJURIES

❓ *During overhead strokes, a tennis player has severe pain that is progressively getting worse. The player is unable to actively abduct the arm between 70 and 120° without excruciating pain. What structures may be injured? How can you determine if it is muscular or ligamentous?*

During abduction, the strong deltoid muscle pulls the humeral head superiorly, relative to the glenoid fossa. The rotator cuff muscles are critical in counteracting this migration. If the tendons are weak, they are incapable of depressing the humeral head in the glenoid fossa during overhead motions, leading to impingement of the supraspinatus tendon and subacromial bursa between the acromion, the coracoacromial ligament, and the greater tubercle of the humerus. This compressive action can lead to a rotator cuff strain, impingement syndrome, bursitis, and bicipital tendinitis.

The infraspinatus, teres minor, and subscapularis prevent the humeral head from migrating upward and impinging the supraspinatus tendon and subacromial bursa between the acromion, the coracoacromial ligament, and the greater tubercle of the humerus

Rotator Cuff/Impingement Injuries

Chronic rotator cuff tears result from repetitive microtraumatic episodes that primarily impinge the supraspinatus tendon just

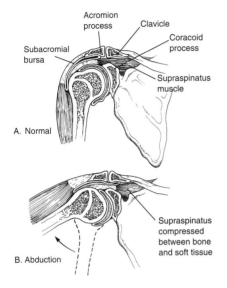

Figure 11.16. Supraspinatus tendon during abduction. **A.** Normal position. **B.** Abducted position. Repetitive overhead motions can impinge the muscle or tendon between nonyielding bony and soft tissue structures, resulting in a chronic rotator cuff injury.

Labels in figure:
- Acromion process
- Clavicle
- Coracoid process
- Subacromial bursa
- Supraspinatus muscle
- A. Normal
- Supraspinatus compressed between bone and soft tissue
- B. Abduction

proximal to the greater tubercle of the humerus **(Fig. 11.16)**. Partial tears are usually seen in young individuals, with total tears occurring in adults over 30 years of age (11). **Impingement syndrome** implies that, in addition to damage to the supraspinatus tendon, the glenoid labrum, long head of the biceps brachii, and subacromial bursa are also injured.

Initially, there is pain with activity, usually only in the impingement position. As repetitive trauma continues, however, pain becomes progressively worse, particularly between 70° and 120° of active and resisted abduction (7). Because forced scapular protraction leads to further impingement and pain in the structures, the individual may be unable to sleep at night on the involved side. Occasionally, a defect or crepitus in the supraspinatus tendon may be palpated just anterior to the acromion process when the arm is extended at the glenohumeral joint. Depending on the severity, positive results may be elicited in the supraspinatus test, "empty can test," and impingement test (see Assessment).

Treatment will involve cryotherapy, NSAIDs, pain-relieving medication, rest, and activity modification. Short arc exercises with abduction and forward flexion up to 90° are initiated early in the rehabilitation process. Lateral rotation exercises can facilitate clearance of the greater tuberosity under the coracoacromial ligament (4). When the condition is severe, all painful activities should be avoided until the individual is pain-free. Maintain mobility with mild stretching exercises, particularly in external rotation at 90°, 135°, and 180° of abduction. Examples of several range-of-motion exercises for the shoulder can be seen later in the chapter in **Field Strategy 11.7**. In addition, scapular retraction, depression, and rotation, and the rotator cuff should be strengthened. The infraspinatus muscle, in particular, is the only muscle in a position to generate a significant inferior pull on the humeral head. In terms

Impingement syndrome
Chronic condition caused by repetitive overhead activity that damages the glenoid labrum, long head of the biceps brachii, and subacromial bursa

Because of forced scapular protraction, the individual may be unable to sleep at night on the involved side

of strength about the shoulder, adduction should be the strongest, followed by extension, flexion, abduction, internal, and external rotation (4). **Field Strategy 11.8** demonstrates several strengthening exercises for the region.

Bursitis

The subacromial bursa is the largest and most commonly injured bursa in the shoulder region

Bursitis is not generally an isolated condition, but is usually associated with a rotator cuff tear, impingement syndrome, or, in older individuals, with pre-existing degenerative changes in the rotator cuff. The subacromial bursa is the largest and most commonly injured bursa in the shoulder region. Frequently, sudden shoulder pain is reported during the initiation and acceleration of the throwing motion. Point tenderness can be elicited on the anterior and lateral edges of the acromion process. A painful arc will exist between 70° and 120° of passive abduction. Treatment is the same as for a rotator cuff strain or impingement syndrome.

Bicipital Tendon Injuries

With bicipital tendinitis, pain is present over the bicipital groove when the tendon is passively stretched, and during resisted supination and elbow flexion

Injury to the biceps brachii tendon often occurs from repetitive overuse during rapid overhead movements involving excessive elbow flexion and supination activities, such as in racquet sports, shot-putters, baseball/softball pitchers, football quarterbacks, swimmers, and javelin throwers. Irritation of the tendon occurs as it passes back and forth in the intertubercular (bicipital) groove of the humerus and it may partially sublux. Pain and tenderness is present over the bicipital groove when the tendon is passively stretched, and during resisted supination and elbow flexion.

Treatment involves restriction of rotational activities that exacerbate symptoms, cryotherapy, and NSAIDs to control inflammation. Ice before and after activity can be combined with a gradual program of stretching and strengthening, as soon as pain subsides.

Prolonged tendinitis can make the tendon vulnerable to forceful rupture during repetitive overhead motions, commonly seen in swimmers, or in forceful flexion activities against excessive resistance, as in weight lifters or gymnasts. The individual will often hear and feel a snapping sensation and experience intense pain. Ecchymosis and a visible, palpable defect can be seen in the muscle belly when the individual flexes the biceps. This individual should be referred immediately to a physician.

💡 *The tennis player had pain during active movement between 70° and 120° of abduction. A possible impingement syndrome may have occurred because of the repetitive overhead strokes. If the supraspinatus tendon is injured, pain will occur during active and resisted shoulder abduction, and the drop arm test and "empty can" test will be positive (see Assessment). If ligaments are involved, pain will also be present during passive abduction.*

FRACTURES

❓ *A young gymnast lost her balance on a dismount and fell onto the point of the right shoulder. The shoulder is sagging down and forward. There is a noticeable bump in the midclavicular region. Shoulder movement is limited because of severe pain. What possible condition might you suspect?*

Most fractures to the shoulder region result from a fall on the point of the shoulder, rolling over onto the top of the shoulder, or, indirectly, falling on an outstretched arm. Clavicular fractures are more common than fractures to the scapula and proximal humerus, with nearly 80% occurring in the midclavicular region **(Fig. 11.17)**. The sternocleidomastoid muscle pulls the proximal bone fragment superiorly, allowing the distal shoulder to droop downward and medially from the force of gravity and pull of the pectoralis major muscle. Swelling, ecchymosis, and a deformity may be visible and palpable at the fracture site. Immediate treatment involves immobilization in a sling and swathe. After assessment by the physician, a figure-8 brace or strapping is used to pull the shoulders backward and upward for 4 to 6 weeks in young adults and 6 or more weeks in older adults **(Fig. 11.18)** (9).

Scapular fractures may involve the body, spine and acromion process, coracoid process, or glenohumeral joint. Most fractures result in minimal displacement and exhibit localized hemorrhage, pain, and tenderness. The individual is reluctant to move the injured arm and prefers to maintain it in adduction. The arm should be immediately immobilized with a sling and swathe and the individual should be referred to a physician. Cryotherapy is used during the first 48 hours to minimize hematoma formation. Fractures to the glenoid area are associated with shoulder subluxations and dislocations and, therefore, treatment is dictated by the shoulder dislocation rather than the fracture.

Epiphyseal centers around the shoulder region remain unfused for a longer span of time than is typically seen at other epiphyseal

> Epiphyseal centers around the shoulder region remain unfused for a longer time than is typically seen at other epiphyseal sites

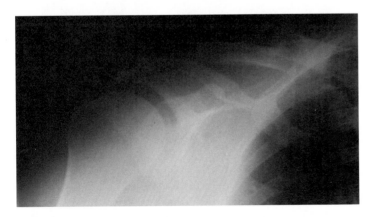

Figure 11.17. Midclavicular fracture.

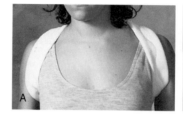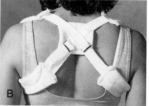

Figure 11.18. Figure-8 clavicular straps. **A.** Anterior view. **B.** Posterior view.

Little league shoulder
Fracture of the proximal humeral growth plate in adolescents caused by repetitive rotational stresses during the act of pitching

sites. For example, the proximal humeral epiphysis does not close until ages 18 to 21, thus predisposing an individual to this injury throughout the competitive high school and collegiate years (12). An epiphyseal fracture at this site, called **little league shoulder**, is often caused by rotation and compressive forces **(Fig. 11.19)**. Whereas the fracture may occur during one throw, more commonly it occurs from repetitive rotational stresses placed on the shoulder during pitching (13). Catchers may also get this fracture, since they throw the ball as hard and as often as pitchers, but with less of a windup. Pain may be elicited with deep palpation in the axilla. Radiographs are necessary to see the widened epiphyseal line and demineralization. Treatment is conservative, with symptoms disappearing after 3 to 4 weeks of rest. If activity is resumed too quickly, the condition may recur.

Humeral fractures result from violent compressive forces as a result of a direct blow, a fall on the upper arm, or a fall on an outstretched hand with the elbow extended. The surgical neck is

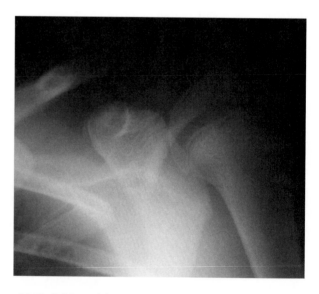

Figure 11.19. Epiphyseal fracture to the proximal humeral growth center is often seen in adolescent pitchers and catchers.

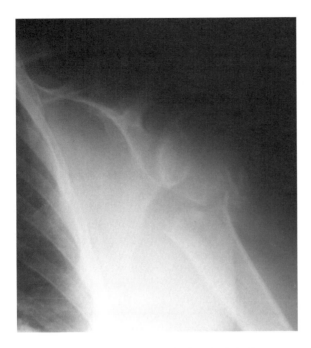

Figure 11.20. Fracture to the surgical neck of the humerus.

the most common site for proximal humeral fractures, and may display an appearance similar to a dislocation **(Fig. 11.20)**. Pain, swelling, hemorrhage, discoloration, an inability to move the arm, and possible paralysis may be present. The arm is often held splinted against the body (13). Fortunately, these fractures are often impacted, which facilitates closed reduction and allows early movement after 3 to 4 weeks of immobilization.

During the throwing motion, the pectoralis major or latissimus dorsi can cause excessive rotational torque through the muscular attachments, fracturing the midportion of the humerus. These spiral fractures are commonly seen in softball players (13). Fractures to this area can be very serious, because of the close proximity of major nerves and vessels running along the bone that may be damaged from jagged bone fragments. As such, immobilization of the limb should be in a rigid or vacuum splint. Assess the neural integrity by stroking the skin on the palm and dorsum of the hand. Ask the individual if it feels bilaterally the same on both sides of the hands. Take a radial pulse, check skin temperature at the hand, and blanch the finger nails and note capillary refill. Immediate referral to a physician is indicated.

> Fractures in the midportion of the humerus can damage major nerves and vessels running along the bone

After a fall on the point of the shoulder, the arm of the gymnast appeared to sag downward and forward, and had a visible bump in the midclavicular region. Any shoulder movement caused severe pain. If you determined a possible clavicular fracture, you are correct. How should the arm be immobilized?

ASSESSMENT OF THE SHOULDER

? *A baseball player is complaining of pain in the right arm every time the arm is abducted above 90°. Pain is localized on the anterior shoulder and aggravated with horizontal adduction. What structures may be injured in this injury? How will you assess the individual?*

The shoulder complex is a complicated region to assess because of the number of important structures located in such a small area. Furthermore, the biomechanical demands on each structure during overhead motion is not fully understood, so identification of all injured structures is difficult. As a result, each joint must be methodically assessed to determine limitation of function in an injured individual. The emphasis, however, remains the same: perform a thorough, complete, objective assessment of the area.

HISTORY

? *What information should be gathered from the baseball player complaining of anterior shoulder pain during shoulder abduction and horizontal adduction?*

Questions about a shoulder injury should focus on the current primary complaint, past injuries to the region, and other factors that may have contributed to the current problem (referred pain, alterations in posture, change in technique, or overuse). Many conditions may be related to improper execution of skills and recent changes in training programs. Keep questions open-ended to allow the individual to fully describe the injury. In addition to the general questions discussed in Chapter 4, specific questions related to the shoulder region can be seen in **Field Strategy 11.5**.

💡 *The baseball player has averaged six games per week for the past 2½ months. During the day he directs the swimming program at a local health club and swims three to five miles/day. The pain started gradually 2 months ago. It hurts to raise the arm and he wakes up at night when he sleeps on the affected side. Although he has had a sore shoulder before, he has never seen a physician.*

OBSERVATION AND INSPECTION

? *After taking a thorough history, what specific factors should be observed in the postural exam and during inspection of the injury site?*

On-the-field assessment may be somewhat limited due to uniforms and protective equipment that may obstruct the region from observation and inspection. Initially, you may have to slide your hands under the pads to palpate the region to determine the presence of a possible fracture or major ligament damage. If necessary, the pads should be cut and gently removed to more fully expose the area. After the initial exam, the individual may

Field Strategy 11.5. Developing a History of the Injury

Current Injury Status

1. How did the injury occur (mechanism)?
2. Ask about the pain location, severity, onset (sudden or gradual), and type (sharp, aching, burning, radiating). Did you hear any sounds during the incident, such as a snap, pop, or crack?
3. Was there any swelling, discoloration, muscle spasms, or numbness with the injury?
4. What actions or motions replicate the pain? Does it wake you up at night? In what part of the arm motion does it hurt the worst? Does it tire easily?
5. Are there certain activities you cannot perform because of the pain? How old are you? (Remember that many shoulder problems are age-related.)

Past Injury Status

1. Have you ever injured your shoulder before? When? How did that occur? What was done for the injury?
2. Have you had any medical problems recently? (You are looking for possible referred pain from the cervical neck, heart, lungs, or visceral organs.) Are you on any medication? Do you have any musculoskeletal problems elsewhere in the body? (These may result in changes in gait or technique that transfer abnormal forces to structures in the shoulder.)

need to be removed from the field to complete a more comprehensive assessment in the training room.

In an ideal situation, women should wear a bathing suit or halter top so the entire shoulder and arm can be fully exposed. Complete a general postural exam, looking for faulty posture or congenital abnormalities that could place additional strain on the anatomical structures. The individual should be viewed from the anterior, lateral, and posterior views. During movement, look for symmetry and fluid scapular motion. Inspect the specific injury site for obvious deformity, swelling, discoloration, symmetry, hypertrophy, muscle atrophy, or previous surgical incisions. Compare the affected limb with the unaffected limb. Specific areas to focus on in this region are summarized in **Field Strategy 11.6**.

No anomalies are observed during the postural exam. Slight swelling is present on the anterior lip of the acromion process and over the bicipital groove.

PALPATIONS

Pain and swelling appear to be confined to the anterior shoulder. Where should palpations begin, and what specific factors are you looking for?

Bilateral palpations can determine temperature, swelling, point tenderness, crepitus, deformity, muscle spasm, and cutaneous sensation. Increased skin temperature could indicate inflammation or infection. Decreased skin temperature could indicate a reduction in circulation. Vascular pulses can be taken at the radial and ulnar arteries in the wrist, brachial artery on the medial arm, or axillary artery in the armpit.

Fractures can be assessed through palpation of pain at the fracture site, compression of the humeral head against the glenoid fossa, compression along the long axis of the humerus, and with percussion and vibration on a specific bony landmark. If a fracture or dislocation is suspected, immediately assess circulatory and neural integrity distal to the site. Take a pulse at the sites indicated above and stroke the palm and dorsum of both hands to see if it feels the same bilaterally. Immobilize the extremity in an appropriate sling or splint, monitor vital signs, and refer the individual to the nearest medical facility. Stand behind the individual to begin bilateral palpations moving proximal to distal. Leave the most painful area until last.

 Field Strategy 11.6. Postural Assessment of the Upper Extremity

Anterior View

1. Check that the neck and head are in the midline of the body
2. Note any clavicular deformity that may indicate a possible fracture
3. Both shoulders should have a rounded, deltoid cap with no prominent acromion process
4. The dominant shoulder will usually be lower than the nondominant side
5. Note any muscular atrophy
6. Are both hands held in the same position. Note the color of the hands. This may indicate a vascular problem

Posterior View

1. Note any abnormal bony prominence or muscle atrophy, particularly the supraspinatus, infraspinatus, or deltoid. Are the scapula at the same height, angle, and distance away from the vertebral column?
2. Are the spines and inferior angles of the two scapula at the same height?
3. Note any "winging" of the scapula during a wall push-up
4. Is scoliosis (abnormal lateral curvature of the spine) present?
5. Is there any swelling or discoloration?

Lateral View

1. Note the attitude of the head and neck in relation to the shoulders. Is the head jutting forward or backward?
2. Is kyphosis (rounded shoulders) or lordosis (hollow back) present?
3. Do the arms appear relaxed and flexed at the same angle?

Bony Palpations

1. Clavicle, acromion process, coracoid process
2. Greater tubercle of the humerus, bicipital groove, and humeral shaft
3. Scapula

Soft Tissue Palpations

1. SC joint and sternocleidomastoid muscle
2. AC joint, subacromial bursa, and coracoacromial ligament
3. Rotator cuff muscles, pectoralis major, deltoid muscle, and biceps brachii muscle and tendon
4. Trapezius, rhomboid muscles, latissimus dorsi, and serratus anterior

💡 *Crepitus and point tenderness were elicited just anterior to the acromion process when the arm was passively flexed and extended. The bicipital groove was also point tender. The anterior shoulder was warm to the touch and swelling was noted anterior to the acromion process and over the bicipital groove.*

Special Tests

❓ *There are several painful areas. How will you determine what structures have been injured, and how severe this injury is?*

Perform special tests in a comfortable position for the patient and begin with gentle stress. It is common at the shoulder to have painful arcs. Note what range of motion is the most painful. Do not force the limb through any sudden motions, nor cause undue pain. Proceed cautiously through the assessment.

Joint Range of Motion

Because pain is frequently referred from the cervical region into the shoulder, perform active range of motion at the neck first. Neck flexion, extension, rotation, and lateral flexion should be assessed for fluid motion and presence of pain. If pain is present at the neck, immediately complete a full neck evaluation. If necessary, immobilize the neck in a cervical collar and refer the individual to a physician.

If no problems are noted during neck movement, continue with the shoulder evaluation. Ask the individual to perform gross movement patterns at the shoulder. Watch the arms from an anterior and posterior view. When standing behind the individual, make sure the scapula and humerus move together in a freely coordinated motion. Move the unaffected arm first to determine what is normal motion. The following gross movement patterns are collectively referred to as Apley's Scratch Test.

1. **Medial rotation and adduction.** Reach in front of the head and touch the opposite shoulder **(Fig. 11.21A)**

> Because pain is frequently referred from the cervical region into the shoulder, perform active range of motion at the neck first

> During gross movement patterns, make sure the scapula and humerus move together in a freely coordinated motion

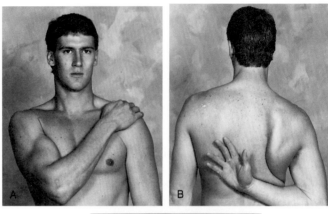

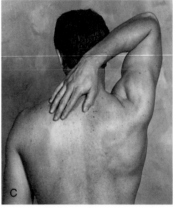

Figure 11.21. Apley's scratch test to determine range of motion. **A.** Internal rotation and adduction. **B.** Internal rotation, extension, and adduction. **C.** Abduction, flexion, and external rotation.

2. **Medial rotation and adduction.** Reach behind the back and touch the inferior angle of the opposite scapula **(Fig. 11.21B)**
3. **Abduction, flexion, and lateral rotation.** Reach behind the head and touch the superior angle of the opposite scapula **(Fig. 11.21C)**

Resisted Manual Muscle Testing

Stabilize the hip and trunk during testing to prevent muscle substitution. Begin with the muscle on stretch and apply resistance throughout the full range of motion. Note any lag, muscle weakness, or painful arc. **Figure 11.22** demonstrates scapular motions to be tested, including:

1. Elevation
2. Depression
3. Protraction
4. Retraction

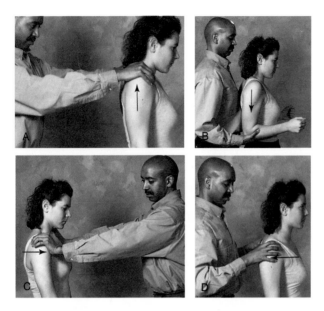

Figure 11.22. Manual muscle testing for the scapula. **A.** Elevation. **B.** Depression. **C.** Protraction. **D.** Scapular retraction. Arrows indicate the direction the athlete moves the scapula against applied resistance.

Figure 11.23 demonstrates glenohumeral motions at the shoulder to be tested, including:

1. Forward flexion
2. Extension
3. Abduction
4. Adduction
5. Lateral rotation
6. Medial rotation

Neurologic Assessment

Neurologic integrity is assessed with manual muscle testing (already completed), reflex testing, and cutaneous sensation. Reflexes in the upper extremity include the biceps (C_5 to C_6), brachioradialis (C_6), and triceps (C_7) (**Fig. 11.24**). The respective tendons are struck with the reflex hammer, using a quick wrist flexion action. A normal response is a slight jerk. To test cutaneous sensation, run the open hand and fingernails over the neck, shoulder, anterior and posterior chest walls, and down both sides of the arms to determine if sensation has been altered.

Reflexes in the upper extremity include the biceps, brachioradialis, and triceps reflex

Stress and Functional Tests

At this point in the assessment, you should have a strong suspicion of what structures may be damaged. In using stress and functional tests, perform only those tests that are absolutely necessary.

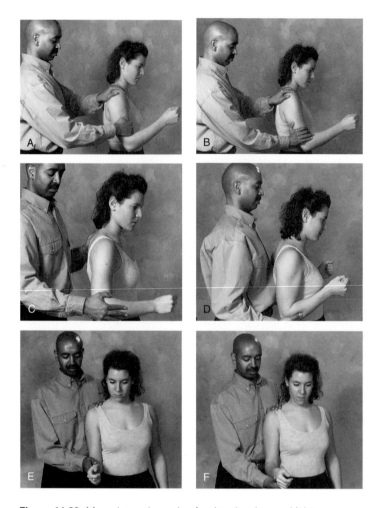

Figure 11.23. Manual muscle testing for the glenohumeral joint.
A. Flexion. **B.** Extension. **C.** Abduction. **D.** Adduction. **E.** External or lateral rotation. **F.** Internal or medial rotation. Arrows indicate the direction the athlete moves the body segment against applied resistance.

Serratus Anterior Weakness

Weakness of the serratus anterior, often called winging of the scapula, is determined by having the individual perform a push-up against the wall **(Fig. 11.25)**. If the muscle is weak, the medial border of the scapula will pull away from the chest wall.

Acromioclavicular (AC) Distraction/Compression

If the AC joint is unstable, traction on the arm will lead to distraction of the acromion process away from the clavicle. Grasp the arm while palpating the joint with the other hand. Apply steady downward traction **(Fig. 11.26A)**. A positive test will produce pain and/or joint movement. Horizontal adduction of the humerus

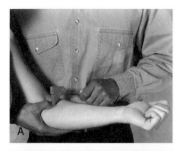

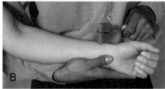

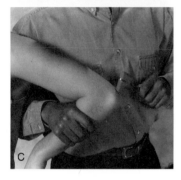

Figure 11.24. Reflex testing.
A. Biceps reflex (C_5, C_6).
B. Brachioradialis reflex (C_6).
C. Triceps reflex (C_7).

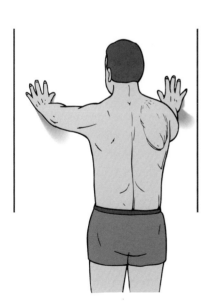

Figure 11.25. Winging of the scapula can result from weakness in the serratus anterior or injury to the long thoracic nerve.

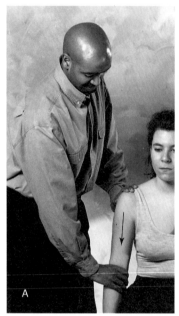

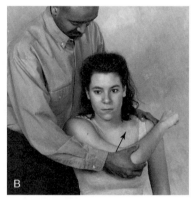

Figure 11.26. Acromioclavicular testing. **A.** Acromioclavicular traction. **B.** Acromioclavicular compression. Arrows indicate the direction the clinician applies the force.

across the chest will also increase pain as the AC joint is compressed (**Fig. 11.26B**).

Apprehension Test for Anterior Shoulder Dislocation

Slowly abduct and externally rotate the individual's humerus (**Fig. 11.27**). If the individual will not allow passive movement to the extremes of motion, or apprehension or alarm is shown in the facial expression, it is a positive sign. This motion should always be done slowly to prevent recurrence of a dislocation.

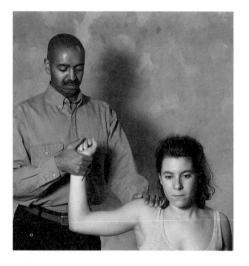

Figure 11.27. To perform the apprehension test, gently abduct and externally rotate the individual's humerus (indicated by the arrow).

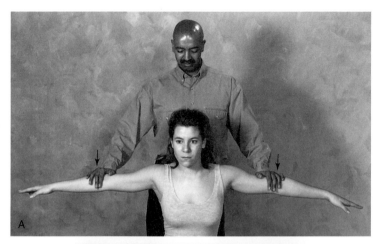

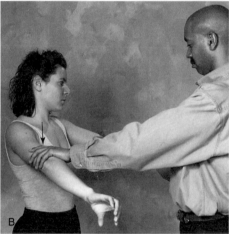

Figure 11.28. Supraspinatus testing. **A.** To perform the drop-arm test, abduct the humerus to 90°. Apply mild downward pressure on the distal humerus. **B.** To perform the "empty-can" or Centinela test, horizontally adduct the arm approximately 30 to 60°, with the humerus internally rotated. Apply mild downward pressure on the distal humerus.

Supraspinatus Testing

To test the integrity of the supraspinatus muscle and tendon, two tests may be used: the drop arm test and the "empty can" test. To perform the drop arm test, abduct the shoulder to 90° with no humeral rotation. Ask the individual to slowly lower the arm to the side. If positive, the arm will not lower smoothly, or increased pain will occur during the motion. An alternative test is to abduct the arm again at 90°, with no rotation, and ask the individual to hold that position. Apply downward resistance to the distal end of the humerus **(Fig. 11.28A)**. A positive test is indicated if the individual is unable to maintain the arm in the abducted position.

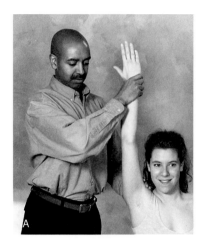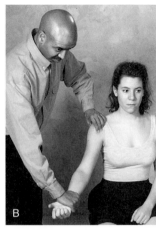

Figure 11.29. A. Anterior impingement test. Internally rotate and passively move the humerus through shoulder flexion while depressing the scapula. Pain or apprehension indicates a possible injury to the supraspinatus or biceps brachii tendon. **B.** Speed's test. With the arm in the same starting position, do resisted forward flexion (indicated by the arrow) while you palpate the bicipital groove. Pain over the bicipital groove indicates bicipital tendinitis.

To perform the "empty can" or Centinela test, place the arm in 90° of abduction, 30° to 60° of horizontally adduction, and point the thumbs downward ("empty can position") **(Fig. 11.28B)**. Apply downward pressure proximal to the elbows and look for pain and/or weakness. The arms should rebound to the 90° abducted position. A positive test indicates a tear to the supraspinatus muscle or tendon.

Anterior Impingement Test

Internally rotate and abduct the humerus through shoulder flexion while depressing the scapula, thus jamming the greater tubercle underneath the anteroinferior border of the acromion process **(Fig. 11.29A)**. Pain or apprehension on the individual's face may indicate an overuse injury to the supraspinatus or biceps brachii tendon.

Speed's Test for Bicipital Tendinitis

Supinate the arm with the elbow fully extended. Place one hand over the bicipital groove and resist forward flexion of the arm with the other hand. A positive test will result in tenderness over the groove, indicating bicipital tendinitis **(Fig. 11.29B)**.

Functional Tests

Occasionally, functional movements are the only activities that reproduce the signs and symptoms. Throwing a ball, performing a swimming stroke, or doing an overhead serve or spike may replicate the painful pattern. These movements are also commonly used to determine when the individual can return to sport participation. All functional patterns should be fluid and pain-free.

💡 *You found a painful arc of motion between 60° and 120° of abduction and flexion at the glenohumeral joint during active and resisted motion. Pain increased when the arm was horizontally adducted as the greater tubercle of the humerus moved under the acromion process. Positive results were found with the drop-arm test, "empty can" test, impingement test, and Speed's test. Neurologic tests were normal. If you determined this individual has an impingement syndrome involving the supraspinatus tendon, subacromial bursa, and long head of the biceps brachii, you are correct.*

REHABILITATION

❓ *The baseball player has a painful shoulder due to an impingement syndrome. What will be your priority of care to rehabilitate this injury and return the player to full functional status?*

Rehabilitation of the shoulder region must involve range-of-motion and strengthening exercises for the entire shoulder complex in a functional progression. Progress within any program is dictated by the type and severity of injury, amount of immobilization, and the supervising physician's treatment plan.

In a general sense, restoration of active range of motion should precede strengthening exercises that focus on specific strength deficits. Codmans' circumduction and pendulum swings are often used immediately after injury. The exercise is performed by making small circles and a pendulum motion in flexion and extension, and horizontal abduction and adduction. Other exercises to improve range of motion were demonstrated in **Field Strategy 11.1**, or may include T-bar exercises, such as those illustrated in **Field Strategy 11.7**. In throwing activities, the range of motion needed to adequately complete the cocking phase exceeds 90° of external rotation when the arm is abducted 90° (7). Special attention should be focused on regaining this additional range of motion.

Gentle isometric exercises can begin immediately after injury or surgery, while the arm is still immobilized. Because strength gains are relatively specific to the joint angle, isometric contractions must be performed at multiple positions. Once range of motion approximates normal for the individual, free weights may be used in a progressive resistance program. Several specific exercises are demonstrated in **Field Strategy 11.8**. The individual should complete 50 to 100 repetitions with a one-pound weight, and should not progress in resistance until 100 repetitions are achieved. Resistance should be limited to five pounds, as this decreases the chance of rotator cuff inflammation during the strengthening program (14).

Closed-chain exercises to regain proprioception may be performed immediately after injury and may include an isometric

Perform the exercises two to three times daily, holding each stretch for 5 to 10 seconds. Repeat each exercise 10 to 20 times per session

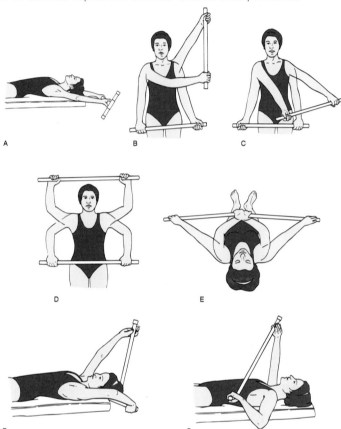

A. Shoulder flexion. Grasp the wand palm down at waist height. Raise the wand directly overhead, leading with the uninvolved arm until a stretch is felt in the involved shoulder. If an impingement syndrome is present, do the exercise palm up

B. Shoulder abduction. Hold the wand with the involved arm palm up, uninvolved arm palm down. Push the wand laterally and upward toward the involved side until a stretch is felt in the involved shoulder

C. Shoulder adduction/horizontal adduction. Reverse hand positions from exercise B. Pull the wand toward the uninvolved side until a stretch is felt in the involved shoulder

D. Shoulder internal/external rotation. With both palms down and elbows flexed, externally rotate the shoulders, then return to waist level

E. Shoulder horizontal abduction/adduction. With both palms down, push the wand across the body with the uninvolved arm, then pull back across the body. Do not twist the trunk

F. Supine external rotation. Abduct the shoulder and flex the elbow to 90°. Grip the T-bar in the hand on the involved arm. Use the opposite arm to push the involved arm into external rotation. Perform external rotation with the arm abducted at 135° and 180°

G. Supine internal rotation. With the arms in the same position as in exercise F, use the uninvolved arm to push the involved arm into internal rotation

Field Strategy 11.8. Rehabilitation Exercises for the Shoulder Complex

Progressive resistance exercises should begin when pain subsides. Exercises should be controlled while focusing on the line of movement. Begin with gravity as resistance, progress to light dumbbells or sandbags, then incorporate the exercises listed in Field Strategy 11.2.

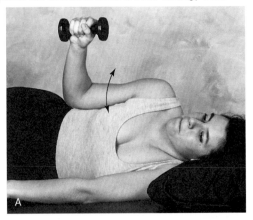

A. Sidelying medial and lateral rotation. With the elbow flexed, perform lateral and medial rotation

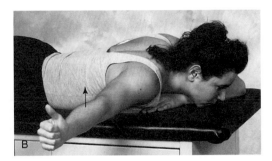

B. Prone horizontal abduction (90°). With the arm over the table and the thumb pointing up, raise the arm and laterally rotate the humerus until it is parallel to the floor

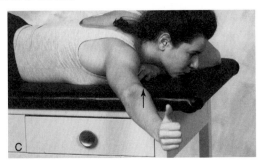

C. Prone horizontal abduction (100°). With the arm abducted at 100°, raise the arm and laterally rotate the humerus

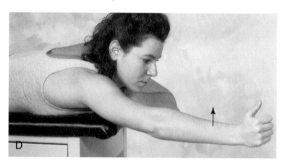

D. Prone flexion and extension. With the thumb pointing up, raise the arm forward into flexion. Repeat, moving the arm into extension

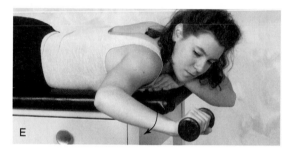

E. Prone medial and lateral rotation. With the shoulder abducted 90° and the elbow flexed, perform lateral and medial rotation. Repeat in the supine position

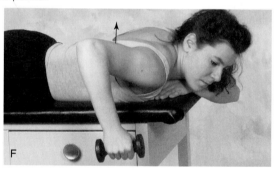

F. Prone rows (scapular adduction). With the shoulder abducted 90° and the elbow flexed, raise the arm off the table as if pinching the shoulder blades together. Do not raise the chest off the table

press-up, isometric weight bearing and weight shifts, and axial compression against a table or wall (15). Shifting body weight from one hand to the other may be done on a wall, table top, or unstable surface, such as a foam mat or BAPS board, from side to side, forward to backward, and diagonally on and off the affected

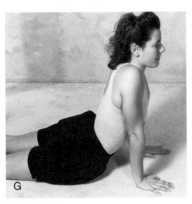

G. Press-ups and wall push-ups

side. Push-ups and exercises in a frontal and sagittal plane can be performed on a ProFitter or slide board, if available. In advanced stages, push-ups can be done with the hands placed on a ball, a balance system, or on a movable platform with the feet elevated on a physioball (15). Other exercises to improve general strength in the shoulder region were demonstrated in **Field Strategy 11.2**.

PNF exercises in resisted diagonal patterns can mimic functional skills, or surgical tubing may be used. As strength, balance, and coordination are developed, it is imperative to make the transference of proprioceptive training to the actual throwing motion. This is accomplished with a slow, deliberate rehearsal of the throwing motion. As motion improves and biomechanical errors are corrected, speed of movement and distance of throw is gradually increased.

Plyometric exercises may involve catching a weighted ball, utilizing a quick eccentric stretch of the muscle to facilitate a concentric contraction in throwing the ball. The exercise can progress through various one- and two-arm chest passes and overhead passes. A mini tramp may also be used to do plyometric bounding push-ups.

General cardiovascular fitness should be maintained throughout the rehabilitation program. Several examples of programs were provided in **Field Strategy 5.7**, and included the use of a jump rope, Stair Master, treadmill, and upper body ergometer (UBE).

The baseball player should increase range of motion in external rotation, restore strength in the rotator cuff and scapulothoracic musculature, regain proprioception and balance, and restore proper throwing mechanics through a functionally progressive throwing program.

> PNF and surgical tubing exercises in diagonal patterns can help to transfer proprioceptive training to the actual throwing motion or functional skill

Field Strategy 11.9. Shoulder Evaluation

History

Primary complaint and mechanism of injury
Onset of symptoms, including pain and discomfort
Disability and functional impairments from the injury
Previous injuries to the area and family history

Observation and Inspection

Observe general posture

Inspect:
Muscle symmetry	Hypertrophy or muscle atrophy
Swelling	Visible congenital deformity
Discoloration	Surgical incisions or scars

Palpation

Bony structures, to determine a possible fracture

Soft tissue structures, to determine:
Temperature	Deformity
Swelling	Muscle spasm
Point tenderness	Cutaneous sensation
Crepitus	Vascular pulses

Special Tests

Joint range of motion, with gross motor movement
Resisted manual muscle testing
Neurologic testing
Stress and functional tests
    Serratus anterior weakness
    Acromioclavicular (AC) distraction/compression
    Apprehension test for anterior dislocation
    Supraspinatus testing
      Drop-arm test
      Empty can test (Centinela test)
    Anterior impingement test
    Speed's test for bicipital tendinitis
    Functional tests

SUMMARY

The extreme mobility needed to perform common athletic skills and techniques, coupled with a lack of stability in the glenohumeral joint, sets the stage for many acute and chronic shoulder injuries. The shoulder complex functions as a series of joints working together in a coordinated manner to allow complicated patterns of motion. Because of this, injury to one structure can affect other structures. This makes assessment of a shoulder injury very complicated. **Field Strategy 11.9** demonstrates the progression of a shoulder assessment.

Always keep in mind that pain may be referred from other areas of the body, particularly the cervical neck, heart, lungs, and visceral organs. Any significant finding should be referred to a physician. Examples of these significant injuries may include: obvious deformity suggesting a suspected fracture or dislocation, significant loss of motion or muscles weakness, joint instability, abnormal cutaneous sensation, absent or weak pulse distal to the injury, or any significant unexplained pain.

If you refer the individual to a physician, immobilize the limb in a sling and swathe, or another commercial product that adequately pads and supports the limb. Apply cryotherapy to reduce inflammation and swelling, and transport the individual in an appropriate manner.

Functional tests should be performed before clearing the individual for re-entry into sport participation. Upper extremity sport-specific skills should be performed pain, free in all movements. In addition, the individual should have bilateral equal strength, flexibility, muscular endurance, and a high cardiovascular fitness level before returning to participation. Whenever possible, protective equipment or padding should be used to prevent reinjury.

REFERENCES

1. Johnson RE, and Rust RJ. 1985. Sports related injury: an anatomic approach, part 2. Minn Med 68:829–831.
2. McMaster WC, and Troup J. 1993. A survey of interfering shoulder pain in United States competitive swimmers. Am J Sports Med 21(1):67–70.
3. Fleisig GS, Escamilla RF, and Andrews JR. Biomechanics of throwing. In *Athletic injuries and rehabilitation,* edited by JE Zachazewski, DJ Magee, and WS Quillen. Philadelphia: WB Saunders, 1996.
4. Magee DJ, and Reid DC. Shoulder injuries. In *Athletic injuries and rehabilitation,* edited by JE Zachazewski, DJ Magee, and WS Quillen. Philadelphia: WB Saunders, 1996.
5. Hamill J, and Knutzen KM. *Biomechanical basis of human movement.* Baltimore: Williams & Wilkins, 1995.
6. Tibone JE. Shoulder problems of adolescents: how they differ from those of adults. In *Clinics in sports medicine,* edited by FV Jobe, vol. 2, no. 2. Philadelphia: WB Saunders, 1983.
7. Irrgang JJ, Witney SL, and Harner CD. 1992. Nonoperative treatment of rotator cuff injuries in throwing athletes. J Spt Rehab 1(3):197–222.
8. Reid DC. *Sports injury assessment and rehabilitation.* New York: Churchill Livingstone, 1992.
9. Hutchinson MR, and Ahuja GS. 1996. Diagnosing and treating clavicle injuries. Phys Sportsmed 24(3):26–36.
10. Wroble RR. 1995. Sternoclavicular injuries: managing damage to an overlooked joint. Phys Sportsmed 23(9):19–26.
11. Warren RF. Surgical considerations for rotator cuff tears in athletes. In *Shoulder surgery in the athlete,* edited by DW Jackson. Rockville, MD: Aspen Systems, 1985.
12. Ireland ML, and Hutchinson NR. Upper extremity injuries in young athletes. In *Clinics in sports medicine,* edited by LJ Micheli, vol 14, no. 3. Philadelphia: WB Saunders, 1995.
13. Julin MJ, and Mathews M. Shoulder injuries. In *The team physician's handbook,* edited by MB Mellion, WM Walsh, and GL Shelton. Philadelphia: Hanley and Belfus, 1990.
14. Stone JA, Lueken JS, Partin NB, Timm KE, and Ryan EJ. 1993. Closed kinetic chain rehabilitation for the glenohumeral joint. J Ath Train 28(1):34–37.
15. Wilk KE, Arrigo CA, and Andrews JR. 1996. Closed and open kinetic chain exercise for the upper extremity. J Spt Rehab 5(1):88–102.

Upper Arm, Elbow, and Forearm Injuries

After completing this chapter, you should be able to:

- Locate the important bony and soft tissue structures in the upper arm, elbow, and forearm

- Describe the motions at the elbow and identify muscles that produce them

- Describe measures used to prevent injuries to the upper arm, elbow, and forearm

- Recognize and manage common injuries in the upper arm, elbow, and forearm

- Demonstrate a basic assessment of the elbow region

- Demonstrate common rehabilitation exercises for the elbow

Key Terms:

Ectopic bone	**Malaise**
Epicondylitis	**Resting position**
Little league elbow	**Volkmann's contracture**

The arms perform lifting and carrying tasks, cushion the body during collisions, and lessen body momentum during falls. Performance in many sports is also contingent on the ability of the arms to effectively swing a racquet or club, or to position the hands for throwing and catching a ball. The elbow is second only to the shoulder as the most commonly dislocated joint, and in children under 10 years of age, it is the most dislocated joint (1). Furthermore, the elbow is believed to be second only to the knee in overuse injuries, with lateral **epicondylitis**, or "tennis elbow," being the most frequent overuse injury in athletes (2,3). Medial epicondylitis, or "little league elbow," is another overuse injury commonly seen in adolescent athletes.

This chapter begins with a review of anatomy and the major muscle actions of the upper arm, elbow, and forearm. Discussion on measures to prevent injury to the region is followed by information on common injuries and their management. Finally, the injury assessment process is presented, followed by examples of rehabilitation exercises.

Epicondylitis
Inflammation and microrupturing of the soft tissues on the epicondyles of the distal humerus

429

An adolescent baseball pitcher is complaining of pain on the medial side of the elbow while practicing the curve ball. What anatomical structures might be inflamed?

Although the elbow may be generally thought of as a simple hinge joint, the elbow actually encompasses three articulations—the humeroulnar, humeroradial, and proximal radioulnar joints **(Fig. 12.1)**. Several strong ligaments bind these articulations together and a single joint capsule surrounds all three joints.

Bony Structure of the Elbow

> The humeroulnar hinge joint is considered to be *the* elbow joint

The hinge joint at the elbow is the humeroulnar joint, where the trochlea of the humerus articulates with the reciprocally shaped trochlear fossa of the ulna. Motion capabilities are primarily flexion and extension, although, in some individuals, particularly women, a small amount of overextension is allowed. The humeroradial joint, just lateral to the humeroulnar joint, is a gliding joint with motion restricted to the sagittal plane by the adjacent humeroulnar joint. The annular ligament binds the head of the radius to the radial notch of the ulna forming the proximal radioulnar joint. This is a pivot joint with forearm pronation and supination occurring as the radius rolls medially and laterally over the ulna **(Fig. 12.2)**.

Ligaments of the Elbow

The elbow is reinforced by the ulnar (medial) and radial (lateral) collateral ligaments and by the annular ligament. The two collateral ligaments are strong and fan-shaped. The annular ligament provides support for the adjacent proximal radioulnar joint.

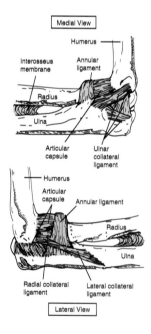

Figure 12.1. The bones and major ligaments of the elbow.

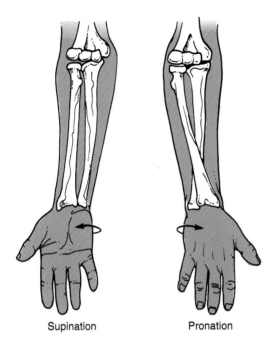

Supination   Pronation

Figure 12.2. Pronation involves the rotation of the radius around the ulna.

Muscles of the Elbow

A number of muscles cross the elbow, including several that also cross the shoulder, or extend down into the hand and fingers. The tendinous attachments of muscles near the medial and lateral aspects of the elbow are often irritated and inflamed by repetitive stresses associated with poor technique or overtraining in sports such as tennis, golf, and baseball pitching. The muscles considered to be primary movers of the elbow are summarized in **Table 12.1**.

Nerves and Blood Vessels of the Elbow

The major nerves of the elbow region descend from the brachial plexus and include the musculocutaneous, median, ulnar, and radial nerves (**Fig. 12.3**). The musculocutaneous nerve provides motor supply to the flexor muscles of the anterior arm and sensory innervation to the skin of the lateral forearm. The median nerve supplies most of the flexor muscles of the anterior forearm. The ulnar nerve innervates the flexor carpi ulnaris and the medial half of the flexor digitorum profundus. The radial nerve, the largest branch of the brachial plexus, divides into the superficial and deep branches to continue to supply all the arm and forearm extensor muscles and the skin on the posterior aspect of the arm and forearm. Specific nerve-muscle associations are shown in **Table 12.1**.

Table 12.1. Muscles of the Elbow

Muscle	Proximal Attachment	Distal Attachment	Primary Action(s)	Nerve Innervation
Biceps brachii		Tuberosity of the radius	Flexion; assists with supination	Musculocutaneous
Long head	Superior rim of the glenoid fossa			
Short head	Coracoid process of the scapula			
Brachioradialis	Upper two-thirds lateral supracondylar ridge of humerus	Styloid process of the radius	Flexion	Radial
Brachialis	Anterior lower half of the humerus	Anterior coronoid process of ulna	Flexion	Musculocutaneous
Pronator Teres		Lateral midpoint of the radius	Assists with flexion and pronation	Median
Humeral head	Medial epicondyle of the humerus			
Ulnar head	Coronoid process of the ulna			
Pronator quadratus	Lower fourth of the anterior ulna	Lower fourth of the anterior radius	Pronation	Anterior interosseus
Triceps brachii		Olecranon process of the ulna	Extension	Radial
Long head	Just inferior to the glenoid fossa			
Lateral head	Upper half of the posterior humerus			
Medial head	Lower two-thirds of posterior humerus			
Anconeus	Posterior, lateral epicondyle of the humerus	Lateral olecranon and posterior ulna	Assists with extension	Radial
Supinator	Lateral epicondyle of humerus and adjacent ulna	Lateral upper third of radius	Supination	Posterior interosseus

The brachial artery supplies blood to the elbow

The major arteries of the elbow and forearm region are the brachial, ulnar, and radial arteries (**Fig. 12.4**). The brachial artery supplies blood to the elbow joint and the flexor muscles of the arm and can be easily palpated in the anterior elbow. Distal to the elbow, the brachial artery splits into the ulnar and radial arteries to supply the medial forearm and lateral forearm, respectively. Pulses can be taken for both arteries on the anterior aspect of the wrist.

The proximal common flexor–pronator tendinous attachment on the medial epicondyle of the humerus is often inflamed during improper technique or repetitive overuse. This growth site is highly vulnerable in adolescents.

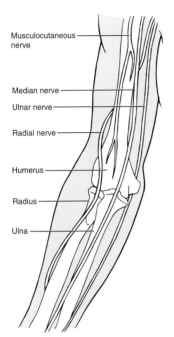

Musculocutaneous nerve

Median nerve

Ulnar nerve

Radial nerve

Humerus

Radius

Ulna

Figure 12.3. The nerves of the elbow region.

MAJOR MUSCLE ACTIONS OF THE ELBOW

? *Why is the effectiveness of some elbow flexor muscles affected by the position of the radioulnar joint?*

The three associated joints at the elbow allow motion in two planes. Flexion and extension are sagittal plane movements that occur at the humeroulnar and humeroradial joints and pronation

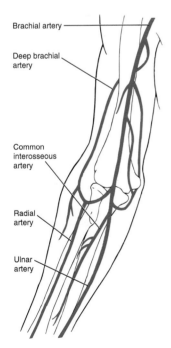

Brachial artery

Deep brachial artery

Common interosseous artery

Radial artery

Ulnar artery

Figure 12.4. The arteries of the elbow region.

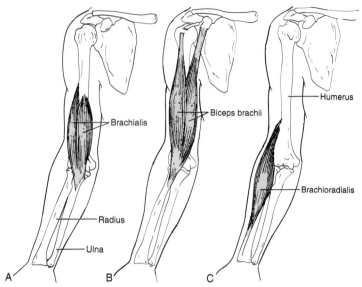

Figure 12.5. The primary flexor muscles of the elbow. **A.** Brachialis. **B.** Biceps brachii. **C.** Brachioradialis.

and supination are longitudinal rotational movements that take place at the proximal radioulnar joint.

Flexion and Extension

The elbow flexors include those muscles crossing the anterior side of the joint (**Fig. 12.5**). The primary elbow flexor is the brachialis. The biceps brachii also contributes to flexion when the arm is supinated, because the muscle is slightly stretched. When the forearm is pronated, the muscle is less taut and, consequently,

> The primary elbow flexor is the brachialis

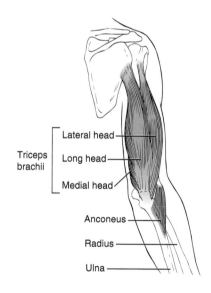

Figure 12.6. The primary extensor muscles of the elbow are the triceps brachii and anconeus.

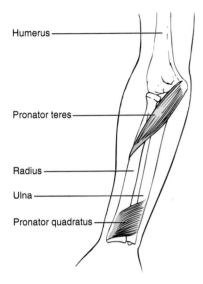

Figure 12.7. The primary pronators of the elbow are the pronator quadratus and pronator teres.

less effective. The brachioradialis, a third elbow flexor, is most effective when the forearm is in a neutral position (midway between full pronation and full supination).

The triceps is the major elbow extensor (**Fig. 12.6**). Although the three heads have separate proximal attachments, they attach to the olecranon process of the ulna through a common distal tendon. The small anconeus also assists with extension at the elbow.

Pronation and Supination

Pronation and supination of the forearm occur when the radius rotates around the ulna. The pronator quadratus, the primary pronator muscle, is assisted by the pronator teres (**Fig. 12.7**).

As the name suggests, the supinator is the muscle primarily

Pronation and supination of the forearm involves the pivoting of the radius around the ulna

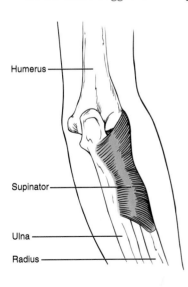

Figure 12.8. The primary supinator of the elbow is the supinator muscle.

responsible for supination (**Fig. 12.8**). During resistance and/or when the elbow is flexed, the biceps also participates in supination.

Muscles function most effectively when slightly stretched. Thus, the biceps brachii is most effective when the forearm is fully supinated and the brachioradialis is most effective when the forearm is in a neutral position.

PREVENTION OF INJURIES

The arms perform lifting and carrying tasks, cushion the body during collisions, and lessen body movements during falls. What measures can be taken to protect the region from injury?

The elbow is often subjected to compressive forces when the arm is placed in such a position to cushion a fall or lessen body impact with another object. Although football, hockey, and lacrosse do require specific pads to protect the upper arm, elbow, and forearm, most sports do not require any protection for the region. Several padded sleeves and braces were illustrated in Chapter 6 that can be purchased to protect the elbow from direct trauma and reduce tensile forces on joint structures.

Many of the muscles that move the elbow also move the shoulder or wrist. Therefore, flexibility and strength exercises must focus on the entire arm. Exercises illustrated in **Field Strategy 12.1** improve general strength at the elbow and wrist and can be combined with strengthening exercises for the shoulder complex illustrated in the previous chapter. Begin with light resistance, progressing to a heavier resistance.

Nearly all overuse injuries at the elbow are directly related to repetitive throwing-type motions that produce microtraumatic tensile forces on the surrounding soft tissue structures. Children who pitch sidearm motions are three times more likely to develop problems than those who use a more overhand technique (2). Movement analysis can detect improper technique in the acceleration and follow-through phase that contribute to these excessive tensile forces. Another preventative measure, already discussed in the shoulder chapter, is teaching sport participants the shoulder roll method of falling. Falling on an extended hand or flexed elbow is one of the most common mechanisms for acute injuries in the upper extremity. Excessive compressive forces can be transmitted along the long axis of the bones, leading to a fracture or dislocation.

Strengthening the musculature at the shoulder, elbow, and wrist, along with using the proper throwing technique, falling correctly, and wearing protective pads, can prevent many injuries from occurring.

CONTUSIONS

A basketball player was struck by an opponent's elbow on the belly of the biceps brachii. Discoloration is present and resisted elbow flexion is somewhat uncomfortable. How would you

Movement analysis can detect improper technique in the acceleration and follow-through phase of throwing that can contribute to excessive tensile forces at the elbow

manage this injury? What potentially serious condition might develop if repeated blows occur to the same area?

Direct blows to the arm and forearm are frequently associated with contact and collision sports. Contusions occur most commonly at the bony prominences (1). For volleyball players, the very nature of the sport leads to forearm trauma **(Fig. 12.9)**. Bruising can lead to internal hemorrhage, rapid swelling, and hematoma formation that can limit range of motion. Chronic blows to the anterior arm or near the distal attachment of the deltoid muscle may, however, result in the development of **ectopic bone** in either the belly of the muscle (myositis ossificans) or as a bony outgrowth (exostosis) of the underlying bone. Standard shoulder pads do not extend far enough to protect the area, and the edge of the pad itself may contribute to the injury. The developing mass can become painful and disabling; however, surgical excision of the calcification is necessary only if function is impaired.

Treatment for contusions will involve ice, compression, elevation, and rest, followed by nonsteroidal anti-inflammatory drugs (NSAIDs) and gentle, pain-free active range-of-motion exercises. Aggressive stretching and strengthening exercises should be

Ectopic bone
Proliferation of bone ossification in an abnormal place

 Field Strategy 12.1. Exercises to Prevent Injury to the Elbow Region

Begin all exercises with light resistance, using dumbbells or surgical tubing.
A. Biceps curl. Fully flex the elbow. This can be performed bilaterally in a standing position with a barbell
B. Triceps curl. Raise the involved arm over the head and extend the involved arm at the elbow. This can be performed bilaterally in a supine or standing position with a barbell

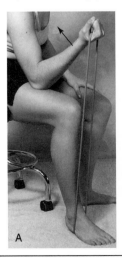
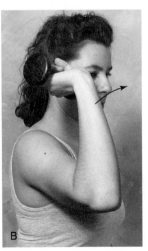

C. Wrist flexion. With the palm facing up, slowly do a full wrist curl and return to the starting position

D. Wrist extension. With the palm facing down, slowly do a full reverse wrist curl and return to the starting position

E. Forearm pronation/supination. With surgical tubing or a hand dumbbell, roll the forearm into pronation, then return to supination. Adjust the surgical tubing and repeat the exercise stressing the supinators. Be sure the elbow remains stationary

F. Ulnar/radial deviation. With surgical tubing or a hand dumbbell, contract the appropriate muscle group. An alternate method is to stand with the arm at the side holding a hammer or weighted bar. Raise the wrist in ulnar deviation/radial deviation

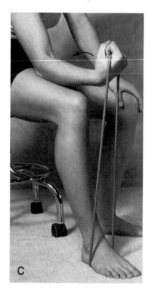

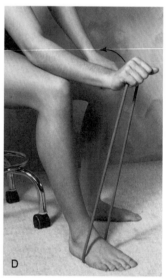

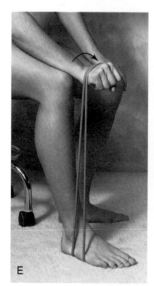

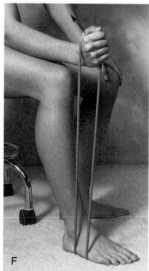

G. Wrist curl-ups. To exercise the wrist extensors, grip the bar with both palms facing down. Slowly wind the cord onto the bar until the weight reaches the top, then slowly unwind the cord. Reverse hand position to work the wrist flexors

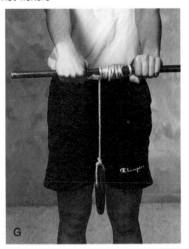

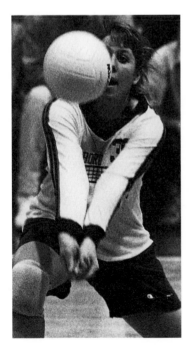

Figure 12.9. Volleyball players contuse the forearms during the early part of the season from repetitive compression on soft tissue structures.

avoided so as not to further injure muscle tissue (4). If conservative measures do not alleviate the condition, refer the individual to a physician for radiographs.

💡 *The contusion to the basketball player can be treated with ice therapy, compression, and elevation. If repeated blows occur to the same spot, myositis ossificans may develop. Should this occur, immediate referral to a physician is necessary for further assessment and possible radiographs.*

OLECRANON BURSITIS

❓ *A wrestler was thrown down onto the mat and now has acute swelling about an inch in diameter on the proximal posterior ulna. What condition is present and how will you manage it?*

The olecranon bursa is the largest bursa in the elbow region. Injury may occur during a fall on a flexed elbow, by constantly leaning on one's elbow ("student's elbow"), by repetitive pressure and friction (as is common in wrestling), or by infections. The acutely inflamed bursa will present with rapid swelling, although it may be relatively painless (**Fig. 12.10**). The swelling may stem from bleeding or seepage of fluid into the bursal sac. Depending on the degree of acute inflammation, there may be heat and redness associated with the swelling. Acute management involves ice, rest, and a compressive wrap applied for the first 24 hours.

Occasionally, the bursa can become infected, regardless of acute trauma to the area. This may result from skin breakdown and a poor blood supply to the area. In this case, the area will be hot to the touch and inflamed. The individual will show traditional signs of infection, including **malaise**, fever, pain, restricted motion, tenderness, and swelling at the elbow. Refer this individual to a physician.

> Olecranon bursitis can occur with direct trauma, repetitive pressure and friction, or by infection

Malaise
Lethargic feeling of general discomfort; out-of-sorts feeling

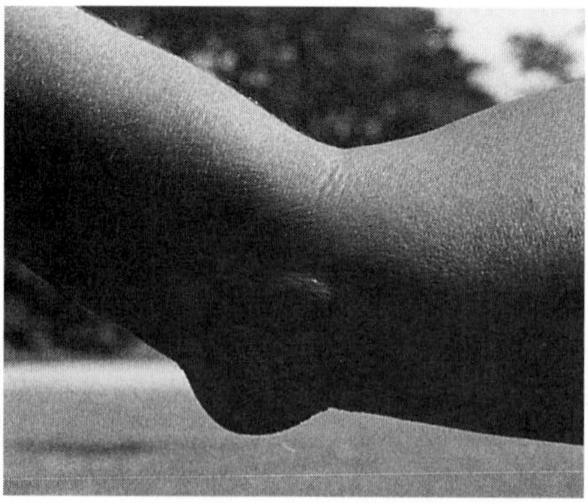

Figure 12.10. When the olecranon bursa ruptures, a discrete, sharply demarcated goose egg is visible directly over the olecranon process.

Did you determine that the wrestler had acute olecranon bursitis? Standard acute care should resolve the condition; however, additional padding can prevent recurrence.

SPRAINS AND DISLOCATIONS

After practice, a javelin thrower is complaining of acute pain on the medial aspect of the elbow. Palpation reveals point tenderness over the medial joint line, but only mild discomfort during active and passive movement. How can you determine if the ulnar collateral ligament is injured?

At the elbow, acute tears to ligamentous and joint structures are rare, but may occur during a fall on an extended hand, producing a hyperextension injury, or through a valgus/varus tensile force. More commonly, however, repetitive tensile forces irritate and tear the ligaments, particularly the ulnar collateral ligament. If the ulnar collateral ligament is damaged, the ulnar nerve may also be affected. A history of pain localized on the medial aspect of the elbow during the late cocking and acceleration phases of throwing is common. Examination will reveal point tenderness on the joint line, and increased pain and instability with the valgus stress test applied to the elbow at 15 to 20° flexion (see Assessment). Ice, compression, NSAIDs, and rest are followed by early range-of-motion exercises to stretch the forearm flexor–pronator group and the forearm extensors.

In adolescents, subluxation or dislocation of the proximal radial head is often associated with an immature annular ligament. Distraction with rotation, such as when a young child is swung by the arms, can cause the radial head to slip out of the supporting annular ligament. If an individual is unable to pronate and supinate the forearm without pain, refer them to a physician.

Most ulnar dislocations occur in individuals younger than 20, with a peak incidence in late adolescence (5). The mechanism of injury is usually hyperextension, or a sudden, violent, unidirectional valgus force that drives the ulna posterior or posterolateral (1). Immediately on impact, a snapping or cracking sensation is followed by severe pain, rapid swelling, total loss of function, and an obvious deformity **(Fig. 12.11)**. The ulnar collateral ligament is usually ruptured, and there may be an associated joint fracture. The arm is frequently held in flexion, with the forearm appearing shortened. The olecranon and radial head are palpable posteriorly and a slight indentation in the triceps is visible just proximal to the olecranon. Damage to the ulnar nerve may lead to numbness in the little finger. Immediate immobilization and transportation to the nearest medical facility is warranted, since early reduction minimizes muscle spasm. Management of an elbow dislocation is discussed in **Field Strategy 12.2**.

Dislocations of the elbow may result from hyperextension, or a sudden, violent, unidirectional valgus or varus blow, driving the ulna posterior or posterolateral

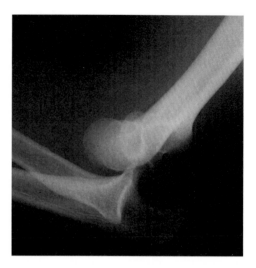

Figure 12.11. Posterior dislocations produce a snapping or cracking sensation, followed by immediate severe pain, rapid swelling, and total loss of function.

 During the assessment, a positive valgus stress test at 15 to 20° of elbow flexion can indicate a tear to the ulnar collateral ligament. Standard acute care is followed by early range-of-motion exercises to minimize disability.

Field Strategy 12.2. Management of a Posterior Elbow Dislocation

Signs and Symptoms

Snapping or cracking sensation
Immediate severe pain, rapid swelling, and total loss of function
An obvious deformity is present as the olecranon is pushed posteriorly, leaving the elbow slightly flexed
If there is an associated fracture, crepitation may be palpated

Management

This injury should be regarded as an emergency!
Immediately apply ice to limit pain and swelling
Assess the radial pulse, skin color, and blanching of the nails to determine possible circulatory impairment
Assess sensory function by stroking the palm and dorsum of the hand with a blunt and sharp object. Ask the individual if it is sharp or dull, and does it feel normal
Immobilize the elbow with a vacuum splint or other appropriate splint and treat for shock
Transport immediately to the nearest medical facility

STRAINS

A rower is complaining of vague anterior arm pain aggra-vated during the pull portion of the stroke. Palpation elicits point tenderness on the distal anterior arm. Pain increases with resisted elbow flexion and supination. What muscles may be in-volved here?

Muscular strains commonly result from inadequate warm-up, excessive training past the point of fatigue, and inadequate rehabil-itation of previous muscular injuries. Less commonly, they may occur as a result of a single massive contraction or sudden over-stretching.

Injury to the elbow flexors (brachialis, biceps brachii, and brach-ioradialis) will result in point tenderness on the anterior distal arm. Pain will increase with passive elbow extension and resisted elbow flexion. With a triceps strain, passive flexion and resisted elbow extension will produce discomfort. Strains to the common flexor/extensor group of the forearm muscles are usually self-limiting, requiring only modified rest, ice, compression, and activ-ity modification. Major tears or ruptures seldom occur. If so, the athlete will have considerable ecchymosis, a palpable defect, and limited, weak motion.

Treatment involves standard acute care with ice, compression, elevation, and protected rest. If a palpable defect is noted or an

> With triceps strains, passive flexion and resisted elbow extension will produce pain

Field Strategy 12.3. Management of Muscular Strains

Acute Management

Apply ice, compression, and elevation to control pain and inflammation
Use of NSAIDs, activity modification, biomechanical analysis of skill
  performance, or equipment modification may be helpful

Rehabilitation

Use cryotherapy prior to exercise
Restore range of motion at the elbow and shoulder region
Perform isometric exercises throughout a pain-free range of motion
Progress to surgical tubing or light hand-held weights, building from 1 to
  5 lbs throughout a pain-free range
Ice the injured muscle after each exercise session, followed by stretching
  exercises
Improve proprioception through closed kinetic chain exercises, such as
  shifting a weighted ball in the hand, push-ups, press-ups, or walking on
  the hands in a push-up position
During gradual return to functional activities, ensure adequate warm-up. If
  the individual is in a throwing activity, begin functional throwing with a
  light toss over a distance of 20 to 30 feet for 5 minutes, progressing to
  15 to 20 minutes. When the individual can throw for 15 to 20 minutes,
  gradually increase the distance to 150 feet. When proper throwing
  mechanics are present, gradually increase velocity

avulsion fracture is suspected, immobilization in a sling is followed by referral to a physician for possible surgical reattachment. Activity modification, NSAIDs, and a gradual active range-of-motion and strengthening exercise program with exercises, such as those listed in **Field Strategy 12.1**, should be initiated as tolerated. **Field Strategy 12.3** summarizes management of muscular strains.

💡 *The rower may have a strain to the biceps brachii or brachialis muscle that is aggravated during elbow flexion on the pull phase of the stroke. Ice, compression, and protected rest should be accompanied with stretching and strengthening exercises for the elbow flexors.*

OVERUSE CONDITIONS

❓ *A tennis player is complaining of pain on the lateral side of the elbow that is aggravated by ground strokes. Palpation reveals point tenderness just distal to the lateral epicondyle of the humerus and pain during active wrist extension and forearm supination. What condition might be present?*

The throwing mechanism discussed in Chapter 11 can also lead to overuse injuries at the elbow. During the initial acceleration phase, the body is brought rapidly forward, but the elbow and hand lag behind the upper arm. This results in a tremendous tensile valgus stress being placed on the medial aspect of the elbow, particularly the ulnar collateral ligament and adjacent tissues. As acceleration continues, the elbow extensors and wrist flexors contract to add velocity to the throw. This whipping action produces significant valgus stress on the medial elbow and concomitant lateral compressive stress in the radiocapitellar joint. At ball release, the elbow is almost fully extended and is positioned slightly anterior to the trunk. At release, the elbow is flexed approximately 20 to 30° (7). As these forces decrease, however, the extreme pronation of the forearm places the lateral ligaments under tension (6). During deceleration, eccentric contractions of the long head of the biceps brachii, supinator, and extensor muscles decelerate the forearm in pronation. Additional stress occurs on structures around the olecranon as pronation and extension jam the olecranon into its fossa. Impingement can occur as the olecranon is forced into the olecranon fossa.

Epicondylitis is a common chronic condition seen in activities involving pronation and supination, such as in tennis, javelin throwing, pitching, volleyball, or golf. Often the individual will reveal a pattern of poor technique, fatigue, and overuse.

Medial Epicondylitis

Valgus forces often produce a combined flexor–pronator muscle strain, ulnar collateral ligament sprain, and ulnar neuritis

Medial epicondylitis is caused by repeated medial tension/lateral compression (valgus) forces placed on the arm during the acceleration phase of the throwing motion **(Fig. 12.12)**. Valgus forces often produce a combined flexor muscle strain, ulnar collateral ligament sprain, and ulnar neuritis. If the medial humeral growth

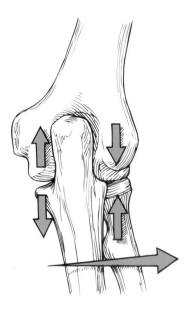

Figure 12.12. An excessive valgus force can lead to both medial tensile stress and lateral compression stress, causing injury to both sides of the joint.

plate is affected, it may be called "**little league elbow**"; however, use of this term negates the fact that other individuals, such as golfers, gymnasts, javelin throwers, tennis players, and wrestlers, are also susceptible to the condition. Simultaneously, lateral compressive forces can damage the lateral condyle of the humerus and radial head. Posterior stresses may lead to triceps strain, olecranon impingement, olecranon fractures, or loose bodies.

Assessment will reveal swelling, ecchymosis, and point tenderness directly over the humeroulnar joint, or on the medial epicondyle. Pain is usually severe and aggravated by resisted wrist flexion and pronation, and by a valgus stress applied at 15 to 20° of elbow flexion. If the ulnar nerve is involved, tingling and numbness may radiate into the forearm and hand, particularly the fourth and fifth fingers. Most conditions can be managed with ice, NSAIDs, and immobilization in a sling for 2 to 3 weeks. Activity should not resume until the individual can complete all functional tests pain-free. A functional brace may limit valgus stress and allow early resumption of strenuous activities. **Field Strategy 12.4** describes basic management of medial elbow pain.

Lateral Epicondylitis

Lateral epicondylitis is the most common overuse injury in the adult elbow. The condition is typically due to eccentric loading of the extensor muscles, predominantly the extensor carpi radialis brevis, during the deceleration phase of the throwing motion or tennis stroke (**Fig. 12.13**). Gripping a racquet too tightly, improper grip size, excessive string tension, excessive racquet weight or stiffness, faulty backhand technique, putting top spin on backhand strokes, or hitting the ball off-center all contribute to this condition (8).

Little league elbow
Tension stress injury of the medial epicondyle, seen in adolescents

Field Strategy 12.4. Management of Epicondylitis

Signs and Symptoms

Initially, pain or spasm will occur only during activity

Later, sharp pain will occur during the throwing motion (medial epicondylitis), or while picking up objects, such as a coffee cup or suitcase (lateral epicondylitis)

Swelling may limit elbow extension

Point tenderness will be over or just distal to the respective epicondyle of the humerus

Pain will increase with resisted wrist flexion or forearm pronation (medial epicondylitis), or resisted wrist extension and supination (lateral epicondylitis)

If the ulnar nerve is involved, numbness and tingling may radiate into the hand, particularly into the fourth and fifth fingers

Management

Ice, compression, elevation, NSAIDs, and rest can limit pain and inflammation

If a fracture of the medial epicondyle is suspected in an adolescent, refer the individual to a physician

Avoid strong gripping activities and painful activities, but allow the individual to perform those activities that do not irritate the region

Rehabilitation

Maintain range of motion and strength at the wrist and shoulder

Stretching exercises within pain-free motions should include elbow flexion/extension, wrist flexion/extension, forearm pronation/supination, and radial/ulnar deviation

Begin pain-free strengthening exercises with fast contractions, using light resistance. Add surgical tubing and tennis ball squeezes as tolerated. Work up to five sets of ten repetitions per session before moving on to heavier resistance

Incorporate early press-ups, wall push-ups, or walking on the hands

Continue to strengthen the shoulder, elbow, and wrist muscles

Do a biomechanical analysis of sport-specific skills to determine proper technique and make adjustments as necessary

After return to protected activity, continue stretching exercises before and after practice, ice after practice to control any inflammation, and return to full activity as tolerated

Pain will be anterior or just distal to the lateral epicondyle and may radiate into the forearm extensors during and after activity. Pain increases with resisted wrist extension, the "coffee cup" test (pain increases while picking up a full cup of coffee), and with the tennis elbow test (see Assessment). Initially ice, compression, NSAIDs, rest, and support will alleviate symptoms. Rehabilitation should focus on increasing the strength, endurance, and flexibility of the extensor muscle group. A counterforce strap placed 2 to 3 inches distal to the elbow joint can limit excessive muscular tension placed on the epicondyle, and is usually sufficient to eliminate symptoms (see Chapter 6). **Field Strategy 12.4** describes management of common extensor tendinitis.

Increased pain, with resisted wrist extension, a coffee cup test, and the tennis elbow test, indicates lateral epicondylitis

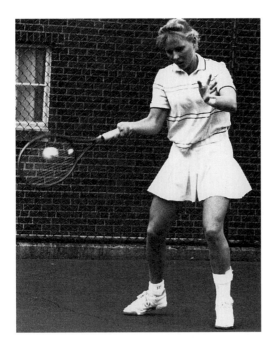

Figure 12.13. Eccentric loading of the elbow extensor muscles occurs with excessive forearm pronation and wrist flexion during the deceleration phase of a tennis stroke or a throwing motion.

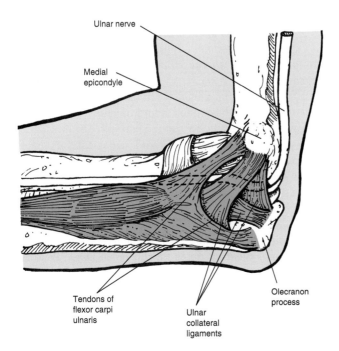

Ulnar nerve

Medial epicondyle

Tendons of flexor carpi ulnaris

Ulnar collateral ligaments

Olecranon process

Figure 12.14. As the ulnar nerve passes through the ulnar groove between the ulnar collateral ligament and the olecranon fossa, it passes under the two heads of the flexor carpi ulnaris. This tendon is slack during extension, but becomes taut during flexion, contributing to ulnar nerve compression.

Impingement of the Ulnar Nerve

The ulnar nerve passes behind the medial epicondyle of the humerus via the ulnar groove, through the cubital tunnel, and underneath the ulnar collateral ligament to enter the forearm (**Fig. 12.14**). Here the nerve is vulnerable to compression and tensile stress. The individual will complain of sharp pain along the medial aspect of the elbow, radiating as if they were "hitting their crazy bone." Palpation in the ulnar groove will generally reproduce symptoms that differentiate this injury from a strain or sprain. Tingling and numbness is typically felt in the ring and little finger. Because the ulnar nerve innervates several intrinsic muscles of the hand, grip strength may be weak. Treatment depends on the frequency, duration, intensity, and cause of the problem. If recognized early, complete rest and NSAIDs can help acute cases and, if the injury was secondary to direct blows, a pad can protect the area. In chronic nerve damage, surgery is usually required to release any pressure or constriction on the nerve.

> *The tennis player may have lateral epicondylitis due to the eccentric loading of the extensor muscles, predominantly the extensor carpi radialis brevis, during the deceleration phase of the tennis stroke. Standard acute care is followed by early range-of-motion and strengthening exercises.*

FRACTURES

> *A gymnast lost his grip on the horizontal bar and fell to the floor on a flexed elbow. Immediate pain and deformity is evident just proximal to the elbow. How will you immobilize this fracture?*

Stress fractures to the ulna and radius can occur during intensive weightlifting and have been found in young individuals who lift heavy weights or lose control of the barbells, resulting in added shear stress (10). In adolescents, a rapid, strong contraction of the flexor–pronator muscle group can lead to an avulsion fracture of the medial epicondyle of the humerus. Pain is severe, with point tenderness, swelling, and ecchymosis directly on the medial epicondyle.

The head of the radius may be fractured as a result of a valgus stress that tears the ulnar collateral ligament, leading to traumatic compressive and shearing stress on the radial head. Tenderness can be elicited on palpation of the radial head, and pronation and supination will be painful and restricted. Early range-of-motion exercises can prevent joint stiffness. Surgery, however, may be necessary if an angulated or displaced fracture if present.

Displaced and undisplaced fractures to the humerus, radius, and ulna usually result from violent compressive forces from direct trauma, such as impact with a helmet or implement, a fall on a flexed elbow or outstretched hand, with or without a valgus/varus stress, or tensile forces associated with throwing. Supracondylar fractures, in particular, account for two-thirds of all elbow fractures

Entrapment of the ulnar nerve may lead to a sharp pain radiating down the medial aspect of the forearm, as if you had "hit your crazy bone"

With a fracture of the radial head, pronation and supination will be very painful and limited

occurring in children, and are seen frequently in children involved in sports activities. The most common complication of elbow fractures is decreased range of motion or stiffness, often manifested by loss of terminal extension (11). A catastrophic complication from a fracture is ischemic necrosis of the forearm muscles, known as **Volkmann's contracture**. The brachial artery or median nerve can be damaged by the fractured bone ends, leading to major circulatory or neural impairment to the forearm and hand. As a result, the hand is cold, white, and numb. Passive extension of the fingers leads to severe pain. These symptoms indicate a serious problem.

Fractures should be suspected in all elbow and forearm injuries, particularly in adolescents. Methods to determine a possible fracture are explained in **Field Strategy 12.6** within the Assessment section. In addition, a neurologic and circulatory assessment should be conducted. If a nerve is damaged, muscle weakness and sensory changes will occur in the hand. Pulses can be taken at the wrist at the ulnar and radial arteries, or blanch the fingernails and note capillary refill. A suspected fracture should be immobilized in a vacuum splint, and the individual referred to a physician immediately.

💡 *You suspect a fracture just proximal to the elbow. Immobilize the arm in a vacuum splint and take a pulse at the radial and ulnar artery, check capillary refill at the fingernails, and check bilateral sensation on the palm and dorsum of the hand to rule out any neurovascular damage.*

Volkmann's contracture
Ischemic necrosis of the forearm muscles and tissues, caused by damage to the blood flow

Any fracture to the humerus, ulna, or radius should involve a full neurologic and circulatory assessment

ASSESSMENT OF THE ELBOW

❓ *One week ago a football player landed on an outstretched hand. Although he didn't think it was too serious to discuss the injury with you, he is now complaining of sharp pain when he fully extends his elbow. How will you conduct the evaluation?*

The elbow's primary role is to position the forearm and hand in the most appropriate position to perform efficient motion. If the individual uses any equipment, such as a bat, racquet, or field hockey or lacrosse stick, check for proper grip size, excessive string tension, and excessive weight or stiffness, and assess skill technique to rule out possible contributing factors. During the evaluation, keep in mind that pain may be referred from the cervical region, shoulder, or wrist. As in any assessment, both elbows should be fully visible to allow for bilateral comparison.

HISTORY

❓ *What questions need to be asked to determine the athlete's primary complaint? Could age, gender, or the sport-specific skills be a factor in this injury?*

To gather information about the primary complaint, ask questions that focus on the individual's perception of pain, weakness, or sensory changes. When was the problem first noticed? Is the injury acute or chronic? Ask specific questions related to equipment, technique, recent changes in training intensity, frequency, or duration. Is there any noticeable locking, catching, or general muscle weakness? Are there specific actions that aggravate the condition, such as throwing? In addition to the general questions discussed in Chapter 4, specific questions to ask in an elbow evaluation are listed in **Field Strategy 12.5**.

 The 16-year-old lineman has fallen several times on an outstretched hand, but this is the first time it has really bothered him. Flexion is somewhat restricted, but not too painful. Full extension, however, is limited and very painful.

OBSERVATION AND INSPECTION

What specific factors should be observed during the assessment? Would it be advantageous to also assess the shoulder and wrist?

Both arms should be clearly visible for bilateral comparison. With an acute injury, it is critical early in the assessment to recognize possible fractures and dislocations. If the individual is in great pain, unable or unwilling to move the elbow, complete the assessment in a position most comfortable for the individual. First observe the position of the arm. Is there a noticeable deformity? How is the individual holding the arm? If swelling is present in the joint, the individual may be unable to fully extend the elbow, resulting in a slightly flexed position. This **resting position** allows

Resting position
Slightly flexed position of a joint that allows for maximal volume to accommodate any intra-articular swelling

---

Field Strategy 12.5. Developing a History of the Injury

Current Injury Status

1. How did the injury occur (mechanism)? If acute, what was the direction of the force?
2. Ask about the pain location, severity, onset (sudden or gradual), and type (sharp, aching, burning, radiating). Did you hear any sounds during the incident, such as a snap, pop, or crack?
3. Was there any swelling, discoloration, muscle spasms, or numbness with the injury?
4. What actions or motions replicate the pain? Do they use a racquet, bat, or stick in their sport? In what part of the arm motion does it hurt the worst?
5. Are there certain activities you cannot perform because of the pain? How old are you? (Remember that apophyseal injuries and dislocations of the radial head are seen in young children; chronic muscle strains related to tennis elbow are seen in older individuals.)

Past Injury Status

1. Have you ever injured your elbow or shoulder before? When? How did that occur? What was done for the injury?
2. Have you had any medical problems recently? (You are looking for possible referred pain from the cervical neck, shoulder, or wrist.)

the joint to have maximal volume to accommodate intra-articular swelling. Any positive sign that indicates a possible fracture should be treated accordingly. When no possible fracture or dislocation is present, inspect the region for symmetry, any abnormal deformity, muscle atrophy, hypertrophy, swelling, discoloration, or previous surgical incisions.

💡 *No visible deformities, muscle atrophy, hypertrophy, or discoloration is apparent on the injured arm. Joint effusion and swelling, however, are visible on the medial and posteromedial humerus.*

PALPATIONS

❓ *The individual reported pain and limitation in motion during extension, and swelling was visible on the medial and posteromedial aspect of the humerus. Where will you begin palpations so that the discomfort is not compounded?*

Bilateral palpations should determine temperature, swelling, point tenderness, crepitus, deformity, muscle spasm, and cutaneous sensation. Vascular pulses can be taken at the radial and ulnar arteries at the wrist **(Fig. 12.15)**. Begin palpations proximal to distal, leaving the most painful areas to last. Support the injured arm during palpations and compare bilaterally. To determine a possible fracture, refer to **Field Strategy 12.6**.

Bony Palpations

1. Medial and lateral supracondylar ridges of the humerus
2. Medial and lateral epicondyles of the humerus
3. Head of the radius and annular ligament. This is facilitated by supination and pronation of the forearm

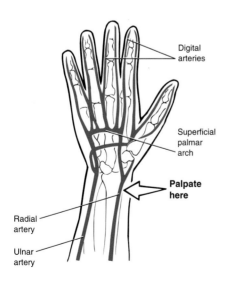

Figure 12.15. A pulse may be taken at the radial artery on the wrist.

Field Strategy 12.6. Determining a Possible Fracture in the Upper Arm and Forearm

A. Compression. Palpate the region for pain, deformity, crepitus, or loose bodies. Ask the individual if they heard any cracking sounds that might indicate a possible fracture. Apply gentle compression along the long axis of the bone, then encircle the distal ulna and radius with your hand and give mild compression. This produces distraction at the proximal ulna and radius. Increased pain indicates a possible fracture

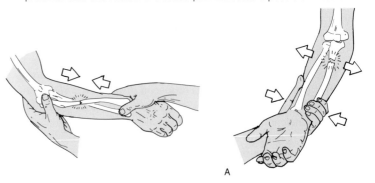

A

B. Distraction. Slowly distract the bones. If pain is eased, this may indicate a possible fracture. If pain increases, it indicates soft tissue damage

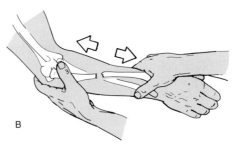

B

C. Percussion. Gently tap the superficial bony landmarks. Vibrations will travel along the bone and cause increased pain at the fracture site. For example, tap the following sites:

    Humerus—medial and lateral epicondyles
    Ulna—olecronan process and distal styloid process
    Radius—distal styloid process

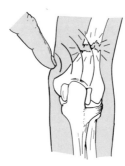

C

D. Vibrations. Tap a tuning fork and place the base on the superficial bone sites mentioned above. Increased pain indicates a possible fracture

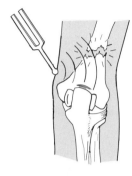

D

If a fracture is suspected, immobilize the limb in a vacuum splint or other appropriate splint or sling, and transport the individual to the nearest trauma center

---

4. Olecranon process, olecranon fossa, and ulna. This is facilitated with the elbow flexed at 45° to relax the triceps

Soft Tissue Palpations

1. Common wrist flexor–pronator tendons and muscles
2. Ulnar (medial) collateral ligament
3. Ulnar nerve in the ulnar groove
4. Common wrist extensors and brachioradialis muscle
5. Radial (lateral) collateral ligament
6. Biceps brachii and brachialis muscles
7. Biceps brachii tendon and brachial artery in cubital fossa
8. Triceps muscle and olecranon bursa. Grasp the skin overlying the olecranon process and note any thickening

💡 *Sharp pain was elicited on the lateral border of the olecranon process and on the corresponding ridge of the olecranon fossa. Palpation over the medial joint line also produced mild pain.*

SPECIAL TESTS

❓ *Swelling and sharp pain appear to be centered on the postero-lateral aspect of the olecranon process and olecranon fossa. Furthermore, it appears the medial collateral ligament may also be involved. How will you proceed to confirm your suspicions about the extent of this injury?*

If a fracture or dislocation is suspected, do not attempt any special tests. Immobilize the arm in an appropriate splint and refer the individual to a physician. For other injuries, do only those tests necessary to assess the current injury.

Joint Range of Motion

As with previous assessments, bilateral comparison with the uninvolved arm should always be completed. In addition, painful active movements should be performed last to prevent painful symptoms from overflowing into the next movement. The following movements should be assessed:

1. Flexion and extension at the elbow
2. Supination and pronation of the forearm
3. Flexion and extension of the wrist

During elbow extension, remember that some females can extend as much as 5 to 15° below the straight line. Bilateral comparison will verify if this extra motion is normal for this individual. In performing active pronation and supination, instruct the individual to flex the elbow to 90° and secure the elbow next to the body to avoid any glenohumeral motion. The individual can hold a pencil in the closed fist and perform both motions in a continuous pattern.

Resisted Manual Muscle Testing

Stabilize the individual's elbow against the body. Begin with the muscle on stretch and apply resistance proximal to the wrist throughout the full range of motion. Instruct the individual to keep the thumb and fingers relaxed, and do bilateral comparison with the uninvolved side. As always, painful motions should be delayed until last. **Figure 12.16** demonstrates motions that should be tested and includes those listed above with active range of motion.

Neurologic Testing

At the elbow and forearm, test the biceps, brachioradialis, and triceps reflexes

Neurologic integrity can be assessed with manual muscle testing (already completed), reflexes, and cutaneous sensation. Reflexes in the upper extremity include the biceps (C_5 to C_6), brachioradialis (C_6), and triceps (C_7), and were demonstrated in Chapter 11. Cutaneous sensation can be assessed bilaterally by determining altered sensation through sharp and dull touch. Run the open hand and fingernails over the neck, shoulder, anterior, and posterior chest walls, and down both sides of the arms and hands. Ask the individual if they can feel it, and does it feel the same on both sides?

Stress and Functional Tests

Stress tests are performed when you have a clear indication of what structures may be damaged. Use only those tests deemed relevant and always compare the results to the uninvolved arm.

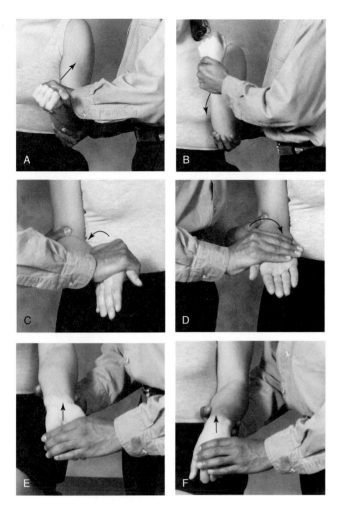

Figure 12.16. Resisted manual muscle testing for the elbow. **A.** Elbow flexion. **B.** Elbow extension. **C.** Forearm supination. **D.** Forearm pronation. **E.** Wrist flexion. **F.** Wrist extension. Arrows indicate the direction the athlete moves the body segment against applied resistance.

Ligamentous Instability Tests

With the individual seated, stabilize the arm and apply a valgus force to the distal forearm to stress the ulnar collateral ligament **(Fig. 12.17A)**. A varus force is then applied at the forearm to stress the radial collateral ligament **(Fig. 12.17B)**. Perform these tests at full extension, and again at 20 to 30° of flexion, to "unlock" the joint and isolate the ligamentous structures. Note any pain or joint laxity.

> Perform ligament instability tests at multiple angles, from full extension to 20 to 30° of flexion, to "unlock" the joint and isolate the ligamentous structures

Tennis Elbow Test for Lateral Epicondylitis

Stabilize the individual's flexed elbow and palpate the lateral epicondyle. Have the individual make a fist and pronate the forearm.

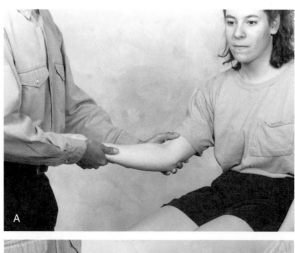

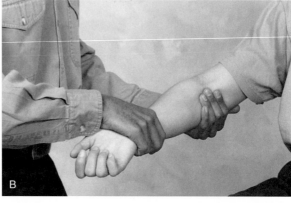

Figure 12.17. Ligamentous instability tests. **A.** To stress the ulnar collateral ligament, apply a valgus force at multiple angles. **B.** To stress the radial collateral ligament, apply a varus force at multiple angles.

Ask them to radially deviate and extend the wrist while you resist the motion (**Fig. 12.18A**). A positive sign is indicated if severe pain is present over the lateral epicondyle of the humerus. The same results can be elicited by stretching the wrist extensor muscles by slowly pronating the forearm, flexing the wrist, and extending the elbow simultaneously (**Fig. 12.18B**).

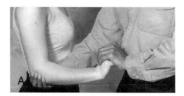 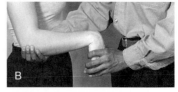

Figure 12.18. Tests for lateral epicondylitis. **A.** Resisted extension and radial deviation of the wrist. **B.** Passive stretching of the wrist extensors.

Medial Epicondylitis Test

Stabilize the flexed elbow and palpate the medial epicondyle. Supinate the forearm and extend the wrist. Have the individual perform pronation and wrist flexion against resistance. A positive sign is indicated by pain over the medial epicondyle of the humerus.

Tinel's Sign for Ulnar Neuritis

The ulnar groove is tapped on the posteromedial side of the elbow. The test is positive if a tingling sensation travels down the ulnar aspect of the forearm into the fourth and fifth finger (**Fig. 12.19**).

Functional Tests

Remember that the elbow is in the middle of the upper extremity kinetic chain. Therefore, it must function properly to position the hand so that daily activities can be performed smoothly and efficiently. Activities such as combing the hair, throwing a ball, lifting an object, or pushing an object should be performed pain-free. Ask the individual to perform those skills needed to complete their daily living activities and to perform skills specific to their sport. Each movement should be pain-free and fluid.

Active elbow flexion is limited by about 10°, which may be due to intra-articular swelling. Passive terminal extension was painful, but all other motions are within normal limits. Valgus stress produced only mild pain and laxity, so the ulnar collateral ligament has been involved. The major complaint, however, of sharp pain on the olecranon process and in the olecranon fossa dictates referral to a physician for radiographs to rule out a possible fracture.

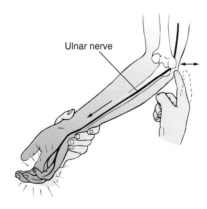

Figure 12.19. Tapping over the ulnar groove will produce a tingling sensation down the ulnar nerve into the forearm and hand. A positive Tinel's sign indicates ulnar nerve entrapment.

? *The football player was seen by the physician. Although no fracture was present, the elbow was immobilized in a sling until the pain subsided. The sling has been removed and you have been instructed to develop a rehabilitation program for the elbow to regain range of motion and strength in the extremity. What exercises should be included in this program?*

Although traumatic injuries to the elbow often require immobilization, early range-of-motion and strengthening exercises can be conducted at the wrist, hand, and shoulder. In overuse injuries in which immobilization is usually not present, pain may be exacerbated by certain motions. The exercise program should focus on early mobilization in the available pain-free motions, and expand to the other motions once pain has subsided. Individuals who are involved in throwing-like activities should also be sure to include scapular stabilization exercises, along with strengthening exercises for the shoulder. The reader should refer to Chapter 11 for appropriate shoulder exercises. Hand and finger exercises are discussed in Chapter 13.

Range-of-motion exercises at the elbow should include elbow flexion and extension, forearm pronation and supination, wrist flexion and extension, and wrist radial and ulnar deviation. The individual can use the opposite hand to apply a low-load, prolonged stretch in the various motions to minimize joint trauma and increase flexibility **(Fig. 12.20)**.

Closed-chain exercises may be performed by shifting body weight from one hand to the other on a wall, table top, or unstable surface, such as a foam mat or BAPS board. Push-ups and exercises in a frontal and sagittal plane can be performed on a ProFitter or slide board, if available. Step-ups can be completed on a box, stool, or Stair Master. As with the shoulder injury, the throwing motion should be rehearsed through the use of mirrors or video-

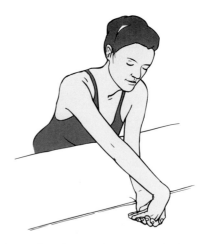

Figure 12.20. Range-of-motion exercises can be facilitated by using the opposite hand to apply a sustained stretch.

tape. As the motion is performed, biomechanical errors at the elbow are corrected. When motion is perfected, speed of movement and distance of throw are gradually increased.

Gentle resisted exercises with surgical tubing or hand-held weights can begin immediately after the initial pain and swelling have subsided. Many of these exercises were shown in **Field Strategy 12.1**. As the individual improves, a more moderate overload is applied. The individual should complete 30 to 50 repetitions with a one-pound weight, and should not progress in resistance until 50 repetitions are achieved. Plyometric exercises may involve catching a weighted ball and utilizing a quick, eccentric stretch of the muscle to facilitate a concentric contraction in throwing the ball. The exercise can progress through various one- and two-arm chest passes and overhead passes. A mini-tramp may also be used to do plyometric bounding push-ups.

General body conditioning should be maintained throughout the rehabilitation program. Several programs were explained in **Field Strategy 5.9**, and included use of a jump rope, Stair Master, treadmill, and upper body ergometer (UBE).

The athlete should focus on restoration of motion in elbow flexion/extension, forearm pronation/supination, wrist flexion/extension, and radial/ulnar deviation. Gentle resisted strengthening exercises should begin immediately after pain and swelling are under control. The program should also include general body conditioning and strengthening exercises for the shoulder and wrist.

SUMMARY

The elbow is constantly subjected to various forces and stresses during normal daily activity. In sports, excessive force can lead to contusions, joint sprains, muscle strains, fractures, or neurovascular impairment. Although attention is often focused on acute injuries, this joint is very susceptible to overuse conditions. Often these injuries result from inadequate warm-up, excessive training past the point of fatigue, inadequate rehabilitation of previous injuries, or neglect of seemingly minor conditions that progress to major complications. Because the elbow works with the shoulder and wrist to provide complex patterns of motion, an injury to one structure can affect other joints. **Field Strategy 12.7** demonstrates a basic assessment of the upper arm, elbow, and forearm.

Keep in mind during the assessment that pain may be referred from other areas of the body, particularly the cervical neck, shoulder, and wrist. With a significant finding, refer the individual to a physician for further evaluation. Examples of these conditions might include: obvious deformity, suggesting a dislocation or fracture; significant loss of motion or unexplained muscle weakness; excessive joint swelling; possible epiphyseal or apophyseal injuries; gross joint instability; abnormal or absent reflexes; abnormal cutaneous sensation; absent or weak pulse; or any unexplained pain.

Field Strategy 12.7. Elbow Evaluation

History

Primary complaint and mechanism of injury
Onset of symptoms, including pain and discomfort
Disability and functional impairments from the injury
Previous injuries to the area, and family history

Observation and Inspection

Observe general posture
Inspect:

Muscle symmetry	Hypertrophy or muscle atrophy
Swelling	Visible congenital deformity
Discoloration	Surgical incisions or scars

Palpation

Bony structures, to determine possible fracture
Soft tissue structures, to determine:

Temperature	Deformity
Swelling	Muscle spasm
Point tenderness	Cutaneous sensation
Crepitus	Vascular pulses

Special Tests

Joint range of motion with gross motor movement
Resisted manual muscle testing
Neurologic testing
Stress and functional tests
  Ligamentous instability tests
  Tennis elbow test for lateral epicondylitis
  Medial epicondylitis test
  Tinel's signs for ulnar neuritis
  Functional tests

Should a decision be made to refer an individual to a physician for care, immobilize the limb in a comfortable position. This may be accomplished by wrapping the arm to the body, or using a sling and swathe, posterior splint, vacuum splint, or a commercial product that can pad and protect the area. Apply cryotherapy to control inflammation and swelling, and transport the individual in an appropriate manner. Follow up with the physician to obtain instructions for further care of the injury. When appropriate, protective braces or padding should be worn to prevent reinjury.

REFERENCES

1. Sobel J, and Nirschl RP. Elbow injuries. In *Athletic injuries and rehabilitation*, edited by AE Zachazewski, DJ Magee, and WS Quillen. Philadelphia: WB Saunders, 1996.
2. Stanitski CL. 1993. Combating overuse injuries: a focus on children and adolescents. Phys Sportsmed 21(1):87–106.

3. Rettig AC, and Patel DV. Epidemiology of elbow, forearm, and wrist injuries in the athlete. In *Clinics in sports medicine*, edited by KD Plancher, vol. 14, no. 2. Philadelphia: WB Saunders, 1995.

4. De Carlo MS, Carrell KR, Misamore GW, and Sell KE. 1992. Rehabilitation of myositis ossificans in the brachialis muscle. J Ath Train 27(1):76–79.

5. Hoffman DF. 1993. Elbow dislocations: avoiding complications. Phys Sportsmed 21(11):56–67.

6. Ireland ML, and Hutchinson MR. Upper extremity injuries in young athletes. In *Clinics in sports medicine*, edited by LJ Micheli, vol. 14, no. 3. Philadelphia: WB Saunders, 1995.

7. Fleisig GS, Escamilla RF, and Andrews JR. Biomechanics of throwing. In *Athletic injuries and rehabilitation*, edited by AE Zachazewski, DJ Magee, and WS Quillen. Philadelphia: WB Saunders, 1996.

8. Garrick JG, and Webb DR. *Sports injuries: diagnosis and management*. Philadelphia: WB Saunders, 1990.

9. Johnston J, Plancher KD, and Hawkins RJ. Elbow injuries to the throwing athlete. In *Clinics in sports medicine*, edited by KD Plancher, vol. 15, no. 2. Philadelphia: WB Saunders, 1996.

10. Weber J. Gymnastics. In *The team physician's handbook*, edited by MB Mellion, WM Walsh, and GL Shelton. Philadelphia: Hanley & Belfus, 1990.

11. Griggs SM, and Weiss AC. Bony injuries of the wrist, forearm, and elbow. In *Clinics in sports medicine*, edited by KD Plancher, vol. 15, no. 2. Philadelphia: WB Saunders, 1996.

Wrist and Hand Injuries

After completing this chapter, you should be able to:

- Locate the important bony and soft tissue structures of the wrist and hand

- Describe the motions of the wrist and hand and identify the muscles that produce them

- Describe measures that can be taken to prevent injuries at the wrist and hand

- Recognize and manage specific injuries to the wrist and hand

- Demonstrate a basic assessment of the wrist and hand

- Demonstrate general rehabilitation exercises for the wrist and hand

Key Terms:

Anatomical snuff box	**Ganglion cyst**
Aseptic necrosis	**Hypothenar**
Bennett's fracture	**Intrinsic muscles**
Boutonniere deformity	**Jersey finger**
Brachial plexus	**Mallet finger**
Carpal tunnel syndrome	**Paronychia**
Circumduction	**Saddle joint**
Colles fracture	**Smith fracture**
Cyclist's palsy	**Stenosing**
de Quervain's tenosynovitis	**Subungual hematoma**
Dorsal	**Thenar**
Extrinsic muscles	**Volar**
Gamekeeper's thumb	

The wrist and hand are used extensively in activities of daily living and in nearly all sport skills. Injuries to the region often result from the natural tendency to sustain the force of a fall on the hyperextended wrist **(Fig. 13.1)**. Pubescent and adolescent athletes have a higher incidence of hand and wrist injuries than adult athletes (1). Many of these injuries are directly related to specific sports. For example, in wrestling, football, hockey, and skiing, forced abduction of the thumb can damage the ulnar collateral ligament of the thumb, leading to an injury called a gamekeeper's thumb. Receivers in football, basketball players, pitchers, and

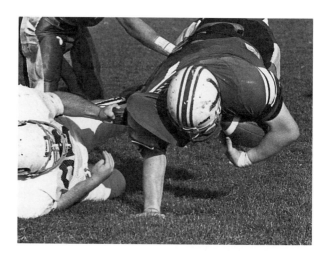

Figure 13.1. Falling on a hyperextended wrist can result in serious injuries to the wrist and hand.

catchers are subject to a "mallet" deformity of the finger caused when a ball hits the end of the finger and avulses an extensor tendon from its distal attachment.

This chapter will begin with a review of the anatomy and major muscle actions of the wrist and hand. Discussion on prevention of injury will be followed by information on common injuries to the wrist and hand and their management. Finally, assessment techniques and rehabilitation exercises are presented.

ANATOMY REVIEW OF THE WRIST AND HAND

? *A basketball player was accidentally struck on the end of the finger by the ball, and now has pain and swelling at the proximal interphalangeal joint of the middle finger. What anatomical structure(s) are likely to have been injured?*

The wrist and hand are composed of numerous small bones and articulations. These function effectively to enable the dexterous movements performed by the hands during both daily living and sport activities.

Bones and Articulations of the Wrist and Hand

The wrist consists of a series of radiocarpal and intercarpal articulations (**Fig. 13.2**). Most wrist motion, however, occurs at the radiocarpal joint, a condyloid joint where the radius articulates with the scaphoid, lunate, and triquetrum. The joint allows sagittal plane motions (flexion, extension, and hyperextension) and frontal plane motions (radial deviation and ulnar deviation), as well as circumduction.

The distal radioulnar joint is immediately adjacent to the radiocarpal joint. A cartilaginous disk separates the distal ulna and radius from the lunate and triquetral bones. Although the two

> The radiocarpal joint is the major joint of the wrist

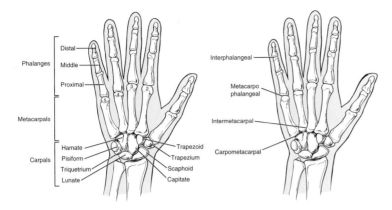

Figure 13.2. The bones and joints of the wrist and hand.

joints share the articular disk, they have separate joint capsules. The **volar** radiocarpal, **dorsal** radiocarpal, radial collateral, and ulnar collateral ligaments reinforce the radiocarpal joint capsule.

A large number of joints are required to provide the extensive motion capabilities of the hand. Included are the carpometacarpal (CM), intermetacarpal (IM), metacarpophalangeal (MP), and interphalangeal (IP) joints **(Fig. 13.2)**. The fingers are numbered digits one through five, with the first digit being the thumb.

The CM joint of the thumb is a classic **saddle joint**. The CM joints of the four fingers are essentially gliding joints. The CM and IM joints of the fingers are mutually surrounded by joint capsules that are reinforced by the dorsal, volar, and interosseous CM ligaments.

The knuckles of the hand are formed by the MP joints. These are condyloid joints, each enclosed in a capsule that is reinforced by strong collateral ligaments.

The proximal interphalangeal (PIP) and distal interphalangeal (DIP) joints of the fingers, and the single IP joint of the thumb, are all hinge joints. An articular capsule joined by volar and collateral ligaments surrounds each IP joint.

Muscles of the Wrist and Hand

Given the numerous highly controlled precision movements that the hand and fingers are capable of doing, it is no surprise that a relatively large number of muscles are responsible. There are nine **extrinsic muscles** that cross the wrist and ten **intrinsic muscles** that have both of their attachments distal to the wrist. The muscles of the wrist and hand are shown in **Figures 13.3** and **13.4**, and their locations and actions are summarized in **Table 13.1**.

Nerves and Blood Vessels of the Wrist and Hand

The median, ulnar, and radial nerves are major terminal branches of the **brachial plexus** that provide motor and sensory innervation

Volar
Referring to the palm of the hand

Dorsal
Referring to the back of the hand

Saddle joint
Joint at which one bone surface has a convex, saddle-like shape, and the articulating bone surface is reciprocally shaped

The interphalangeal joints are stabilized by volar and collateral ligaments

Extrinsic muscles
Muscles with attachments located both proximal and distal to the wrist

Intrinsic muscles
Muscles with attachments located distal to the wrist

Brachial plexus
Large mass of interwoven spinal nerves (C_5 to T_1) that innervate the upper extremity

Table 13.1. Major Muscles of the Hand and Fingers

Muscle	Proximal Attachment	Distal Attachment	Primary Action(s)	Nerve Innervation
Extrinsic Muscles				
Extensor pollicis longus	Middle dorsal ulna	Dorsal distal phalanx of thumb	Extension at MP & IP joints of thumb	Radial
Extensor pollicis brevis	Middle dorsal radius	Dorsal proximal phalanx of thumb	Extension at MP & CM joints of thumb	Radial
Flexor pollicis longus	Middle palmar radius	Palmar distal phalanx of thumb	Flexion at IP & MP joints of thumb	Median
Abductor pollicis longus	Middle dorsal ulna and radius	Radial base of 1st metacarpal	Abduction at CM joint of thumb	Radial
Extensor indicis	Distal dorsal ulna	Ulnar side of the extensor digitorum tendon	Extension at MP joint of 2nd digit	Radial
Extensor digitorum	Lateral epicondyle of humerus	Base of 2nd & 3rd phalanges, digits 2–5	Extension at MP, proximal & distal IP joints, digits 2–5	Radial
Extensor digiti minimi	Proximal tendon of extensor digitorum	Tendon of extensor digitorum distal to 5th MP joint	Extension at 5th MP joint	Radial
Flexor digitorum profundus	Proximal 3/4 ulna	Base of distal phalanx, digits 2–5	Flexion at distal & proximal IP joints and MP joints, digits 2–5	Ulnar & median
Flexor digitorum superficialis	Medial epicondyle of humerus	Base of middle phalanx, digits 2–5	Flexion at proximal IP and MP joints, digits 2–5	Median
Intrinsic Muscles				
Flexor pollicis brevis	Ulnar side, 1st metacarpal	Ulnar, palmar base of proximal phalanx of the thumb	Flexion at MP joint of the thumb	Median
Abductor pollicis brevis	Scaphoid & trapezium bones	Radial base of 1st phalanx of thumb	Abduction at 1st CM joint	Median
Opponens pollicis	Scaphoid bone	Radial side 1st metacarpal	Opposition at CM joint of the thumb	Median
Adductor pollicis	Capitate, distal 2nd & 3rd metacarpals	Ulnar proximal phalanx of thumb	Adduction & flexion at CM joint of thumb	Ulnar
Abductor digiti minimi	Pisiform bone	Ulnar base of proximal phalanx, 5th digit	Abduction & flexion at 5th MP joint	Ulnar
Flexor digiti minimi brevis	Hamate bone	Ulnar base of proximal phalanx, 5th digit	Flexion at 5th MP joint	Ulnar
Opponens digiti minimi	Hamate bone	Ulnar metacarpal of 5th metacarpal	Opposition at 5th CM joint	Ulnar
Dorsal interossei (four muscles)	Sides of metacarpals, all digits	Base of proximal phalanx, all digits	Abduction at 2nd & 4th MP joints, radial & ulnar deviation of 3rd MP joint, flexion of MP joints 2–4	Ulnar
Palmar interossei (three muscles)	2nd, 4th, & 5th metacarpals	Base of proximal phalanx, digits 2, 4, & 5	Adduction & flexion at MP joints, digits 2, 4, & 5	Ulnar
Lumbricales (four muscles)	Tendons of flexor digitorum profundus, digits 2–5	Tendons of extensor digitorum, digits 2–5	Flexion at MP joints of digits 2–5	Median & ulnar

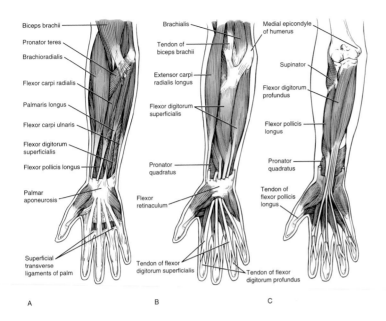

Figure 13.3. A–C. The anterior muscles of the wrist and hand.

to the wrist and hand (**Fig. 13.5**). The median nerve supplies the majority of the flexor muscles of the wrist and hand, the intrinsic flexor muscles on the radial side of the palm, and cutaneous sensation to the skin on the lateral two-thirds of the palm of the hand and the dorsum of the second and third fingers. The ulnar nerve innervates the flexor carpi ulnaris and the ulnar portion of the flexor digitorum profundus, along with most of the intrinsic muscles of the hand. It also provides cutaneous sensation to the fifth and half of the fourth finger on both dorsal and palmar sides. The radial nerve innervates most of the extensor muscles of the forearm, and provides cutaneous sensation to the skin on the dorsum of the hand. Specific nerve–muscle associations are presented in **Table 13.1**.

The major vessels supplying the muscles of the wrist and hand are the radial and ulnar arteries (**Fig. 13.6**). The radial artery supplies the muscles on the radial side of the forearm, as well as the thumb and index finger. The ulnar artery divides into anterior and posterior interosseous arteries to supply the deep flexor muscles and extensor muscles of the forearm, respectively. In the palm, the radial and ulnar arteries merge to form the superficial and deep palmar arches. Digital arteries branch from the palmar arches to supply the fingers. The radial artery is superficial on the anterior aspect of the wrist, where the pulse is readily palpable.

Retinacula of the Wrist

The fascial tissue surrounding the wrist is thickened into strong fibrous bands called retinacula that form protective passageways

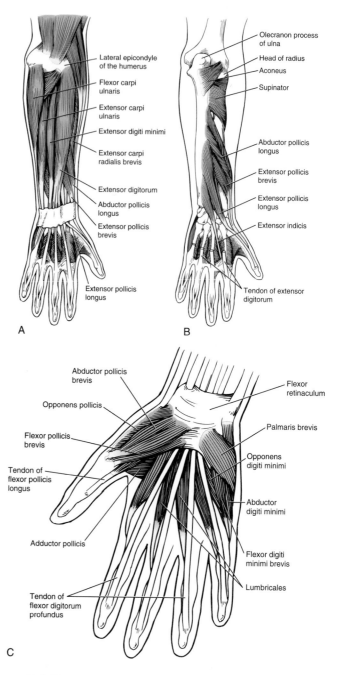

Figure 13.4. The posterior muscles of the wrist and hand, **A** and **B**. Intrinsic muscles of the palm, **C**.

through which tendons, nerves, and blood vessels pass. On the palmar side of the wrist, the flexor retinaculum protects the extrinsic flexor tendons and the median nerve. On the dorsal side of the wrist, the extensor retinaculum provides a passageway for the extrinsic extensor tendons.

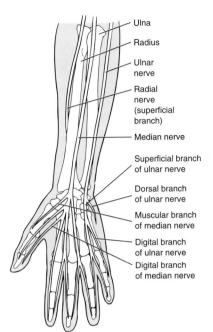

Figure 13.5. The nerve supply to the wrist and hand.

Did you determine what structures may have been damaged on the basketball player's finger? If you concluded possible damage to the bones, joint capsule, collateral ligaments, or the volar plate, you are correct.

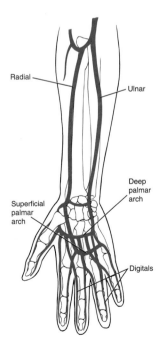

Figure 13.6. The blood supply to the wrist and hand.

The radial pulse should be palpated with the fingers rather than the thumb, because a pulse can sometimes be felt in the examiner's thumb

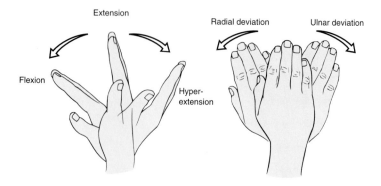

Figure 13.7. Directional movement capabilities at the wrist.

MAJOR MUSCLE ACTIONS OF THE WRIST AND HAND

? *Why is the range of motion permitted by the CM joint of the thumb so much greater than the ranges of motion allowed at the CM joints of the second through fifth digits?*

The wrist is capable of sagittal and frontal plane movements, as well as rotary motion (**Fig. 13.7**). Flexion occurs when the palmar surface of the hand is moved toward the anterior forearm. Extension involves the return of the hand to anatomical position from a position of flexion, and hyperextension occurs when the dorsal surface of the hand is brought toward the posterior forearm. Movement of the hand toward the radial side of the arm is radial deviation, with movement in the opposite direction known as ulnar deviation. Rotational movement of the hand through all four directions is termed **circumduction**.

Circumduction
Circular motion of a body segment resulting from sequential flexion, abduction, extension, and adduction, or vice versa

Flexion

The major flexor muscles of the wrist are the flexor carpi radialis and flexor carpi ulnaris (**Fig. 13.3**). The palmaris longus, which is often absent in one or both forearms, contributes to flexion when present. The flexor digitorum superficialis and flexor digitorum profundus assist with flexion at the wrist when the fingers are completely extended, but when the fingers are in flexion these muscles cannot develop sufficient tension to assist.

Extension and Hyperextension

Extensor carpi radialis longus, extensor carpi radialis brevis, and extensor carpi ulnaris produce extension and hyperextension at the wrist (**Fig. 13.4**). The other posterior wrist muscles may also assist with extension movements, particularly when the fingers are in flexion. Included are the extensor pollicis longus, extensor indicis, extensor digiti minimi, and extensor digitorum (**Fig. 13.4**).

Radial and Ulnar Deviation

The flexor and extensor muscles of the wrist cooperatively develop tension to produce radial and ulnar deviation of the hand at the wrist. The flexor carpi radialis and extensor carpi radialis act to produce radial deviation, and the flexor carpi ulnaris and extensor carpi ulnaris cause ulnar deviation (**Figs. 13.3 and 13.4**).

Carpometacarpal Joint Motion

The CM joint of the thumb allows a large range of movement, comparable to that of a ball and socket joint. The fifth CM joint permits significantly less range of motion, however, and only a very small amount of motion is allowed at the second through fourth CM joints, due to the presence of restrictive ligaments.

Metacarpophalangeal Joint Motion

The MP joints of the fingers allow flexion, extension, abduction, adduction, and circumduction (**Fig. 13.8**). Among the fingers, abduction is defined as movement away from the middle finger and adduction is movement toward the middle finger. The MP joint of the thumb functions more as a hinge joint, with the primary movements being flexion and extension.

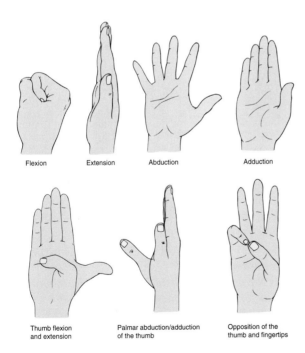

Flexion   Extension   Abduction   Adduction

Thumb flexion and extension   Palmar abduction/adduction of the thumb   Opposition of the thumb and fingertips

Figure 13.8. Directional movement capabilities at the fingers and thumb.

Interphalangeal Joint Motion

The IP joints permit flexion and extension and, in some individuals, slight hyperextension. These are classic hinge joints.

There are actually two reasons why the thumb possesses a greater range of CM joint motion than the other digits. As discussed, ligaments restrict the range of motion across the CM joints of digits two to five. Also remember that the CM joint of the thumb is a classic saddle joint that allows greater freedom of motion than the modified saddle joints of the other digits.

PREVENTION OF INJURIES

The wrist, hand, and fingers must be positioned to perform intricate tasks, yet must sustain tremendous loads to cushion the body during collisions, or lessen body movement during falls. What measures can be taken to protect and strengthen the region to prevent injuries?

The very nature of many contact and collision sports places the wrist and hand in an extremely vulnerable position for injury. The hand is almost always the first point of contact to cushion the body during collisions, deflect flying objects, or to lessen body impact during a fall. Falling on an outstretched hand is the leading cause of fractures and dislocations at the distal forearm, wrist, and hand. As such, practicing the shoulder roll method of falling can lessen the risk for injury in the entire upper extremity. Other preventative strategies include the regular use of padded gloves and a complete conditioning program for the upper extremity.

Goalies, baseball/softball catchers, and field players in many sports, such as hockey and lacrosse, are required to wear wrist and hand protection (See **Figure 6.9**). The padded gloves prevent direct compression from a stick, puck, or ball. Several other gloves have extra padding on high impact areas, aid in gripping, and protect the hand from abrasions, particularly when playing on artificial turf or on a baseball/softball field. Whenever possible, protective pads and gloves should be worn during sport participation to lessen the risk for injury.

Several muscles that move the wrist and hand cross the elbow. As such, flexibility and strengthening exercises for the wrist and hand must also include exercises for the elbow, which were illustrated in **Field Strategy 12.1**. Other exercises, such as squeezing a tennis ball or a spring-loaded grip device, can be used to strengthen the finger flexors.

Physical conditioning should include exercises for the shoulder, elbow, wrist, and hand. Specialized padded gloves are available for a variety of sports and should be worn whenever possible. One of the key elements, however, in preventing injury to the wrist and hand is learning how to fall properly to avoid direct impact on an extended wrist.

CONTUSIONS AND ABRASIONS

? *A track athlete hit a hurdle and fell onto the track, sustaining an abrasion on the palm of the hand. What factors should be considered in cleansing this wound?*

Direct impact to the hand can produce a soft, painful, bluish-colored contusion. Although many are minor, always be cautious of an underlying fracture. Initial treatment involves ice, compression, elevation, and rest. Symptoms should disappear in 2 to 3 days. If not, refer the individual to a physician for follow-up care.

Abrasions must be thoroughly cleansed of all foreign matter. A soap wash for 10 minutes using surgical soap, with a water-soluble iodine solution and brush, can remove imbedded foreign matter. Once cleansed, an antiseptic is applied and the wound is covered with a nonocclusive dressing. Inspect the wound daily for signs of infection. If the wound appears red, swollen, purulent, or is hot and tender, refer the individual to a physician.

⚡ *After cleansing the abrasion on the palm of the hand, apply an antiseptic and a nonocclusive dressing. Check the wound daily for signs of infection.*

> Always determine the possibility of an underlying fracture in a contusion or abrasion of the hand

SPRAINS

? *A soccer player fell on the turf and landed on his outstretched hand to cushion the fall. Radiographs and muscle testing did not show anything conclusive, and the physician diagnosed the injury as a wrist sprain. How would you treat this condition to help facilitate safe return to activity?*

Ligamentous sprains in the wrist and hand are the result either of a single episode of trauma or from repetitive stress. When due to a single episode, the severity of the injury is dependent on: 1) characteristics of the injury force (its point of application, magnitude, rate, and direction); 2) position of the hand at impact; and 3) relative strength of the carpal bones and ligaments (2). Most injuries to the region result from a compressive load applied while the hand is in some degree of extension, although hyperflexion or rotation may also lead to injury. Unfortunately, most individuals do not allow ample time for healing, due to the need to perform simple daily activities. Consequently, many sprains are neglected, leading to chronic instability.

Wrist Sprains

Axial loading on the proximal palm during a fall on an outstretched hand is the leading cause of wrist sprains. Assessment will reveal point tenderness on the dorsum of the radiocarpal joint. Pain increases with active or passive extension. After a fracture or carpal dislocation has been ruled out through a radiograph, treatment involves decreasing intensity of training; cryotherapy before and after practice; nonsteroidal anti-inflammatory drugs (NSAIDs);

> Wrist sprains commonly result from axial loading on the proximal palm during a fall on an outstretched hand

and the use of an appropriate bandage, taping technique, or splint to prevent excessive hyperextension. As pain decreases, range-of-motion exercises and wrist- and hand-strengthening exercises, such as those listed in **Field Strategy 12.1** can begin.

Gamekeeper's Thumb

The thumb is exposed to more force than the fingers by the very virtue of its position on the hand. Integrity of the ulnar collateral ligament at the MP joint is critical for normal hand function, as it stabilizes the joint as the thumb is pushed against the index and middle fingers while performing many pinching, grasping, and gripping motions. **Gamekeeper's thumb** occurs when the MP joint is near full extension and the thumb is forcefully abducted away from the hand, tearing the ulnar collateral ligament at the MP joint **(Fig. 13.9)**.

The palmar aspect of the joint is painful, swollen, and may have visible bruising. Instability is detected by replicating the mechanism of injury or by stressing the thumb in flexion. Initial treatment includes ice, compression, elevation, and referral to a physician to rule out an undisplaced avulsion fracture. With no instability, treatment involves early mobilization accompanied with cryotherapy, contrast baths, and NSAIDs. Strapping or taping the thumb can prevent reinjury. If there is joint instability, a thumb spica cast may be applied for 3 to 6 weeks, followed by further taping for another 3 to 6 weeks during risk activities. Severe cases require surgical repair.

Interphalangeal Collateral Ligament Sprains

Excessive varus/valgus stress and hyperextension can damage the collateral ligaments of the fingers. Hyperextension of the proximal phalanx can stretch or rupture the volar plate on the palmar side of the joint **(Fig. 13.10)**. An obvious deformity may not be present, unless there is a fracture or total rupture of the supporting tissues leading to a dorsal dislocation. Rapid swelling makes assessment

Gamekeeper's thumb
Rupture of the volar ligament at the MP joint, due to forceful abduction of the thumb while the thumb is extended

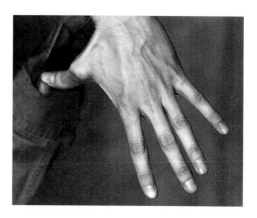

Figure 13.9. Clinical appearance of a Gamekeeper's thumb.

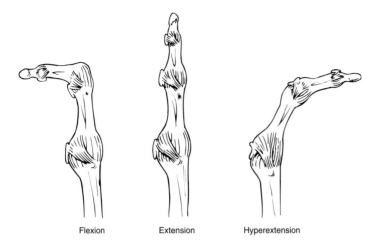

Flexion   Extension   Hyperextension

Figure 13.10. Hyperextension and a varus/valgus force stress can damage the collateral ligaments and volar plates of the fingers.

difficult. A radiograph is needed to rule out an associated dislocation or fracture.

After standard acute care, a mild sprain can be treated by taping the injured finger to an adjacent finger (buddy taping—see **Figure 7.28**). This provides some support and mobility, but should not be used in an acutely swollen, painful finger because of possible constriction to the vascular flow. If more support is needed, the involved joint can be splinted in extension with a molded polypropylene splint to avoid flexion contractures.

Dislocations

Because of the shape of the lunate and its position between the large capitate and lower end of the radius, this carpal bone is particularly prone to dislocation during axial loading (**Fig. 13.11**).

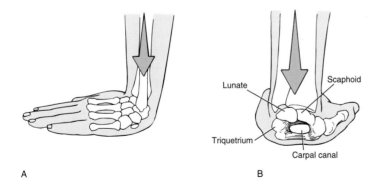

A   B

Figure 13.11. During a fall on an outstretched hand, the lunate can dislocate when the radius drives the lunate in a volar direction (**A**). If the bone moves into the carpal tunnel, the median nerve can become compressed, leading to sensory changes in the first and second fingers (**B**).

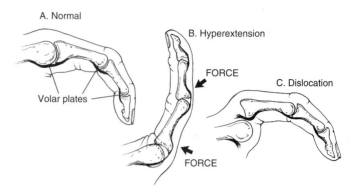

A. Normal

B. Hyperextension

FORCE

C. Dislocation

Volar plates

FORCE

Figure 13.12. The volar plates protect the anterior joint capsules of the fingers (**A**). Hyperextension can tear the anterior capsule and supporting ligaments (**B**). As the force continues, the capsule ruptures, dislocating the phalanx (**C**). The resulting deformity signals a serious dislocation that needs immediate referral to a physician for reduction.

Dislocations at the wrist commonly involve the lunate, which can move into the carpal tunnel, thereby compressing the median nerve, leading to paresthesia in the first and second fingers

The most common finger dislocation occurs at the PIP joint

The dorsum of the hand will be point tender, and a thickened area on the palm can be palpated just distal to the end of the radius, if not obscured by swelling. Passive and active motion may not be painful. If the bone moves into the carpal tunnel, compression of the median nerve leads to pain, numbness, and tingling in the first and second fingers.

MP joint dislocations are rare, but readily recognizable as a serious injury. Hyperextension causes the anterior capsule to tear, allowing the proximal phalanx to move backward over the metacarpal to stand at a 90° angle to the metacarpal (**Fig. 13.12**).

The most common dislocation in the body occurs at the PIP joint (**Fig. 13.13**). Because digital nerves and vessels run along the sides of the fingers and thumb, dislocations here can be potentially serious. The mechanism of injury is usually hyperextension and axial compression, such as when a ball hits the end of the finger, forcing it into hyperextension (3). A swollen, painful finger caused by a ball striking the extended finger is the most frequent initial complaint. Pain will be present at the joint line and will increase when the mechanism of injury is reproduced.

Because of the probability of entrapping the volar plate in an IP joint, which can lead to permanent dysfunction of the finger, no attempt should be made to reduce a finger dislocation by

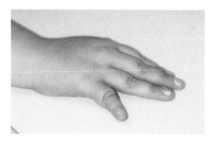

Figure 13.13. The most common finger dislocation occurs at the proximal interphalangeal (PIP) joint.

an untrained individual. Immediate treatment for all dislocations involves immobilization in a wrist or finger splint, application of ice to reduce swelling and inflammation, and referral to a physician. The prognosis and rehabilitation program will depend on the extent of tissue damage and instability.

💡 *The soccer player had a mild wrist sprain and was allowed to participate in activity, as tolerated. Activity should be supplemented by ice treatments, NSAIDs, and gentle stretching. A wrist splint or other appropriate strapping may be worn to alleviate any mild discomfort.*

STRAINS

❓ *A catcher was hit on the tip of the finger by a foul ball. While palpating the distal finger in a supine position, you find increased pain over the distal phalanx. What must you keep in mind when palpating the hand for possible injury?*

Muscular strains occur as a result of excessive overload against resistance, or overstretching the tendon beyond its normal range. In mild or moderate strains, pain and restricted motion may not be a major factor. In many injuries, muscular strains occur simultaneously with a joint sprain. The joint sprain takes precedence in priority of care, especially with an associated dislocation. As a result, tendon damage may go unrecognized and untreated.

> Muscular strains occur as a result of excessive overload against resistance, or overstretching the tendon beyond its normal range

Jersey Finger (Profundus Tendon Rupture)

This injury typically occurs when an individual grips an opponent's jersey while the opponent simultaneously twists and turns to get away. This jerking action may force the fingers to rapidly extend, rupturing the flexor digitorum profundus tendon from its attachment on the distal phalanx, hence the name "**jersey finger**". The ring finger is more commonly involved (3). If avulsed, the tendon can be palpated at the proximal aspect of the involved finger and the individual will be unable to flex the DIP joint against resistance. After standard acute care, the individual should be referred to the physician for possible surgical repair of the tendon.

> **Jersey finger**
> Rupture of the flexor digitorum profundus tendon from the distal phalanx, due to rapid extension of the finger while actively flexed

> If the flexor digitorum profundus tendon is avulsed, the individual will be unable to flex the DIP joint against resistance

Mallet Finger

Mallet finger occurs when an object hits the end of the finger while the extensor tendon is taut, such as when catching a ball. The resulting forceful flexion of the distal phalanx avulses the lateral bands of the extensor mechanism from its distal attachment, leaving a characteristic mallet deformity **(Fig. 13.14)**. In nearly 25% of all cases, an avulsion fracture to the distal phalanx occurs (4). With this injury, the DIP joint is immobilized in extension, with the PIP joint left free to move for 6 to 8 weeks. An additional 6 to 8 weeks of splints should be employed during athletic participation (3).

> **Mallet finger**
> Rupture of the extensor tendon from the distal phalanx, due to forceful flexion of the phalanx

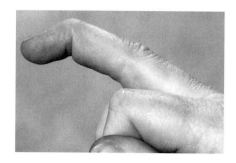

Figure 13.14. Mallet finger is caused when the extensor tendon avulses from its attachment on the distal phalanx.

Boutonniere Deformity

Boutonnière deformity
Rupture of the central slip of the extensor tendon at the middle phalanx, resulting in no active extensor mechanism at the PIP joint

Because the head of the proximal phalanx protrudes through the split in the extensor hood, this condition is sometimes referred to as a "buttonhole rupture"

A **boutonniere deformity** is caused by blunt trauma to the dorsal aspect of the PIP joint or by a rapid, forceful flexion of the joint against resistance. The central slip of the extensor tendon ruptures at the middle phalanx, leaving no active extensor mechanism intact over the PIP joint. The ruptured middle slip allows the lateral slips to move in a palmar direction, resulting in hyperextension at the MCP joint, flexion at the PIP joint, and hyperextension at the DIP joint (**Fig. 13.15**). Because the head of the proximal phalanx protrudes through the split in the extensor hood, this condition is sometimes referred to as a "buttonhole rupture." The PIP joint will be swollen and lack full extension. Any injury that lacks greater than 30° of PIP extension, along with dorsal tenderness over the base of the middle phalanx, should be treated as an acute tendon rupture and should be immediately referred to a physician (3).

Tendinitis and Stenosing Tenosynovitis

Individuals involved in strenuous and repetitive training often inflame tendons and tendon sheaths in the wrist and hand. Tendinitis in the wrist flexors or extensors leads to stiffness and an aching pain that is aggravated by activity. It may appear several hours after participation in sports. Pain is usually localized over

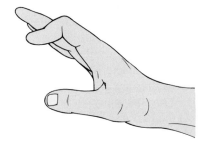

Figure 13.15. With a boutonniere deformity, the proximal joint flexes while the distal joint hyperextends.

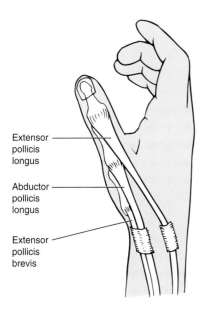

Extensor pollicis longus

Abductor pollicis longus

Extensor pollicis brevis

Figure 13.16. The abductor pollicis longus and extensor pollicis brevis share the same synovial sheath. Excessive friction between the tendons, sheath, and bone lead to tenosynovitis of the tendons.

the involved tendons and is aggravated with passive stretching and resisted motion of the affected tendons.

In the wrist, the abductor pollicis longus and extensor pollicis brevis are commonly affected. These two tendons share a single synovial tendon sheath that turns sharply, as much as 105°, to enter the thumb when the wrist is in radial deviation (**Fig. 13.16**). Friction between the tendons, the **stenosing** sheath, and bony process lead to a condition called "**de Quervain's tenosynovitis.**" The individual will complain of pain over the radial styloid process and during thumb movement. Treatment involves ice, rest, and NSAIDs as prescribed by a physician. If symptoms are not relieved, steroid injections or immobilization with a thumb spica for 3 weeks, or both, may be helpful.

Ganglion Cysts

Ganglion cysts are benign tumor masses typically seen on the dorsal aspect of the wrist. Associated with tissue sheath degeneration, the dorsal cyst contains a jelly-like colorless fluid of mucin and is freely mobile and palpable between the extensor tendons. Occurring spontaneously, there may be localized tenderness and maximal aggravation of pain during wrist flexion. Treatment involves splinting, NSAIDs, and steroid injection; however, surgical excision may be necessary.

In assessing the catcher who was struck on the end of the finger, it is important to palpate the hand in both the supine and prone position. In this particular injury, the extensor mechanism may have been avulsed from the distal phalanx and would not be apparent unless viewed in a prone position.

Stenosing
Narrowing of an opening or stricture of a canal

de Quervain's tenosynovitis
An inflammatory stenosing tenosynovitis of the abductor pollicis longus and extensor pollicis brevis tendons

Ganglion cyst
Benign tumor mass commonly seen on the dorsal aspect of the wrist

FINGERTIP INJURIES

> A water polo player pinched a finger between the pool deck and weighted base of a goal cage, causing blood to accumulate under the fingernail. The fingertip is extremely painful from the increasing pressure. What must you keep in mind in deciding whether or not to relieve the pressure?

Subungual hematoma
Collection of blood under the fingernail, caused by direct trauma

Direct trauma to the nail bed can result in blood forming under the fingernail and is called a **subungual hematoma**. Increasing pressure can lead to throbbing pain. After determining the possibility of an underlying fracture, soak the finger in ice water for 10 to 15 minutes to numb the area and reduce bleeding under the nail bed. If it is not absolutely necessary to relieve the pressure, do not do so, as this opens an avenue for infection. If, however, discomfort is so great the individual is unable to perform, drain the hematoma under the direction of a physician. Cut a hole through the nail with a rotary drill, a number 11 surgical blade, or melt a hole through the nail with the end of a paper clip heated to a bright red color. **Field Strategy 13.1** explains how to properly care for a subungual hematoma. After draining the blood, check the area daily for signs of infection.

Paronychia
A fungal/bacterial infection in the folds of skin surrounding a fingernail or toenail

Paronychia is an infection along the nail fold, commonly seen with a hangnail. The nail fold becomes red, swollen, painful, and can produce purulent drainage. The condition is treated with warm water soaks and germicide. In more severe cases, the physician may recommend systemic antibiotics and drainage of localized pus (5). The area is then protected with a dry, sterile dressing.

> The water polo player has a subungual hematoma. If it is not absolutely necessary to relieve pressure under the nail, do not do so, as this opens an avenue for infection. Any drainage of fluid should be done under the supervision of a physician, and should follow universal safety precautions.

NERVE ENTRAPMENT SYNDROMES

> A long-distance cyclist is complaining of bilateral numbness in the little finger and an inability to adduct the little finger. The individual cannot recall an incident that could have caused this condition, but stated that training distance has significantly increased this past week. What possible factors are involved in this condition, and what suggestions can be made to alleviate the symptoms, yet still allow this cyclist to continue training?

Neurovascular syndromes in the wrist and hand are seen in several activities, including bowling, cycling, karate, rowing, baseball/softball, field hockey, lacrosse, rugby, weightlifting, and handball, and in wheelchair athletes. The two most common nerve entrapment syndromes are carpal tunnel syndrome and ulnar entrapment (commonly associated with "cyclist's palsy").

Field Strategy 13.1. Management of a Subungual Hematoma

Under the Direction of a Physician

1. Soak the finger in ice water for 10 to 15 minutes to numb the area and reduce hemorrhage
2. Cleanse your hands thoroughly with antiseptic soap and water and apply latex gloves
3. Thoroughly cleanse the finger with antiseptic soap or an antibacterial solution
4. Use a sterile number 11 surgical blade, clean rotary drill, or melt a hole through the nail bed with the end of a paper clip heated to a bright red color

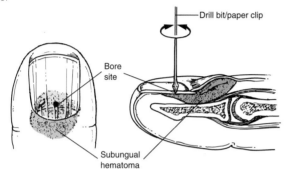

5. After the hole has been made, have the individual exert mild pressure on the distal pulp of the finger to drive excess blood through the hole
6. Watch the individual carefully for signs of shock as it sometimes occurs in minor injuries. Treat accordingly
7. Soak the finger in an iodine solution for 10 minutes. Heat should not be applied for 48 hours
8. Cover the phalanx with a sterile dressing and apply a protective splint. Check the finger daily for signs of infection. If any appear, refer the individual to a physician

---

Carpal Tunnel Syndrome

Carpal tunnel syndrome is caused by direct trauma or repetitive overuse. The condition is three times more common in women and peaks between ages 30 and 50, with the right hand being more affected (6). This higher incidence may be largely due to occupational tasks that demand repetitive digital manipulations, such as typing or computer keyboard work. Sporting activities that predispose athletes to carpal tunnel syndrome include those that involve repetitive or continuous flexion and extension of the wrist, as in cycling, throwing sports, racquets sports, archery, and gymnastics (7).

The carpal tunnel runs between the floor of the volar wrist capsule and the transverse retinacular ligament that courses from the hamate and pisiform on the lateral side to the trapezium and scaphoid on the medial side. This unyielding tunnel accommodates

Carpal tunnel syndrome
Compression of the median nerve as it passes through the carpal tunnel, leading to pain and tingling in the hand

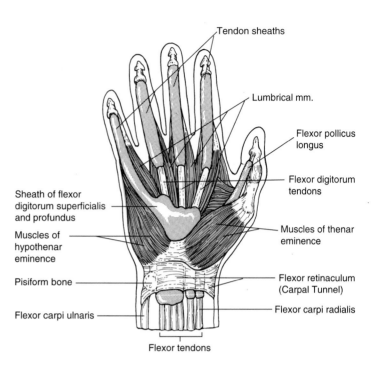

Tendon sheaths

Lumbrical mm.

Flexor pollicus longus

Flexor digitorum tendons

Muscles of thenar eminence

Flexor retinaculum (Carpal Tunnel)

Flexor carpi radialis

Sheath of flexor digitorum superficialis and profundus

Muscles of hypothenar eminence

Pisiform bone

Flexor carpi ulnaris

Flexor tendons

Figure 13.17. The flexor tendons of the fingers pass through the carpal tunnel in a single synovial sheath.

the median nerve, the finger flexors in a common sheath, and the flexor pollicis longus in an independent sheath **(Fig. 13.17)**. Therefore, any irritation of the synovial sheath covering these tendons can produce swelling or edema that can put pressure on the median nerve.

The individual will report that pain wakes them in the middle of the night and is often relieved by shaking the hands (7). Pain and numbness may be felt only in the fingertips on the palmar aspect of the thumb, index, and middle finger. Grip strength and pinch strength may be limited. Symptoms are reproduced when direct compression is applied over the carpal tunnel for about 30 seconds (8). Individuals with suspected carpal tunnel syndrome should be referred to a physician for care. Conservative care involves splinting, NSAIDs, and cessation of any activity that contributes to the nerve compression.

Ulnar Neuropathy

The ulnar nerve can become entrapped between the hook of the hamate and pisiform, which is frequently seen in cycling, racquet sports, and in baseball/softball catchers that experience repetitive trauma to the palm. The individual will have numbness in the ulnar nerve distribution, particularly the little finger, and may have a weakened grip strength and atrophy of muscles in the **hypothenar** mass. Treatment involves cessation of activities that

With carpal tunnel syndrome, the hand pain and numbness will often wake an individual in the middle of the night, but it is relieved by shaking the hands

Ulnar neuropathy is frequently seen in activities involving repetitive trauma to the palm of the hand

Hypothenar
Mass of intrinsic muscles of the little finger, including the abductor digiti minimi, flexor digiti minimi brevis, and opponens digiti minimi

contribute to the compression, rest, cryotherapy, and NSAIDs to minimize pain and inflammation; however, surgical decompression may be necessary to alleviate symptoms.

Cyclist's palsy occurs when a biker leans on the handlebar for an extended period of time, leading to temporary swelling in the hypothenar area. Symptoms mimic the more serious ulnar nerve entrapment syndrome, but usually disappear rapidly after completion of the ride. Properly padding the handlebars, wearing padded gloves, varying hand position, and properly fitting the bike to the rider can greatly reduce the incidence of this condition (9).

💡 *The cyclist may have compressed the ulnar nerve while leaning on the handlebars during the recent increased training. To alleviate symptoms, suggest padding the handlebars, wearing padded gloves, varying hand position, and properly fitting the bike to the rider.*

FRACTURES

❓ *A gymnast lost her balance on a dismount and fell onto an outstretched hand. There is noticeable swelling on the thenar mass and intense pain during palpation of the anatomical snuffbox and with mild compression along the long axis of the first metacarpal. What should you suspect? How will you immobilize the hand?*

The majority of wrist and hand fractures are simple and nondisplaced. With the advent and fabrication of external orthoses, many fractures can be immobilized adequately to allow individuals to continue with sport participation. Specific rules governing special protective equipment, however, require that braces, casts, or any unyielding substances on the elbow, forearm, wrist, or hand be padded on all sides so as not to endanger other players. Once the fracture has reached a stage where external support is no longer necessary, a splint may be worn just during sport participation.

Distal Radial and Ulnar Fractures

Fractures to the distal forearm may involve one or both bones. A **Colles fracture** occurs within one-and-one-half inches of the wrist joint, and results in a "dinner-fork" deformity when the distal segment displaces in a dorsal and radial direction **(Fig. 13.18A)**. A reverse of this fracture is the **Smith fracture** that tends to move in a volar direction **(Fig. 13.18B)**. Swelling and hemorrhage may lead to circulatory impairment or the median nerve may be damaged as it passes through the forearm. As a result, immediate immobilization and referral to a physician is necessary. In many instances, open reduction and internal fixation with rigid plates and screws is necessary to restore function (10).

Carpal Fractures

Often an individual will fall on the wrist, have normal radiographs, and be discharged with a diagnosis of a wrist sprain without further

Thenar
Mass of intrinsic muscles of the thumb, including the flexor pollicis brevis, abductor pollicis brevis, and opponens pollicis

Cyclist's palsy
Seen when bikers lean on the handlebars for an extended period of time, resulting in paresthesia in the ulnar nerve distribution

The majority of hand and wrist fractures are simple and nondisplaced and, if properly immobilized, sport participation can continue

Colles' fracture
Fracture of the radius and ulna, just proximal to the wrist, that results in the distal segment displacing in a dorsal and radial direction

Smith's fracture
Fracture of the radius and ulna, just proximal to the wrist, that results in the distal segment displacing in a volar direction; opposite of Colles' fracture

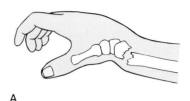

A

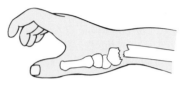

Figure 13.18. Fractures of the forearm may result in the wrist and hand angulating in a dorsal direction, called a Colles fracture (**A**), or in a volar direction, called a Smith fracture (**B**).

B

Aseptic necrosis
The death or decay of tissue due to a poor blood supply in the area

care. Several months later, however, the individual will continue to experience persistent wrist pain. Radiographs at this time may reveal an established nonunion fracture of the scaphoid (**Fig. 13.19**). Because of a poor blood supply to the area, **aseptic necrosis** is a common complication with this fracture.

Scaphoid fractures account for 70% of all carpal fractures (3). Assessment will reveal a history of falling on an outstretched hand.

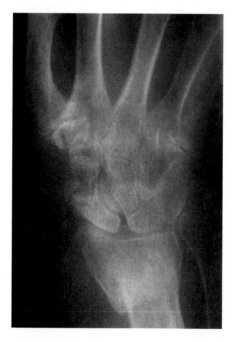

Figure 13.19. Nonunion fractures of the scaphoid occur when there is a poor blood supply to the area. Note this individual also has a fractured radius.

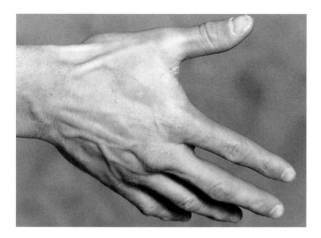

Figure 13.20. The scaphoid forms the floor of the anatomical snuff box and is bounded by the extensor pollicis brevis medially, and the extensor pollicis longus laterally.

If pain is present in the "**anatomical snuff box**" **(Fig. 13.20)**, which lies directly over the scaphoid, or with inward pressure along the long axis of the first metacarpal bone, suspect a fracture. Pain will also increase during wrist extension and radial deviation. Because of the critical role the thumb plays in hand function, any pain in the anatomical snuff box should be evaluated by a physician. Treatment involves ice, compression, immobilization in an appropriate splint, and referral to a physician.

Direct impact to the hamate may also lead to a nonunion fracture. This typically occurs when an athlete strikes a stationary object with a racquet or club in full swing (10). The hypothenar muscle mass will be painful and the individual will have decreased grip strength. Care is usually symptomatic with a protective orthosis worn for 4 to 6 weeks until tenderness subsides.

Anatomical snuff box
Region directly over the scaphoid bone bounded by the extensor pollicis brevis medially and the extensor pollicis longus laterally

Metacarpal Fractures

Uncomplicated fractures to the metacarpals result in severe pain, dorsal swelling, and deformity. Proper immobilization, followed by an early exercise program, can help prevent an extension contracture (3). **Bennett's fracture** is a more serious articular fracture to the proximal end of the first metacarpal. During axial compression, such as when a punch is thrown with a closed fist, the abductor pollicis longus tendon pulls the metacarpal shaft proximally. A small medial fragment, however, is held in place by the deep volar ligament, leading to a fracture-dislocation **(Fig. 13.21)**. Pain and swelling is localized, but deformity may or may not be present. **Field Strategy 13.4** in the Assessment section demonstrates how to determine a possible metacarpal fracture. These techniques can also detect possible fractures in the carpals and phalanges. Acute care involves ice, compression, immobiliza-

Bennett's fracture
Fracture-dislocation to the proximal end of the first metacarpal at the carpal-metacarpal joint

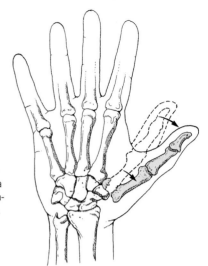

Figure 13.21. A Bennett's fracture is usually associated with a dislocation of the metacarpophalangeal (MP) joint of the thumb. An avulsion fracture, however, occurs when a segment of the metacarpal is held in place by the deep volar ligament.

tion in a wrist splint, with the palm face down and fingers slightly flexed, and referral to a physician.

Phalangeal Fractures

Fractures of the phalanges are very common in sport participation and may be caused by having the fingers stepped on, having them impinged between two hard objects, or hyperextending them, leading to a fracture-dislocation (**Fig. 13.22**). Immobilize a suspected fracture in a full wrist splint and place gauze pads or a gauze roll under the fingers to produce about 30° finger flexion, to reduce the pull of the flexor tendons. Refer the individual to a physician for care. Immobilization will depend upon the type of fracture and its location, and may vary from 2 to 4 weeks.

💡 *The gymnast may have fractured the scaphoid. Immobilize the hand with a wrist splint, apply ice to reduce swelling, and transport the individual to the physician.*

ASSESSMENT OF THE WRIST AND HAND

❓ *A diver has pain on the anterior wrist during entry. Pain increases with resisted wrist and finger flexion, and passive wrist and finger extension. How will you assess this injury?*

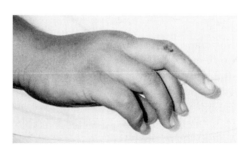

Figure 13.22. This finger was crushed between two football helmets during a tackle, fracturing the phalanx.

The wrist and hand are difficult to evaluate because of the number of anatomical structures providing motor and sensory function to the region. Although many injuries can be handled on-site, any injury that impairs the function of the hand or fingers should be referred to a physician for more extensive evaluation. Also keep in mind that if the mechanism of injury involves axial loading at the wrist, additional assessment may be necessary at the elbow or shoulder.

HISTORY

What information must be gathered from the diver to identify the primary complaint and ascertain if other factors, such as sport-specific skills, contributed to this injury?

Questions about the wrist injury should focus on the primary complaint, past injuries, and other factors that may have contributed to the current problem (demands of the sport, changes in technique, equipment, overuse, occupational requirements, or referred pain). For example, ask how the injury occurred. Is the region subjected to repetitive trauma, such as from constant impact from a ball, racquet, bat, or stick? Determine what symptoms are currently present and how they progressed. Is the pain localized, general, or does it radiate into the forearm? What activities increase or decrease pain? What recent changes, if any, have occurred in the training program? In addition to general questions discussed in Chapter 4, specific questions for the wrist and hand region are listed in **Field Strategy 13.2**.

 Field Strategy 13.2. Developing a History of the Injury

Current Injury Status

1. How did the injury occur (mechanism)? Is the region subjected to multiple impact from a ball, bat, racquet, or stick?
2. Ask about the pain location, severity, onset (sudden or gradual), and type (sharp, aching, burning, radiating). Does it wake you up at night (possible carpal tunnel syndrome)? Did you hear any sounds during the incident, such as a snap, pop, or crack?
3. Was there any swelling, discoloration, muscle spasms, or numbness with the injury?
4. Are there certain activities you cannot perform because of the pain? What actions or motions replicate the pain? At what angle of wrist or finger motion does it hurt the worst? Does your elbow or shoulder bother you?

Past Injury Status

1. Have you ever injured your wrist or fingers before? When? How did that occur? What was done for the injury?
2. Have you had any medical problems recently? (You are looking for possible referred pain from the cervical neck, shoulder, or elbow.)

The 19-year-old diver has been working quite extensively on several new dives on the 3-meter board in preparation for an upcoming competition. Pain on the anterior wrist started 3 weeks ago, when both wrists were hyperextended during entry on a dive. Pain has continued to persist, increasing as the practice session progresses. It now hurts to pick up a book bag or to hook an object with the fingers.

OBSERVATION AND INSPECTION

What specific factors should be observed at the injury site? Since pain is present in both wrists, can you still do bilateral comparison?

The entire arm should be exposed for observation and inspection. Although the individual may have a wrist injury, the elbow and shoulder region may also need to be evaluated, depending on the mechanism of injury. First observe the position of the wrist, hand, and fingers. Is there a noticeable deformity? How is the individual holding the wrist and hand? If swelling is present in a specific joint, the individual may be unable to fully extend that joint, supporting it in a slightly flexed position. Inspect the specific injury site for obvious abrasions, deformity, swelling, discoloration, symmetry, muscle hypertrophy or atrophy, or previous surgical incisions. **Field Strategy 13.3** summarizes observations at the wrist and hand from a dorsal and palmar view.

Bilateral comparison reveals slight redness and swelling over the carpal tunnel on both hands; however, it is greater on the right hand. No bilateral differences are visible in the thenar or hypothenar muscle masses. The fingers appear to be normal with no discoloration or swelling present.

PALPATIONS

Pain and swelling are confined over the carpal tunnel on both wrists. Where will you begin palpations? What specific factors are you looking for?

With an acute injury, determine the possibility of a fracture or dislocation before moving the wrist or hand. If the individual is in great pain, unable or unwilling to move the wrist or hand, perform the fracture tests listed in **Field Strategy 13.4**. If a fracture is suspected, treat accordingly. Immobilize the wrist and hand in a vacuum splint or wrist splint, apply ice to control pain and inflammation, and transport the individual to a physician.

Palpate the wrist and hand proximal to distal, beginning on the dorsal aspect, then move to the palmar aspect. Support the individual's hand throughout the palpations. Bilateral palpations can determine temperature, swelling, point tenderness, crepitus, deformity, muscle spasm, and cutaneous sensation. Circulation can be assessed by blanching the fingernails. Squeeze the nail. Initially the nail should turn white, but color should return imme-

Field Strategy 13.3. Observation and Inspection of the Wrist and Hand

Dorsal View

1. Check bilateral shape and contour of the bony and soft tissue structures of the forearm, wrist, and hand. Note how the individual moves the hand into the requested positions
2. Note skin color, presence of ganglions, or muscle wasting. Do the hands appear healthy?
3. Note any localized swelling, effusion, or synovial thickening at the MP or IP joints
4. Observe for any angular deformities of the fingers that may indicate a fracture or dislocation
5. With the forearm in pronation, note whether or not the distal phalanx fails to remain in an extended position (possible mallet finger)
6. Observe the fingernails for any abnormality or change in color during blanching

Palmar View

1. Check the smooth contours of the bony and soft tissue structures of the forearm, wrist, and hand
2. Look for muscle wasting in the thenar eminence (median nerve) and hypothenar eminence (ulnar nerve) that may indicate a nerve injury
3. Have the individual flex the MP and PIP joints and keep the DIP joint extended. Note any angular deformity that may indicate a previous fracture
4. Note any localized swelling, effusion, or synovial thickening at the MP, PIP, and DIP joints. (This may be more visible on the dorsal view)
5. Check skin color and presence of any abrasions or scars. Scars may decrease the mobility of a joint because of the formation of scar tissue around the tendons and joint

diately upon release of pressure. Vascular pulses can also be taken at the radial and ulnar arteries in the wrist.

Bony Palpations

1. Radius and ulna
2. Carpal bones and "anatomical snuffbox"
3. Metacarpal bones and phalanges. Palpate the MP, PIP, and DIP joints for synovial thickening, swelling, and tenderness

Soft Tissue Palpations

1. Finger and thumb extensors and thumb abductor
2. Carpal tunnel and flexor tendons
3. Palmar fascia and intrinsic muscles within the thenar and hypothenar muscle masses

Swelling and exquisite point tenderness were apparent over the flexor tendons and carpal tunnel on both hands, particularly the right hand. Slight crepitation was felt during passive flexion and extension of the wrist flexors on the right hand. Circulation was normal.

Field Strategy 13.4. Determining a Possible Fracture to a Metacarpal

History
  Determine mechanism of injury
  Primary complaint (severe pain and/or loss of motion)
  Disability from injury (limited or loss of function)
Observation and inspection
  Obvious deformity or angulation
  Swelling or discoloration directly over the bone
Palpation
  Pain along the shaft of the bone
  Pain on compression of soft tissue around the bone
Stress tests for fracture
  Compression along the long axis of the bone **(A)**
  Percussion or vibration at the end of the bone **(B)**
  Positive sign occurs if pain is felt at the fracture site
  Distraction at the end of the bone **(C)**
  Positive sign occurs if pain is decreased (increased pain may indicate a
    ligamentous injury)

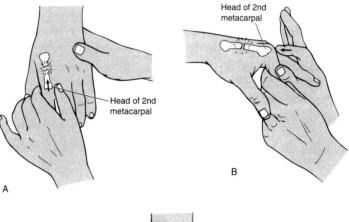

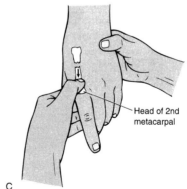

Management

Check the ABC's. Shock may set in, particularly if there is angulation and
  deformity
If any positive signs are noted, immobilize the joint above and below the
  fracture site with a wrist or finger splint, apply ice to reduce
  hemorrhage and swelling, and refer the individual to a physician

? *Although the right hand appears to be more seriously injured, it is imperative that both hands continue to be assessed. What specific tests should be performed to determine the extent and seriousness of this injury?*

Perform special tests in a comfortable position and begin with gentle stress. Note what range of motion is the most painful. Do not force the wrist or hand through any sudden motions, nor cause undue pain. Proceed cautiously through the assessment.

Joint Range of Motion

In determining active movements at the wrist and hand, perform the most painful movements last. Finger active motion is usually done in a continuous pattern. Ask the individual to (a) make a tight fist (flexion), (b) straighten the fingers (extension), (c) spread the fingers (abduction), and (d) bring the fingers together (adduction). Note how fluid each digit moves throughout the range of motion. If one finger does not move through the full ROM, that finger can be evaluated separately. The following movements at the wrist and hand should be assessed:

1. Forearm pronation and supination
2. Wrist flexion and extension
3. Wrist radial and ulnar deviation
4. Finger flexion and extension
5. Finger abduction and adduction
6. Thumb flexion, extension, abduction, and adduction
7. Opposition of the thumb and little finger (tip to tip)

Resisted Manual Muscle Testing

Active movements are tested using resisted movements throughout the full range of motion. The proximal joint is stabilized and a mild resistance is applied to the distal joint. The following movements can be tested (**Fig. 13.23**):

1. Forearm pronation and supination
2. Wrist flexion and extension
3. Wrist ulnar and radial deviation
4. Finger flexion and extension
5. Finger abduction and adduction
6. Thumb flexion and extension
7. Thumb abduction and adduction
8. Opposition of the thumb and little finger

Neurologic Testing

Neurologic integrity is assessed with resisted manual muscle testing (already completed), reflexes, and cutaneous sensation. Reflexes in the upper extremity were discussed and demonstrated in Chapter 11, and include the biceps (C_5 to C_6), brachioradialis

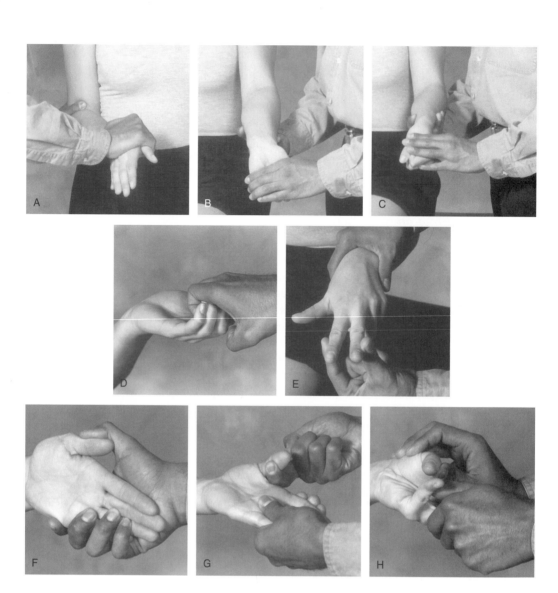

Figure 13.23. Resisted manual muscle testing. **A.** Wrist pronation and supination. **B.** Wrist flexion and extension. **C.** Wrist ulnar and radial deviation. **D.** Finger flexion and extension. **E.** Finger abduction and adduction. **F.** Thumb flexion and extension. **G.** Thumb abduction and adduction. **H.** Opposition.

(C_6), and triceps (C_7). Test bilaterally for altered sensation with sharp and dull touch by running the open hand and fingernails over the shoulder and down both sides of the arms and hands. Ask if it feels the same on both sides of the limb.

Stress and Functional Tests

Stress tests are performed when you have a clear indication of what structures may be damaged. Because of the complexity of

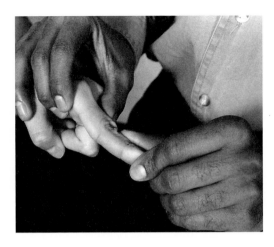

Figure 13.24. To stress the ligamentous structures, apply a varus and valgus force at the specific joint.

the wrist and hand, and basic level of information in this text, any impairment in motor or sensory function should be referred to a physician for a more complete evaluation. Only basic tests can be presented here.

Ligamentous Instability Tests

Stabilize the thumb or finger with one hand proximal to the joint being tested. Apply a valgus and varus stress to the joint to test the integrity of the collateral ligaments (**Fig. 13.24**). Do bilateral comparison with the uninvolved hand. This test is used for gamekeeper's thumb or joint sprains of the fingers.

Carpal Tunnel Compression Test

Exert even pressure with both thumbs directly over the carpal tunnel and hold for at least 30 seconds (**Fig. 13.25A**). A positive test produces numbness or tingling into the palmar aspect of the thumb, index finger, and middle finger.

Phalen's (Wrist Flexion) Test

Place the dorsum of the hands together to maximally flex the wrists. Hold this position for 1 minute by gently pushing the wrists together (**Fig. 13.25B**). A positive test, indicating either median nerve or ulnar nerve compression, produces numbness or tingling into the fingers.

Functional Tests

Because the wrist, hand, and fingers are vital to perform activities of daily living, the individual should be assessed for manual dexterity and coordination. Can they hook, pinch, and grasp an object?

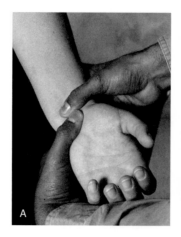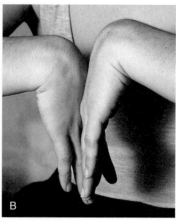

Figure 13.25. Compression of nerves can be detected by either (**A**) compression over the carpal tunnel or by (**B**) maximally flexing the wrists together (Phalen's test). A positive test will lead to tingling or numbness in the palm, fingers, or thumb.

Can they comb their hair, hold a fork, brush their teeth, or pick up a book bag? Prior to return to sport, the individual should be able to perform these simple functional skills, in addition to having bilateral range of motion and strength in the wrist and fingers.

The diver had pain on active and resisted wrist and finger flexion, particularly with the right hand. There was a slight sensory change on the palmar aspect of the thumb, second, and third fingers that was reproduced with the carpal tunnel compression test. This individual has strained the flexor muscles of the wrist and fingers. The resulting inflammation has added compression to the median nerve in the carpal tunnel. How will you manage this condition?

REHABILITATION

The diver has a flexor wrist strain and mild carpal tunnel syndrome. After the physician assesses and treats the individual, what exercises should be included in the general rehabilitation program for this wrist injury?

Traumatic injuries to the wrist and hand often require immobilization; however, early range-of-motion and strengthening exercises should be conducted at the elbow and shoulder. Many of the exercises for the wrist and hand were discussed in Chapter 12, because they are often combined with elbow rehabilitation.

Immobilization typically results in joint contractures and stiffness in the fingers; therefore, active range-of-motion exercises should begin as soon as possible. In the acute phase, exercises can be performed using cryokinetic techniques. Ice immersion is alternated with active range-of-motion exercises. The individual can use the opposite hand to apply a low-load, prolonged stretch in the various motions to minimize joint trauma and increase flexibility. As inflammation decreases, a warm whirlpool or paraffin bath may be used to facilitate motion. Precision techniques to restore dexterity can be performed by picking up and manipulating: (a) coins of differing thicknesses; (b) playing cards; (c) small objects of differing shapes; (d) large, light objects; and (e) large, heavy objects. In addition, the individual can tear tape, use scissors to cut paper, or juggle balls of different sizes.

Closed-chain exercises may involve shifting body weight from one hand to the other on a wall, table top, or unstable surface, such as a foam mat or BAPS board. Push-ups and step-ups on a box, stool, or Stair Master can also be used. Several strengthening exercises involving light-weight dumbbells and surgical tubing were explained in **Field Strategy 12.1**. Plyometric exercises may involve catching a weighted ball in a single hand and throwing it straight up and down, or using a mini-tramp to do bounding push-ups.

General body conditioning should be maintained throughout the rehabilitation program. Several examples of programs were provided in **Field Strategy 5.9**, and included use of a jump rope, Stair Master, treadmill, and upper body ergometer (UBE).

The diver should restore motion at the wrist and fingers, and begin early strengthening exercises using light resistance, gripping exercises, PNF-resisted exercises, and surgical tubing. Precision skills can be done to improve dexterity. The program should also include general body conditioning and strengthening exercises for the shoulder and elbow.

SUMMARY

The hands of sport participants have special requirements for strength and dexterity, and can ill-afford casual assessment and inadequate treatment. Although many injuries can be managed without seeking medical assistance, any injury that does not show an improvement within a week should be seen by a physician. Hand and wrist injuries that demand immediate attention by a physician include: a suspected fracture or dislocation, significant pain, pain in the anatomical snuffbox, excessive swelling in soft tissues or around joints, joint instability, loss of motion, or the presence of sensory changes. **Field Strategy 13.5** outlines a basic wrist and hand assessment.

If a decision is made to refer the individual to a physician, immobilize the area in a wrist or finger splint, apply ice to control edema, and transport the individual in an appropriate manner. Follow up with the physician to obtain instructions for further care of the injury. When appropriate, protective braces or padding should be worn to prevent reinjury.

Field Strategy 13.5. Wrist and Hand Evaluation

History

Primary complaint and mechanism of injury
Onset of symptoms, including pain and discomfort
Disability and functional impairments from the injury
Previous injuries to the area and family history

Observation and Inspection

Observe general shape, contour, and posture of the hand
Inspect:

Muscle symmetry	Hypertrophy or muscle atrophy
Swelling	Visible congenital deformity
Discoloration	Surgical incisions or scars

Palpation

Bony structures, to determine possible fracture
Soft tissue structures, to determine:

Temperature	Deformity
Swelling	Muscle spasm
Point tenderness	Cutaneous sensation
Crepitus	Vascular pulses

Special Tests

Joint range of motion
Resisted manual muscle testing
Neurologic testing
Stress and functional tests
  Ligamentous instability tests
  Carpal tunnel compression test
  Functional tests

REFERENCES

1. Rettig AC, and Patel DV. Epidemiology of elbow, forearm, and wrist injuries in the athlete. In *Clinics in sports medicine*, edited by KD Plancher, vol. 14, no. 2. Philadelphia: WB Saunders, 1995.
2. Halikis MN, and Taleisnik J. Soft-tissue injuries of the wrist. In *Clinics in sports medicine*, edited by KD Plancher, vol. 15, no. 2. Philadelphia: WB Saunders, 1996.
3. McCue FC, Hussamy OD, and Gieck JH. Hand and wrist injuries. In *Athletic injuries and rehabilitation*, edited by JE Zachazewski, DJ Magee, and WS Quillen. Philadelphia: WB Saunders, 1996.
4. Garrick JG, and Webb DR. *Sports injuries: diagnosis and management.* Philadelphia: WB Saunders, 1990.
5. Canales FL, Newmeyer WL, and Kilgore ES. 1989. The treatment of felons and paronychias. Hand Clin 5(4):515–523.
6. Bravaccio F, Trabucco M, Ammendola A, and Cantore R. 1990. Carpal tunnel syndrome: a clinical electrophysiological study of 84 cases. Neurophysio Clin 20(4):269–281.
7. Plancher KD, Peterson RK, and Steichen JB. Compressive neuropathies and tendinopathies in the athletic elbow and wrist. In *Clinics in sports medicine*, edited by KD Plancher, vol. 15, no. 2. Philadelphia: WB Saunders, 1996.

8. Durkan JA. 1991. A new diagnostic test for carpal tunnel syndrome. J Bone Joint Surg, Am 73A(4):535–538.

9. Mellion MB. 1991. Common cycling injuries: management and prevention. Sports Med 11(1):52–70.

10. Griggs SM, and Weiss AC. Bony injuries of the wrist, forearm, and elbow. In *Clinics in sports medicine*, edited by KD Plancher, vol. 15, no. 2. Philadelphia: WB Saunders, 1996.

Injuries to the Axial Region

Chapter 14: **Head and Facial Injuries**

Chapter 15: **Injuries to the Spine**

Chapter 16: **Throat, Thorax, and Visceral Injuries**

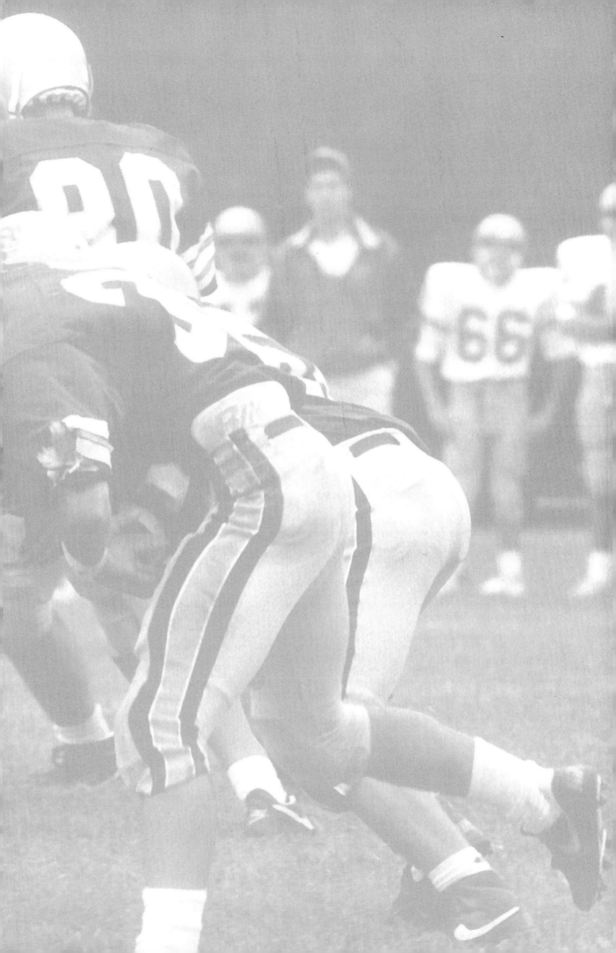

Maria Hutsick, MS, LATC

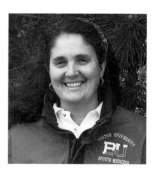

I went to Ithaca College in New York to become a teacher. After fracturing my ankle in competition and observing what went on in the training room, however, I immediately switched over to the athletic training program. I did my master's work at Indiana University, but in the early 1970s, women did not work with many of the men's sports. After coaching a year at Cortland, I landed my first training job at Yale University and worked there for 3 years with Daphne Benas. She was great and helped me perfect many of my evaluation skills. Boston University hired me in 1980 as the Women's Athletic Trainer, and I eventually moved into the head athletic training position. Today, we take care of over 500 athletes with four staff trainers and one graduate assistant. Because of our NATA curriculum program, thankfully, we also have the assistance of 25 student athletic trainers. We could not provide the quality care without these students.

As Head Athletic Trainer, I am directly responsible for administering the budget; ordering all the protective equipment; hiring, supervising, and evaluating personnel; developing policies and procedures for the training room; doing physical exams; drug testing; supervising the treatment plans for rehabilitation and use of the modalities; assessing the clinical supervision of the student athletic trainers; and doing individual referrals to other medical professionals on campus.

I require the staff and student athletic trainers to wear a designated uniform and follow a strict conduct code, which includes not dating an athlete. I think this diminishes the professional standards we must maintain to carry out our role as part of the medical staff. Every time an athlete walks in the door, that visit is logged in and recorded in the athlete's S.O.A.P. notes in their permanent medical files. We have an excellent medical staff that respects the work the trainers do. The physicians and specialists contact me daily to discuss specific cases and treatment of the athletes.

When I was first appointed head trainer, the hardest thing to deal with was getting the football coaches and officials to recognize that I was the boss and that they had to communicate with me. The players never blinked twice about having women in the locker room. They always respected and appreciated the care we provided, but the old football staff just couldn't accept it. Needless to say, they aren't with us anymore. Our current staff is excellent, but it's really a shame that women have to continually prove themselves in football, despite the fact we are fully qualified.

Another realization about working at a big-time Division I school is the long hours. You have to be prepared to work ten hours a day, seven days a week, and no time off between seasons. For a woman, that means a limited social or personal life, especially if you are thinking of having a family. It's real tough, but it can be done. I require my staff to take one morning off a week just to get their errands done. Hopefully, this will avoid some burnout. All of us work out regularly, and recognize the need to stay healthy and fit.

Working on the university level is personally gratifying when you see these young women and men achieve success in their sport. But to be a trainer at this level, you have to be sharp, professional, and a cut above the next person. A master's degree in athletic training is almost essential. The job is exciting because you're always meeting new people and facing new challenges. You see people at their worst and most vulnerable state, yet you are the one to work with them and help them return safely to their sport. It's just neat to have that kind of positive impact on a person's well-being, and I love it. You just can't find a more challenging and satisfying career.

Maria Hutsick is Head Athletic Trainer at Boston University in Boston, Massachusetts. As one of the few women who serve as the head athletic trainer at a Division I institution, Maria has established herself as an outstanding role model and professional in the field of athletic training.

500

Head and Facial Injuries

After completing this chapter, you should be able to:

- Locate the important bony and soft tissue structures of the head and facial region

- Recognize the importance of wearing protective equipment to prevent injury to the head and facial region

- Identify forces responsible for cranial injuries

- Recognize important signs and symptoms that indicate a cranial injury

- Demonstrate a basic assessment of a cranial injury

- Identify common facial injuries, their assessment and management

Key Terms:

Battle's sign	Malocclusion
Cauliflower ear	Meninges
Concussion	Meningitis
Conjunctivitis	Myopia
Contrecoup injuries	Nystagmus
Decompression	Periorbital ecchymosis
Detached retina	Photophobia
Diffuse injuries	Postconcussion syndrome
Diplopia	Posttraumatic memory loss
Dural sinuses	Raccoon eyes
Epistaxis	Retrograde amnesia
Focal injuries	Subconjunctival hemorrhage
Hyphema	Tinnitus

The head and facial areas are frequent sites for minor injuries, including lacerations, contusions, and mild concussions. Although intracranial injuries have been associated with sport-related fatalities, measures, such as increased standards in protective equipment, rule changes that prohibit leading with the head for contact, and the development and use of the face mask, have significantly decreased the incidence of these injuries since the mid-1970s (1). A significant decrease has also been seen in eye, ear, and dental injuries when protective equipment is worn.

This chapter begins with a review of the anatomy of the head and facial region. Discussions on preventive measures are followed by information on cranial injuries, their management, and protocol for a basic assessment of a head injury. The final section discusses common injuries to the facial area and their management.

ANATOMY REVIEW OF THE HEAD AND FACIAL REGION

? *A diver struck the board during a dive and sustained a superficial cut to the back of the head. The cut is bleeding profusely. What anatomical structure(s) are likely to have been damaged? How serious is this injury?*

The anatomy review will focuses on bony structure, the brain and its coverings, the eye, and the nerve and blood supply to the region. Although the numerous muscles of the face and jaw enable speaking, chewing, and facial expression, and because these muscles are not commonly involved in sport injuries, they are not discussed in this chapter.

Bones of the Skull

> The cranium is divided from the face by an imaginary line that runs above the eyes and around the back of the ears

The skull is primarily composed of flat bones that interlock at immovable joints called sutures (**Fig. 14.1**). The bones that form the portion of the skull referred to as the cranium protect the brain. These thin bones include the frontal, occipital, sphenoid, and ethmoid bones, as well as two parietal bones and two temporal

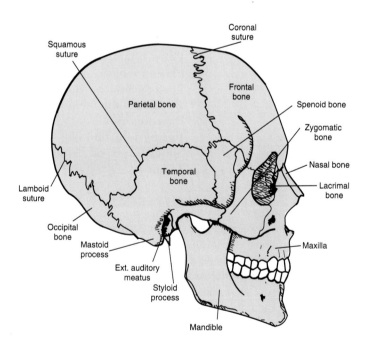

Figure 14.1. The bones of the skull.

bones. The facial bones provide the structure of the face and form the sinuses, orbits of the eyes, nasal cavity, and mouth. These bones include the paired maxilla, zygomatic, palatine, nasal, lacrimal, and inferior nasal concha bones, along with the bridge and mandible. The large opening at the base of the skull that sits atop the spinal column is called the foramen magnum.

The Scalp

The scalp is composed of three layers: the skin, subcutaneous connective tissue, and the pericranium. The protective function of these tissues is enhanced by the hair and the looseness of the scalp that enables some dissipation of force when the head sustains a glancing blow. The scalp and face have an extensive blood supply, which is why even superficial lacerations tend to bleed profusely.

The Brain

The four major regions of the brain are the cerebral hemispheres, diencephalon, brainstem, and cerebellum. The entire brain and spinal cord are enclosed in three layers of protective tissue known collectively as the **meninges (Fig. 14.2)**. The outermost membrane is the dura mater, a thick, fibrous tissue containing **dural sinuses** that act as veins to transport blood from the brain to the jugular veins of the neck. The arachnoid mater is a thin membrane internal to the dura mater, separated from the dura mater by the subdural space. Beneath the arachnoid mater is the subarachnoid space, which is filled with cerebrospinal fluid (CSF) and contains the largest of the blood vessels supplying the brain. The arachnoid mater is connected to the inner pia mater by web-like strands of connective tissue. Whereas the dura mater and arachnoid mater

Meninges
Three protective membranes that surround the brain and spinal cord

Dural sinuses
Formed by tubular separations in the inner and outer layers of the dura mater, these sinuses function as small veins for the brain

The meninges include the dura mater, arachnoid mater, and pia mater

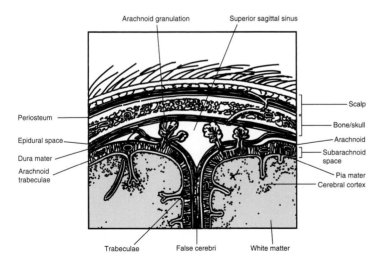

Figure 14.2. The meninges.

are rather loose membranes, the pia mater is in direct contact with the cerebral cortex. The pia mater contains numerous small blood vessels.

The Eyes

The eye is a hollow sphere, approximately 2.5 cm (1 in) in diameter in adults (**Fig. 14.3**). The anterior eye surface receives protection from the eyelids, eyelashes, and the attached conjunctiva. The conjunctiva lines the eyelids and external surface of the eye and secretes mucus to lubricate the external eye. The lacrimal glands, located above the lateral ends of the eyes, continually release tears across the eye surface through several small ducts. The lacrimal ducts, located at the medial corners of the eyes, serve as drains for the moisture. These ducts funnel the moisture into the lacrimal sac and eventually into the nasal cavity.

The anterior eye receives protection from the eyelids, eyelashes, and the attached conjunctiva

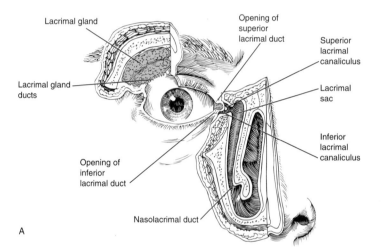

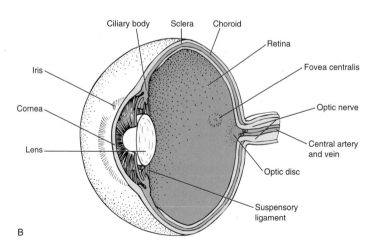

Figure 14.3. A, B. The eye.

Like the brain, the eye is surrounded by three protective tissue layers. The outer thick, white connective tissue is the sclera that forms the "white of the eye." The cornea, found in the central anterior part of the sclera, is clear to permit passage of light into the eye. The choroid, the middle covering, is a highly vascularized tissue, which, on the anterior eye, usually appears blue or brown and contains the pupil. The iris controls the size of the pupil, regulating the amount of light that enters the eye. The internal protective layer is the retina, which contains light-sensitive photoreceptor cells that stimulate nerve endings to provide sight.

Nerves and Blood Vessels of the Head and Face

Twelve pairs of cranial nerves emerge from the brain, some with motor functions, some with sensory functions, and some with both. The cranial nerves are numbered and named in accordance with their functions, as listed in **Table 14.1**.

The major vessels supplying the head and face are the common carotid and vertebral arteries (**Fig. 14.4**). The common carotid artery ascends through the neck on either side to divide into an external and internal carotid artery just below the level of the jaw. The external carotid artery and its branches supply most regions of the head external to the brain. Of particular importance, the middle meningeal artery supplies the skull and dura mater and, if damaged, serious epidural bleeding can result. The internal carotid arteries send branches to the eyes and supply portions of the cerebral hemispheres and the parietal and temporal lobes of the cerebrum. The left and right vertebral arteries and their branches supply blood to the posterior region of the brain.

The common carotid artery is superficial on the lateral anterior aspect of the neck just below the jaw, where it may be readily palpated. Severance of this major artery can result in death in a matter of minutes

Table 14.1. The Cranial Nerves

Number	Name	Sensory	Motor	Function
I	Olfactory	X		Sense of smell
II	Optic	X		Vision
III	Oculomotor		X	Control of some of the extrinsic eye muscles
IV	Trochlear		X	Control of other of the extrinsic eye muscles
V	Trigeminal	X	X	Sensation in the facial region and movement of the jaw muscles
VI	Abducens		X	Control of lateral eye movement
VII	Facial	X	X	Control of facial movement, taste, and secretion of tears and saliva
VIII	Vestibulocochlear	X		Hearing and equilibrium
IX	Glossopharyngeal	X	X	Taste, control of the tongue and pharynx, secretion of saliva
X	Vagus	X		Taste, sensation to the pharynx, larynx, trachea, and bronchioles
XI	Accessory		X	Control of movements of the pharynx, larynx, head, and shoulders
XII	Hypoglossal		X	Control of tongue movements

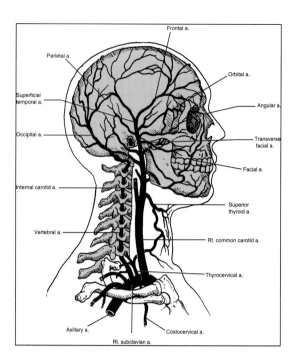

Figure 14.4. The blood supply to the head—right lateral view.

💡 *Because the scalp and face have an extensive blood supply, superficial lacerations of the head tend to bleed profusely. If there are no signs of a concussion (discussed later in this chapter), the injury is probably a superficial cut of the scalp.*

PREVENTION OF INJURIES

❓ *What steps can a football player take to prevent head and facial injuries?*

In reviewing measures normally taken to prevent injuries at the joints (i.e., protective equipment, physical conditioning, and proper skill technique), the most important preventative measure for the head and facial area, by far, is use of protective equipment. Many sports require some type of head or facial protective equipment. Protective equipment, when properly used, can protect the head and facial area from accidental or routine injuries. Even regular use, however, cannot prevent all injuries. To be effective, equipment must be properly fitted, clean, in good condition, utilized regularly, and used in a manner for which it was designed. Refer to Chapter 6 to review head and facial protection.

> To be effective, equipment must be properly fitted, clean, in good condition, utilized regularly, and used in a manner for which it was designed to be used

💡 *A football player can protect the head and facial region by wearing a face guard and helmet that is approved by the National Operating Committee for Athletic Equipment (NOC-SAE). In addition, protective eye wear and a mouthguard can be worn to protect the eyes and oral region.*

CRANIAL INJURY MECHANISMS

If a batter is struck in the head by a baseball, what happens to the skull and brain during impact? Will damage be limited to the area directly under the point of impact?

The occurrence of a skull fracture or intracranial injury is dependent on the material properties of the skull, thickness of the skull in the specific area, magnitude and direction of impact, and size of the impact area (2). In Chapter 2, you learned that direct impact causes two phenomena to occur—deformation and acceleration. When a blow impacts the skull, the bone deforms and bends inward, placing the inner border of the skull under tensile strain, whereas the outer border is placed in compression **(Fig. 14.5A)**. If impact is of sufficient magnitude and the skull is thin in the region of impact, a skull fracture will occur at the site where tensile loading occurs. In contrast, if the skull is thick and dense enough at the area of impact, it may sustain inward bending without fracture. Fracture may then occur some distance from the impact zone in a region where the skull is thinner **(Fig. 14.5B)**.

On impact, shock waves pass through the skull to the brain, causing acceleration. This acceleration can lead to shear, tensile, and compression strains within the brain substance, with shear

> Skull fractures are dependent on the material properties of the skull, thickness of the skull in various areas, magnitude and direction of impact, and size of the impact area

> Acceleration forces cause shear, tensile, and compression strains within the brain substance, with shear being the most serious

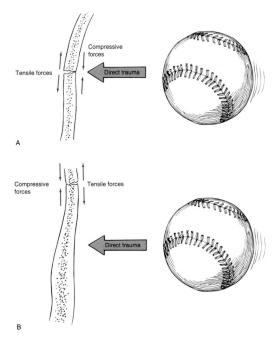

Figure 14.5. Mechanical failure in bone. When a blow impacts the skull, the bone deforms and bends inward, placing tensile stress on the inner border of the skull. **A.** If impact is of sufficient magnitude and the skull is thin in the region of impact, a skull fracture occurs at the impact site. **B.** If the skull is thick and dense enough at the area of impact, it may sustain inward bending without fracture. However, the fracture may occur some distance from the impact zone, in a region where the skull is thinner.

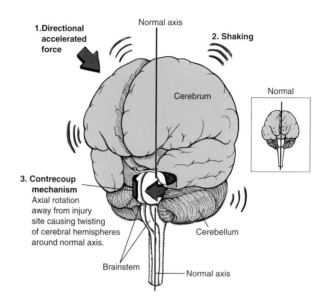

Figure 14.6. Axial rotation coupled with acceleration is called a contrecoup injury and can lead to injuries away from the actual injury site.

Contrecoup injuries
Injuries away from the actual injury site due to axial rotation and acceleration

Focal injuries
Injuries in a small, concentrated area, usually due to high-velocity–low-mass forces

Diffuse injuries
Injury over a large body area, usually due to low-velocity–high-mass forces

being the most serious (2). Axial rotation coupled with acceleration can lead to **contrecoup injuries (Fig. 14.6)**, or injuries away from the actual injury site.

Cerebral trauma may lead to **focal injuries** involving only localized damage (i.e., epidural, subdural, or intracerebral hematomas), or **diffuse injuries** that involve widespread disruption and damage to the function and/or structure of the brain, such as a cerebral concussion (3). Although diffuse injuries account for only one-quarter of the fatalities due to head trauma, they are the most prevalent cause of long-term neurologic deficits in individuals (2).

Impact forces cause skull deformation and shock waves to pass through the skull to the brain. Rotation, coupled with acceleration, causes shear, tensile, and compression strains elsewhere in the brain. As such, the probability exists that damage will occur at the point of impact and at a point away from the site of impact as a contrecoup injury.

SKULL FRACTURES

During hitting practice, a foul tip struck the head of another baseball player standing near the dugout. The skin is not broken, but the individual is complaining of an intense headache, disorientation, blurred vision, and cannot recall what happened. Do these signs indicate that a skull fracture may be present?

Skull fractures may be *linear* (in a line), *comminuted* (in multiple pieces), *depressed* (fragments are driven internally toward the brain), or *basilar* (involving the base of the skull) **(Fig. 14.7)**. If there is a break in the skin adjacent to the fracture site and a tear

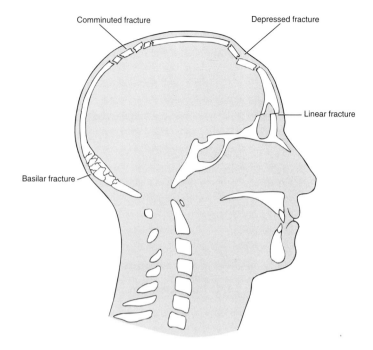

Figure 14.7. Fractures of the skull are categorized as linear, comminuted, depressed, or basilar.

Labels on figure:
- Comminuted fracture
- Depressed fracture
- Linear fracture
- Basilar fracture

to the underlying dura mater, there is a high risk of bacterial infection into the intracranial cavity, which can result in septic **meningitis**. Whenever a severe blow to the head occurs, a skull fracture should always be suspected.

Depending on the fracture site, different signs may appear. For example, a fracture at eyebrow level may travel into the anterior cranial fossa and sinuses, leading to discoloration around the eyes (**raccoon eyes**). Blood or CSF may leak from the nose. Bony fragments may damage the optic or olfactory cranial nerves, leading to blindness or loss of smell. A basilar fracture above and behind the ear may lead to **Battle's sign**, a discoloration that can appear within minutes behind the ear. In addition, blood or CSF may leak from the ear canal and a hearing loss or facial paralysis may be present. A fracture to the temple region may damage the meningeal arteries, causing epidural bleeding between the dura mater and skull (epidural hematoma). This can be life-threatening and will be discussed in more detail in the section on cerebral injuries. **Table 14.2** summarizes signs and symptoms indicating a possible skull fracture.

A suspected skull fracture requires immediate action. Immediately initiate the emergency care plan and summon an ambulance. If fluids from the ears or nose are present, do not apply any pressure bandage or attempt to restrict the flow, as it may increase intracranial pressure, complicating the injury. Cover open wounds with a sterile dressing but do not apply pressure. Stabilize the

Meningitis
Inflammation of the meninges of the brain and spinal column

A danger with open fractures is the risk of bacterial infection that can result in septic meningitis

Raccoon eyes
Delayed discoloration around the eyes from anterior cranial fossa fracture

Battle's sign
Delayed discoloration behind the ear due to basilar skull fracture

Table 14.2. Identifying Possible Skull Fractures

Suspect a Skull Fracture if Any of the Following Are Present

Deep laceration or severe bruise to the scalp
Visible deformity
Bleeding or clear fluid (CFS) from the nose and/or ear
Discoloration under both eyes (raccoon eyes) or behind the ear (Battle's sign)
Unequal pupils
Palpable depression or crepitus is present
Loss of smell, sight, or major vision disturbances
Individual is unconscious for more than 2 minutes after direct trauma to the head

---

 Field Strategy 14.1. Management of a Suspected Skull Fracture

Stabilize the head and neck
Check the ABCs
Initiate emergency care plan and summon EMS
Take vital signs
Observe for:
 Swelling or discoloration around the eyes or behind the ears
 Blood or CSF leaking from the nose or ears
 Pupil size, pupillary response to light, and eye movement
Palpate for depressions, blood, and crepitus. Palpate cervical vertebrae for associated neck injury
Cover any open wounds with a sterile dressing, but do not apply pressure
Treat for shock and monitor ABCs every 5 minutes, until ambulance arrives

---

neck region, as it may also be injured. Monitor vital signs, initiate any emergency procedures (artificial ventilation or CPR), and treat for shock until help arrives. **Field Strategy 14.1** suggests management of a suspected skull fracture.

Signs that indicate a possible skull fracture include deformity, unequal pupils, discoloration around both eyes or behind the ears, bleeding or CSF leaking from the nose and/or ear, and any loss of sight or smell. If any of these signs are present, summon an ambulance immediately.

CEREBRAL HEMATOMAS

A soccer goalie collided with the goal post and is dazed and shaking the head. After removing the player to ice the region, the athlete is complaining of an increasing headache and is feeling nauseous. The player appears lethargic, disoriented, and sensitive to sunlight. What might be happening?

A hematoma is a collection of blood, or a blood clot, in a localized area. Within the skull there is no room for additional accumulation of blood or fluid. Any additional matter within the cranial cavity increases pressure on the brain, leading to significant alterations in neurologic function. Depending on the location of the accumulated blood relative to the dura mater, these hematomas are classified as epidural (outside the dura mater), or subdural (deep to the dura mater).

Hematomas within the skull are classified in relation to the dura mater and include epidural (outside the dura mater) or subdural (inside the dura mater)

Epidural Hematoma

An epidural hematoma, typically caused by a direct blow to the side of the head, is almost always associated with a skull fracture **(Fig. 14.8A)**. If the middle meningeal artery or its branches are severed, the subsequent arterial bleeding will lead to a "high-pressure" epidural hematoma. The athlete will have an initial loss of consciousness at the time of injury, followed by a lucid interval in which the athlete feels relatively normal, but within 10 to 20 minutes, a decline in mental status occurs (4). Signs and symptoms may include increased headache, drowsiness, nausea, vomiting, a decreased level of consciousness, a dilated pupil on the side of the hematoma, and contralateral extremity weakness or decerebrate posture (3,4). Immediate surgery is needed to **decompress** the hematoma and control arterial bleeding.

Epidural hematomas frequently involve tearing the middle meningeal artery, leading to high-pressure bleeding, whereas subdural hematomas resulting from contrecoup injuries tear bridging veins, leading to low-pressure venous bleeding

Decompression
Surgical release of pressure caused by fluid or blood accumulation

Subdural Hematoma

Subdural hematomas occur at approximately three times the rate of epidural hematomas and are a result of the acceleration forces of the head and not of the impact of the force (4). Hemorrhaging occurs deep to the dura mater and involves bleeding from a cerebral vein rather than an artery **(Fig. 14.8B)**. As impact occurs, the brain is thrust against the point of impact, tearing veins on the opposite side, causing low-pressure venous bleeding that clots very slowly. Signs and symptoms may not become apparent for hours, days, or even weeks after injury, when the clot absorbs fluid and expands (5). Because of delayed signs and symptoms, this injury is the most prevalent cause of death from trauma in contact sports. Thus, the coach or athletic trainer must be suspicious of a blow to the head and carefully watch the person for delayed complications. **Table 14.3** is an example of an information sheet that can be given to parents of minor children who have sustained a head injury. This information should inform parents of danger signs that indicate a serious problem and can alert parents to seek immediate medical treatment should the condition deteriorate.

The soccer goalie is experiencing an increase in intracranial pressure, possibly due to an epidural hematoma. Disorientation, headache, and nausea are red flags indicating serious intracranial hemorrhage. Summon EMS to transport this individual to the nearest medical facility.

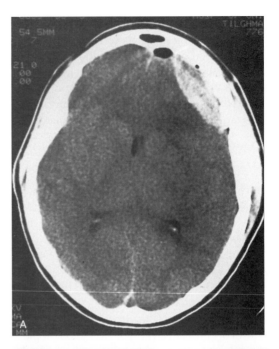

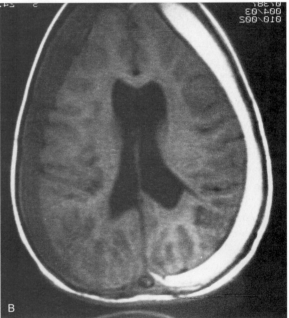

Figure 14.8. Cerebral hematomas. **A.** This epidural hematoma resulted from a fracture that extended into the orbital roof and sinus area, leading to rapid hemorrhage in the right frontal lobe of the brain. **B.** The subdural hematoma on the right side of the brain is fairly evident; however, note the darkened area on the far left side of the brain. This indicates bilateral subdural hematomas of different ages.

Table 14.3. Information Sheet on Follow-up Care for a Head Injury

_____ has recently received a head injury during an interscholastic athletic practice. Often many signs and symptoms from a head injury do not become apparent until hours after the initial trauma. As such, we want to alert you to possible signs and symptoms that may indicate a significant head injury. If you observe any of these symptoms, please seek medical help immediately.

Persistent or increasing headache, nausea, and/or vomiting
Restless and irritable, or drastic changes in emotional control
Increasing mental confusion, dizziness, or drowsiness
Difficulty speaking, or slurring of speech
Loss of appetite
Unequal pupils or dilated pupils
Bleeding and/or clear fluid from the nose or ears
Alterations in breathing pattern
Progressive or sudden impairment of consciousness

For the rest of the day _____ should:

Rest quietly
Not consume any medication except Tylenol as prescribed
Not consume alcohol
Not drive a vehicle

She/He should not participate or play again without medical clearance by a doctor.

Emergency Phone Numbers:
Ambulance   911
Hospital _____
Remember: If any of the symptoms or signs listed above become apparent, do not delay seeking medical treatment.

CONCUSSIONS

? _A swimmer misjudged the distance to the wall and collided head-first into the wall. The individual was momentarily stunned, "saw stars," and had blurred vision for about 30 seconds. After 3 or 4 minutes, the individual reports feeling much better, except for a slight headache. Can this individual return to activity?_

A "**concussion**" literally means a violent shaking or jarring action that can result in immediate or transient impairment of neurological function. This condition does not always involve loss of consciousness. Under normal conditions, the brain balances a series of electrochemical events in billions of brain cells. When shaken or jarred, brain function can be disrupted temporarily without causing injury or damage to the brain tissue. For example, with mild trauma, cerebral function is first interrupted. Signs and symptoms range from mild to moderate, and are transient and reversible, since damage to soft tissue structures is minimal. As impact magnitude increases with an acceleration injury, both cerebral function and structural damage occurs, resulting in more serious signs and symptoms. These include varying degrees of consciousness, headache, memory loss, nausea, **tinnitus**, pupillary changes, confusion, dizziness, and loss of coordination. Concus-

Concussion
Violent shaking or jarring action of the brain, resulting in immediate or transient impairment of neurologic function

Concussions are graded by the length of mental impairment and loss of memory before and after the injury

Tinnitus
Ringing or other noises in the ear due to trauma or disease

sions are graded by the length of mental impairment and loss of memory before and after injury. The various grades of concussions are summarized in **Table 14.4**. Grades I and II are mild concussions, grade III is a moderate concussion, and grades IV and V are severe concussions. Grade VI concussions are associated with death.

Grade I Concussion

A grade I concussion involves no loss of consciousness, but there may be slight mental confusion, dizziness, unsteadiness, and a brief loss of judgement. The individual may simply report "I had my bell rung." Usually the state of confusion is over within 5 to 15 minutes and the individual can return to sport participation, but should be carefully watched for any signs of deterioration. Symptoms such as an unsteady gait, headache, nausea, or **photophobia** should preclude the individual from returning to activity

Photophobia
Abnormal sensitivity to light

Table 14.4. Signs and Symptoms of Concussions

Degree of Concussion	Mild		Moderate	Severe	
	Grade I	Grade II	Grade III	Grade IV	Grade V
Loss of consciousness	None	Few seconds up to 3 to 4 minutes	Unconscious for 2 to 5 minutes, or may appear normal, then suddenly collapse	Involves being "knocked-out." May appear in paralytic coma and pass through stages of stupor	Person in paralytic coma. May need CPR
Headache	None	Mild	Moderate	Severe	Convulsions may occur
Confusion	Slight	Mild	Moderate	Severe	Initially severe; then may become alert
Dizziness	Slight	Moderate	Moderate	Severe	Severe
Memory loss	None	Posttraumatic amnesia is transient and reversible	Posttraumatic amnesia and 5 to 15 minutes retrograde amnesia present	Posttraumatic amnesia and retrograde amnesia present	Posttraumatic amnesia, retrograde amnesia, and postconcussion syndrome present
Nausea	None	Slight	Present	Present	Present
Tinnitus	None	Slight	Moderate	Severe	Severe
Pupils/vision	Normal	Normal pupils; blurred vision	One or both pupils dilated; nystagmus and photophobia present	One or both pupils dilated; nystagmus and photophobia present	Both pupils dilated initially, but may appear unequal later
Balance problems	Slight	Mild with positive special tests	Moderate with positive special tests	Severe with positive special tests	

(3,4). A second mild concussion during the same game, or within a few days, should mandate removal from activity for about 2 weeks (6). All symptoms should be absent for 1 week before the individual is allowed to return to participation.

Grade II Concussion

With a grade II concussion, there is a transitory loss of consciousness lasting from a few seconds up to 3 to 4 minutes, followed by mental confusion, moderate dizziness, unsteady gait, blurred vision, tinnitus, and headache. **Posttraumatic memory loss**, a very common symptom, develops after 5 to 15 minutes. This athlete should not continue to play that day. They may develop "**postconcussion syndrome**," which can last for several weeks and may involve persistent headaches, blurred vision, irritability, and an inability to concentrate even on the simplest task. This individual should be thoroughly evaluated by a physician.

Grade III Concussion

With a grade III concussion, the individual will experience many of the symptoms in a grade II concussion. Unconsciousness will last more than 2 minutes and can extend up to 5 minutes. If examined immediately after injury, the individual may have total recall of events prior to the injury, but as the condition deteriorates, **retrograde amnesia** develops (3,4). One or both eyes may appear dilated or irregular, be sensitive to light, and exhibit involuntary eye movement (**nystagmus**). The individual may appear fine during the evaluation, but later may suddenly collapse. An individual who is unable to remember events leading up to the injury or events following the injury should not be permitted to continue play, and should be referred immediately to a physician.

Grade IV Concussion

A grade IV concussion is characterized as being "knocked out." An inability to stimulate movement can last a few seconds to several minutes. When they regain consciousness, they appear confused, then pass through a lucid state before becoming fully alert and oriented to the surroundings. Posttraumatic memory loss or retrograde amnesia may also be present. In addition, convulsions may occur (6). If unconsciousness lasts greater than 5 minutes or if other neurologic deficits become apparent, summon EMS to place the athlete on a spineboard or stretcher, and transport them to the nearest medical facility.

Grade V Concussion

Impact, acceleration, and shearing forces can lead to severe diffuse cerebral injuries when the blood vessels rupture within the cranial cavity. The resulting coma may be associated with altered vital signs, unequal pupils, partial paralysis on one side of the body,

Posttraumatic memory loss
Forgetting events after an injury

Postconcussion syndrome
Delayed condition characterized by persistent headaches, blurred vision, irritability, and inability to concentrate

Retrograde amnesia
Forgetting events that happened before an injury

Nystagmus
Abnormal jerking or involuntary eye movement

An individual who cannot remember events leading up to the injury or after the injury should be referred immediately to a physician

body posturing (see **Fig. 3.7**), or cardiorespiratory impairment. Summon EMS for immediate transportation to the nearest medical facility.

Grade VI Concussion

Severe head trauma in a grade V concussion can lead to massive intracranial bleeding, total cardiorespiratory collapse, and death.

Second Impact Syndrome

Second impact syndrome (SIS) occurs when an athlete who has sustained an initial head injury, usually a concussion, sustains a second head injury before the symptoms associated from the previous injury have totally resolved. Although the condition is often linked to football, it can occur in any contact sport. In the initial injury, visual, motor, or sensory changes occur, and the individual may have difficulty with thought and memory. Before these symptoms resolve, which may take days or weeks, the individual returns to competition and receives a second blow to the head (7). This second blow may be relatively minor. The athlete may appear stunned, but often completes the play and sometimes walks off the field under his or her own power. As the vascular engorgement within the cranium increases the intracranial pressure, the brainstem becomes compromised. The athlete collapses with rapidly dilating pupils, loss of eye movement, coma, and respiratory failure ensues. The usual time from second impact to brainstem failure is rapid, usually 2 to 5 minutes (7). It is imperative that any athlete who complains of headache, light-headedness, visual disturbances, or other neurologic symptoms should not be allowed to participate in any athletic event in which head trauma may occur until they are totally asymptomatic.

The individual was momentarily stunned, "saw stars," and had blurred vision. This is not uncommon in a grade I concussion. A lingering headache, however, should signal caution. This individual can return to activity, but should be watched for any deterioration of symptoms.

SCALP INJURIES

An individual has a scalp laceration that is bleeding freely. What concerns must be kept in mind when dealing with an open head wound?

The scalp is the outermost anatomical structure of the cranium and is the first area of contact to receive trauma. It is highly vascular and bleeds freely, making it a frequent site for abrasions, lacerations, contusions, or hematomas between the layers of tissue. The primary concern with any scalp laceration is to control bleeding, prevent contamination, and determine if it is a possible skull fracture. As with any open wound, latex gloves should be worn as part of universal precautions. Apply mild, direct pressure with sterile gauze until bleeding has stopped. Inspect the wound for any foreign bodies or signs of a skull fracture. If a skull fracture is ruled out, cleanse the wound with surgical soap or saline solution, cover the wound with a sterile dressing, and refer the individual to a physician for possible suturing.

Abrasions and contusions can be treated with gentle cleansing, topical antiseptics, and ice to control hemorrhage. Hematomas, or "goose eggs," require a more thorough assessment. These injuries involve a collection of blood between the layers of the scalp and skull. Treatment with ice and a pressure bandage to control hemorrhage is usually sufficient to care for the injury. With a possible skull fracture, use of a pressure bandage is contraindicated. The individual should be referred to a physician for examination.

The primary concern with any scalp laceration is to control bleeding, prevent contamination, and determine a possible skull fracture. If you suspect a possible skull fracture, summon EMS to transport the individual to the nearest medical facility.

> With lacerations of the scalp, control bleeding, prevent contamination, and determine a possible skull fracture

ASSESSMENT OF CRANIAL INJURIES

A gymnast fell from the parallel bars and hit the head on a support. The individual is somewhat disoriented, dizzy, and has a slight headache, but vision appears to be normal. How will you assess the severity of this injury?

Head trauma demands immediate assessment for life-threatening conditions. In Chapter 3, primary and secondary assessment included establishing and maintaining the ABCs and determining the level of consciousness. In head injuries, this encompasses gathering a history, observing and inspecting the head and facial area, and assessing motor control. These components are not separate and distinct, but rather occur simultaneously. For matters of clarity, these components are presented in separate parts of this section.

Because significant head trauma may also cause cervical injury, always assume a cervical neck injury is present. As you approach the individual, gather a brief history of the mechanism of injury, duration of unconsciousness, and any other pertinent information from individuals at the scene. Never place ammonia capsules under the nose to arouse the person, as they may jerk the head and neck, leading to serious complications if a spinal injury is present. Establish and maintain an open airway. If the individual is face down, stabilize the head and neck, and log roll the individual to a supine position and stabilize the cervical spine. A face mask should be removed but do not remove the helmet or chin strap. Any mouth guard, dentures, or partial plates should be removed to prevent occluding the airway. Begin rescue breathing and CPR as needed.

> Because significant head trauma may also cause cervical injury, always assume a cervical neck injury is present

Vital signs, history of the injury, observation, inspection, and general assessment are then used to judge the magnitude of a cerebral injury. A practical measure commonly used to quantify

> Vital signs, history of the injury, observation, inspection, and general assessment are used to judge the magnitude of a cerebral injury

the level of consciousness in head trauma is the Glasgow Coma Scale (**Table 14.5**). This scale measures the individual's ability to open and move the eyes, talk to you, and do voluntary muscle movement on command. A numerical score is given for the best response. For example, eyes that open spontaneously are given a score of 4; to a verbal command, a 3; to pain, a 2; and no response, with the eyes remaining closed, a score of 1. Motor response is given a 6 if the person responds to a verbal command. Otherwise, values are assessed depending on how the individual responds to painful stimuli (e.g., pinching under the arms, or knuckle to the sternum). Verbal response that is coherent and clear is given a 5, with the remaining values dependent on quality of speech or sentence structure. Total scores range from 3 to 15. A score of 12 or more is considered to be a mild injury, 9 to 11 is a moderate injury, and 8 or less is considered a serious head injury.

Vital Signs

Vital signs should be taken early in the assessment to establish a baseline of information that can be periodically rechecked to determine if the individual's status is improving or deteriorating. Vital signs include pulse, respiration, blood pressure, and body temperature; however, with head trauma, body temperature is not as critical as the others. In addition, skin color, pupillary response to light, and eye movement should be documented and

Table 14.5. Glasgow Coma Scale[a]

Eyes	Open	Spontaneously	4
		To verbal command	3
		To pain	2
		No response	1
Best motor response	To verbal commands	Obeys	6
	To painful stimulus[b]	Localizes pain	5
		Flexion—withdrawal	4
		Flexion—abnormal (decorticate rigidity)	3
		Extension (decerebrate rigidity)	2
		No response	1
Best verbal response[c]		Oriented and converses	5
		Disoriented and converses	4
		Inappropriate words	3
		Incomprehensible sounds	2
		No response	1
Total			3–15

[a]The Glasgow Coma Scale is based on eye opening, motor, and verbal response, and is used to monitor changes in level of consciousness. If response on the scale is given a number, then responsiveness of the injured party can be expressed by totalling the figures. Lowest score is 3; highest is 15. A score of 12 or greater is considered to be a mild injury, 9 to 11 is a moderate injury, and 8 or less is a severe head injury
[b]Squeeze trapezius, pinch soft tissue between thumb and forefinger or in the axilla, knuckle to sternum; observe arms
[c]Arouse injured party with painful stimulus if necessary

will be discussed in the following sections. Any abnormal variations indicate a serious injury. Summon EMS and proceed with the secondary assessment.

History

While gathering information on the mechanism of injury and symptoms, assess the level of consciousness, ability to recall events (amnesia), and pupil abnormalities. Remember to stabilize the head and neck throughout the assessment. Call the person's name, gently tap them on the cheek, or touch the arm. You may have to shout loudly to get a response.

1. **Mechanism of injury**. Ask the individual what happened. Can the individual remember what position they were in and the direction of impact? If the individual is unable to respond or is confused, ask others what happened.
2. **Loss of consciousness**. Did the individual lose consciousness? How long were they unconscious? Did it occur immediately or did the person progress to unconsciousness? Is the individual unresponsive, confused, or disoriented? Do they respond to painful stimuli (e.g., squeezing the trapezius, pinching soft tissue between the thumb and index finger in the axilla, knuckle to the sternum, or squeezing the Achilles tendon)? Has the individual ever had a head injury before? When? How bad was it?
3. **Amnesia.** Start with simple questions, then progress to more difficult questions (e.g., date, time, what they had for breakfast, or what play was called before the injury). Confusion indicates a grade I concussion. Loss of memory for events immediately after the injury (posttraumatic amnesia) indicates a grade II concussion. Loss of memory for events prior to (retrograde amnesia) and immediately after the injury indicate a grade III concussion. Amnesia may not become apparent until 5 to 15 minutes after trauma, so continue to reassess the status of the individual.
4. **Pupil abnormalities**. Note pupil size and accommodation to light; both should be equal. A one-sided dilated pupil may indicate a subdural or epidural hematoma. Bilateral dilated pupils indicates severe cranial injury with death imminent. Ask the individual to look up, down, and sideways, while you observe the fluid motion of both eyes. Is there blurred or double vision? Did the person see "stars" or flashes of light on impact? Vision difficulties indicate the cranial nerves that innervate the eye and eye muscles are affected.

> Blurred or double vision, or uncoordinated eye movement, indicates disturbance to the cranial nerves that innervate the eye and eye muscles

5. **Headache**. Does the individual have a headache or ringing in the ears? Progressive headaches indicate increasing intracranial pressure and signal danger.
6. **Nausea and/or vomiting**. Intracranial pressure can stimulate the reflex onset of nausea and vomiting and signals a fairly serious injury.

7. **Associated neck injury**. Is there pain, numbness, or weakness elsewhere in the body? Is grip strength bilaterally equal? Can sharp and dull sensations be distinguished?

Observation and Inspection

Observe facial expression and function. Cranial nerve integrity can be assessed through sense of smell, vision, eye tracking, smiling, clenching the jaw, hearing, balance, taste, speaking, and strength of shoulder shrugs. Watch the face and note any slurred speech, difficulty in constructing sentences, or inability to understand commands. Continue to watch the eyes for neurologic signs indicating increasing intracranial pressure.

1. **Leakage of cerebrospinal fluid (CSF).** CSF is a clear, colorless fluid that protects and cushions the brain and spinal cord. A basilar fracture may result in bleeding and CSF leaking from the ear. A fracture in the anterior cranial area may result in bleeding and CSF leaking from the nose.
2. **Signs of trauma**. Look for discoloration around the eyes (raccoon's eyes) and behind the ears (Battle's sign) that may indicate a skull fracture. Note any depressions, elevations, or bleeding indicating a skull fracture, laceration, or hematoma. Listen for snoring, which may occur as a result of a fracture to the anterior cranial floor.
3. **Skin color**. Note skin color and presence of moisture. If shock is setting in, the skin may appear ashen or pale, and may be moist and cool.
4. **Loss of emotional control**. Irritability, aggressive behavior, or uncontrolled crying should signal immediate referral to a physician.

Palpation

Most of the vital information will be gained in the vital signs, history, and observation portion of the assessment. Palpations can help pinpoint possible skull or facial fractures. Palpate for point tenderness, crepitus, depressions, elevations, swelling, blood, or changes in skin temperature. The following sites can be palpated:

1. Scalp and hair
2. Cervical spinous process
3. Base of the skull and around the external ear
4. Frontal bone, eye orbit, and bridge of the nose
5. Zygomatic arch (cheek)
6. Upper and lower jaw

Special tests assess coordination, balance, depth perception, and logical thought processes by having the individual respond to simple commands

Special Tests

These special tests assess brain function through coordination, balance, depth perception, and logical thought processes by having the individual respond to simple commands. If the assessment has already determined a possible intracranial or spinal injury, do not subject the individual to these tests. Immobilize the head and neck and transport the individual to the nearest medical facility. The following tests may be performed:

1. **100 minus 7 test**. This tests one's ability to concentrate. The individual is asked to start at 100 and subtract 7, then subtract 7 from that number, and so on. This can be adapted to other mathematical problems. Start with 3 and multiply by factors of 3, or start at 100 and subtract by 5 each time.
2. **Finger to nose test**. To test depth perception and the ability to focus on an object, hold a finger in front of the injured individual. Ask the individual to reach out and touch it, alternating touching between the right and left hand (**Fig. 14.9**). Change the position of your finger after two or three touches. A variation is to ask the individual to touch their nose between each touch of your finger. Progressively increase the speed of touch between the nose and your finger.
3. **Romberg test**. Ask the individual to stand with the feet together, arms at the side, and eyes closed while maintaining balance (**Fig. 14.10**). Variations include raising the arms at 90°, standing on the toes, or touching the nose with the hand while the eyes are closed. From an anterior view, observe if a body sway occurs, indicating a positive test.
4. **Stork stand**. With the eyes closed, have the individual stand on one leg.
5. **Heel/toe walking**. Ask the individual to walk on the toes, then the heels. Note any swaying or inability to walk in a straight line.

Determination of Findings

If the individual is not in a crisis situation, vital signs and special tests should be completed every 5 to 7 minutes to determine progress of the condition. If physical signs and symptoms improve

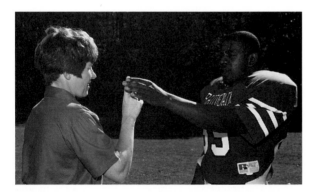

Figure 14.9. Finger to nose test. Ask the person to alternately touch their nose and touch your finger. Progressively increase the speed of touch.

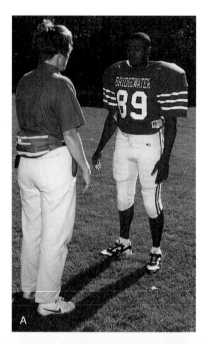

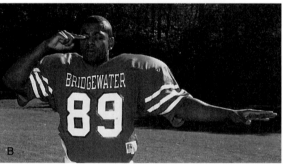

Figure 14.10. To perform the Romberg test, the person should be able to maintain balance while standing with the eyes closed (**A**). Variations may include raising the arms to the side, standing on the toes, or touching the nose with a finger (**B**). A tendency to sway is a positive sign.

or appear normal, the individual may return to play. If signs and symptoms linger but appear minor, an individual close to the injured party, such as a parent or roommate, should be informed of the injury and told to look for changes in behavior, unsteady gait, slurring of speech, a progressive headache or nausea, restlessness, mental confusion, or drowsiness. These danger signs should be fully explained to the observer orally and documented on an information sheet, such as the one demonstrated in **Table 14.2**. **Field Strategy 14.2** summarizes a cranial injury assessment and lists signs that indicate emergency action is needed.

Field Strategy 14.2. Cranial Injury Evaluation

Primary Survey

Stabilize head and neck and check the ABCs
If a helmet is worn, remove the face mask, but do not remove the helmet
   or chin strap
Determine initial level of consciousness

Secondary Survey

Vital signs. Check pulse, respiration, and blood pressure
History
   Mechanism of injury
   Loss of consciousness (dizziness, disorientation, confusion)
   Presence of posttraumatic and/or retrograde amnesia
   Pupil abnormalities (pupil size, response to light, eye movement, blurred
      vision)
   Headache, tinnitis, nausea and/or vomiting
Observation and inspection
   Obvious deformities and body posturing
   Discoloration around the eyes and behind the ears, bleeding and/or CSF
      from ears or nose, depressions or elevations, and skin color
   Observe facial expression and behavior of the individual (irritability or
      uncontrolled crying)
   Listen for snoring, slurred speech, or inability to organize thoughts
   Observe voluntary or involuntary movements in the extremities
Palpation
   Bony and soft tissue structures for point tenderness, crepitus,
      depressions, elevations, swelling, blood, or changes in skin
      temperature
Special tests
   Check for spinal injury (response to verbal commands, painful stimuli,
      grip strength, sensory ability)
   100 minus 7 test, or multiply by factors of 3
   Finger/nose coordination test, Romberg test, stork stand, and heel/toe
      walking
   Take vital signs and recheck every 5 minutes

Danger Signs that Indicate Emergency Action

Possible skull fracture:
   Bleeding and/or CSF from the ears or nose
   Raccoon eyes or Battle's sign
Persistent or increasing headache, nausea, and/or vomiting
Drastic changes in emotional control
Unequal pupils or dilated pupils that fail to react to light
Increasing mental confusion, dizziness, drowsiness, or prolonged amnesia
Difficulty speaking or slurring of speech
Progressive or sudden impairment of consciousness
Alterations in breathing pattern
Gradual increase in systolic blood pressure, or a decrease in diastolic
   blood pressure or pulse rate

Did you determine how to assess the gymnast with the head injury? Danger signs include progressive headache, amnesia, disorientation, or an unsteady gait. Refer to **Field Strategy 14.2** *for more danger signs.*

FACIAL INJURIES

A basketball player was accidentally struck in the jaw by an opposing player's elbow. Although the player was wearing a mouth guard, bleeding from the mouth is apparent and they are unable to close the jaw. What injury may have occurred?

Injuries to the cheek, nose, lips, and jaw are very common in sports with moving projectiles (sticks, racquets, bats, balls), in contact sports (football, rugby, or ice hockey), or in sports where collisions with objects occur (diving, skiing, hockey, swimming). Many of these injuries can be prevented by wearing properly fitted face masks and mouth guards. Because the facial area has a vast arterial system, lacerations bleed freely and rapid swelling often hides the true extent of injury.

Many jaw injuries can be prevented by wearing properly fitted face masks and mouth guards

Facial Soft Tissue Injuries

Facial contusions, abrasions, and lacerations are managed the same as elsewhere on the body. Contusions are treated with ice to control swelling and hemorrhage. With abrasions and lacerations, cleanse the wound with a saline solution, apply an antibiotic ointment, and cover with a sterile gauze dressing. In minor lacerations (less than 1 inch long and an eighth of an inch deep), application of butterfly bandages or Steri-strips can facilitate wound closure (see **Field Strategy 14.3**). Protect the area with sterile gauze and tape. The individual can return to participation, but, at the conclusion of the event, refer the individual to a physician to determine if sutures are needed. Larger and more complicated injuries, such as those with jagged edges or damage to nerves, veins, or bony structures, should be immediately referred to a physician.

Facial Fractures

Fractures to the mandible often involve a double fracture or a fracture-dislocation

Mandibular fractures are the third most common facial fracture associated with sports participation, behind nasal and zygomatic fractures (6). They seldom occur as an isolated single fracture, but rather occur as a double fracture or fracture-dislocation. The most common fracture site is near the angle of the lower jaw, which leads to **malocclusion**. Because the articulation of words is impossible, changes in speech are apparent. Oral bleeding may occur even though a mouth guard is properly fitted and worn.

Malocclusion
Inability to bring the teeth together in a normal bite

If the upper jaw, or maxilla, is fractured, the maxilla may be mobile, giving the appearance of a longer face. Nasal bleeding is also commonly seen. With direct impact forces, a fracture to the zygomatic arch (cheek bone) may result in the cheek appearing flat or depressed. Swelling and ecchymosis about the eye may occlude vision and hide damage to the eye orbit. Occasionally, the eye on the side of the fracture may appear sunken in, or the

A fractured cheek will appear flat or depressed

Field Strategy 14.3. Wound Care Using Steri-Strips or Butterfly Bandages

1. Put on latex gloves
2. Control bleeding with direct compression using a sterile gauze pad
3. Clean the wound with a saline solution and antiseptic, such as Betadine
4. Spray tape adherent on a cotton-tipped applicator and dab below and above the wound
5. Beginning in the middle of the wound, bring the edges together and secure the Steri-Strip below the wound. Lift up against gravity and secure above the wound. Make sure the edges of the wound are approximated

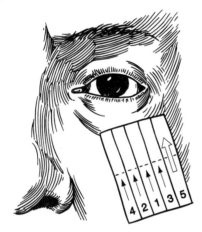

6. Apply the second Steri-Strip in a similar manner immediately adjacent to one side of the original strip. Apply the third strip on the other side. Alternate sides until the entire wound is covered
7. Cover the wound with a sterile dressing and secure in place
8. After the contest, refer the athlete to a physician for medical care if the wound is greater than 1 inch long or ⅛ inch deep
9. Check the wound daily for signs of infection. Keep it clean and protected for at least 1 week

eye opposite the fracture may appear to be raised. Double vision is common and numbness may be present on the affected cheek.

In all fractures, it is important to maintain an open airway. Dress any open wounds, immobilize the jaw with an elastic wrap that runs from under the chin over the top of the head, and refer the individual to a physician.

Because of the malocclusion, you should suspect a fractured jaw. Immobilize the jaw with an elastic wrap and refer this person to a physician.

NASAL INJURIES

A third baseman covering a hit was struck on the side of the nose when the ball bounced unexpectedly. The nose is bleeding and appears to be swollen at the top. What assessment and management protocol will you follow?

Nasal injuries are common in sports where protective face guards are not worn. Nosebleeds (epistaxis) and nasal fractures are traumatic injuries frequently seen.

Epistaxis

Epistaxis
Profuse bleeding from the
nose; nosebleed

Epistaxis, or a nosebleed, occurs when superficial blood vessels on the anterior septum are lacerated. In most cases, bleeding will stop spontaneously by applying mild pressure at the nasal bone; however, ice may be applied to stop more persistent bleeding. A nasal plug or pledget may be used, although this is seldom needed. If used, the plug should protrude from the nostrils at least one-half inch to facilitate removal. If bleeding continues for more than 5 minutes in spite of manual pressure and ice, refer the individual to a physician.

Nasal Fractures

Fractures to the nasal bone are the most common facial fracture in sport and it is particularly susceptible to lateral displacement (**Fig. 14.11A**). The nose may appear flattened and lose its symmetry. Deformity is usually present, particularly with a lateral force, and epistaxis is almost always seen. Stand behind and above the individual, and look down an imaginary line to determine if the nose is centered (**Fig. 14.11B**). Hand a small mirror to the athlete and have them look at the nose to determine if it appears normal. There may be crepitus over the nasal bridge and ecchymosis under the eyes. Control bleeding, apply ice to limit swelling and hemorrhage, and refer the individual to a doctor for further examination. A nose guard can be worn after a few days to protect the area from additional injury. **Field Strategy 14.4** suggests assessment and care of a fractured nose.

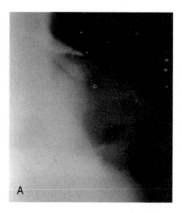
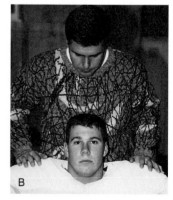

Figure 14.11. A. Nasal deformity from a nasal fracture. **B.** A nasal deformity can best be seen by standing behind the injured person and looking down an imaginary line to determine if the nose is centered.

Field Strategy 14.4. Management of a Nasal Injury

Primary Survey

Check ABCs. Bony fragments may occlude the airway
Check for signs of a concussion and/or skull fracture

Secondary Survey

History
  Determine mechanism of injury
  Primary complaint (pain, dizziness, nausea, or vision disturbances)
  Presence of posttraumatic and/or retrograde amnesia
  Disability from injury (inability to breathe through one side of nose)
Observation and inspection
  Obvious deformity or abnormal deviation
  Bleeding and/or CSF from the nose
  Check pupil size, pupillary response to light, eye movement, and visual
    acuity
  Stand behind the individual and look down an imaginary line to see if
    the nose is deviated
Palpation
  Palpate the two nasal bones with the forefinger and thumb (swelling,
    depressions, crepitus, mobility, etc.)
  Control any bleeding
After bleeding is controlled, inspect the internal structures for any
  abnormalities
Apply ice to control hemorrhage and refer the individual for medical care if
  necessary

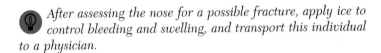

After assessing the nose for a possible fracture, apply ice to control bleeding and swelling, and transport this individual to a physician.

ORAL AND DENTAL INJURIES

A rugby player was struck in the mouth by an elbow. The inside of the upper lip is bleeding. At least two teeth are loose and one tooth appears to be chipped. How will you manage this injury? Can the chipped tooth be repaired?

Approximately 15% of school-aged children will have serious dental injuries before the age of 18 (8). For athletes, nearly all are preventable through regular use of mouth guards. These guards provide protection to the lips, teeth, and gums by absorbing shock, dispersing impact, cushioning the contact between the upper and lower jaw, and keeping the upper lip away from the edges of teeth (9).

Lacerations of the Mouth

Treatment for minor mouth lacerations is the same as in other lacerations. Apply direct pressure to stop bleeding, cleanse the area with a saline solution, apply Steri-strips if needed, and cover the wound with a dry sterile dressing. Mouth lacerations that

> Mouth guards protect the lips, teeth, and gums by absorbing shock, dispersing impact, cushioning the contact between the upper and lower jaw, and keeping the upper lip away from the incisal edges of teeth

extend completely through the lip, or involve the outer lip or large tongue lacerations, necessitate special suturing. Cleanse the wound with water or mouthwash and refer for possible suturing. The individual should not be returned to participation until the wound is healed.

Dental Injuries

When a loose tooth is displaced outward or laterally, try to place the tooth back into its normal position

When the tooth has been displaced outwardly or is laterally displaced, try to place the tooth back into its normal position. Teeth that are driven inward should be left alone, as any attempt to move the tooth may result in permanent loss of the tooth or damage underlying permanent teeth. Immediately transport the individual to the dentist for follow-up treatment. A dental radiograph can rule out damage under the gum line and ensure the tooth is properly replaced. The damaged tooth is then splinted to surrounding teeth for 2 to 3 weeks.

Teeth that have been totally avulsed from their socket can often be located in the individual's mouth or on the ground. These teeth can be saved, but speed is of the essence. Do not touch the root of the tooth or brush the tooth off. If the tooth is rinsed in milk, saline, or Hank's solution and replaced intraorally with 30 minutes, the prognosis for successful replanting is 90%. Replanting that occurs after 2 hours results in a 95% failure rate (10). If it is properly placed, the individual should be able to close the jaw normally. If the tooth cannot be replaced by gentle pressure, place it under the individual's tongue and transport the individual to a dentist. Tap or drinking water will damage the periodontal ligament cells on the root surface and compromise the replanting procedure, and therefore, should not be used (10).

Fractures may occur through the enamel, dentin, pulp, or root of the tooth (**Fig. 14.12**). Fractures involving the enamel cause no symptoms and can be smoothed to prevent further injury to the lips and inner lining of the oral cavity. Fractures extending into the dentin cause pain and increased sensitivity to cold and heat. The individual should be referred to a dentist, who will apply a sedative dressing over the exposed area. The tooth can then have a permanent composite resin crown attached. Fractures exposing the pulp lead to severe pain and sensitivity, and involve more extensive dental work. Root fractures are commonly seen in male athletes in contact and collision sports. The predominant sign is a mobile tooth. A tooth with a horizontal fracture can be successfully splinted to the surrounding teeth for 6 weeks (9). Vertical fractures along the length of the tooth require extraction.

With the rugby player, you should put on latex gloves, stop the bleeding with a sterile gauze pad and compression, cleanse the mouth with a saline solution, and refer the individual immediately to a dentist. The dentist may be able to apply a permanent composite resin crown to the tooth.

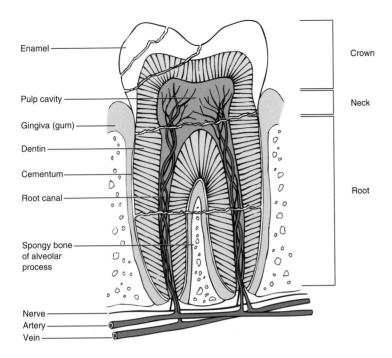

Enamel

Pulp cavity

Gingiva (gum)

Dentin

Cementum

Root canal

Spongy bone
of alveolar
process

Nerve
Artery
Vein

Crown

Neck

Root

Figure 14.12. Tooth fractures may occur through the enamel, dentine, pulp, or root of the tooth.

EAR INJURIES

> ⓘ *A boxer was not wearing protective headgear during sparring, and is now complaining about a burning, aching feeling on the outer ear. The ear is inflamed and sensitive to touch, but no swelling is present. How will you manage this injury?*

Several conditions may affect the ear. Foreign bodies in the ear are usually harmless and easily removed with a speculum. Trauma to the external ear can lead to auricular hematoma or "cauliflower ear," rupture of the eardrum, localized inflammation of the auditory canal, and swimmer's ear.

External Ear Injury

Auricular hematoma, or "**cauliflower ear**," is a relatively minor injury caused when repeated blunt trauma pulls the cartilage away from the perichondrium. A hematoma forms between the perichondrium and cartilage of the ear, and compromises blood supply to the cartilage. The hematoma must be aspirated by a physician to avoid pressure and permanent cartilage damage. If left untreated, the hematoma forms a fibrosis in the overlying skin, leading to necrosis of the auricular cartilage, resulting in the characteristic "cauliflower ear" appearance (**Fig. 14.13**). Protective headgear in sports such as boxing, wrestling, water polo, baseball, and softball is designed to prevent trauma to the ear, but must be worn regularly to be effective.

Cauliflower ear
Hematoma between the perichondrium and cartilage of the outer ear; auricular hematoma

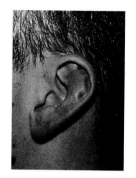

Figure 14.13. Cauliflower ear deformity. Note how the hematoma has pulled the skin away from the ear cartilage.

Internal Ear Injury

An individual with intense pain in the ear, a feeling of fullness, nausea, tinnitus, dizziness, or a hearing loss should be immediately seen by a physician

A blow to the ear, pressure changes (seen in diving and scuba diving), and infection may injure the eardrum. Although typically seen in water sports, damage to the internal ear may occur in any sport, such as in soccer, when a player is hit on the ear by a ball. Any individual with intense pain in the ear, a feeling of fullness, nausea, tinnitus, dizziness, or a hearing loss should be evaluated immediately by a physician. If the eardrum is ruptured, most minor ruptures heal spontaneously. Larger ruptures may necessitate surgical repair.

Localized infections of the middle ear are often secondary to upper respiratory infections. Swelling of the mucous membranes may cause a partial or complete block of the eustachian tube (the connection between the middle ear and pharynx). When the mastoid area is pressed, the individual will complain of pain, the "ears popping," and a sense of fullness in the ear. The supervising physician may prescribe an antibiotic for the infection, or decongestants to shrink the swollen mucous membranes.

Swimmer's ear is a bacterial infection involving the lining of the auditory canal. It frequently occurs in individuals who fail to dry the canal after being in water, thereby changing the pH of the ear canal's skin. The individual will feel itching and intense pain in the ear. Gentle pressure around the external auditory opening and pulling on the pinna will increase the pain. If left untreated, the infection can spread to the middle ear, causing balance disturbances or a hearing loss.

Commercial ear plugs may not be helpful in preventing swimmer's ear. Custom ear plugs from an otolaryngologist may be necessary. The condition can also be prevented by using ear drops to dry the canal. A weak solution of either 2% vinegar (acetic acid), 70% alcohol, or 3% boric acid in isopropyl alcohol will reestablish the proper pH (11). If no improvement is seen, refer the individual to a physician.

Place ice on the boxer's ear to control swelling. If you notice any hemorrhage or edema between the perichondrium and cartilage that flattens the wrinkles or creases of the ear, refer the individual to a physician for follow-up care.

> A softball player was struck in the eye by a deflected ground ball. The eye is swollen and closed. Attempts to open the eye produce excessive tearing and discomfort for the individual. How will you assess this injury and rule out a serious underlying condition?

The eyes are exposed daily to potential trauma and injury, yet many eye injuries could be prevented if protective eyewear is worn. This is especially true in racquetball and squash, when players are confined to a limited space with swinging racquets and balls traveling at high speeds. Athletes who require corrective lenses should use strong plastic or semirigid rubber frames, and impact-resistant lenses. If glasses are not required, protective eyewear and/or face masks should be worn in sports in which risk of injury is high. Sport participants with only one good eye should consult an ophthalmologist to determine if they should participate in a specific activity and, if so, what protective eyewear can be worn to prevent injury.

Periorbital Ecchymosis (Black eye)

Impact forces can cause significant swelling and hemorrhage in the surrounding eyelids, leading to **periorbital ecchymosis (Fig. 14.14)**. Inspect the eye for obvious abnormalities and palpate the eye orbit for a possible orbital fracture. Check pupillary response to light by shining a concentrated light beam into the eye and note the bilateral rate of constriction. Ask the individual if they can focus clearly on an object. Inspect the anterior chamber of the eye for any obvious bleeding (refer to Hemorrhage into the Anterior Chamber). Control swelling and hemorrhage by using crushed ice or ice water in a latex surgical glove. Make sure the glove does not have rosin or other powdered substances on it. Do

Periorbital ecchymosis
Swelling and hemorrhage into the surrounding eyelids; black eye

Control swelling and hemorrhage by using crushed ice or ice water in a latex surgical glove. Make sure the glove does not have rosin or other powdered substances on it

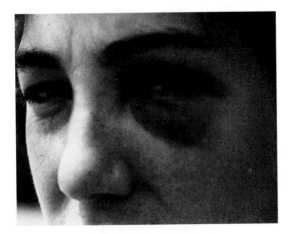

Figure 14.14. Periorbital ecchymosis caused by direct trauma to the eye.

not use chemical ice bags, as they may leak. Refer the individual to an ophthalmologist for further examination and x-rays to rule out an underlying fracture or injury to the globe.

Foreign Bodies

Dust or dirt in the eyes can lead to intense pain and tearing. The foreign body, if not imbedded or on the cornea, should be removed and the eye inspected for any scratches, abrasions, or lacerations (see **Field Strategy 14.5**). If the foreign object is impaled or embedded, however, do not touch or attempt to remove the object. Summon EMS. Medically-trained technicians will stabilize the object and provide rigid protection for the orbit.

 Field Strategy 14.5. Removing a Foreign Body from the Eye

1. In an upright position, examine the lower lid by gently pulling the skin down below the eye. Ask the individual to look up and inspect the lower portion of the globe and eyelid for any foreign object
2. Examine the upper lid by asking the individual to look downward
3. Grasp the eyelashes and pull downward
4. Place a cotton-tipped applicator on the outside portion of the upper lid
5. Pull the lid over the applicator and hold the rolled lid against the upper bony ridge of the orbit
6. Remove the foreign body with a sterile, moist gauze pad. If you are unable to successfully remove the foreign object, patch both eyes with a sterile, nonpressure oval gauze pad and refer the individual to a physician

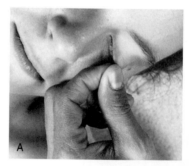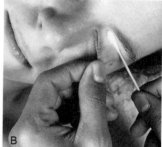

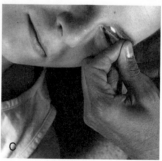

Conjunctivitis (Pinkeye)

Conjunctivitis is an inflammation or bacterial infection of the conjunctiva, the membrane between the inner lining of the eyelid and anterior eyeball. The infection leads to itching, burning, and watering of the eye, causing the conjunctiva to become inflamed and red, giving a pinkeye appearance. This condition can be highly infectious and, therefore, the individual should be referred immediately to a physician for medical treatment.

Conjunctivitis
Bacterial infection leading to itching, burning, watering, and inflamed eye; pinkeye

Corneal Abrasion

Occasionally, a foreign body will scratch the cornea, resulting in a sudden onset of pain, tearing, and photophobia. Blinking and movement of the eye only aggravates the condition. Examination may not reveal a foreign object, but the individual continues to complain that something is in the eye. A corneal abrasion is best seen by using a fluorescein dye strip. The orange color of the dye is augmented by using a blue light, changing the orange dye to a bright green, illuminating the abrasion. Treatment usually involves a prescribed topical ointment to reduce pain and relax ciliary muscle spasms, and an antibiotic ointment to prevent secondary bacterial infection. An eye patch may be worn for 24 to 48 hours. Make sure soft contacts are removed before applying the dye, as they will absorb the dye and be ruined.

Subconjunctival Hemorrhage

Direct trauma can also lead to **subconjunctival hemorrhage**. Several small capillaries rupture making it look much worse than it is. This relatively harmless condition requires no treatment and resolves spontaneously in 1 to 3 weeks. If blurred vision, pain, limited eye movement, or blood in the anterior chamber are present, however, immediate referral to an ophthalmologist is warranted.

Subconjunctival hemorrhage
Minor capillary ruptures in the eye globe

Hemorrhage into the Anterior Chamber

Hemorrhage into the anterior chamber (**hyphema**) usually results from blunt trauma from a small ball (squash or racquetball), hockey puck, stick (field hockey or ice hockey), or swinging racquet (squash or racquetball). The small size of the object can fit within the confines of the eye orbit, thereby inflicting direct damage to the eye. Initially, a red tinge in the anterior chamber may be present, but within a few hours, blood will begin to settle into the anterior chamber, giving a characteristic meniscus appearance. If this is present, immediate referral to a physician is warranted.

Hyphema
Hemorrhage into the anterior chamber of the eye

Detached Retina

Damage to the posterior segment of the eye can occur with or without trauma to the anterior segment. A **detached retina** oc-

Detached retina
Neurosensory retina is separated from the retinal epithelium by swelling

curs when fluid seeps into the retinal break and separates the neurosensory retina from the retinal epithelium. This can occur days or even weeks after the initial trauma. The individual frequently describes the condition with phases like, "a curtain fell over my eye," or "I keep seeing flashes of light going on and off." Floaters and light flashes are early signs that the retina is damaged. Immediately refer this person to an ophthalmologist, as surgery is often necessary.

Floaters and light flashes are early signs that the retina is damaged

Orbital "Blowout" Fracture

A blowout fracture is caused by impact from a blunt object, usually larger than the eye orbit. Upon impact, forces drive the orbital contents posteriorly against the orbital walls. This sudden increase in intraorbital pressure is released in the area of least resistance, typically the orbital floor. The globe descends into the defect in the floor. Examination may reveal **diplopia**, absent eye movement, numbness on the side of fracture below the eye, and a recessed, downward displaced globe. The lack of eye movement becomes evident when the individual is asked to look up, and only one eye is able to move (**Fig. 14.15**). Tomograms or radiographs are necessary to confirm a fracture, and surgery is indicated to repair the defect in the orbit floor.

Diplopia
Double vision

Displaced Contact Lens

Hard contact lenses are frequently involved in corneal abrasions. Foreign objects get underneath the lens and damage the cornea or the cornea may be injured while putting in or taking out the lens. If irritation is present, the lens should be removed and cleaned. Hard contact lenses can slow the progression of **myopia**; however, in sports, soft contact lenses are preferred. This is because eye accommodation and adjustment time are less, they can be easily replaced, and can be worn for longer periods of time. In an eye injury, individuals may be able to remove the lens themselves. However, pain or photophobia (sensitivity to light) may preclude them from doing this, and it may become necessary to assist them. **Field Strategy 14.6** demonstrates a full assessment of an eye injury.

Myopia
Nearsightedness

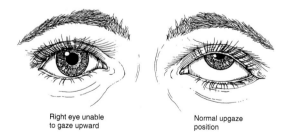

Right eye unable to gaze upward

Normal upgaze position

Figure 14.15. An orbital fracture can entrap the inferior rectus muscle, leading to an inability to voluntarily elevate the eye.

Field Strategy 14.6. Eye Evaluation

Check ABCs
Determine responsiveness

Secondary Survey

History
  Determine mechanism of injury (objects larger than the eye orbit may
    lead to orbital fracture; objects smaller than the eye orbit may lead to
    direct trauma to the eye globe
  Primary complaint (pain, discomfort, eye movement, and vision
    problems)
  Eye irritation from a foreign body and blurring vision that clears quickly
    with blinking can be managed on-site
Observation and inspection
  Look for obvious deformity or depressions around the eye orbit
  Observe ecchymosis and swelling in the eyelids and surrounding tissue.
    If the eyelid is swollen shut and the individual cannot open it, do not
    force it open, as it may cause further damage
  Observe and control any bleeding around the eye
  Observe the level of both pupils and eye globe for any corneal
    lacerations, abrasions, or bleeding in the anterior chamber
  Inspect pupil size, accommodation to light, and sensitivity to light with a
    penlight
Palpation
  Palpate the bony rim of the eye orbit for any swelling, depressions,
    crepitus, or mobility
  Control any bleeding
Special tests
  Determine eye vision. Is it blurred, sensitive to light, or does the
    individual have double vision? Can the individual distinguish how
    many fingers you are holding up?
  Determine eye movement. Move your finger and watch if the eyes
    move in a coordinated manner. If one eye moves upward and the
    other remains in a stationary position, the inferior rectus muscle may
    be entrapped to an orbital fracture

**Vision disturbances, such as persistent blurred vision, diplopia,
sensitivity to light, loss of all or part of a field of vision, dilated
pupils, any abnormal eye movement, and throbbing pain or
headache indicate a serious eye injury that warrants immediate
referral.**

*With the softball player, did you rule out an orbital fracture,
check pupillary response to light and vision acuity, and look
for possible blood in the anterior chamber? If so, you did the
right thing.*

SUMMARY

The head and facial region are frequent sites for injury. Wearing
protective equipment can significantly reduce the incidence and
severity of head and facial injuries. Minor injuries, such as nosebleeds, contusions, abrasions, lacerations, and grade I concussions,

can easily be handled on the field by the coach, athletic trainer, or sport supervisor. Injuries that require referral to a physician are listed in **Table 14.6.** In evaluating any head or facial injury, it is always best to error on the conservative side and refer questionable injuries to a physician or appropriate specialist. If a decision is made to refer an individual for medical care, control any bleeding, cover the area with a sterile gauze pad, maintain an open airway, and treat for shock.

Table 14.6. Signs and Symptoms that Indicate Immediate Medical Referral

Facial bones

Obvious deformity, crepitus, or increased pain on palpation
Malocclusion of the teeth

Nasal region

Bleeding or CSF from the nose
Loss of smell
Nasal deformity or fractures
Nosebleeds that do not stop within 5 minutes
Foreign objects that cannot be easily removed

Oral and dental region

Lacerations involving the lip, outer border of the lip, or tongue
Loose, chipped, cracked, fractured, or dislodged teeth
Persistent toothache or sensitivity to heat and cold
Malocclusion of the teeth

Ear

Bleeding or CSF from the ear canal
Bleeding or swelling behind the ear (Battle's sign)
Hematoma or swelling that removes the creases of the outer ear
Tinnitis, hearing impairment, or pain when the ear lobe is pulled
Feeling of fullness in the ear, "popping," or itching in the ear
Foreign body in ear that cannot be easily removed

Eye

Visual disturbances or loss of vision
Unequal pupils or dilated pupils
Irregular eye movement or failure to accommodate to light
Severe ecchymosis and swelling (raccoon eyes)
Suspected imbedded foreign body, corneal abrasion, or corneal laceration
Blood in the anterior chamber
Individual complaining of floaters, light flashes, or a "curtain falling over the eye"
Itching, burning, watery eye that appears pink
Dislodged contact lens that cannot be easily removed

Skin

Lacerations longer than 1 inch or deeper than ⅛ inch

REFERENCES

1. Clarke KS. An epidemiologic view. In *Athletic injuries to the head, neck, and face*, edited by JS Torg. St. Louis: Mosby-Year Book, 1991.
2. Gennarelli TA. Head injury mechanisms. In *Athletic injuries to the head, neck, and face*, edited by JS Torg. St. Louis: Mosby-Year Book, 1991.
3. Bruno LA, Gennarelli TA, and Torg JS. Management guidelines for head injuries in athletics. In *Clinics in sports medicine*, edited by JS Torg, vol. 6, no. 1. Philadelphia: WB Saunders, 1987.
4. Kinderknecht JJ. Head injuries. In *Athletic injuries and rehabilitation*, edited by JE Zachazewski, DJ Magee, and WS Quillen. Philadelphia: WB Saunders, 1996.
5. Vegso JJ, and Torg JS. Field evaluation and management of intracranial injuries. In *Athletic injuries to the head, neck, and face*, edited by JS Torg. St. Louis: Mosby-Year Book, 1991.
6. Tu HK, Davis LF, and Nique TA. Maxillofacial injuries. In *The team physician's handbook*, edited by MB Mellion, WM Walsh, and GL Shelton. Philadelphia: Hanley & Belfus, 1990.
7. Cantu RC, and Voy T. 1995. Second impact syndrome: a risk in any contact sport. Phys Sportsmed 23(6):27–34.
8. Bishop BM, Davies EH, and von Fraunhofer JA. 1985. Materials for mouth protectors. J Prosthet Dent 53:256–261.
9. Greenberg MS, and Springer PS. Diagnosis and management of oral injuries. In *Athletic injuries to the head, neck, and face*, edited by JS Torg. St. Louis: Mosby-Year Book, 1991.
10. Kumamoto DP, Jacob M, and Nickelsen D. 1995. Oral trauma: on-field assessment. Phys Sportsmed 23(5):53–62.
11. Hammer RW. Swimming and diving. In *The team physician's handbook*, edited by MB Mellion, WM Walsh, and GL Shelton. Philadelphia: Hanley & Belfus, 1990.

Chapter 15

Injuries to the Spine

After completing this chapter, you should be able to:

- Locate and explain the functional significance of the important bony and soft tissue structures of the spine

- Describe the motion capabilities in the different regions of the spine

- Specify strategies in activities of daily living to reduce spinal stress

- Identify anatomical variations that may predispose individuals to spine injuries

- Explain important measures used to prevent injury to the spinal region

- Recognize and describe common sports injuries to the spine and back

- Demonstrate a basic assessment of the spine

- Demonstrate rehabilitative exercises for the region

Key Terms:

Annulus fibrosus	**Nucleus pulposus**
Burner	**Osteopoenia**
Cauda equina	**Prolapsed disc**
Extruded disc	**Reflex**
Idiopathic	**Sciatica**
Ipsilateral	**Scoliosis**
Kyphosis	**Spondylolisthesis**
Lordosis	**Spondylolysis**
Motion segment	**Wedge fracture**

The spine transfers loads between the upper and lower extremities, enables motion of the trunk in all three planes, and protects the delicate spinal cord. Most sports injuries to the back are relatively minor, consisting of contusions, muscle strains, and ligament sprains. Acute spinal fractures and dislocations, however, are extremely serious and can lead to paralysis or death. Although sports-related cervical injuries account for only 15 percent of all spinal cord injuries annually, nearly 92% of these injuries result in quadriplegia (1). Unfortunately, with the increasing prevalence of leisure time in recent years, there has been a concomitant increase in spinal injuries and low back pain. Low back problems are especially common in equestrian sports, weightlifting, ice hockey, gymnastics, diving, football, wrestling, and aerobics (2).

This chapter begins with a review of the anatomy and major muscle actions that move the spine, followed by a discussion of anatomical variations that may predispose individuals to spinal injuries. Strategies to prevent injury is then followed by discussion of common spinal injuries. Finally, a basic spinal injury assessment is presented and general rehabilitation exercises are provided.

ANATOMY REVIEW OF THE SPINE

 How is vertebral structure related to the function of the cervical, thoracic, and lumbar regions of the spine?

The five regions of the spine—cervical, thoracic, lumbar, sacral, and coccygeal—are all structurally and functionally distinct. There are four normal spinal curves (**Fig. 15.1**). As viewed from the side, the thoracic and sacral curves are convex posteriorly and the lumbar and cervical curves are concave posteriorly. These curves constitute posture and can be modified by a host of factors, including heredity, pathological conditions, and forces acting on the spine. Abnormal spinal curves are referred to as curvatures and are discussed later in this chapter.

> The spinal curves constitute posture and can be modified by heredity, pathological conditions, and forces acting on the spine

Vertebrae and Intervertebral Discs

The vertebral column consists of 33 vertebrae, most of which are separated and cushioned by discs composed of fibrocartilage (**Fig. 15.1**). There are five regions of the spine based on vertebral

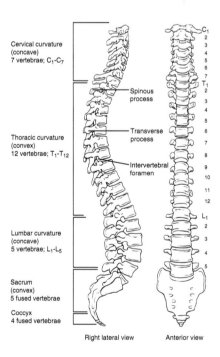

Cervical curvature
(concave)
7 vertebrae; C_1-C_7

Spinous process

Transverse process

Intervertebral foramen

Thoracic curvature
(convex)
12 vertebrae; T_1-T_{12}

Lumbar curvature
(concave)
5 vertebrae; L_1-L_5

Sacrum
(convex)
5 fused vertebrae

Coccyx
4 fused vertebrae

Right lateral view   Anterior view

Figure 15.1. The vertebral column has four characteristic curves of the spine when viewed from the lateral aspect.

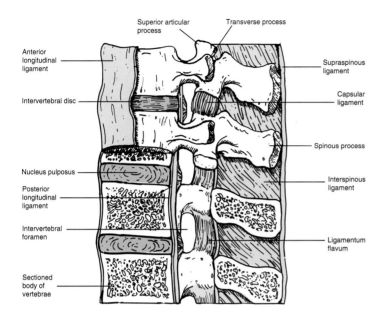

Figure 15.2. A motion segment of the spine includes two adjacent vertebrae and the intervening soft tissues. The motion segment is considered to be the functional unit of the spine.

structure and function. These regions include 7 cervical vertebrae, 12 thoracic vertebrae, 5 lumbar vertebrae, 5 fused sacral vertebrae, and 4 small, fused coccygeal vertebrae. The bony structures of the vertebrae and ribs govern the varying amounts of spinal motion permitted throughout the cervical, thoracic, and lumbar regions. Within these regions, any two adjacent vertebrae and the soft tissues between them are collectively referred to as a **motion segment**. The motion segment is the functional unit of the spine (**Fig. 15.2**).

A typical vertebra consists of a body, a hollow ring known as the vertebral arch, and several bony processes (**Fig. 15.3**). The superior and inferior articular processes mate with the articular process of adjacent vertebrae to form the facet joints. Forming a stacked column, the neural arches, posterior sides of the bodies, and the intervertebral discs form a protective passageway for the spinal cord and associated blood vessels. There is a progressive increase in vertebral size from the cervical region down through the lumbar region. This serves a functional purpose, because when the body is in an upright position, each vertebra must support the weight of not only the arms and head, but all the trunk positioned above it.

Fibrocartilaginous discs provide cushioning between the articulating vertebral bodies. In the intervertebral disc, a thick ring of fibrous cartilage, the **annulus fibrosus**, surrounds a gelatinous material known as the **nucleus pulposus**. The discs serve as shock absorbers and also allow the spine to bend.

The bony structures of the vertebrae and ribs govern the amount of motion allowed at each motion segment

Motion segment
Two adjacent vertebrae and the intervening soft tissues; the functional unit of the spine

Annulus fibrosus
Tough outer covering of the intervertebral disc, composed of fibrocartilage

Nucleus pulposus
Gelatinous-like material comprising the inner portion of the intervertebral disc

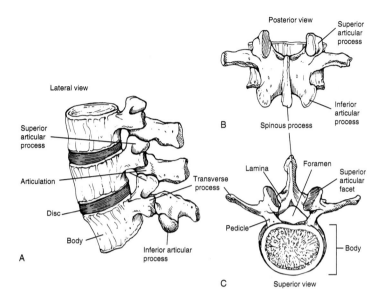

Figure 15.3. The structure of a typical vertebra. **A.** Lateral view. **B.** Posterior view. **C.** Superior view.

Ligaments of the Spine

A number of ligaments support the spine **(Fig. 15.2)**. Anterior and posterior longitudinal ligaments connect the vertebral bodies in the cervical, thoracic, and lumbar regions. The supraspinous ligament attaches to the spinous processes throughout the length of the spine and is enlarged in the cervical region, where it is known as the ligamentum nuchae or "ligament of the neck." Another major ligament, the ligamentum flavum, connects the pedicles of adjacent vertebrae and is important in maintaining spinal stability. The interspinous ligaments, intertransverse ligaments, and ligamenta flava, respectively, link the spinous processes, transverse processes, and laminae of adjacent vertebrae.

> The ligament flavum is constantly in tension, thereby serving as a major contributor to spinal stability

Muscles of the Spine and Trunk

Muscles of the neck and trunk are paired, with one on the left and one on the right side of the body. These muscles cause lateral flexion and/or rotation of the trunk when they act unilaterally and trunk flexion or extension when acting bilaterally. Collectively, the primary movers for back extension are called the erector spinae muscles **(Fig. 15.4)**. The attachments, actions, and innervations of the major muscles of the trunk are summarized in **Table 15.1**.

Spinal Cord and Spinal Nerves

The brain and spinal cord make up the central nervous system. The spinal cord extends from the brainstem to the level of the first or second lumbar vertebrae **(Fig. 15.5)**. Like the brain, the spinal cord is encased in the three meninges. Thirty-one pairs of

Table 15.1. Muscles of the Spine

Muscle	Proximal Attachment	Distal Attachment	Primary Action(s)	Nerve Innervation
Prevertebral muscles Rectus capitis anterior, rectus capitis lateralis, longus capitis, longus coli	Anterior aspect of occipital bone and cervical vertebrae	Anterior surfaces cervical and first three thoracic vertebrae	Flexion, lateral flexion, rotation to opposite side	Cervical nerves (C_1 to C_6)
Rectus abdominis	Costal cartilage of ribs 5 to 7	Pubic crest	Flexion, lateral flexion	Intercostal nerves (T_6 to T_{12})
External oblique	External surface of lower eight ribs	Linea alba and anterior iliac crest	Flexion, lateral flexion, rotation to opposite side	Intercostal nerves (T_7 to T_{12})
Internal oblique	Linea alba and the lower four ribs	Inguinal ligament, iliac crest, and the lumbodorsal fascia	Flexion, lateral flexion, rotation to same side	Intercostal nerves (T_7 to T_{12}, L_1)
Splenius Capitis and cervicis	Mastoid process of the temporal bone, transverse processes of C_1 to C_3 vertebrae	Lower half of the ligamentum nuchae, spinous processes of C_7 to T_6 vertebrae	Extension, lateral flexion, rotation to same side	Middle and lower cervical nerves (C_4 to C_8)
The suboccipitals Obliquus capitus superior and inferior, rectus capitis posterior major and minor	Occipital bone, transverse process of C_1 vertebra	Posterior surfaces, C_1 to C_2 vertebrae	Extension, lateral flexion, rotation to same side	Suboccipital nerve (C_1)
Erector spinae Spinalis, longissimus, and iliocostalis	Lower part of the ligamentum nuchae, posterior cervical, thoracic, and lumbar spine, lower 9 ribs, iliac crest, posterior sacrum	Mastoid process of the temporal bone, posterior cervical, thoracic, and lumbar spine, 12 ribs	Extension, lateral flexion, rotation to opposite side	Spinal nerves (T_1 to T_{12})
Semispinalis Capitis, cervicis, and thoracis	Occipital bone, spinous processes of T_2 to T_4 vertebrae	Transverse process, C_7 to T_{12} vertebrae	Extension, lateral flexion, rotation to opposite side	Cervical and thoracic spinal nerves (C_1 to T_{12})
The deep spinal muscles Multifidi, rotators, interspinales intertransversarii, levatores costarum	Posterior processes of all vertebrae, posterior sacrum	Spinous and transverse processes and laminae of vertebrae below those of the proximal attachment	Extension, lateral flexion, rotation to opposite side	Spinal and intercostal nerves (T_1 to T_{12})
Sternocleidomastoid	Mastoid process of the temporal bone	Superior sternum, inner third of the clavicle	Flexion of the neck, extension of the head, lateral flexion, rotation to opposite side	Accessory nerve and C_2 spinal nerve
Levator scapulae	Transverse process of the first four cervical vertebrae	Vertebral border of the scapula	Lateral flexion	C_3 to C_4 spinal nerves, dorsal scapular nerve (C_3 to C_5)

Table 15.1. Muscles of the Spine (continued)

Muscle	Proximal Attachment	Distal Attachment	Primary Action(s)	Nerve Innervation
The scaleni Scalenus anterior, medius, and posterior	Transverse processes, C_1 to C_7 vertebrae	Upper two ribs	Flexion, lateral flexion	Cervical nerves (C_3 to C_8)
Quadratus lumborum	Last rib, transverse processes of L_1 to L_4 vertebrae	Iliolumbar ligament, adjacent lumbar iliac crest	Lateral flexion	T_{12} to L_4 spinal nerves
Psoas major	Sides of twelfth thoracic and all lumbar vertebrae	Lesser trochanter of the femur	Flexion	Femoral nerve (L_1 to L_3)

Cauda equina
Lower spinal nerves, resembling a horse's tail, that course through the lumbar spinal canal

Reflex
Action involving stimulation of a motor neuron by a sensory neuron in the spinal cord without involvement of the brain

spinal nerves emanate from the cord, including 8 cervical, 12 thoracic, 5 lumbar, 5 sacral, and 1 coccygeal. A bundle of spinal nerves extends downward through the vertebral canal from the end of the spinal cord at the L_1 to L_2 level. This nerve bundle is known collectively as the **cauda equina,** after its resemblance to a horse's tail.

The spinal cord serves as the major neural pathway for conducting sensory impulses to the brain and motor impulses from the brain. It also provides direct connections between sensory and motor nerves inside the cord, enabling **reflex** activity. Reflex actions occur very quickly, before there is time for the brain to process a sensory input and respond with an appropriate motor

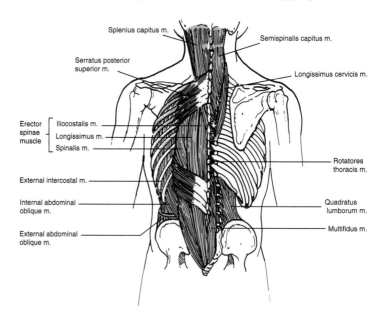

Figure 15.4. The deep posterior back muscles attaching to the spine.

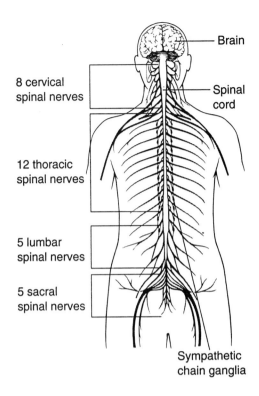

 placed above — diagram labels:

Brain

8 cervical
spinal nerves

Spinal
cord

12 thoracic
spinal nerves

5 lumbar
spinal nerves

5 sacral
spinal nerves

Sympathetic
chain ganglia

Figure 15.5. The spinal cord and spinal nerves.

signal. An example of a reflex is removing a hand from a source of extreme heat through reflex action before the sensory information that the hand is being burned even reaches the brain. Deep tendon reflexes are used consistently in injury assessment to determine possible spinal nerve damage. Exaggerated, distorted, or absent reflexes indicate damage to the nervous system, often before other signs are apparent.

Structure and function are intimately related in the spinal column. The size of each vertebral body is proportional to the amount of weight that it must support and the orientation of the facet joints governs available range of motion.

MAJOR MUSCLE ACTIONS OF THE SPINE

Which regions of the spine allow the freest motion? Can you speculate as to what implications this might have for injury potential?

The vertebral joints enable motion in all planes of movement, as well as circumduction (**Fig. 15.6**). Because the motion allowed between any two adjacent vertebrae is small, however, spinal movements always involve a number of motion segments. The available range of motion is governed by anatomical constraints that vary through the cervical, thoracic, and lumbar regions of the spine.

> Deep tendon reflexes are used consistently in injury assessment to determine possible spinal nerve damage

> Spinal movements always involve a number of motion segments

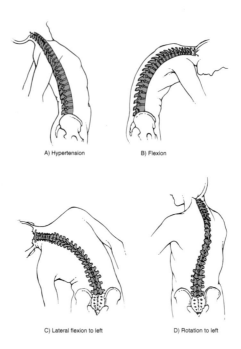

A) Hypertension   B) Flexion

C) Lateral flexion to left   D) Rotation to left

Figure 15.6. A-D. Motions of the trunk.

Flexion, Extension, and Hyperextension

Spinal flexion is anterior bending of the spine in the sagittal plane, with extension being the return to anatomical position. The flexion/extension capability of the motion segments at all levels of the spine is relatively small. When the spine is extended backward past anatomical position in the sagittal plane, the motion is termed hyperextension. The capability for hyperextension is greatest in the cervical region, followed by the lumbar region, followed by the thoracic region (3).

Lateral Flexion and Rotation

Movement of the spine away from anatomical position in a lateral direction in the frontal plane is termed lateral flexion and is predominantly carried out in the thoracic region, followed by the lumbar and cervical regions. Spinal rotation capability is greatest in the cervical region. Rotation is also permitted to some degree in the upper six thoracic motion segments; however, from T_7 to T_8 downward, range of motion in rotation progressively decreases. At the lumbosacral joint, about 5° of rotation is allowed (3).

Motion capability of the cervical, thoracic, and lumbar regions varies with the direction of movement. Mobility often translates to greater activity in the surrounding muscles and, subsequently, to higher intra-joint forces, which increases the potential for injury.

Spinal rotation is greatest in the cervical region, with up to 50° of motion at C_1 to C_2

ANATOMICAL VARIATIONS PREDISPOSING INDIVIDUALS TO SPINE INJURIES

❓ *The normal anatomical curves of the spine vary in size among individuals. Can extreme variations in these curves predispose an individual to a back injury?*

Excessive spinal curvatures can be congenital or acquired through weight training or sport participation. Defects in the pars interarticularis of the neural arch can be caused by mechanical stress, also placing an individual at risk for serious spinal injury.

Spinal Curvatures

Accentuation of the thoracic curve is called **kyphosis (Fig. 15.7).** This condition has been called "rounded back" or "swimmer's back" because it can be caused by overtraining with the butterfly stroke, particularly among adolescents (4). Athletes such as weight lifters, gymnasts, and football linemen, who over-develop the pectoral muscles, are also prone to this condition.

Lateral curvature of the spine is known as **scoliosis (Fig. 15.7).** The lateral deformity, coupled with rotational deformity of the involved vertebrae, may range from mild to severe. Scoliosis may appear as either a "C" or an "S" curve involving the thoracic spine, the lumbar spine, or both. Although congenital abnormalities, selected cancers, and leg length discrepancy may lead to scoliosis, approximately 70 to 90% of all cases are **idiopathic**, which means that the cause is unknown (5). Idiopathic scoliosis is more commonly diagnosed between the ages of 10 and 13 years, and is more common in females.

Abnormal exaggeration of the lumbar curve, or **lordosis**, is often associated with weakened abdominal muscles and anterior pelvic tilt **(Fig. 15.7)**. Causes include congenital spinal deformity, weakness of the abdominal muscles, poor postural habits, and

Kyphosis
Excessive curve in the thoracic region of the spine

Swimmers, weight lifters, gymnasts, and football linemen who over-develop the pectoral muscles are prone to kyphosis, or "rounded back"

Scoliosis
Lateral rotational spinal curvature

Idiopathic
Of unknown origin

Lordosis
Excessive convex curve in the lumbar region of the spine

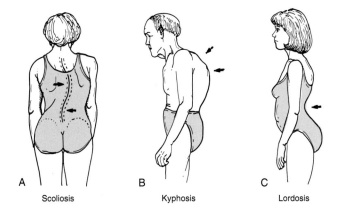

Figure 15.7. Spinal anomalies. **A.** Scoliosis. **B.** Thoracic kyphosis. **C.** Lordosis.

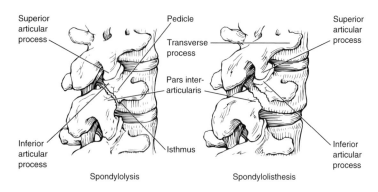

Figure 15.8. Spondylolysis is a stress fracture of the pars interarticularis (**A**). Spondylolisthesis is a bilateral fracture of the pars interarticularis accompanied by anterior slippage of the involved vertebra (**B**).

overtraining in sports requiring repeated lumbar hyperextension, such as gymnastics, figure skating, football (linemen), javelin throwing, or swimming the butterfly stroke. Lordosis is seen in many adolescent athletes, predisposing them to low back injuries (6).

Pars Interarticularis Fractures

The pars interarticularis is the weakest bony portion of the vertebral neural arch, the region between the superior and inferior articular facets. A fracture in this region is termed **spondylolysis** (**Fig. 15.8**). Although some pars defects may be congenital, they may also be caused by mechanical stress from axial loading of the lumbar spine during repeated flexion, hyperextension, and twisting (2). These repetitive movements cause a shearing stress to the vertebrae, resulting in a stress fracture.

A bilateral separation in the pars interarticularis, called **spondylolisthesis**, results in an anterior displacement of a vertebra with respect to the vertebra below it (**Fig. 15.9**). The most common site for this injury is the lumbosacral joint, with 90% of the slips occurring at this level. Spondylolisthesis is often diagnosed in children between the ages of 10 and 15 years, and is more common in boys (7).

Unlike most stress fractures, spondylolysis and spondylolisthesis do not typically heal with time, but tend to persist, particularly when there is no interruption in sport participation. Those individuals particularly susceptible to this condition include female gymnasts, interior football linemen, weight lifters, tennis players, volleyball players, hurdlers, pole vaulters, wrestlers, divers, and rowers. The individual may complain of a dull backache aggravated by activity. There is demonstrable muscle spasm in the lumbosacral region and flattening of the lumbosacral curve, but there are usually no sciatic nerve symptoms. Pain may radiate into the buttock region or down the sciatic nerve if the L_5 nerve root is

Spondylolysis
A stress fracture of the pars interarticularis

Spondylolisthesis
Anterior slippage of a vertebra, resulting from a complete bilateral fracture of the pars interarticularis

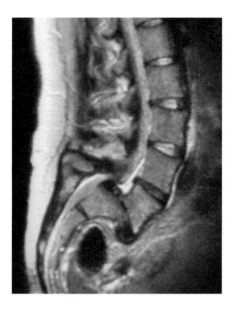

Figure 15.9. In this MRI of spondylolisthesis, note the anterior shift of the L₅ vertebra.

compressed. Muscle spasm may occur in the erector spinae muscles or hamstrings. This individual should be referred to a physician. Modifications can be made in training and technique to permit the individual to continue to participate if the slip is not too great. A lumbosacral orthosis may also be prescribed to decrease lumbar lordosis.

Spine anomalies can predispose an individual to injury; however, training modifications, correction of technique, and muscle strengthening can permit individuals to continue participating in sport. Each case must be evaluated by a physician on an individual basis.

PREVENTION OF INJURIES

The spine is a complex linkage system that transfers loads between the upper and lower extremities, enables motion of the trunk in all three planes, and protects the delicate spinal cord. What measures can be taken to protect this vulnerable region?

In an upright position, body weight, the weight of any load held in the hands, and tension in the surrounding ligaments and muscles all contribute to spinal compression. Intra-abdominal pressure, on the other hand, works like a balloon inside the abdominal cavity to support the adjacent lumbar spine by creating a tensile force that partially offsets the axial compressive load. Although most of the load on the spine is borne by the vertebral bodies and discs, the facet joints do assist with some load bearing. As with other body regions, protective equipment can prevent some injuries from occurring, particularly at the cervical, sacrum, and coccyx regions. Physical conditioning, however, plays a more important role in preventing injuries to the overall region.

Several pieces of protective equipment can be used to protect the spinal region. In the cervical region, a neck roll or a posterolateral pad can be attached to shoulder pads to limit motion of the cervical spine and this has been shown to reduce the incidence of repetitive burners and stingers. In the upper body, shoulder pads extend over and protect the upper thoracic region. Rib protectors can protect a limited region of the thoracic spine. Weight training belts, abdominal binders, and other similar lumbosacral supportive devices are used to support the abdominal contents, stabilize the trunk, and prevent spinal deformity and damage. They place the low back in a more vertical lifting posture, decrease lumbar lordosis, limit pelvic torsion, and lessen axial loading on the spine by increasing intra-abdominal pressure, which, in turn, reduces compressive forces in the vertebral bodies (2). Many of these protective devices were discussed and demonstrated in Chapter 6.

Flexibility of the back muscles is imperative to stabilize the spinal column. Stretching exercises should increase range of motion in the cervical, thoracic, lumbar, and hip regions. In the cervical region, the hands are used to provide a slow, prolonged stretch in the various motions. Exercises, such as those shown in **Field Strategy 15.1**, can be used to stretch the thoracic, lumbar, and hip regions.

Strengthening exercises for the cervical region may involve isometric contractions, manual resistance, use of surgical tubing, or weight training with free weights or specialized machines. Exercises should include neck flexion, extension, lateral flexion, and rotation, as well as scapular elevation. Stabilization of the cervical spine is particularly important to wrestlers and football lineman, who are consistently subjected to the extremes of motion at the neck. Exercises to strengthen the thoracic and low back area should involve back extension, lateral flexion and rotation, abdominal strengthening, and exercises for lower trapezius and latissimus dorsi. Many of these exercises are demonstrated in **Field Strategy 15.1**.

Proper skill technique is vital to prevent spinal injuries. Helmets are designed to protect the cranial region from injury, but do not prevent axial loading on the cervical spine. Since the 1976 rule change banning spearing in high school football, there has been a large reduction in the incidence of catastrophic spinal injuries, although the incidence of spearing continues to occur (8).

Proper lifting technique can also affect spinal loading. It has been shown that executing a lift in a very rapid, jerking fashion dramatically increases compression and shear forces on the spine, as well as tension in the paraspinal muscles (5). For this reason, isotonic resistance exercises should always be performed in a slow, controlled fashion, inhaling deeply as the lift is initiated and exhal-

Field Strategy 15.1. Prevention of Spinal Injuries

Flexibility Exercises

A. **Single knee to chest stretch.** In a supine position, pull one knee toward the chest with the hands. Keep the back flat. Switch to the opposite leg and repeat

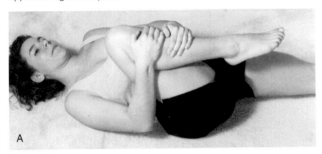

A

B. **Double knee to the chest stretch.** In a supine position, pull both knees to the chest with the hands. Keep the back flat

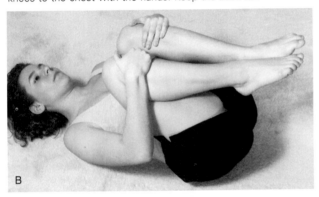

B

C. **Hamstring stretch.** See Field Strategy 9.1

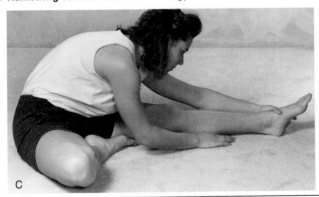

C

Field Strategy 15.1. Prevention of Spinal Injuries (continued)

Flexibility Exercises

D. **Hip flexor stretch.** See Field Strategy 10.1

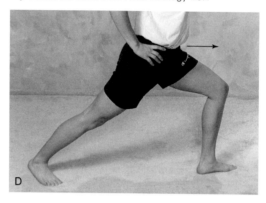

E. **Lateral rotator stretch.** See Field Strategy 10.1

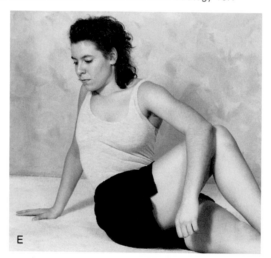

F. **Lower trunk rotation stretch.** In a supine position, rotate the flexed knees to one side, keeping the back flat and the feet together

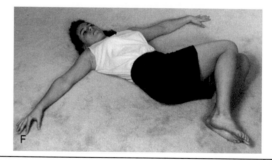

Field Strategy 15.1. Prevention of Spinal Injuries (continued)

Flexibility Exercises

G. **Angry cat stretch (posterior pelvic tilt).** Kneel on all fours with knees hip-width apart. Tighten the buttocks and arch the back upward while lowering the chin and tilting the pelvis backward. Relax the buttocks and allow the pelvis to drop downward and forward

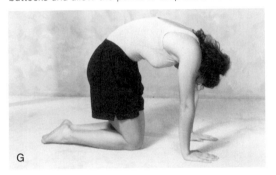

G

Strengthening Exercises

H. **Crunch curl-up.** In a supine position, with the knees flexed and the arms diagonally across the chest, flatten the back and curl up to elevate the head and shoulders from the floor. Alternate exercises include diagonal crunch curl-ups and hip crunches

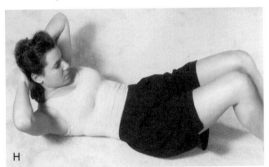

H

I. **Prone extension.** In a prone position, raise up on the elbows. Progress to raising up onto the hands

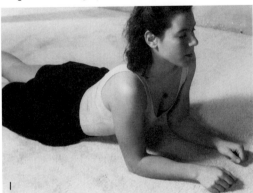

I

Flexibility Exercises

J. **Alternate arm and leg lift.** In a fully extended prone position, lift one arm and the opposite leg off the surface at least 3 inches. Repeat with the opposite arm and leg

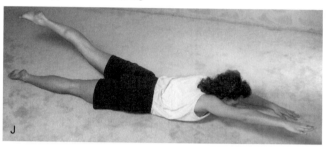

K. **Double arm and leg lift.** In a fully extended prone position, lift both arms and legs off the surface at least 3 inches. Hold and return to starting position

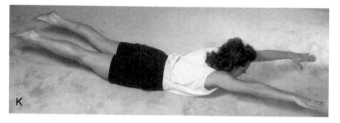

L. **Alternate arm and leg extension on all fours.** Kneel on all fours, raise one leg behind the body while raising the opposite arm in front of the body. Ankle and wrist weights may be added for additional resistance

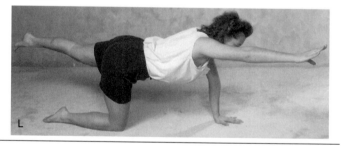

ing forcefully and smoothly at the end of the lift. In addition, use of a supportive weight training belt and a spotter can prevent injury to the lumbar region.

Poor posture during walking, sitting, standing, lying down, and running may lead to chronic low back strain or ligamentous sprains. All cases of postural deformity should be assessed to determine the cause and an appropriate exercise program should be developed to address the deficits.

Field Strategy 15.1. Prevention of Spinal Injuries (continued)

Flexibility Exercises

M. **Back extension.** Using a back extension machine or having another individual stabilize the feet and legs, raise the trunk into a slightly hyperextended position

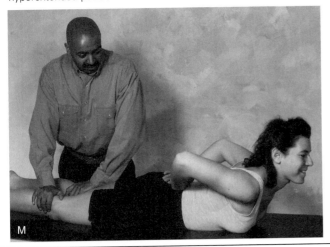

Although protective equipment can protect limited portions of the spine, improved flexibility and strength in the spinal musculature, and proper technique and posture, can be more effective at limiting the risk for injury.

CERVICAL SPINE INJURIES

A gymnast is complaining of a stiff neck. There is full range of motion, but he is more comfortable with the head slightly rotated to the right. Point tenderness is present in the muscle mass on the left anterolateral neck. Resisted neck lateral flexion to the left and rotation to the right increase the pain. No change in sensation or grip strength is evident. What injury might you suspect, and how would you manage it?

The cervical spine is the most mobile region of the spinal column. This, combined with the small mass of the neck as compared to the trunk, makes the cervical spine especially vulnerable to injury. Because range of motion in the cervical spine is greatest in flexion, a head position of extreme flexion generates the largest bending moment. When combined with axial compressional loading, the leading mechanism of injury for severe cervical spine injuries is generated (9). For example, when a tackle in football is executed with the head in a flexed position, the cervical spine

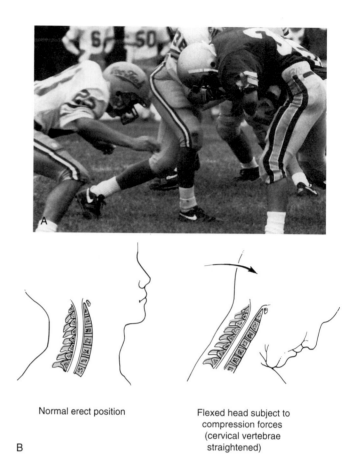

Figure 15.10. A, B. In a normal erect position, the cervical spine is slightly extended. When a tackle in football is executed with the head flexed at about 30°, the cervical vertebrae are in a column and subject to compressional forces generated by the cervical muscles and to axial loading.

Normal erect position

Flexed head subject to
compression forces
(cervical vertebrae
straightened)

is aligned in a segmented column and subjected to large compressional forces generated by the cervical muscles and axial impact forces **(Fig. 15.10)**. Impact causes loading along the longitudinal axis of the cervical vertebrae, leading to compression deformation. The intervertebral discs can initially absorb some energy; however, as continued force is exerted, further deformation and buckling occurs, leading to failure of the intervertebral discs, cervical vertebrae, or both **(Fig. 15.11)**. This results in a possible subluxation, disc herniation, facet dislocation, or fracture-dislocation at one or more spinal levels (9).

Axial loading with the cervical spine slightly flexed is the leading mechanism of injury for severe cervical spine injuries

Cervical Strains and Sprains

Cervical strains usually involve the sternocleidomastoid or upper trapezius, although other muscles may be involved. Strains typically occur at the extremes of motion, or in association with a violent muscle contraction or external force. Symptoms include

Cervical strains occur at the extremes of motion, or in association with a violent muscle contraction or external force

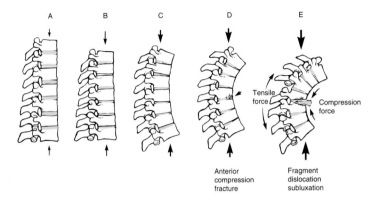

Figure 15.11. Axial loading on the vertebral column causes compressive deformation of the intervertebral discs (**A, B**). As load continues and maximum compression deformation is reached, angular deformation and buckling occurs (**C, D**). Continued force results in an anterior compression fracture, subluxation, or dislocation (**E**).

pain, stiffness, and restricted range of motion. Palpation will reveal muscle spasms and increased pain during active contraction or passive stretching of the involved muscle. Generally, symptoms subside within 3 to 7 days.

Sprains can occur to major ligaments traversing the cervical spine, as well as to the capsular ligaments surrounding the facet joints. The same mechanisms that cause cervical strains also lead to cervical sprains. Both injuries often occur simultaneously. Minor activity, such as maintaining the head in an uncomfortable posture or sleeping position, can also produce sprains of the neck. Symptoms mirror those seen in cervical strains; however, with severe sprains, symptoms tend to persist longer. In cases when pain or numbness radiates into the back of the head or extremities, referral to a physician is warranted to rule out a possible spinal fracture, dislocation, or disc injury.

> Symptoms for a cervical sprain mirror those in a cervical strain, but tend to persist longer

Initial treatment includes rest, cryotherapy, prescribed non-steroidal anti-inflammatory drugs (NSAIDs), and use of a cervical collar for support. Follow-up treatment may involve continued cryotherapy or use of superficial heat, gentle stretching, and isometric exercises. Individuals participating in contact sports should strengthen the neck muscles through appropriate resistance exercise.

Cervical Fractures and Dislocations

Unsafe practices, such as diving into shallow water, spearing in football, or landing on the posterior neck during gymnastics or trampoline activities, can lead to cervical fractures and dislocations from the axial loading and violent neck flexion. In sports, these serious injuries commonly occur at the fourth, fifth, and sixth cervical vertebrae. Because neural damage can range from none

Table 15.2. Danger Signs Indicating a Possible Cervical Spine Injury

Pain over the spinous process with or without deformity
Unrelenting neck pain or muscle spasm
Abnormal sensations on the head, neck, trunk, or extremities
Muscular weakness in the extremities
Loss of coordinated movement
Paralysis or inability to move a body part
Absent or weak reflexes
Loss of bladder or bowel control

to complete severance of the spinal cord, there is a range of accompanying symptoms. Painful palpation over the spinous processes, muscle spasm, or a defect indicates a possible fracture or dislocation. Radiating pain, numbness, muscle weakness, paralysis, or loss of bladder or bowel control are all critical signs of neural damage. Many of the serious signs and symptoms are summarized in **Table 15.2**.

Because of possible spinal cord damage leading to paralysis or death, any suspected unstable neck injury should be treated as a medical emergency. An unstable neck injury should be suspected in an unconscious athlete, an athlete who is awake but has numbness and/or paralysis, and in a neurologically intact athlete who has neck pain or pain with neck movement (10). Without moving the head or neck out of alignment, apply light cervical traction while the neck is being stabilized, then conduct a primary survey to recognize and manage any life-threatening situation. Summon EMS and assist the technicians in immobilizing the injured athlete on a spine board.

Did you determine the gymnast had a muscle strain of the left sternocleidomastoid muscle? If so, you are correct. Cryotherapy and support from a cervical collar will alleviate some of the discomfort. A mild stretching program and isometric strengthening should be initiated immediately.

BRACHIAL PLEXUS INJURIES

A defensive lineman charged the quarterback preparing to throw a pass, and struck the throwing arm, forcing it into excessive abduction and external rotation. An immediate burning sensation traveled down the length of the quarterback's arm and now his thumb is tingling. What might have happened here? Is this a serious injury?

The brachial plexus is a complex neural structure that innervates the upper extremity and is typically damaged in two manners. A stretch injury may be caused when a tensile force leads to forceful downward traction of the clavicle while the head is distracted in

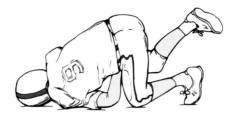

Figure 15.12. Common mechanism of a brachial plexus stretch.

the opposite direction, such as when an individual is tackled and subsequently rolls onto the shoulder with the head turned to the opposite side (**Fig. 15.12**). A stretch-injury may also occur when the arm is forced into excessive external rotation, abduction, and extension. This injury usually affects the upper trunk (C_5, C_6) of the brachial plexus, which will lead to a sensory loss or paresthesia in the thumb and index finger. The other mechanism of injury may involve compression of the fixed plexus between the football shoulder pad and the superior medial scapula, where the brachial plexus is most superficial (11).

Acute symptoms involve a burning or stinging pain that radiates from the clavicular area down the arm into the hand, hence the nickname "**burner**" or "stinger." Pain is usually transient and subsides in 5 to 10 minutes, but tenderness over the clavicular area may persist. Often the individual will try to shake the arm to "get the feeling back." Muscle weakness is evident in shoulder abduction and external rotation. When weakness is present, the individual should be removed from competition. If strength and function return completely in 1 to 2 minutes, the athlete can return to play. If any neurologic symptoms persist after this time, the athlete should not be allowed to return to play until full strength, range of motion, and sensation are restored in the cervical spine and extremity (12).

Chronic burners, however, are characterized by more frequent acute episodes that may not produce areas of numbness. Muscle weakness in the shoulder muscles may develop hours or days after the initial injury and may result in a dropped shoulder or visible atrophy in the shoulder muscles (11). These individuals should be examined after the game, during the week, and again the following week, because weakness may not become apparent until days after the initial injury. The use of high shoulder pads supplemented by a cervical collar may limit excessive lateral neck flexion and extension.

Did you determine the quarterback experienced a brachial plexus stretch injury? The pain and tingling in the thumb should resolve in a few minutes. If it lingers and/or muscular weakness becomes evident in shoulder abduction or external rotation, this person should be referred to a physician for further examination.

Brachial plexus injuries usually affect the upper trunk (C_5, C_6), leading to sensory loss or paresthesia in the thumb and index finger

Burner
Burning or stinging sensation characteristic of a brachial plexus injury

With a burner, pain is usually transient and resolves itself in 5 to 10 minutes, but local tenderness over the clavicular area may persist

? *A 15-year-old butterfly-stroke swimmer is complaining of localized pain and tenderness in the mid-back region over the thoracic spine. The pain came on gradually and only hurts during the execution of the stroke. Fracture tests are negative. What other condition(s) might be suspected?*

The protective rib cage serves to limit movement in the thoracic motion segments. The thoracolumbar junction, however, is a region of potentially high stress during flexion–extension movements of the trunk. Injuries here may involve contusions, strains, sprains, fractures, and apophysitis.

Thoracic Contusions, Strains, and Sprains

Direct blows to the back during contact sports frequently yield contusions to the muscles in the thoracic region. Such injuries range in severity but are generally characterized by pain, ecchymosis, spasm, limited swelling, and pain.

> Thoracic strains result from either overstretching or overloading muscles in the region through violent or sustained muscle contractions

Thoracic sprains and strains result from either overloading or overstretching muscles in the region through violent or sustained muscle contractions. Painful spasms and knot-like contractions of the back muscles serve as a protective mechanism to immobilize the injured area and may develop as a sympathetic response to sprains (13). The presence of such spasms, however, makes it difficult to determine whether the injury is actually a sprain or strain. Dramatic improvement in a thoracic sprain can be seen in 24 to 48 hours. Severe strains, however, may require 3 or 4 weeks to heal.

Initial treatment for soft tissue injuries consists of cryotherapy, prescribed NSAIDs, and activity modification. Follow-up management may include application of superficial heat, ultrasound, massage, and appropriate stretching and resistance exercise, as needed, to recondition the individual.

Thoracic Spinal Fractures and Apophysitis

> Large compressive loads, such as those sustained during heavy weightlifting or head-on contact in football or rugby, can cause fractures of the vertebral end plates

The rib cage stabilizes and limits motion in the thoracic spine, thereby lessening the likelihood of injury to this area. Thoracic fractures, subsequently, tend to be concentrated at the lower end of the thoracic spine in the transition region between the thoracic and lumbar curvatures.

Wedge fracture
A crushing compression fracture that leaves a vertebra narrowed anteriorly

Osteopoenia
Condition of reduced bone mineral density that predisposes the individual to fractures

Large compressive loads, such as those sustained during heavy weightlifting, head-on contact in football or rugby, or landing on the buttock area during tobogganing or snowmobiling, can fracture the vertebral end plates or lead to a **wedge fracture**, named after the shape of the deformed vertebral body (**Fig. 15.13**). Females with **osteopoenia**, a condition of reduced bone mineralization, are particularly susceptible to these fractures. More commonly, however, compressive stress during small, repetitive loads in an activity, such as running, leads to a progressive compression frac-

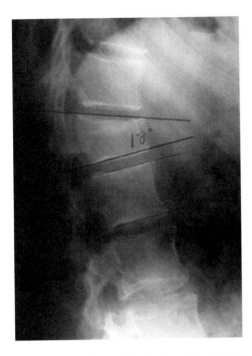

Figure 15.13. A compression wedge fracture in the thoracic region.

ture of a weakened vertebral body. In addition, repeated flexion–extension of the thoracic spine, such as what occurs during the butterfly and breast strokes, can inflame the apophyses, or the growth centers of the vertebral bodies. Apophysitis is a progressive condition characterized by local pain and tenderness. Treatment for apophysitis includes elimination of the flexion–extension stress and strengthening abdominal and other trunk muscles.

💡 *Did you determine that the swimmer may have possible apophysitis because of the repeated flexion–extension motions executed during the butterfly stroke? This individual should be referred to a physician for further examination.*

LUMBAR SPINE INJURIES

❓ *A distance runner is experiencing chronic low back pain during the workout. What advice might you provide to reduce stress on the low back during running?*

When the body is in an upright position, the line of gravity passes anterior to the spinal column (**Fig. 15.14**). As a result, the spine is under a constant forward bending moment. As the trunk is progressively flexed, the line of gravity shifts farther away from the spine, increasing the moment arm. To maintain body position, this action must be counteracted by tension in the back muscles. The more muscle tension required to maintain body position, the greater the compressional load on the spine. In comparison to the load present during upright standing, compression on the

When the trunk is erect, the back muscles must develop tension to balance the spinal moment—the product of weight and distance from the spine. Thus, the heavier an object, or the farther it is held from the body, the more the back muscles must work to maintain an upright position

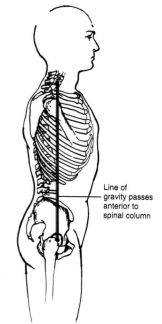

Line of gravity passes anterior to spinal column

Figure 15.14. The line of gravity for the head and trunk passes anterior to the spinal column during upright standing. The moment arm for head/trunk weight at any given vertebral joint is the perpendicular distance between the line of gravity and the spinal column.

lumbar spine increases with sitting, increases more with spinal flexion, and increases still further with a slouched sitting position. During lifting and carrying, holding the load as close to the trunk as possible minimizes the load on the back. **Field Strategy 15.2** provides several guidelines to reduce spinal stress in daily activities to prevent low back injuries.

Low Back Pain

An estimated 60 to 80% of the population experiences low back pain (LBP) at some time. Although LBP typically strikes individuals between the ages of 25 and 60 years, with frequency peaking at about age 40, it also occurs in as many as 25% of adolescents and children, ranging down to age 10 (14,15). Males and females appear to be equally susceptible (15,16).

Although several known pathologies may cause LBP, most cases are idiopathic, brought on by repetitive microtraumatic stress. Low back pain is common in running activities, because many runners have muscle tightness in the hip flexors and hamstrings. Tight hip flexors produce a forward body lean, leading to anterior pelvic tilt and hyperlordosis of the lumbar spine. This, coupled with tight hamstrings, can lead to a shorter stride. To decrease the incidence of LBP, training techniques should allow for adequate progression of distance, speed, and hill work, and include extensive flexibility exercises for the hip and thigh region. **Field Strategy 15.3** outlines suggestions for reducing the incidence of LBP in runners.

Low back pain is found in as many as 25% of adolescents and children, but typically strikes individuals between the ages of 25 and 60

Many runners have muscle tightness in the hip flexors and hamstrings, leading to anterior pelvic tilt and increased lordosis

Field Strategy 15.2. Preventing Low Back Injuries in Activities of Daily Living

Sitting

Sit on a firm, straight-back chair
Place the buttocks as far back into the chair as possible to avoid slouching
Sit with the feet flat on the floor
Avoid sitting for long periods of time, particularly with the knees fully
   extended

Driving

Place the seat forward so the knees are level with the hips and you do
   not have to reach for the pedals
If the left foot is not working the pedals, place it flat on the floor
Keep the back of the seat in a nearly upright position to avoid slouching or
   leaning forward

Standing

If you must stand in one area for an extended time:
   Shift body weight from one foot to the other
   Elevate one foot on a piece of furniture to keep the knees flexed
   Do toe flexion and extension inside the shoes
Hold the chin up, keep the shoulders back, and relax the knees

Lifting and Carrying

Use a lumbosacral belt or have assistance when lifting heavy objects
To lift an object:
   Place the object close to the body
   Bend at the knees, not the waist, and keep the back erect
   Tighten the abdominal muscles and inhale while lifting the object
   Exhale at the end of the lift; do not hold your breath
   Do not twist while lifting
To carry a heavy object:
   Hold the object close to the body at waist level
   Carry the object in the middle of the body, not to one side

Sleeping

Sleep on a firm mattress. If needed, place a sheet of ¾ inch plywood
   under the mattress
Sleep on your side and place pillows between the legs
If you sleep supine, place pillows under the knees. Avoid sleeping in the
   prone position
Because waterbeds support the body curves more evenly, they may
   relieve low back pain

Lumbar Contusions, Strains, and Sprains

Soft tissue injuries are the most frequent injuries in the lumbar region. The injuries and mechanisms are the same as those described in the thoracic region. Because the lumbar muscles must develop tension to counteract the forward bending moment of the entire trunk when the trunk is in flexion, these muscles are particularly susceptible to strain. Symptoms include localized pain

Field Strategy 15.3. Reducing Low Back Pain in Runners

Wear properly fitted shoes that control heel motion and provide maximum shock-absorption

Increase flexibility in the muscles of the hip and thigh, ankle plantar flexors, and the trunk extensors

Increase strength in the abdominal and trunk extensor muscles

Avoid excessive body weight

Warm up and stretch thoroughly before and after running

Run with an upright stance rather than a forward lean

Avoid excessive side-to-side sway

Run on even terrain and limit hill work; avoid running on concrete

Avoid overstriding to increase speed, as this increases leg shock

Gradually increase distance, intensity, and duration. Do not increase any one parameter more than 10% in one week

If orthoses are worn and pain persists, check for wear and rigidity

Consider alternatives to running, such as cycling, rowing, or swimming

---

that increases with active and resisted motion, but radiating pain and neurologic deficits will not be present. Treatment includes rest, cryotherapy, and prescribed NSAIDs. A lumbar support brace may help alleviate some stress on the region (see **Fig. 6.13**). If symptoms do not improve within a week, refer the individual to a physician to rule out a more serious underlying condition.

Sciatica

Sciatica is an inflammatory condition of the sciatic nerve, resulting from a herniated disc, a muscle-related or facet joint disease, or compression of the nerve between the two parts of the piriformis muscle (17). If related to a herniated disc, radiating leg pain is greater than back pain and increases with sitting and leaning forward, coughing, sneezing, and straining. Pain is reproduced during an **ipsilateral** straight-leg raising test (see **Fig. 15.21**). Morning pain and muscular stiffness are characteristic of a muscle-related disease. If the facet joint is involved, pain will be localized over the joint on spinal extension and is exacerbated with ipsilateral lateral flexion. If the sciatic nerve is compressed between the piriformis muscle, pain increases during internal rotation of the thigh (17).

Referral to a physician is necessary to determine the presence of a serious underlying condition. Under normal circumstances, bed rest is usually not indicated, although side-lying with the knees flexed may relieve some symptoms. Lifting, bending, twisting, and prolonged sitting and standing may aggravate the condition and, therefore, should be avoided. When asymptomatic, abdominal and extensor muscle strengthening exercises can begin with gradual return to activity. If symptoms resume, stop activity and refer the individual back to the physician. Occasionally, extended rest is

Sciatica
Compression of a spinal nerve due to a herniated disc, a muscle-related or facet joint disease, or compression between the two parts of the piriformis muscle

Ipsilateral
Situated on, pertaining to, or affecting the same side, as opposed to contralateral

needed for symptoms to totally resolve or, if a significant disc protrusion is present, surgery may be indicated.

Lumbar Disc Injuries

Prolonged mechanical loading of the spine can lead to microruptures in the annulus fibrosus, resulting in degeneration of the disc. When the nucleus of the disc works its way through the fibers of the annulus, it is called a **prolapsed disc**. It is called an **extruded disc** when the material moves into the spinal canal, where it runs the risk of impinging adjacent nerve roots. The most commonly herniated discs are the lower two lumbar discs between L_4 to L_5 and L_5 to S_1, with most ruptures moving in a posterior or posterolateral direction as a result of torsion and compression, not just compression (2).

Because the intervertebral discs are not innervated, the sensation of pain will not occur until the surrounding soft tissue structures are impinged. Symptoms include sharp pain and muscle spasms at the site of the herniation that often shoot down the sciatic nerve into the lower extremity. The individual may walk in a slightly crouched position, leaning away from the side of the lesion. Forward trunk flexion or a straight-leg raising test (see **Fig. 15.21**) may exacerbate pain and increase distal symptoms. Significant signs indicating the need for immediate referral to a physician include muscle weakness, sensory changes, diminished reflexes in the lower extremity, and abnormal bladder or bowel function.

In mild cases, treatment consists of minimizing load on the spine by avoiding activities that involve impact, lifting, bending, twisting, and prolonged sitting and standing. Painful muscle spasms can be eliminated with ice and/or heat, administration of prescribed NSAIDs and/or muscle relaxants, and gentle stretching. Following resolution of spasm and acute pain, rehabilitation should include spine and hamstring flexibility, spinal strength and stabilization exercises, and functional stabilization control in sports and daily activities (2).

Lumbar Fractures and Dislocations

As mentioned earlier, fractures more commonly involve the L_1 vertebra at the thoracolumbar junction. Hyperflexion, or jack-knifing of the trunk, crushes the anterior aspect of the vertebral body. The primary danger with this injury is the possibility of bony fragments moving into the spinal canal to damage the spinal cord or spinal nerves. Symptoms will include localized, palpable pain that may radiate down the nerve root if a bony fragment compresses a spinal nerve. Because the spinal cord ends at about the L_1 or L_2 level, fractures of the lumbar vertebrae below this point do not pose a serious threat, but should still be handled with care to minimize potential nerve damage to the cauda equina. Confirmation of a possible fracture is made with an radiograph or CT scan.

Prolapsed disc
Condition when the eccentric nucleus produces a definite deformity as it works its way through the fibers of the annulus fibrosus

Extruded disc
Condition in which the nuclear material moves into the spinal canal and runs the risk of impinging adjacent nerve roots

The most commonly herniated discs are the lower two lumbar discs between L_4 to L_5 and L_5 to S_1 vertebrae

Forward trunk flexion or a straight-leg raising test may lead to excruciating pain and an increase in distal symptoms

Compression fractures at the thoracolumbar junction are typically caused by violent hyperflexion, or jack-knifing of the trunk, which crushes the anterior aspect of the vertebral body

💡 *To reduce low back pain, you might advise the runner to incorporate a regular flexibility program for the hip flexors, hip abductors, hamstrings, and Achilles tendon. In addition, they should avoid running with a forward body lean, avoid overstriding and excessive side-to-side sway, and should run on even terrain, gradually increasing the distance of the workout. For other suggestions, see* **Field Strategy 15.3.**

SACRUM AND COCCYX INJURIES

❓ *An individual is complaining of sharp pain in the sacral region when running on uneven terrain. After sitting for an extended period of time, pain begins to ache in the posterior pelvic region. What might you suspect is injured? What would you recommend for this person?*

Because the sacrum and coccyx are essentially immobile, the potential for mechanical injury to these regions is dramatically reduced. Sprains of the sacroiliac (SI) joint, however, can lead to localized pain and stiffness. The injury may result from a single traumatic episode involving bending and/or twisting, repetitive stress from lifting, a fall on the buttocks, excessive side-to-side or up-and-down motion during running and jogging, running on uneven terrain, suddenly slipping or stumbling forward, or wearing new shoes or orthotics (2,17). Symptoms may involve unilateral dull pain in the sacral area that extends into the buttock and posterior thigh. Muscle spasm is not often seen. Standing on one leg and climbing stairs may also increase the pain. Treatment for sacroiliac sprains includes cryotherapy, prescribed NSAIDs, and gentle stretching to alleviate stiffness. Flexibility, pelvic stabilization exercises, mobilization of the affected joint, and strengthening exercises for the low back can then begin.

> Sacroiliac sprains may be caused by a single traumatic episode involving bending and/or twisting, repetitive stress from lifting, or excessive side-to-side or up-and-down motion during running and jogging

Direct blows to the region can produce contusions and fractures of the coccyx. Pain resulting from a fracture may last for several months. Treatment for coccygeal pain includes analgesics and use of padding for protection and a ring seat to alleviate compression during sitting.

💡 *The runner has probably irritated the sacroiliac joint from repeated stress while running on uneven terrain. This individual should ice the region to control inflammation and pain, stretch the low back and buttock region, and run on more even terrain. If conditions do not improve, refer the individual to a physician for further assessment.*

ASSESSMENT OF THE SPINE

❓ *A 17-year-old female high jumper is complaining of pain in the low back and sacroiliac region, aggravated by flexion and hyperextension of the trunk during jumping. How will you progress through the assessment to determine the extent and severity of injury?*

Injury assessment of the spine is complex and cannot be rushed. It is uncommon in a traumatic episode when a conscious individual is lying on the field or court, to have a significant spinal injury without severe pain, spasm, or tenderness. It is very common, however, for an individual with a minor injury, such as a muscular strain, to have only mild to moderate pain and tenderness. The severity of pain and presence or absence of neurological symptoms, neck spasm, and tenderness can indicate when a backboard and neck stabilization is needed (10,19). When in doubt, always assume a severe spinal injury has occurred and initiate the emergency care plan. Do not remove the helmet or move the individual's head, neck, or spine. Once a significant physical finding indicates possible nerve involvement, immediate transportation to the nearest medical facility is warranted, regardless of whether a total assessment is completed. Immobilization of the individual should be completed under the direction of trained personnel.

In nontraumatic injuries, when the individual walks into the training room complaining of neck or back pain, it is relatively safe to assume that a serious spinal injury is not present. Because of the high incidence of referred pain, a quick scan exam can be performed during observation to determine if other body parts need to be assessed. This section will focus on a spinal assessment of a conscious individual. Specific information related to an acute injury is included where appropriate. To review assessment procedures for the primary survey and for an unconscious individual with a suspected spinal injury, refer to Chapter 3.

> Once a significant physical finding indicates probable nerve involvement, immediate transportation to the nearest medical facility is warranted, regardless of whether a total assessment is completed

HISTORY

> **?** *The high jumper complained of pain in the low back and sacroiliac region, aggravated by flexion and hyperextension of the trunk during jumping. What questions need to be asked to identify the cause and extent of injury?*

A history of the injury should include information on the mechanism of injury; extent of pain; or disability due to the injury, previous injuries to the area, and family history which may have some bearing on this specific condition. In a spinal injury, ask about the location of pain (localized or radiating), type of pain (dull, aching, sharp, burning), presence of sensory changes (numbness, tingling, or absence of sensation), and possible muscle weakness or paralysis. Ask questions to determine both long- and short-term memory loss that may indicate an associated concussion or subdural hematoma. Note how long it takes to respond to the questions. General questions related to an injury to the spine can be seen in **Field Strategy 15.4**.

> In a spinal injury, ask specific information on the location of pain, type of pain, presence of sensory changes, and possible muscle weakness or paralysis

> **💡** *The 17-year-old jumper has been a competitive athlete since seventh grade. The primary complaint is an aching pain when bending over, aggravated with hyperextension and prolonged sitting, that produces sharp, radiating pain into the low*

Field Strategy 15.4. Developing a History for a Spinal Injury

Current Injury Status

1. How did the injury occur (mechanism)? Did the injury involve twisting of the trunk, a violent stretch, or jack-knife maneuver?
2. Ask about the pain location, severity, onset (sudden or gradual), and type (sharp, aching, burning, radiating, deep, or superficial). Does the severity of symptoms change when you change position?
3. Was there any muscle spasm, numbness, or change in sensation anywhere in the body?
4. What different activities have you been doing in the last week? (Look for activities such as lifting or carrying heavy objects, or positions involving bending over for long periods of time)
5. Are there certain activities you cannot perform because of the pain? Note the gender. Females have a higher incidence of low back pain.

Past Injury Status

1. Have you ever injured your back before? When? How did that occur? What was done for the injury?
2. Have you had any medical problems recently? (Look for possible referred pain from visceral organs, heart, and lungs.) Are you on any medication? Do you have any musculoskeletal problems elsewhere in the body? (These may result in changes in gait or technique that transfer abnormal forces to structures in the spinal region.)
3. Has anyone in your family had a similar problem?

---

back and sacroiliac region. The condition has been present for 4 weeks and is not getting better. She cannot recall any traumatic episode that led to the condition.

OBSERVATION AND INSPECTION

? *Would it be appropriate to do a scan exam to rule out other painful areas? What specific factors should be observed to identify the injury?*

Begin observation immediately when the individual enters the room. Body language can signal such factors as pain, disability, and muscle weakness. Note the individual's willingness or ability to move, general posture, ease in motion, and general attitude. Clothing and protective equipment may prevent visual observation of abnormalities in the spinal alignment. As such, the individual should be suitably dressed so the back is exposed as much as possible. For girls and women, a bra, halter top, or swim suit can be worn. Begin with a general postural assessment, progress through a scan exam, and inspect the injury site.

Body language can signal such factors as pain, disability, and muscle weakness

Posture

In assessing the posture, ask the individual to sit down to begin the exam; then stand. Note the head and neck posture. Is the

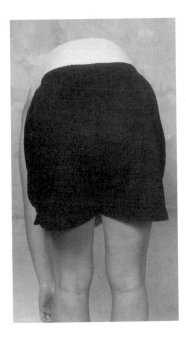

Figure 15.15. Performing the "sky-line" view (Adam's position) of the spine can assess the presence of scoliosis.

head held erect or carried in a forward position? Are any abnormal spinal curvatures present? Ask the individual to lean forward and touch the toes while keeping the knees straight (Adam's position). Observe the vertebrae and contour of the back **(Fig. 15.15)**. Look for a hump or raised scapula on one side (convex side of curve) and a hollow (concave side of curve) on the other, indicating scoliosis. The combination of the hump and hollow is due to vertebral rotation. Are there any noticeable asymmetries, such as discrepancies in shoulder or scapula height, hip height, or patella height? Is the trunk rotated so one shoulder is forward? Are the ribs more prominent on one side?

Scan Exam

A scan exam assesses general motor function and can rule out injury at other joints that may be overlooked due to intense pain or discomfort at the primary injury site. Active movement of the spine may be included in this step prior to palpation, and need not be repeated with special tests. Note if there is any hesitation to move a body part, or if the individual prefers to use one side over the other. Examples of gross motor movements for the spine are listed in **Field Strategy 15.5**. Additional gross motor movements for the upper and lower extremity should also be performed.

Active movement of the spine may be included in a scan exam prior to palpation and need not be repeated again with special tests

Inspection of the Injury Site

Local inspection at the injury site should observe for deformity, swelling, discoloration, muscle spasm, atrophy, hypertrophy, scars that might indicate previous surgery, and general skin condition. A step deformity in the lumbar spine may indicate spondylolisthesis.

Ask the individual to perform the following actions:
1. Touch the chin to the chest
2. Look up at the ceiling, keeping the back straight
3. Turn the head sideways in both directions
4. Try to touch each ear to the shoulder
5. Rotate the trunk sideways, keeping the hips stabilized
6. Lean forward and touch the toes
7. Look up at the ceiling with hyperextension of the trunk
8. Lean sideways and do lateral flexion of the trunk
9. While placing a hand on a table for support, do a straight-leg raise forward, backward, and sideways

Gross Neuromuscular Assessment

In an acute injury, a posture and scan exam is not possible. It would be beneficial, however, to do a neuromuscular assessment prior to palpations to detect any motor and/or sensory deficits. Without moving the individual, ask them to perform a submaximal bilateral hand-squeeze test and ankle dorsiflexion. These two actions assess the cervical and lumbar spinal nerves, respectively. Muscle weakness and/or diminished sensation over the hands and feet indicate a serious injury. If any deficits are noted, initiate the emergency care plan and summon EMS. If no deficits are noted, it does not rule out possible neurological involvement or fracture. Therefore, palpations should be done in the position the individual is found in.

> *Slight lordosis and anterior pelvic tilt is present in the high jumper. During the scan exam, trunk flexion and extension produced a dull pain in the low back. Lateral flexion to the right caused sharp pain to radiate into the right buttock and posterior leg. A forward straight-leg raise with the right leg was limited and could not be performed without bending the knee. Visual inspection showed no abnormalities.*

PALPATIONS

> *The injury is confined to the low back region. What specific structures can be palpated to determine if the injury is bony or soft tissue in origin?*

In injuries that do not involve neural damage, fracture, or dislocation, palpations can proceed in the following manner. Palpate bony and soft tissue structures to detect temperature, swelling, point tenderness, deformity, crepitus, muscle spasm, and cutaneous sensation. Palpations may be done in a seated, standing, or lying position. To relax the neck and spinal muscles, the individual should lie on a table. To palpate posterior neck structures, have the individual supine. Reach around the neck with both hands and palpate either side of the spine with the fingertips. In the

Marginal notes:

Without moving the individual, ask them to do a submaximal bilateral hand-squeeze test and ankle dorsiflexion test

If the individual is lying in a prone position, place a pillow or blanket under the hip region to tilt the pelvis back and relax the lumbar curvature

thoracic and low back region, have the individual prone. Place a pillow or blanket under the hip region to tilt the pelvis back and relax the lumbar curvature. Muscle spasms may indicate dysfunction of the specific spinal region. Palpate the following structures.

Anterior Aspect

1. Anterior throat region
2. Sternocleidomastoid muscle, manubrium, and clavicle
3. Sternum, ribs, and costocartilage
4. Abdomen and inguinal area (note any abnormal tenderness or masses that may indicate internal pathology that is referring pain to the spinal region)
5. Iliac crest

Posterior Aspect

1. Occipital bone
2. Spinous and transverse processes of all vertebrae (any tenderness, crepitus, or deviation from the norm may indicate a fracture or vertebral subluxation)
3. Spinal ligaments
4. Scapula, trapezius, and latissimus dorsi
5. Iliac crest
6. Ischial tuberosity, sciatic nerve, and greater trochanter **(Fig. 15.16)**

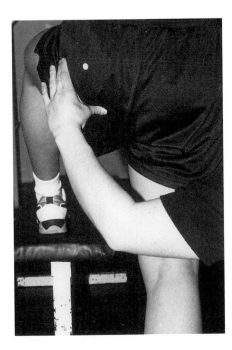

Figure 15.16. To palpate the sciatic nerve, flex the hip and locate the ischial tuberosity and greater trochanter. The sciatic nerve can be palpated at the midpoint, designated here by the dot.

Point tenderness was palpated in the low back region between
L_3 to S_1 vertebrae, with increased pain in the L_4 to L_5 region.
Muscle spasm was present on either side of the lumbar region.
Pain was also elicited with palpation midway between the ischial
tuberosity and greater trochanter.

SPECIAL TESTS

The high jumper has concentrated palpable pain in the L_4
to L_5 region, with associated muscle spasm and pain over
the sciatic nerve as it passes into the posterior thigh. How will
you proceed to determine bony versus soft tissue involvement?

Because injuries to the spinal region can be very complex, it
is imperative to work slowly through the different tests. If, at
anytime, movement leads to increased acute pain, change in sensation, or the individual resists moving the spine, assume that a
significant injury is present and take appropriate measures to refer
this individual to a physician for further evaluation.

Joint Range of Motion

Active movements should not be performed when pain is present
over the vertebrae or when motor/sensory deficits are present. If
active movement of the spine was conducted during the scan
exam, it need not be repeated here. Look for the individual's
willingness to perform the movement. Is the movement fluid and
complete? Does pain, spasm, or stiffness block the full range of
motion? With movements to the left and right, always compare
bilaterally. Spinal movements include:

1. Cervical flexion and extension
2. Cervical lateral flexion (left and right)
3. Cervical rotation (left and right)
4. Trunk forward flexion
5. Trunk extension
6. Trunk lateral flexion (left and right)
7. Trunk rotation (left and right)

Completion of gross movement patterns is adequate enough
to determine normal ranges of motion. If motion is limited, further
assessment can be conducted.

Resisted Manual Muscle Testing

Stabilize the hip and trunk during cervical testing to avoid muscle
substitution. With the individual seated, use one hand to stabilize
the shoulder or thorax while the other hand applies manual overpressure. When testing the thoracic and lumbar regions, the
weight of the trunk will stabilize the hips in a seated position.
Inform the individual not to allow you to move the body part

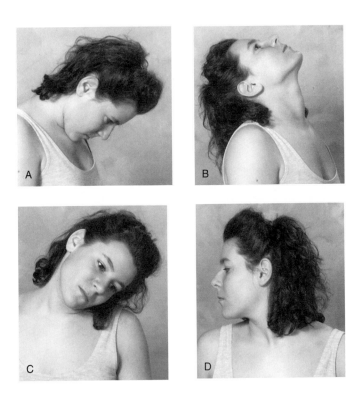

Figure 15.17. Active movements of the cervical spine. **A.** Flexion. **B.** Extension. **C.** Lateral flexion. **D.** Rotation.

being tested. Cervical movements assessed are demonstrated in **Figure 15.17**. Thoracic and lumbar movements are demonstrated in **Figure 15.18**.

Neurologic Assessment

Neurological integrity can be assessed with manual muscle testing (already completed), reflex testing, and cutaneous sensation. Reflexes in the upper extremity include the biceps (C_5 to C_6), brachialis (C_6), and triceps (C_7). In the lower extremity, the two major reflexes are the patella (L_3, L_4) and Achilles tendon reflex (S_1). To test for cutaneous sensory changes, run the open hand and fingernails over the head, neck, back, thorax, abdomen, and upper and lower extremities (front, back, and sides). Ask the person if the sensation feels the same on one body segment as compared to another.

Stress and Functional Tests

Several stress tests may be used in a basic spinal assessment. Only those deemed relevant should be performed. If any increased pain or sensory change occurs, the individual should be referred immediately to a physician.

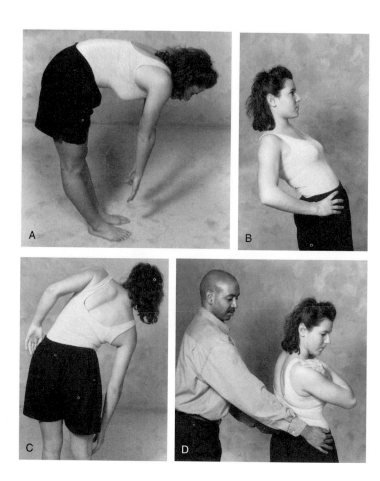

Figure 15.18. Active movements of the thoracic and lumbar regions. **A.** Flexion. **B.** Extension. **C.** Lateral flexion. **D.** Rotation.

Cervical Compression Test

The individual flexes the neck slightly toward one side. Carefully compress straight down on the individual's head while the person is sitting on a stable chair or table **(Fig. 15.19)**. Increased pain or altered sensation is a positive sign indicating pressure on a nerve root.

Cervical Distraction Test

Place one hand under the individual's chin and the other around the occiput. Slowly lift the head **(Fig. 15.20)**. The test is positive if pain decreases or is relieved as the head is lifted, indicating that pressure on the nerve root is relieved. If pain increases with distraction, it indicates ligamentous injury.

Straight-Leg Raising Test

This test indicates stretching of the dura mater of the spinal cord and can be used to assess sacroiliac joint pain or tight hamstrings.

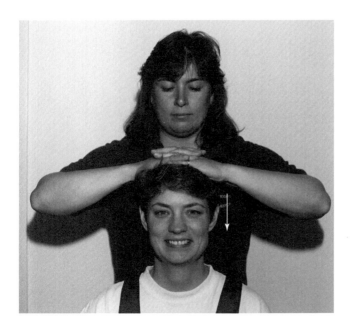

Figure 15.19. To perform the compression test, carefully push straight down on the individual's head. Increased pain or altered sensation is a positive sign indicating pressure on a nerve root.

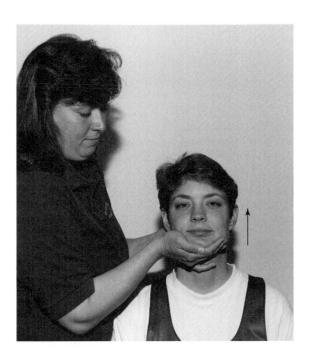

Figure 15.20. To perform the distraction test, lift the head slowly. The test is positive if pain is decreased or relieved as the head is lifted, indicating that pressure on the nerve root is relieved. If pain increases with distraction, it indicates ligamentous injury.

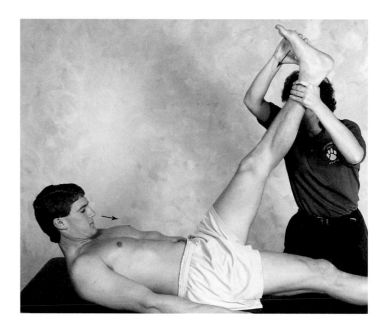

Figure 15.21. Passively flex the individual's hip while keeping the knee extended until pain or tension is felt in the hamstrings. Slowly lower the leg until the pain or tension disappears. Then, dorsiflex the foot, have the individual flex the neck, or do both simultaneously. If pain does not increase with dorsiflexion of the ankle or flexion of the neck, it indicates tight hamstrings.

Pain that increases with neck flexion or dorsiflexion indicates spinal cord involvement. Pain that does not increase with neck flexion or dorsiflexion indicates tight hamstrings

The individual is placed in a relaxed supine position with the hip medially rotated and knee extended. Grasp the individual's heel with one hand and place the other on top of the patella to prevent the knee from flexing. Slowly raise the leg until the individual complains of pain or tightness. Lower the leg slightly until pain is relieved. The individual is then asked to flex the neck onto the chest, or dorsiflex the foot, or do both actions simultaneously **(Fig. 15.21)**. Pain that increases with neck flexion or dorsiflexion indicates stretching of the dura mater of the spinal cord. Pain that does not increase with neck flexion or dorsiflexion indicates tight hamstrings. Pain that occurs opposite the leg lifted indicates a herniated disc. Always compare both legs for any difference.

Functional Testing

Prior to return to play, the individual must have a normal neurologic exam with pain-free range of motion, normal bilateral muscle strength, cutaneous sensation, and reflexes. Axial head compression can be performed on the sideline as an additional safety check. If pain is present, the individual should not return to competition. Other functional tests include walking, bending, lifting, jogging, running, figure-8 running, karioka running, and sport-specific skills. All must be performed pain-free and with no limited movement.

Pain increases in the right lumbar region on resisted trunk extension, lateral flexion, and rotation to the right. The quadriceps reflex is diminished on the right side and muscle weakness is apparent with knee extension and ankle dorsiflexion. Pain was elicited down the right leg during a straight-leg raising test. If you determined a possible sciatica due to an extruded disc at the L_4 level you are correct. What is your course of action?

REHABILITATION

The individual was seen by a physician who prescribed NSAIDs, muscle relaxants, and rest until symptoms subside. When the individual begins rehabilitation, what exercises should be included in the general program?

Rehabilitation programs must be developed on an individual basis and address the specific needs of the patient. Exercises to relieve pain related to postural problems may not address pain emanating from sciatica. Therefore, a variety of exercises are listed in this section, allowing you to select those appropriate for the patient.

Maintaining a prolonged posture can lead to some discomfort. This can be avoided by doing active range-of-motion exercises to relieve stress on supporting structures, promote circulation, and maintain flexibility (20). For example, to relieve tension in the cervical and upper thoracic region, do neck flexion, extension, and lateral flexion, and rotation, shoulder rolls, and glenohumeral circumduction. In the lower thoracic and lumbar region, exercises such as back extension, side bending in each direction, spinal flexion (avoiding hip flexion), trunk rotation, and walking a short distance can relieve discomfort. Other exercises to relieve pain and discomfort in the low back region include bringing both knees to the chest and gently rocking back and forth in a cranial/caudal direction and, in a standing position, shifting the hips from one side to another, lateral trunk flexion, and rotation exercises.

Several preventative exercises were demonstrated in **Field Strategy 15.1**. Other exercises may include single-leg hip extension and double-leg hip extension while holding onto a table, beginning with the knee(s) flexed, then with the knee(s) extended. Exercises to stretch the upper thoracic and pectoral regions, trunk rotators and lateral flexors, and the hip adductors, abductors, extensors, and medial and lateral rotators should also be added to improve flexibility and strength.

Isometric contractions to strengthen the neck musculature can progress to manual resistance, surgical tubing, or use of commercially available machines, as tolerated. Neck strength is particularly important for wrestlers and football lineman, who need added stability and strength in the cervical region. Abdominal strengthening exercises should begin with pelvic tilts, and progress to crunch curl-ups and diagonal crunch curl-ups, to reduce functional lordosis. Progressive prone extension exercises and resisted back extension exercises can increase strength in the erector spinae.

Avoid prolonged standing or sitting positions. Do active range-of-motion exercises in the opposite direction to relieve stress on supporting structures, promote circulation, and maintain flexibility

Proprioception and balance are regained through upper and lower extremity closed-chain exercises. For example, the upper thoracic region can benefit from push-ups, press-ups, and balancing on a wobble board, ball, ProFitter, or slide board, while weight bearing on the hands. Squats, the leg press, lunges, or exercises on a Stair Master, ProFitter, or slide board can restore proprioception and balance in the hip and lower extremity. Use of surgical tubing through functional patterns can also restore proprioception and balance. These exercises should be performed in front of a mirror or videotaped, if available, so the individual can observe proper posture and mechanics. Constant verbal reinforcement from the supervising therapist can also maximize feedback.

Aquatic exercises are very beneficial, because buoyancy can relieve load on sensitive structures. Deep water allows the individual to exercise all muscle groups through a full range of motion without the pain associated with gravity. Performing sport-specific skills against water resistance can apply an equal and uniform force to the muscles similar to isokinetic strengthening. With low back pain, an upper body ergometer, stationary bicycle, Stair Master, or slide board may be incorporated as tolerated to maintain cardiovascular fitness. Jogging can begin when all symptoms have subsided.

After acute symptoms subside, pain and muscle tension should be relieved. Stretching the piriformis, gluteals, and hamstrings should be combined with proprioceptive neuromuscular facilitation (PNF) and Theraband exercises to stretch the lumbar musculature and strengthen the abdominals and low back region. As strength is regained, functional activities can be incorporated with gradual return to full activity.

SUMMARY

The spine is a linkage system that transfers loads between the upper and lower extremities, enables motion in all three planes, and serves to protect the delicate spinal cord. Although most injuries to the back are relatively minor and can be successfully managed using the PRICE principles, spinal fractures and dislocations can occur.

Table 15.3. Conditions that Warrant Immediate Referral to a Physician

Severe pain, point tenderness, or deformity along the vertebral column
Loss or change in sensation anywhere in the body
Paralysis or inability to move a body part
Diminished or absent reflexes
Muscle weakness in a myotome
Radiating pain into the extremities
Trunk or abdominal pain that may be referred from the visceral organs
Any injury with questionable severity or nature

Field Strategy 15.6. Assessment for a Spinal Injury

History

Primary complaint and mechanism of injury
Onset of symptoms, including pain and discomfort
Disability and functional impairments from the injury
Previous injuries to the area, and family history

Observation and inspection

Observe general posture and perform a scan exam
Inspect:

Muscle symmetry	Hypertrophy or muscle atrophy
Swelling	Visible congenital deformity
Discoloration	Surgical incisions or scars

Palpation

Bony structures, to determine a possible fracture
Soft tissue structures, to determine:

Temperature	Deformity
Swelling	Muscle spasm
Point tenderness	Cutaneous sensation
Crepitus	Vascular pulses

Special Tests

Joint range of motion with gross movements
Resisted manual muscle testing
Neurological testing
Stress and functional tests
  Cervical compression and distraction test
  Straight-leg raising test
  Functional testing

In assessing a spinal injury, always begin with a thorough history of the injury and determine possible nerve involvement. The severity of pain and presence or absence of neurological symptoms, neck spasm, and tenderness can indicate when a backboard and neck stabilization are needed. Conditions that warrant special attention and should be referred to a physician are listed in **Table 15.3**. A summary of a full assessment of a spinal injury can be seen in **Field Strategy 15.6**.

If at anytime an individual complains of acute pain in the spine, change in sensation anywhere on the body, or the individual resists moving the spine, assume that a significant injury is present and take appropriate measures to immobilize the spinal region and refer this individual to a physician for further evaluation.

REFERENCES

1. Zachazewski JE, Geissler G, and Hangen D. Traumatic injuries to the cervical spine. In *Athletic injuries and rehabilitation*, edited by JE Zachazewski, DJ Magee, and WS Quillen. Philadelphia: WB Saunders, 1996.

2. Dyrek DA, Micheli LJ, and Magee DJ. Injuries to the thoracolumbar spine and pelvis. In *Athletic injuries and rehabilitation*, edited by JE Zachazewski, DJ Magee, and WS Quillen. Philadelphia: WB Saunders, 1996.
3. Hamill J, and Knutzen KM. *Biomechanical basis of human movement*. Baltimore: Williams & Wilkins, 1995.
4. Shirazi-Adl A, and Drouin G. 1987. Load bearing role of facets in a lumbar segment under sagittal plane loadings. J Biomech 20(6):610–614.
5. Patwardhan AG, et al. Biomechanics of adolescent idiopathic scoliosis—natural history and treatment. In *Biomechanics of the spine: clinical and surgical perspective*, edited by VK Goel and JN Weinstein. Boca Raton: CRC Press, 1990.
6. Goldberg B, and Boiardo R. 1984. Profiling children for sports participation. Clin Sports Med 3(1):153–169.
7. Johnson RJ. 1993. Low-back pain in sports: managing spondylolysis in young patients. Phys Sportsmed 21(4):53–59.
8. Heck JF. 1996. The incidence of spearing during a high school's 1975 and 1990 football seasons. J Ath Train 31(1):31–37.
9. Torg JS, Vegso JJ, O'Neil MJ, and Sennett B. 1990. The epidemiologic, pathologic, biomechanical and cinematographic analysis of football-induced cervical spine trauma. Am J Sports Med 18(1):50–57.
10. Wiesenfarth J, and Briner W. 1996. Neck injuries: urgent decisions and actions. Phys Sportsmed 24(1):35–41.
11. Markey KL, Benedetto MD, and Curl WW. 1993. Upper trunk brachial plexopathy: the stinger syndrome. Am J Sports Med 21(5):650–655.
12. Drye C, and Zachazewski, JE. Peripheral nerve injuries. In *Athletic injuries and rehabilitation*, edited by JE Zachazewski, DJ Magee, and WS Quillen. Philadelphia: WB Saunders, 1996.
13. Rovere GD. 1987. Low back pain in athletes. Phys Sportsmed 15(1):105–117.
14. Spengler DM, et al. 1986. Back injuries in industry: a retrospective study: overview and cost analysis. Spine 11(3):241–245.
15. Kujala UM, et al. 1996. Low-back pain in adolescent athletes. Med Sci Sports Ex 28(2):165–170.
16. Helliovaara M. 1989. Risk factors for low back pain and sciatica. Ann Med 21:257–264.
17. Cox JM. Diagnosis of the patient with low back pain. In *Low back pain: mechanism, diagnosis and treatment*, edited by JM Cox. Baltimore: Williams & Wilkins, 1990.
18. Plowman SA. Physical activity, physical fitness, and low back pain. In *Exercise and sport sciences reviews*, edited by JO Holloszy, vol. 20. Champaign, IL: Human Kinetics, 1992.
19. Anderson C. 1993. Neck injuries: backboard, bench, or return to play? Phys Sportsmed 21(8):23–34.
20. Kisner C, and Colby LA. *Therapeutic exercise: foundations and techniques*. Philadelphia: FA Davis, 1990.

Throat, Thorax, and Visceral Injuries

After completing this chapter, you should be able to:

- Locate the important bony and soft tissue structures of the throat, thorax, and viscera

- Identify measures to prevent injuries to the throat, thorax, and viscera

- Recognize and manage specific injuries of the throat, thorax, and viscera

- Describe life-threatening conditions that can occur spontaneously or as a result of direct trauma to the throat, thorax, and viscera

- Demonstrate a basic assessment of the throat, thorax, and visceral regions

Key Terms:

Alveoli	McBurney's point
Appendicitis	Peristalsis
Atria	Peritonitis
Cardiac tamponade	Pneumothorax
Chyme	Pulmonary circuit
Cirrhosis	Pulmonary contusion
Cyclist's nipples	Runner's nipples
Hematuria	Solar plexus punch
Hemothorax	Stitch in the side
Hepatitis	Subcutaneous emphysema
Hernia	Sudden death
Hypertrophic cardiomyopathy	Systemic circuit
Hyperventilation	Tension pneumothorax
Infectious mononucleosis	Traumatic asphyxia
Kehr's sign	Ventricles

Torso injuries occur in nearly every sport, particularly those involving sudden deceleration and impact. Although protective equipment and padding is available to protect the anterior throat, thorax, and viscera, only football, lacrosse, hockey, fencing, baseball, and softball require specific safety equipment for this vital region. Most injuries are superficial and easily recognized and managed. It is estimated that 7 to 10% of all athletic injuries affect the abdomen, the most commonly injured abdominal organs being the spleen, liver, and kidney (1). Some injuries, however, may involve the respiratory or circulatory system, leading to a life-threatening situation.

This chapter begins with a review of the anatomy of the region and injury prevention, followed by discussion on common injuries and internal complications that may lead to a life-threatening situation. Finally, a step-by-step basic injury assessment is presented that uses the HOPS format to determine the extent and seriousness of injury. Because rehabilitation of the region is usually included with other body regions, specific exercises for the thorax and visceral region will not be discussed.

ANATOMY REVIEW OF THE THROAT

? *Why is a blow to the throat potentially dangerous? Could respiratory arrest be a potential outcome?*

The throat includes the pharynx, larynx, trachea, esophagus, a number of glands, and several major blood vessels (**Fig. 16.1**). The laryngeal prominence on the thyroid cartilage that shields the front of the larynx is known as the "Adam's apple." The epiglottis covers the superior opening of the larynx during swallowing to prevent food and liquids from entering. If a foreign

> The epiglottis covers the superior opening of the larynx during swallowing to prevent food and liquids from entering the larynx

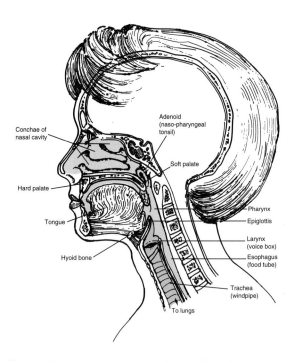

Figure 16.1. Lateral cross-sectional view of the throat region.

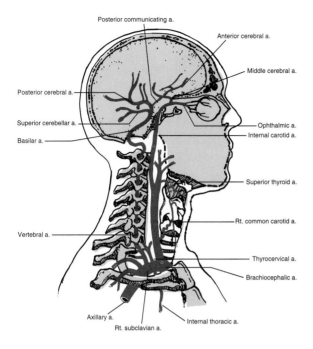

Figure 16.2. The arterial supply to the neck and throat region.

body does slip past the epiglottis, the cough reflex is initiated and the foreign body is normally ejected back into the pharynx. The trachea is formed by C-shaped rings of hyaline cartilage joined by fibroelastic connective tissue. Smooth muscle fibers of the trachealis muscle form the open side of the C and allow for expansion of the posteriorly adjacent esophagus as swallowed food passes through. When empty, the esophagus tube is collapsed.

The largest blood vessels coursing through the neck are the common carotid arteries (**Fig. 16.2**). At the level of the Adam's apple, the common carotid arteries divide into external and internal carotid arteries, which provide the major blood supply to the brain, head, and face.

A blow to the throat can lead to acute coughing, spasm, and an inability to catch one's breath. Because the trachea and superficial carotid arteries course through the neck, severe blows can disrupt the function of one or both of these structures, which can become life-threatening.

> The trachealis muscle allows the trachea to expand and allow food in the adjacent esophagus to pass through to the stomach

ANATOMY REVIEW OF THE THORAX

What anatomical structures protect the heart and lungs?
The thoracic cavity, or chest cavity, lies anterior to the spinal column and extends from the level of the clavicle down to the diaphragm. The bones of the thorax, including the sternum, ribs

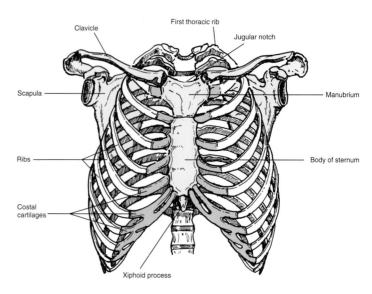

Figure 16.3. The thoracic cage. Note that only the first seven pairs of ribs articulate anteriorly with the sternum through the costal cartilages.

Alveoli
Air sacs at the terminal ends of the bronchial tree, where oxygen and carbon dioxide are exchanged between the lungs and surrounding capillaries

Pulmonary circuit
Blood vessels that transport unoxygenated blood to the lungs from the right heart ventricle and oxygenated blood from the lungs to the left heart atrium

Systemic circuit
Blood vessels that transport unoxygenated blood to the right heart atrium and oxygenated blood from the left heart ventricle

and costal cartilages, and thoracic vertebrae, form a protective cage around the heart and lungs (**Fig. 16.3**). The costal cartilages of the first seven pairs of ribs attach directly to the sternum, and the costal cartilages of ribs 8 to 10 attach to the costal cartilages of the immediate superior ribs. The last two rib pairs are known as floating ribs because they do not attach anteriorly to any structure.

The thoracic cavity is lined with a thin, double-layered membrane called the pleura. The pleural cavity is a narrow space between the pleural membranes that is filled with a pleural fluid secreted by the membranes, which enables the lungs to move against the thoracic wall with minimal friction during breathing.

The primary bronchial tubes branch obliquely downward from the trachea, then branch into approximately 25 subsequent levels until the terminal bronchioles are reached (**Fig. 16.4**). These tiny air sacs are called **alveoli** and serve as diffusion chambers where oxygen from the lungs enter adjacent capillaries, and carbon dioxide from the blood is returned to the lungs.

The heart and lungs have an intimate relationship both physically and functionally. The right side of the heart pumps blood to the lungs, where it is oxygenated and carbon dioxide is given off. The left side of the heart receives the freshly oxygenated blood from the lungs and pumps it out to the systemic circulation. The vessels interconnecting the heart and lungs are known as the **pulmonary circuit**, whereas the vessels that supply the body are known as the **systemic circuit** (**Fig. 16.5**).

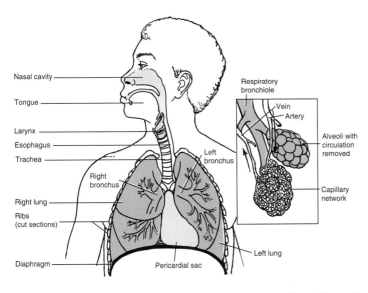

Figure 16.4. The respiratory system. **A.** The trachea, bronchi, and lungs. **B.** The terminal ends of the bronchial tree are alveolar sacs where oxygen and carbon dioxide are exchanged.

In the figure, the following labels appear:
Nasal cavity, Tongue, Larynx, Esophagus, Trachea, Right bronchus, Right lung, Ribs (cut sections), Diaphragm, Pericardial sac, Left lung, Left bronchus, Respiratory bronchiole, Vein, Artery, Alveoli with circulation removed, Capillary network

The heart is divided into four chambers—the right and left **atria,** superiorly, and the right and left **ventricles,** inferiorly **(Fig. 16.6).** The heartbeat consists of a simultaneous contraction of the two atria followed immediately by a simultaneous contraction of the two ventricles. The contraction phase is known as systole. The phase in which the chambers are relaxing and filling with blood is known as diastole.

The locations, primary functions, and innervations of the muscles of the thoracic region are summarized in **Table 16.1 (Figs. 16.7 and 16.8).** The major respiratory muscle is the diaphragm, a powerful sheet of muscle that completely separates the thoracic and abdominal cavities. During relaxation, the diaphragm is dome-shaped. During contraction it flattens, thereby increasing the size of the thoracic cavity. This increase in cavity volume causes a decrease in intrathoracic pressure, resulting in inhalation of air into the lungs.

The heart and lungs lie in the thoracic cavity, where they are protected by the pleural lining of the cavity and, external to the cavity, by the rib cage and sternum.

ANATOMY REVIEW OF THE VISCERAL REGION

An individual is complaining of pain and cramping in the lower right abdominal quadrant. What possible structures might account for this pain?

The visceral region includes all organs and structures between the diaphragm and pelvic floor **(Fig. 16.9).** The solid organs

Atria
Two superior chambers of the heart that pump blood into the ventricles

Ventricles
Two inferior chambers of the heart that pump blood out of the heart, one to the pulmonary circuit and one to the systemic circuit

Blood pressure is read as pressure during systole over pressure during diastole (e.g., 120/80)

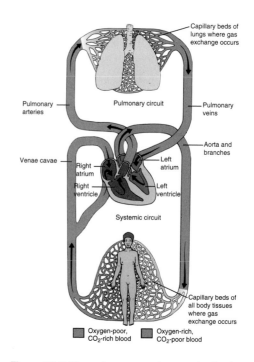

Figure 16.5. The pulmonary and systemic circuits.

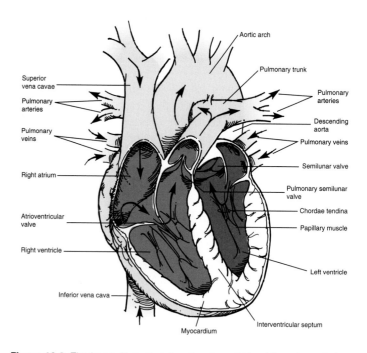

Figure 16.6. The heart. Note that the direction of blood flow through the chambers of the heart is indicated by the arrows.

Table 16.1. Muscles of the Thorax

Muscle	Proximal Attachment	Distal Attachment	Primary Action(s)	Nerve Innervation
Pectoralis minor	Coracoid process of the scapula	Anterior surfaces of ribs 3 to 5	With ribs fixed, pulls scapula forward & downward; with scapula fixed, pulls ribs upward	Medial pectoral
Serratus anterior	Vertebral border of scapula	Ribs 1 to 8 or 9	Protraction & rotation of the scapula	Long thoracic
Subclavius	Groove on inferior surface of clavicle	Costal cartilage of rib 1	Assists with stabilization and depression of shoulder girdle	Nerve to subclavius
Levator scapulae	Transverse process of the first four cervical vertebrae	Vertebral border of the scapula	Lateral flexion of the neck	C_3 to C_4 nerve roots Dorsal scapular
Trapezius	Occipital bone, ligamentum nuchae, C_7 and T_1–T_{12}	Acromion and spine of scapula & lateral clavicle	Stabilizes, elevates, retracts, & rotates scapula, lateral extension of neck	Accessory (cranial nerve XI)
Rhomboids	C_7, T_1–T_5	Medial border of scapula	Retracts, rotates, & stabilizes scapula	Dorsal scapular
External intercostals (11 pairs between ribs)	Inferior border of rib above	Superior border of rib below	Elevation of rib cage; assist the diaphragm with inspiration	Intercostal nerves
Internal intercostals (11 pairs between ribs)	Inferior border of rib above	Superior border of rib below	Depress rib cage; assist with expiration	Intercostal nerves
Diaphragm	Inferior border of rib cage and sternum; costal cartilages of ribs 6–12; lumbar vertebrae	Central tendon	Inspiration	Phrenic nerve

include the spleen, liver, pancreas, kidneys, and adrenal glands. The hollow organs include the stomach, small and large intestines, bladder, and ureters. The pelvic girdle protects the lower abdominal organs.

Food is stored in the stomach for approximately 4 hours, during which time it is broken down into a paste-like substance known as **chyme**. A few substances, including water, electrolytes, aspirin, and alcohol are absorbed into the blood stream across the stomach lining without full digestion. The chyme then moves into the small intestine where it is progressively absorbed. The small intestine, about 2 m (6 ft) long, is responsible for most of the digestion and

Chyme
Paste-like substance that food is churned into in the stomach

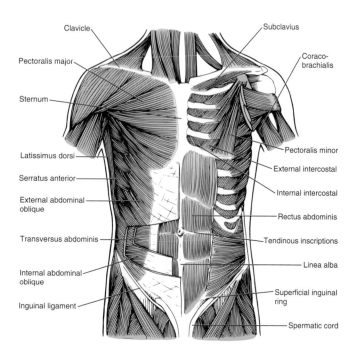

Figure 16.7. Anterior muscles of the trunk.

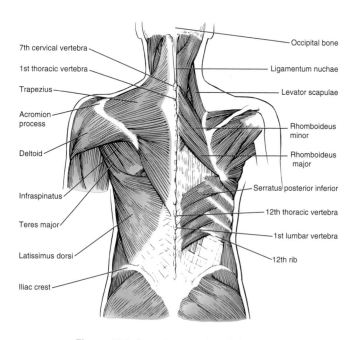

Figure 16.8. Posterior muscles of the trunk.

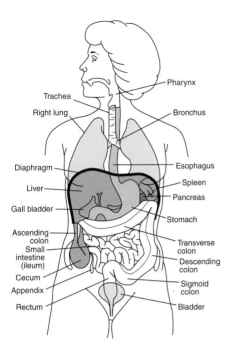

Pharynx

Trachea

Right lung

Bronchus

Diaphragm

Esophagus

Liver

Spleen

Pancreas

Gall bladder

Stomach

Ascending colon

Small intestine (ileum)

Transverse colon

Descending colon

Cecum

Sigmoid colon

Appendix

Rectum

Bladder

Figure 16.9. Anterior view of the visceral organs.

absorption of food as it is propelled through the small intestine in about 3 to 6 hours by a process called **peristalsis**. Water and electrolytes are further absorbed from the stored material in the large intestine during the next 12 to 24 hours. Mass peristaltic movements pass through the intestines several times per day to move the feces to the rectum. The vermiform appendix protrudes from the large intestine in the right lower quadrant of the abdomen, and can become a protected environment for the accumulation of bacteria, leading to inflammation of the appendix, or appendicitis.

The liver, located in the upper right quadrant under the diaphragm, produces bile, a greenish liquid that helps break down fat in the small intestine. The liver also absorbs excess glucose from the blood stream and stores it in the form of glycogen for later use. Among its other functions are processing fats and amino acids, manufacturing blood proteins, and detoxifying certain poisons and drugs. These functions can be severely impaired with alcohol abuse, which can result in **cirrhosis** of the liver. **Hepatitis** is inflammation of the liver caused by a viral infection that can also reduce the liver's efficiency. The gallbladder functions as an accessory to the liver to store concentrated bile on its way to the small intestine.

The spleen, the largest of the lymphoid organs, performs four vital functions: 1) cleansing the blood of foreign matter, bacteria, viruses, and toxins; 2) storing excess red blood cells for later reuse and releasing others into the blood for processing by the liver; 3) producing red blood cells in the fetus; and 4) storing blood plate-

Peristalsis
Periodic waves of smooth muscle contraction that propel food through the digestive system

Cirrhosis
Progressive inflammation of the liver, usually caused by alcoholism

Hepatitis
Inflammation of the liver

The pancreas secretes digestive enzymes into the small intestine, where most of the digestion and absorption of nutrients occur

lets. The pancreas secretes most of the digestive enzymes that break down food in the small intestine and secretes the hormones insulin and glucagon, which, respectively, lower and elevate blood sugar levels.

The kidneys filter and cleanse the blood. They are vital for filtering out toxins, metabolic wastes, drugs, and excess ions that leave the body in urine. The kidneys also return needed substances, such as water and electrolytes to the blood. The urinary bladder is an expandable sac that stores urine.

The major blood vessel of the trunk is the aorta and its numerous branches (**Fig. 16.10**). The distal portion of the descending aorta becomes the abdominal aorta, which divides into the common iliac arteries, then divides into an internal iliac artery to supply the organs of the pelvis, and an external iliac artery, which enters the thigh to become the femoral artery.

As is the case throughout the neck and trunk, muscles in the pelvic region are named in pairs, with one located on the left and the other on the right side of the body. These muscles cause lateral flexion or rotation when they contract unilaterally, but contribute to spinal flexion or extension when bilateral contractions occur. The locations, primary functions, and innervations of the major muscles of the pelvic girdle are summarized in **Table 16.2**.

Pain from the lower right abdominal region may emanate from the appendix or lower intestinal tract. If appendicitis is suspected, the individual should be referred immediately to a physician.

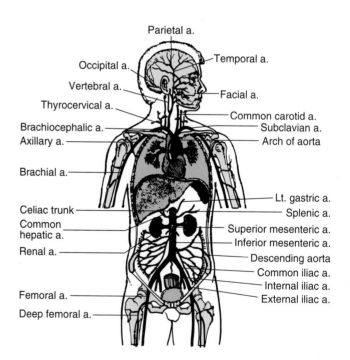

Figure 16.10. Arterial system of the trunk.

Table 16.2. Muscles of the Pelvic Girdle

Muscle	Proximal Attachment	Distal Attachment	Primary Action(s)	Nerve Innervation
Rectus abdominis	Costal cartilage of ribs 5–7	Pubic crest	Flexion, lateral flexion	Intercostal nerves
External oblique	External surface of lower eight ribs	Linea alba and anterior iliac crest	Flexion, lateral flexion, rotation to opposite side	Intercostal nerves
Internal oblique	Linea alba and the lower four ribs	Inguinal ligament, iliac crest, and the lumbodorsal fascia	Flexion, lateral flexion, rotation to same side	Intercostal nerves
Transverse abdominis	Inguinal ligament, lumbodorsal fascia, cartilages of ribs 6–12, iliac crest	Linea alba & pubic crest	Compression of the abdomen	Intercostal nerves
Quadratus lumborum	Last rib, transverse processes of the first four lumbar vertebrae	Iliolumbar ligament, adjacent iliac crest	Lateral flexion	Spinal nerves

PREVENTION OF INJURIES

The throat, thorax, and viscera are vulnerable to direct impact injuries. Because this is such a critical area where injury can lead to a life-threatening situation, what measures can be taken to prevent injuries to this region?

Injuries to the throat, thorax, and abdomen occur in nearly every sport, yet few sports require protective equipment for all players. For example, face masks with throat protectors are required for only fencers, baseball/softball catchers, and for goalies in field hockey, ice hockey, and lacrosse. Many sport participants in collision and contact sports also wear full chest and abdominal protection, such as in fencing, ice hockey, baseball/softball catchers, and goalies in field hockey and lacrosse. In young baseball and softball players (younger than 12 years), it has been suggested that all infield players wear chest protectors. Adolescent rib cages are less rigid, placing the heart at a greater risk from direct impact. In this age group, more deaths occur from impacts to the chest than to the head in baseball and softball (2). Shoulder pads can protect the upper thoracic region and rib protectors can provide protection for rib, upper abdominal, or low back contusions. Body suits made of mesh with pockets can hold rib and hip pads to protect the sides and back. For women, sport bras provide added support to reduce excessive vertical and horizontal breast motion during exercise. Abdominal binders may also be used to reduce the discomfort from hernias. Much of this protective equipment was discussed in detail and illustrated in Chapter 6.

Flexibility and strengthening of the torso muscles should not be an isolated program, but should include a well-rounded conditioning program for the back, shoulder, abdomen, and hip regions. Exercises for the thorax and abdominal regions were included in the chapters on the hip, shoulder, and spine, and will not be repeated here. The reader should review the appropriate Field Strategies in those chapters to develop a conditioning program for the torso.

💡 *Injuries to the throat, thorax, and viscera can be prevented by wearing appropriate protective equipment. Physical conditioning should include a well-rounded flexibility and strengthening program for the shoulder, back, abdominal, and hip regions.*

THROAT INJURIES

❓ *An opponent's elbow inadvertently struck a basketball player's anterior neck. The player is down on the court, coughing and having difficulty swallowing and speaking. How will you control the situation and manage the injury?*

Although uncommon, lacerations to the neck caused by a skate blade can occur. Bleeding is profuse and, if sufficiently deep, can damage the jugular vein or carotid artery as they pass deep on the lateral side of the neck. Immediate control of hemorrhage is imperative. In addition to blood loss, air may be sucked into the vein and carried to the heart as an air embolism, which may be fatal. Management involves providing firm, direct pressure over the wound, followed by an airway assessment. Continuous manual pressure should be applied while the individual is in rapid transit to the nearest medical facility.

Contusions and fractures to the trachea, larynx, and hyoid bone frequently occur during hyperextension of the neck, when the thyroid cartilage (Adam's apple) becomes prominent and vulnerable to direct impact forces. A hockey cross-check or slash, a clothesline tackle in football, or a hit or blow to the neck can injure the cartilage. Immediate symptoms include hoarseness, dyspnea (difficulty breathing), coughing, difficulty in swallowing, and laryngeal tenderness. Often the person becomes agitated and avoids any assistance; therefore, reassuring the individual and maintaining an open airway is a priority.

With severe anterior neck trauma or spasm, it is important to consider an associated injury to the cervical spine. Carefully place and maintain the individual's neck in a neutral position and apply a cervical collar. With the jaw-thrust maneuver (see Chapter 3), the hyoid bone and surrounding ligaments move away from the vocal cords and may open the airway. As the spasm relaxes, usually in a minute, a loud inspiratory crowing sound is often heard (3). The individual should be immediately transported to a medical facility. **Field Strategy 16.1** summarizes signs, symptoms, and management of tracheal and laryngeal injuries.

💡 *In responding to the injured basketball player, did you reassure the individual and attempt to place the chin in a forward position to straighten the airway? It may help to have the individ-*

With a major laceration to the anterior neck, an air embolism can travel to the heart, causing death

Contusions or fractures to the anterior neck produce immediate signs and symptoms, such as a change in voice, dyspnea, coughing, difficulty swallowing, and pain

As the laryngospasm relaxes (usually in a minute), a loud inspiratory, crowing sound is heard

Field Strategy 16.1. Management of Tracheal and Laryngeal Injuries

Signs and symptoms
   Shortness of breath or difficulty when swallowing or coughing
   Hoarseness or loss of voice
   Severe pain and point tenderness
   Presence of hemorrhage with blood-tinged sputum
   Loss of contour of the Adam's apple (thyroid cartilage)
Management
   Talk calmly to the individual and loosen any restrictive clothing or
     equipment
   Reassure the individual you are there to help
   Ensure an open airway
   Place the individual in a chin-up position and apply ice, if appropriate, to
     control swelling
   If a laceration is present, control hemorrhage with firm, manual
     pressure, and maintain it during transportation to the nearest
     medical facility
   If severe anterior throat trauma occurred, assume the presence of a
     possible cervical spinal injury and treat accordingly

ual focus on inhaling and exhaling in a normal breathing pattern. If breathing does not return to normal within a few minutes, summon EMS.

THORACIC INJURIES

? *After being tackled by several opponents, a football player is complaining of a sharp pain on the lower right side of the rib cage. The pain is aggravated with deep breathing and coughing. What possible injury might you suspect?*

Thoracic injuries are frequently caused by sudden deceleration and impact, which can lead to compression and subsequent deformation of the rib cage. The extent of damage depends on the direction, magnitude of force, and the point of impact. For example, a glancing blow may contuse the chest wall, whereas a baseball that directly impacts the ribs may fracture a rib. Recognizing the potential for serious underlying problems is vital to provide emergency care to an injured individual.

> The extent of damage in thoracic injuries is dependent on the direction and magnitude of force and point of impact

Stitch in the Side

A "**stitch in the side**" refers to a sharp pain or spasm in the chest wall, usually on the lower right side, during exertion. Potential causes include trapped colonic gas bubbles, localized diaphragmatic hypoxia with spasm, liver congestion with stretching of the liver capsule, and poor conditioning (1). Most individuals can run through the sharp pain by (a) forcibly exhaling through pursed lips; (b) breathing deeply and regularly; (c) leaning away from the affected side; or (d) stretching the arm on the affected side over the head as high as possible. The frequency of a stitch usually diminishes as the individual becomes more fit.

> **Stitch in the side**
> A sharp pain or spasm in the chest wall, usually on the lower right side, that occurs during exertion

Breast Injuries

Excessive breast motion during activity can lead to soreness, contusions, and nipple irritation. Contusions to the breast may produce fat necrosis or hematoma formation, both of which are painful and may result in the formation of a localized breast mass. Appearance of these lesions on a mammogram may be indistinguishable from a malignant tumor (1). Although immediate management will involve ice and support, direct trauma should always be recorded on a woman's permanent medical records. Nipple irritation is commonly seen in distance runners when the shirt rubs over the nipples. The resulting friction can lead to abrasions, blisters, or bleeding (**runner's nipples**). This condition can be prevented by applying petroleum jelly, band-aids, or tape over the nipples to reduce irritation (1,4). Initial treatment involves cleansing the wound, applying a medicated ointment, and covering the wound with a nonadhering sterile gauze pad. Infection, secondary to the injury, may involve the entire nipple region and may necessitate referral to a physician. **Cyclist's nipples** is a condition not caused by friction, but rather from the combined effects of perspiration and windchill that produce cold, painful nipples that may last for several days. Wearing a wind-proof jacket and rewarming the nipples after completion of the event can prevent the irritation.

Runner's nipples
Nipple irritation due to friction as the shirt rubs over the nipples

Cyclist's nipples
Nipple irritation caused by the combined effects of perspiration and windchill, producing cold, painful nipples

Strain of the Pectoralis Major Muscle

Pectoralis major muscle strains may occur in power lifting, water skiing, football, boxing, wrestling, and basketball, or in sudden violent deceleration maneuvers, such as when punching in boxing or blocking with an extended arm in football (5,6). An aching or fatigue-like pain is more common than a sharp pain, and horizontal adduction and internal rotation of the shoulder will be limited. If the muscle ruptures, a popping or snapping sensation at the time of rupture is the most frequently reported symptom (5). Most of these injuries occur in athletes between the ages of 30 and 40 and involve an avulsion of the tendon from the humerus. The mechanism of injury often involves excessive tension from acute overload of an eccentrically loaded tendon, as occurs in a bench press (6). Having the individual press his or her hands together in front of the abdomen will cause the muscle to bulge medially into the chest region, causing the axillary fold to appear thin.

Weakness and a popping or snapping sensation are common symptoms with a rupture to the pectoralis major muscle

Treatment depends on the extent of damage. Mild and moderate strains (Grades I and II) begin with control of inflammation, protected range-of-motion exercises, and gradual strengthening. Once range of motion as been achieved, strength, endurance, and power are restored. Third degree ruptures of the muscle are treated surgically (6).

Costochondral Injury

Costochondral sprains may occur during a collision with another object or as a result of a severe twisting motion of the thorax.

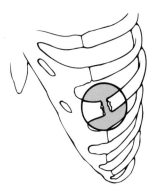

Figure 16.11. Undisplaced costochondral separation.

This action can sprain or separate the costal cartilage where it attaches to the rib or sternum (**Fig. 16.11**). The individual may hear or feel a pop, but the initial localized sharp pain may be followed by intermittent stabbing pain as the displaced cartilage overrides the bone. A visible deformity and localized pain can be palpated at the involved joint. More severe sprains produce pain during deep inhalation. The discomfort usually resolves itself with three or four weeks of rest and anti-inflammatory medication; however, the discomfort may persist for more than six weeks. Occasionally, a physician may choose to inject the site with steroid medication to relieve chronic pain.

> A blow to the anterolateral aspect of the chest can sprain or separate the costal cartilage where it attaches to the rib or sternum

Sternal and Rib Fractures

The sternum is rarely fractured in sports, but this may occur as a result of rapid deceleration and high-impact into an object, leading to an immediate loss of breath. Severe pain is aggravated with deep inspiration if the fracture is incomplete, but pain occurs during normal respiration if the fracture is complete (1). With any suspected fracture, always assess for an underlying cardiac injury, such as a cardiac contusion.

> Severe pain is aggravated with deep inspiration if the fracture is incomplete, but pain occurs during normal respiration if the fracture is complete

Rib fractures may be caused by an indirect force, such as a violent muscle contraction in a golf swing or baseball pitch, or by direct compression of the chest. The fourth through ninth ribs are the most commonly fractured, resulting in intense localized pain aggravated with deep inspiration, coughing, and chest movement at the site of the injury. A visible contusion and crepitus may be present at the impact site. Often, the individual will take shallow breaths and lean toward the fracture site, stabilizing the area with a hand to prevent excessive movement of the chest to ease the pain. Manual compression of the rib cage in an anteroposterior direction and lateral compression will produce pain over the fracture site (see **Fig. 16.14**). Pain tends to be most severe during the first 3 to 5 days following injury, at which time it gradually subsides, and ultimately disappears after 3 to 6 weeks (1). If pain is intense or multiple fractures are suspected, application of a sling and swathe may be used to immobilize the chest. Should any

> With a rib fracture, shallow breathing will be present, because deep inspirations cause intense pain

Field Strategy 16.2. Management of Rib Fractures

Signs and Symptoms

History of direct blow, compression of the chest, or violent muscle
    contraction
Individual may lean toward the fractured side, stabilizing the area with a
    hand to prevent movement of the chest
Localized discoloration or swelling over the fracture site
Slight step deformity may be visible, and palpable pain and crepitus may
    be present at the fracture site
Pain increases with deep inspiration, trunk rotation, and lateral flexion
    away from the fracture site
Pain increases with manual compression of the rib cage in an
    anteroposterior direction, or with lateral compression
Management

Rule out underlying internal complications
    Look for coughing up of any bright red or frothy blood
    Listen for abnormal or absent breathing sounds
    Record rate and depth of respirations
    Record strength and pulse rate
    Note pupillary response to light
Apply sling and swathe
Treat for shock and transport the individual to the nearest medical facility

signs of respiratory distress, cyanosis, or shock appear, a thorough
assessment for an underlying visceral injury should be conducted.

Treatment involves ice and prescribed nonsteroidal anti-
inflammatory drugs (NSAIDs). Depending on the sport, fracture
site, the presence of a displaced or nondisplaced fracture, and the
number of ribs involved, this individual may be excluded from
sport participation during the full healing process. With a simple
fracture, a flak jacket or rib vest can be worn to protect the
area from reinjury. **Field Strategy 16.2** summarizes the signs,
symptoms, and management of rib fractures.

*The football player has ecchymosis on the anterolateral aspect
of the rib cage at the level of the ninth rib. Palpation causes
increased pain and crepitus, as does deep breathing and lateral
flexion away from the injury site. If you determined a possible rib
fracture, you are correct.*

INTERNAL COMPLICATIONS

*The second baseman fielded a line drive and threw the ball
to first base. By accident, the ball struck a runner going to
second base directly on the sternum. The runner immediately
collapsed on the base path. You arrived at the scene to find the
player in obvious pain and gasping for air. How will you manage
this situation? What underlying serious problems can occur as a
result of direct impact to the sternum or ribs?*

Several conditions can alter breathing and cardiac function.
Hyperventilation is associated with an inability to catch one's

breath and, in most instances, is not a serious problem. Direct trauma to the thorax, however, can lead to serious underlying problems, although, in sport participation, these conditions are rare.

Hyperventilation

Hyperventilation is often linked to pain, stress, or trauma in sport participation (7). During activity, the respiratory rate increases. Rapid, deep inhalations draw more oxygen into the lungs. Conversely, long exhalations result in too much carbon dioxide being exhaled. Signs and symptoms include an inability to catch one's breath, chest pain, dizziness, and, occasionally, fainting. Immediately calm the individual, as panic and anxiety can complicate the condition. Although breathing into a paper bag has proven to be quite successful in restoring the oxygen–carbon dioxide balance, many individuals find it embarrassing. An alternative treatment involves concentrating on slow inhalations through the nose and exhaling through the mouth until symptoms have stopped. The use of breathing into a paper bag is not needed, except in severe cases.

Hyperventilation
Respiratory condition in which too much carbon dioxide is exhaled, leading to an inability to catch one's breath

Treatment involves concentrating on slow inhalations through the nose and exhaling through the mouth until symptoms have ceased

Pulmonary Contusion

Pulmonary contusion usually results from nonpenetrating chest trauma, but is rare in sport participation. Force transmitted through the thorax, as in landing on a football or a body slam onto the hard ground, causes bleeding in the alveolar spaces. Breathing may be compromised, and hypoxia may appear 2 to 4 hours after trauma (8). The condition may go undetected until the individual coughs up blood or has other underlying problems, such as pneumothorax, rib fractures, or **subcutaneous emphysema**. Mild contusions heal within days, with the individual returning to full participation in as little as 10 days (9). In more severe cases, the individual is usually hospitalized and monitored with ventilatory support.

Pulmonary contusion
Contusion to the lungs due to compressive force

Subcutaneous emphysema
Presence of air or gas in subcutaneous tissue, characterized by a crackling sensation on palpation

Pneumothorax

Pneumothorax is a condition whereby air is trapped in the pleural space, causing a portion of a lung to collapse. Although a fractured rib is the leading cause, pneumothorax may occur spontaneously. Individuals with spontaneous pneumothorax are commonly male and typically are tall and thin (8). The episode often follows heavy exertion or running (10). In a traumatic injury when lung tissue is lacerated, air escapes into the pleural cavity with each inhalation and prevents the lung from fully expanding **(Fig. 16.12)**. Shortness of breath, cyanosis, severe chest pain on the affected side, and progressive respiratory collapse are the most common symptoms in severe cases.

Pneumothorax
Condition whereby air is trapped in the pleural space, causing a portion of a lung to collapse

Shortness of breath and severe chest pain on the affected side are common symptoms of pneumothorax

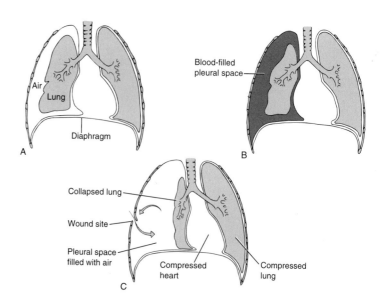

Figure 16.12. Internal complication to the lungs. **A.** Pneumothorax. **B.** Hemothorax. **C.** Tension pneumothorax. Each condition can become life-threatening if the lung collapses.

Tension Pneumothorax

Tension pneumothorax
Condition in which air continuously leaks into the pleural space, causing the mediastinum to displace to the opposite side, compressing the uninjured lung and thoracic aorta

Tension pneumothorax occurs when air progressively accumulates in the pleural space during inspiration and cannot escape on expiration. The pleural space expands with each breath, resulting in the mediastinum being displaced to the opposite side, compressing the uninjured lung and thoracic aorta. Signs and symptoms may include severe difficulty in breathing, absence of breath sounds, distention of neck veins, hypotension, and circulatory compromise leading to cyanosis and possible death. This is a true emergency, with immediate referral to the nearest medical facility necessary to prevent total collapse of the lung.

Traumatic Asphyxia

Traumatic asphyxia
Condition involving extravasation of blood into the skin and conjunctivae due to a sudden increase in venous pressure

Traumatic asphyxia results from massive direct trauma to the thorax. Classic symptoms include a bluish tinge over the neck and facial regions, subconjunctival hemorrhage, ecchymosis, and minute hemorrhagic spots on the face. Loss of vision has also been reported as a result of retinal edema, but vision may promptly improve within hours or days (11). Again, immediate recognition and referral to the nearest medical facility is necessary for prompt care.

Hemothorax

Hemothorax
Condition involving the loss of blood into the pleural cavity, but outside the lung

Hemothorax involves the loss of blood, rather than air, into the pleural cavity. Fractured ribs may tear lung tissue and blood vessels in the chest or chest cavity. Signs and symptoms include severe

Table 16.3. Indications of Severe Blunt Trauma to the Chest

Shortness of breath or difficulty in breathing
Severe chest pain aggravated with deep inspiration
Abnormal or absent breath sounds
Individual may cough up bright red or frothy blood
Eyes may be bulging or bloodshot
Signs of shock

pain during breathing, hypoxia, difficulty breathing, cyanosis, coughing up frothy blood, and shock. This condition is a true medical emergency. Treat for shock and immediately transport this individual to the nearest medical facility. **Table 16.3** lists several signs and symptoms indicating blunt injury to the thorax.

Heart Injuries

Blunt chest trauma can compress the heart between the sternum and spine, leading to myocardial contusion. The right ventricle is often injured because it lies directly posterior to the sternum. Blunt trauma can also lead to **cardiac tamponade**, the leading cause of traumatic death in youth baseball (2,12). This condition has also occurred from projectiles in other sports, such as softball, hockey, and lacrosse (13–15). In nearly all cases, the individual collapses within seconds and goes into respiratory arrest. In many cases, resuscitation is unsuccessful even though it is given immediately after injury. Treatment is the same as for any other chest trauma: maintain an open airway, initiate breathing and chest compressions, if necessary, and immediately transport the individual to the nearest medical facility.

Sudden Death in Athletes

Sudden death is defined as an event that is nontraumatic, unexpected, and occurs instantaneously or within minutes of an abrupt change in an individual's previous clinical state (16). For individuals under 35 years of age, the most common cause is **hypertrophic cardiomyopathy**, with a higher frequency seen in male athletes as compared to female athletes (17). Other causes include abnormalities in the coronary arteries, aortic rupture associated with Marfan's syndrome, and mitral valve prolapse (16,17). In an individual over the age of 35, the most common cause is ischemic coronary artery disease. Symptoms, such as chest pains, sudden onset of fatigue, heartburn or indigestion, and excessive breathlessness during exercise, should signal the need for immediate referral to a physician for further investigation.

💡 *The baseball runner is in obvious respiratory distress. The impact of the ball may have caused hyperventilation or more serious internal complications. Initiate a primary survey, talk to*

Cardiac tamponade
Acute compression of the heart caused by effusion of fluid or blood into the pericardium from rupture of the heart or penetrating trauma

In nearly all cases of cardiac tamponade, the individual collapses within seconds and goes into respiratory arrest

Sudden death
Nontraumatic, unexpected death occurring instantaneously or within a few minutes of an abrupt change in an individual's previous clinical state

Hypertrophic cardiomyopathy
Excessive hypertrophy of the heart, often of obscure or unknown origin

Symptoms such as chest pains, sudden onset of fatigue, heartburn or indigestion, and excessive breathlessness during exercise should signal the need for immediate referral to a physician for further investigation

the individual to calm them down, and assess breathing and circulation. If respirations do not return to normal within minutes, or if respiratory or cardiac irregularities are present, summon EMS.

ABDOMINAL WALL INJURIES

? *A high jumper felt a sharp pain in the abdominal region during a jump. There is marked tenderness and muscle guarding slightly below and to the right of the umbilicus. No swelling or discoloration is visible; however, it hurts to do a modified sit-up. What condition may be present? How will you manage it?*

The muscles of the abdominal wall are strong and powerful, yet flexible enough to absorb impact. Consequently, injuries to the abdominal wall are usually minor; however, other conditions, such as a contusion to the solar plexus and hernias, can affect sport participation.

Skin Wounds and Contusions

> Lacerations that penetrate the abdominal wall muscles or deeper should be referred immediately to the nearest medical facility

With a skin abrasion, cleanse the wound to prevent contamination, cover the area with a sterile nonstick dressing, and secure the dressing to prevent friction directly over the abrasion. Lacerations that penetrate the abdominal wall muscles or deeper should be referred immediately to the nearest medical facility. Because further examination is necessary to rule out intra-abdominal injuries, ointments or creams should not be placed on the wound. Instead, irrigate the wound with sterile water and cover the area with an absorbent pad to control hemorrhage. Simple contusions to the abdominal wall are evident by tenderness over the area of impact, pain during active contraction of the abdominal muscles, and the absence of referred pain (1). Treatment involves ice and compression to limit the amount of hemorrhage. A pressure dressing may be applied if a large hematoma forms.

Muscle Strains

> Marked tenderness and muscle guarding, along with abdominal pain on straight-leg raising or hyperextension of the back, indicates an abdominal muscle strain

Muscular strains may be caused by direct trauma, sudden twisting, or sudden extension of the spine. The rectus abdominis is the most commonly injured muscle. Complications arise when the epigastric artery or intramuscular vessels are damaged, leading to hematoma formation. Nearly 80% of the hematomas occur below the umbilicus. Severe abdominal pain, nausea, vomiting, marked tenderness, and muscle guarding may be present. Straight-leg raising or hyperextension of the back increases the pain. Treatment consists of ice, rest, and early use of NSAIDs for the first 36 to 48 hours. Hydrocollator packs and whirlpools can be used with activity modification until the hematoma and soreness ends. Activities, such as twisting, turning, or sudden stretching should be avoided until painful symptoms subside.

Solar Plexus Contusion ("Wind Knocked Out")

A blow to the abdomen with the muscles relaxed is referred to as a "**solar plexus punch**," and results in an immediate inability to catch one's breath. Fear and anxiety complicate the condition. Assessment should include a thorough airway analysis. Remove any mouth guard or partial plates. Loosen any restrictive equipment and clothing around the abdomen and have the individual flex the knees toward the chest. Paradoxical as it may seem, asking the athlete to take a deep breath and hold it, and to repeat this several times, often restores the athlete's breath more quickly (1). Because a severe blow may lead to an intra-abdominal injury, reassess the individual at the end of the practice session to rule out any injury that may have been overlooked.

Solar plexus punch
A blow to the abdomen that results in an immediate inability to breath freely

Loosen any restrictive equipment and clothing around the abdomen and have the individual flex the knees toward the chest

Hernias

A **hernia** is a protrusion of abdominal viscera through a weakened portion of the abdominal wall and may be classified as indirect, direct, or femoral (**Fig. 16.13**). Indirect inguinal hernias result from a weakness in the peritoneum around the deep inguinal ring that allows the abdominal viscera to protrude through the ring into the inguinal canal. Direct hernias result from a weakness in an area of fascia, bounded by the rectus abdominis muscle, the inguinal ligament, and the epigastric vessels, and allows the abdominal viscera to protrude into the scrotum. Femoral hernias, more commonly seen in women, allows the abdominal viscera to protrude through the femoral ring into the femoral canal, compressing the lymph vessels, connective tissue, and the femoral artery and vein.

Hernia
Protrusion of abdominal viscera through a weakened portion of the abdominal wall

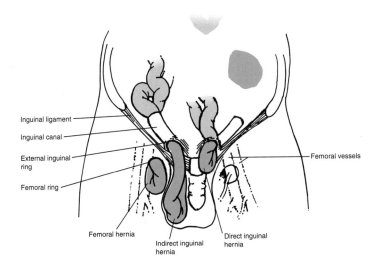

Figure 16.13. A hernia may be classified as indirect, direct, or femoral.

Symptoms vary, but for most hernias the first sign is a visible tender swelling and an aching feeling in the groin. Many hernias are asymptomatic until the preparticipation exam, when the physician palpates the protrusion by invaginating the scrotum with a finger. Protrusion of the hernia increases with coughing. The danger of a hernia lies in continued trauma to the weakened area during falls, blows, or increased intra-abdominal pressure exerted during activity. The hernia can twist on itself and produce a strangulated hernia, which can become gangrenous. As a result, most hernias are surgically repaired.

💡 *The athlete experienced sharp abdominal pain after sudden hyperextension of the back during a jump. No swelling or discoloration is present; however, pain increases with active contraction of the abdominal muscles. If you determined a possible strain of the rectus abdominis, you are correct. Application of ice, compression, and rest will reduce the acute swelling and pain.*

INTRA-ABDOMINAL INJURIES

❓ *A 22-year-old football player was struck in the abdomen with a helmet and experienced a sudden onset of abdominal pain in the upper left quadrant that seemed to radiate into the upper chest and left shoulder. Weakness and a light-headed feeling are also present. Blood pressure is 96/72, and pulse is weak at 96 beats per minute. What possible injury might be present?*

Trauma to the abdomen can lead to severe internal hemorrhage if organs or major blood vessels are lacerated or ruptured. The solid organs are more commonly injured in sport participation. Hollow viscera, if damaged, can leak the contents into the abdominal cavity, causing severe hemorrhage, **peritonitis**, and shock. Many signs and symptoms indicating an intra-abdominal injury are similar in nature regardless of the organ involved. Variations arise in the area of palpable pain and site of referred pain. Signs and symptoms indicating a general intra-abdominal injury include the absence of normal abdominal movement during the respiratory motion; localized tenderness and abdominal rigidity on palpation; rebound tenderness with release of deep pressure; absence of normal bowel sounds; referred pain into the shoulder, back, or groin; decreased blood pressure; and a rapid, weak pulse. **Table 16.4** summarizes the signs and symptoms of intra-abdominal injury.

Acute management of suspected intra-abdominal injuries is also very similar regardless of the injured organ. Initially, keep the individual relaxed while a primary survey is completed, and summon EMS. Place the individual supine and flex the knees. This position relaxes the low back and abdominal muscles. Monitor vital signs regularly and treat for shock. If external bleeding is present, control bleeding and apply an absorbent sterile dressing. **Field Strategy 16.3** summarizes acute management of intra-abdominal injuries.

The solid organs are more commonly injured in sport participation

Peritonitis
Inflammation of the peritoneum that lines the abdomen

Table 16.4. Signs and Symptoms Indicating an Intra-abdominal Injury

Individual may lean forward and bring the knees to the chest to reduce tension in the abdominal muscles
Abdominal pain that rapidly increases in severity
Coughing up or vomiting blood that looks like used coffee grounds
Palpable local tenderness or rigidity over the injured organ
Cramps or muscle guarding (splinting)
Rebound pain on deep palpation
Absence of bowel sounds
Signs of shock

Splenic Rupture

Although rarely injured in sport participation, certain systemic disorders, such as **infectious mononucleosis**, can enlarge the spleen, making it vulnerable to injury. The spleen is the second most commonly injured abdominal organ after the kidneys, and is the most frequent cause of death due to abdominal blunt trauma in sport. The reason is that the spleen can splint itself and stop hemorrhage, only to produce delayed hemorrhage days, weeks, or months later, after a seemingly minor jarring motion, such as a cough. Indications of a splenic rupture include a history of blunt trauma to the left upper quadrant and a persistent dull pain in the left upper quadrant, left lower chest, and left shoulder, referred to as **Kehr's sign**. In addition, the individual is often nauseated, cold, clammy, and will show signs of shock at the time of injury. Acute care can be seen in **Field Strategy 16.3**.

Infectious mononucleosis
Viral condition caused by the Epstein-Barr virus that attacks the respiratory system and leaves the spleen enlarged and weak

Kehr's sign
Referred pain down the left shoulder indicative of a ruptured spleen

With a ruptured spleen, the individual is nauseated, cold and clammy, and will show signs of shock

Liver Contusion and Rupture

A direct blow to the upper right quadrant can contuse the liver, causing significant palpable pain, point tenderness, and hypoten-

 Field Strategy 16.3. Management of Suspected Intra-abdominal Injuries

Lay the individual supine, with the knees flexed to relax the abdominal muscles. *Do not* extend the legs or elevate the feet
Maintain an open airway
Assess vital signs
  Respirations—Rapid, shallow breathing indicates shock
  Pulse—Rapid, weak pulse indicates shock
  Blood pressure—A marked drop in blood pressure indicates shock
  Pupillary response to light—Lackluster, dilated pupils indicate shock
Control any external hemorrhage with a sterile dressing
If the individual vomits, roll the person on their side to allow for excretion, making certain the airway remains open
Treat for shock and give nothing by mouth
Transport immediately to the nearest medical facility

sion (low blood pressure). Shock is also commonly seen. As with the spleen, systemic diseases, such as hepatitis, can enlarge the liver making it more susceptible to injury. Although the lacerated liver, is capable of massive bleeding, often the organ has stopped bleeding by the time the wound is exposed in surgery. As such, there has been an increasing trend toward nonoperative management (18).

Appendicitis

The vermiform appendix is a pouch extending from the cecum (see **Fig. 16.9**). If it becomes obstructed (for example, with hardened fecal material), venous circulation may be impaired, leading to an increase in bacterial growth and the formation of pus. The resulting inflamed appendix, called **appendicitis**, can lead to ischemia and gangrene. If the appendix ruptures, feces containing bacteria are sprayed over the abdominal contents, causing peritonitis. Signs and symptoms include acute abdominal pain in the lower right quadrant, loss of appetite, nausea, vomiting, and a low-grade fever. Rebound pain can be elicited at **McBurney's point**, which is one-third the distance between the anterior superior iliac spine (ASIS) and the umbilicus.

Kidney and Bladder Injuries

The kidney is the most frequently injured organ in sports-related abdominal trauma. Serious injury often occurs when the body is extended and the abdominal muscles are relaxed, such as when a receiver leaps to catch a pass. Suspicion should be high if impact is to the midback region, especially if persistent back or significant flank pain is present. Individuals may complain of blood in the urine (hematuria), although this is not always indicative of the magnitude of injury (19).

Damage to the bladder is rare, although **hematuria** may occur. Most sport participants void prior to running and competition. Running with an empty bladder increases the risk of gross hematuria, because no fluid cushion exists between the posterior wall and base of the bladder. This condition is commonly seen in long distance runners, hence the name "runner's bladder" (20). Hematuria due to running rapidly resolves within 24 to 48 hours of rest.

Treatment for kidney and bladder injuries may involve ice to control inflammation and pain, treating for shock, and if needed, transporting the individual to the nearest medical facility. A radiograph or CT scan may be used to determine the extent of injury. Most injuries are managed conservatively with rest and fluid management.

The football player had a history of direct trauma to the abdomen, pain in the upper left quadrant, referred pain to the left shoulder, and showed signs of shock. This indicates a possible splenic rupture. Summon EMS.

Appendicitis
Inflammation of the appendix

McBurney's point
A site one-third the distance between the ASIS and umbilicus that, with deep palpation, produces rebound tenderness, indicating appendicitis

Blood in the urine is not always indicative of the magnitude of injury

Hematuria
Blood or red blood cells in the urine

Running with an empty bladder can increase the chances of gross hematuria, since no fluid cushion exists between the posterior wall and base of the bladder

ASSESSMENT OF THE THROAT, THORAX, AND VISCERA

? *A 17-year-old wrestler was hurt during practice. He reported hearing a pop and severe pain about five inches lateral to the sternum at the level of the ninth rib. The continuing stabbing pain increases on deep inhalations. How will you progress through this assessment to determine the extent and seriousness of injury?*

Injury assessment for thoracic and visceral injuries should focus on the primary survey, vital signs, and history of the injury. Chest or abdominal trauma, although initially appearing superficial and minor, can mask internal hemorrhage and swelling that can seriously compromise function of the vital organs. In addition, the individual's condition can slowly deteriorate, leading to a life-threatening condition. Although general observations and palpations can confirm the possibility of a serious underlying condition, a good history of the injury and constant monitoring of vital signs will be a stronger assessment tool.

> Chest or abdominal trauma, although initially appearing superficial and minor, can mask underlying complications that can seriously compromise function of the vital organs

While approaching the individual, assess consciousness, respirations, and circulation. If the individual is having difficulty breathing, anxiety and panic may make the task more difficult. After ruling out possible spinal injury, place the individual supine, with the knees flexed to facilitate breathing. Make sure the airway is open and clear of any blood or vomitus. The trachea should be in the middle of the throat and should not move during respirations. Speak in a slow, calm, confident manner. If breathing does not return to normal in a minute or two, summon EMS and take the vital signs, so that a baseline of information is established. Blood pressure, pulse, respirations, and pupillary response to light should be documented, so that comparisons can be made later in the assessment. A decrease in blood pressure may indicate loss of blood volume. It is always better to have EMS en route during the assessment than to wait and see if the condition gets any better. Several conditions intensify in severity with time, thereby seriously compromising the health of the injured party. Remember that with an acute abdominal injury, never give any water or food to the individual. Not only can the condition be aggravated, but, if surgery is needed, any food or fluid in the gastrointestinal tract will make the surgery more dangerous. When the assessment is completed, continue to monitor vital signs, and treat for shock until the ambulance arrives.

> Blood pressure, pulse, respirations, and pupillary response to light should be documented, so that comparisons can be made later in the assessment

> Never give water or food to an individual with an acute abdominal injury

HISTORY

? *You have completed the primary survey on the wrestler. He is obviously conscious, but cannot take a deep breath without stabbing pains. The pulse is somewhat elevated, but you are not sure if this is due to anxiety or an internal injury. What questions can be asked to determine the cause of this condition?*

The history of a chest or abdominal injury is extremely important, because few special tests are available for the region.

Gather information on the cause or mechanism of injury. For example, renal injury is more common in an athlete whose body is extended, with the abdominal musculature relaxed, such as a receiver diving for a ball. The extent and location of pain can also be helpful. Flank and back pain may indicate injury to the kidneys. Left upper quadrant or lower thoracic pain may indicate splenic injury. Right upper quadrant or lower thoracic pain may signal liver injury. Spleen and liver injuries may also refer pain to the left or right shoulder, respectively. Ask the individual what aggravates the pain. Coughing, sneezing, rapid movements, and walking down stairs may indicate peritoneal irritation, while musculoskeletal pain is often relieved by changing body position (21). Disability due to the injury, previous injuries to the area, and family history may have some bearing on this specific condition. In addition to the general questions discussed in Chapter 4, specific questions that can be asked for chest and abdominal injuries can be seen in **Field Strategy 16.4**.

 The wrestler violently twisted away from his opponent, when he felt a pop and sharp pain just lateral to his sternum on the lower chest wall. The stabbing pain intensifies with a deep breath. He does not recall any previous chest trauma, nor does he recall any member of the family having a similar problem.

Field Strategy 16.4. Developing a History of the Injury

Current Injury Status

1. How did the injury occur? What position were you in and from what direction was the force (glancing, direct, or violent muscle contraction)? Does it hurt to take a deep breath?
2. Ask about the pain location, severity, onset (sudden or gradual), and type (sharp, aching, burning, radiating). Did the pain disappear, then gradually increase (spontaneous pneumothorax, ruptured spleen)? Are you nauseous, lightheaded, or weak?
3. Did you hear any sounds during the incident (rib fracture or costochondral separation)? Have you had any muscle spasms or cramps with the injury?
4. What motions aggravate the symptoms? In what position are you most comfortable?
5. Have you noticed blood in the urine? Does it occur after long-distance running? Is it painful to urinate?

Past Injury Status

1. Have you ever been injured this area before? When? How did that occur? What was done for the injury?
2. Do you have a history of any cardiovascular disease, heart conditions, chest pains, or shortness of breath? Have you ever fainted before? Have any of these previous conditions occurred after strenuous exercise? Has anyone in your family had a history of any of these conditions?
3. Have you had any medical problems recently? (Look for problems that may refer pain to the area from visceral organs, heart, and lungs.)

OBSERVATION AND INSPECTION

🔴 *You suspect a rib or costochondral problem because of the mechanism of injury, area of pain, and pain on deep inspiration. You are not sure, however, if other internal complications may also be present. What factors can you observe that might provide clues to help determine if there is an injury to the chest wall or an internal complication?*

Observation of body position can give an indication of the site, nature, and severity of injury. For example, in an acute thoracic injury, the individual may lean toward the injured side, using an arm or hand to stabilize the region. In an acute abdominal injury, the individual may lie on the injured side and bring the knees toward the chest to relax the abdominal muscles. Observe for deformity, edema, bruising, ecchymosis, and skin color. Deformity may indicate a sternal or rib fracture, costochondral separation, or muscle rupture. Coughing up bright blood or frothy blood indicates a severe lung injury. Diffuse bruising in the axilla and chest wall may indicate a ruptured pectoralis major. Distention in the abdomen or flank ecchymosis may indicate bleeding in the abdomen. Pale, cold, and clammy skin is associated with shock. Cyanosis indicates a lack of oxygen due to internal pulmonary or cardiac problems.

Observe the rate and depth of respirations; note any difficulty in catching the breath. If the condition is only transitory, that is, the wind has been knocked out, breathing and color should return to normal quickly. If breathing does not return to normal quickly, or the individual's condition rapidly deteriorates, the injury is significant and EMS should be summoned. Note the symmetrical rise and fall of the chest. **Field Strategy 16.5** provides specific observations that can help determine the extent and severity of thoracic or abdominal injuries.

> If breathing does not return to normal quickly, or the individual's condition rapidly deteriorates, the injury is significant and EMS should be summoned

💡 *The wrestler shows no sign of trauma on the chest wall; however, while sitting, he leans to the right side, using his right arm to stabilize the chest. Breathing is shallow and there appears to be a slight indentation at the level of the ninth rib, about five inches lateral to the sternum.*

PALPATIONS

🔴 *You suspect a rib or costochondral injury to the lower right chest wall, but can not totally rule out internal damage to the organs in the upper right abdominal quadrant. What anatomical structures in this region can be palpated?*

Palpations of the chest and abdominal region should begin away from the painful area, so that pain cannot be carried over into other areas. Begin with gentle circular motions and feel for deformity, crepitus, swelling, rigidity, muscle guarding, or tenderness. Place the individual in a supine position, with the knees flexed for more comfort. Palpate the clavicle, ribs, costochondral cartilage, and sternum for deformity and crepitus. Possible frac-

Field Strategy 16.5. Observation and Inspection of the Thorax and Viscera

In what position is the individual (standing, leaning to one side, knees drawn to the chest, hands stabilizing an area)? Do the facial expressions indicate pain, anxiety, or panic? Is cyanosis present?

Is the trachea centered or deviated to one side (tension pneumothorax)? Does the trachea move during breathing? Are the neck veins distended (traumatic asphyxia)?

Note any bruising, ecchymosis, deformity, or muscular atrophy that may be present in the chest and abdomen

Does the rib cage look symmetrical and move symmetrically with each breath? Is shallow breathing present? Is the individual coughing up a bright red or frothy blood?

Are abrasions, blisters, or bleeding present at the nipples?

Is there any bruising or ecchymosis present in the abdomen (bruising in the umbilical area indicates intraperitoneal bleeding)? Is the discoloration localized or diffuse? Are there any soft tissue protrusions in the lower abdomen or groin (hernia)?

Is the individual pale, cold, clammy, or lethargic (shock)?

---

tures and costochondral separations are assessed with gentle pressure applied to the sternum and vertebrae in an anteroposterior direction (**Fig. 16.14A**). This action causes the rib cage to bow out laterally. Lateral compression on the sides of the rib cage causes strain on the costochondral junctions (**Fig. 16.14B**). Begin compression superiorly and move down in an inferior direction until the entire area is covered. Pain at a specific site indicates a positive sign.

Palpate the abdomen with the hips flexed to relax the abdominal muscles. Use the flat part of several fingers, with both hands moving in small circular motions (**Fig. 16.15**). Move across the abdomen in a straight line. Palpate for tenderness, muscle resistance, muscle guarding, and superficial masses or deficits in the continuity of the abdominal wall. Deeper palpation can detect rigidity, swelling, or masses. If the athlete seems to be apprehensive or overreacts to palpation, ask the athlete questions during

> Compression in an anteroposterior direction can detect possible rib fractures; lateral compression can detect possible costochondral separations

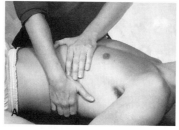
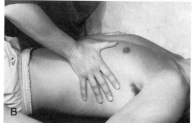

Figure 16.14. Compression of the rib cage in a supine position. **A.** Anteroposterior compression for rib fracture. **B.** Lateral compression for costochondral separation.

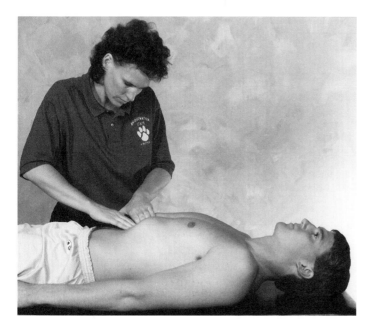

Figure 16.15. Palpation of the abdomen.

palpation. It is difficult to talk and voluntarily guard at the same time. If the pain is genuine, the individual will stop talking during guarding (21). Rebound tenderness at McBurney's point is indicative of appendicitis. The rebounding pain is caused when the inflamed appendix is impacted by the viscera returning to their normal position.

💡 *During palpations, you found extreme pain and deformity at the costochondral joint of the ninth rib. Pain increased at the site with lateral compression of the chest wall.*

SPECIAL TESTS

❓ *You suspect a costochondral separation of the ninth rib. While talking to the athlete, you notice perspiration forming on his forehead and his skin color appears pale. The eyes appear somewhat sunken and dull. What might be occurring? What is your next course of action?*

There are very few special tests for the thorax and visceral area. Many of these tests are too advanced for discussion and demonstration at this fundamental level. Therefore, most of the information on a thoracic or abdominal injury must be gathered during the primary survey, history, observation, and palpation phase of the assessment. Referred pain into the shoulders, abdominal region, or low back area can indicate what visceral organ is injured. **Table 16.5** summarizes the most common sites of referred pain for injury to the internal organs of the torso. If a muscular strain is suspected, active, passive, and resisted muscle

Table 16.5. Common Sites of Referred Pain

Organ	Localization of Pain
Appendicitis	Lower right quadrant
Bladder	Lower pelvic region over pubic bone
Heart	Left shoulder, down medial left arm, or it can extend into neck and jaw
Kidneys	Posterior lumbar region radiating to flanks and groin
Liver and gallbladder	Upper right quadrant or right shoulder
Lung and diaphragm	Upper shoulders and neck
Spleen	Left shoulder or proximal third of left arm (Kehr's sign)

 Field Strategy 16.6. Assessment of the Thorax and Visceral Region

Primary Survey

Assess the ABCs and maintain an open airway
Take vital signs (respirations, pulse, blood pressure, and pupillary response to light)

History

Primary complaint and mechanism of injury
Onset of symptoms, including pain and discomfort
Disability and functional impairments from the injury
Previous injuries or conditions, and family history

Observation and Inspection

Observe general body position that may indicate the injury site, difficulties in breathing, and signs of shock
Inspect the injured area for:

Muscle symmetry	Hypertrophy or muscle atrophy
Swelling	Visible congenital deformity
Discoloration	Surgical incisions or scars

Palpation

Do compressions in an anteroposterior direction (rib fracture) and lateral compression (costochondral separation)
Palpate soft tissue structures to determine temperature, point tenderness, rigidity, rebound tenderness, or muscle spasm

Special Tests

Active and resistive movements for muscular strains
Check change in sensation or areas of referred or radiating pain

Table 16.6. Conditions that Warrant Immediate Action

General body signs and symptoms, including:
   Eyes that are bulging or bloodshot, or distended neck veins
   Deviated trachea or trachea that moves during breathing
   Coughing up bright red or frothy blood, or vomiting blood that looks
      like used coffee grounds
   Signs of shock or cyanosis
   Sudden fatigue, weakness, palpitations, or chest pain during exercise
   Radiating or referred pain to the shoulder tip, back, or groin
Throat signs and symptoms, including:
   Hoarseness, loss of voice, or difficulty swallowing
   Presence of hemorrhage with blood-tinged sputum
   Loss of contour of the Adam's apple
Thoracic conditions, including:
   Shortness of breath, difficulty in breathing, or increased pain on deep
      inspiration
   Suspected rib or sternal fracture
   Abnormal or absent breath sounds
Abdominal conditions, including:
   Severe abdominal pain, nausea, or vomiting
   Distention, tenderness, rigidity, or muscle spasm
   Rebound pain on deep palpation
   Absence of bowel sounds
   Blood in the urine or stool

testing can be performed. **Field Strategy 16.6** lists the steps in a basic injury assessment of the thorax and visceral region.

You determined that muscle testing was not necessary be-cause pain was centered on the costochondral joint of the ninth rib. After immobilization of the region with an elastic wrap, treat for shock and transport the athlete to the nearest medical facility for further examination.

SUMMARY

Severe blunt trauma to the anterior neck region, thorax, and viscera can be devastating and can lead to serious respiratory and circulatory compromise. Certain injuries may not develop until hours, days, or weeks later. As such, the presumption of possible intrathoracic or intra-abdominal injuries necessitates a thorough assessment focusing on the primary survey, vital signs, and history of the injury. Observation, palpation, and sites of referred pain can confirm suspicions of an existing internal injury. If at anytime signs or symptoms indicate an intrathoracic or intra-abdominal injury, summon EMS immediately. Monitor vital signs every 3 to 5 minutes to determine if the individual is improving or deteriorating, and treat for shock. Conditions that warrant immediate action are listed in **Table 16.6**. If in doubt, always assume a serious internal injury is present and refer the individual to a physician.

REFERENCES

1. Nichols AW. Abdominal and thoracic injuries. In *Athletic injuries and rehabilitation* edited by JE Zachazewski, DJ Magee, and WS Quillen. Philadelphia: WB Saunders, 1996.
2. Rutherford GW, Kennedy J, and McGee L. *Hazard analysis: baseball and softball related injuries to children 5–14 years of age.* US Consumer Product Safety Commission, 1984.
3. McCutcheon ML, and Anderson JL. 1985. How I manage sports injuries to the larynx. Phys Sportsmed 13(4):100–112.
4. Haycock CE. 1987. How I manage breast problems in athletes. Phys Sportsmed 15(3):89–95.
5. Kretzler HH, and Richardson AB. 1989. Rupture of the pectoralis major muscle. Am J Spts Med 17(4):453–458.
6. Butcher JD, Siekanowicz A, and Pettrone F. 1996. Pectoralis major rupture: ensuring accurate diagnosis and effective rehabilitation. Phys Sportsmed 24(3):37–44.
7. Karofsky PS. 1987. Hyperventilation syndrome in adolescent athletes. Phys Sportsmed 15(2):133–138.
8. Erickson SM, and Rich BSE. 1995. Pulmonary and chest wall emergencies: on-site treatment of potentially fatal conditions. Phys Sportsmed 23(11):95–104.
9. Wagner RB, Sidhu GS, and Radcliffe WB. 1992. Pulmonary contusion in contact sports. Phys Sportsmed 20(2):126–136.
10. Volk CP, McFarland EG, and Horsmon G. 1995. Pneumothorax: on-field recognition. Phys Sportsmed 23(10):43–46.
11. Lee MC, et al. 1991. Traumatic asphyxia. Ann Thorac Surg 51(1):86–88.
12. King AI, and Viano DC. *Baseball related chest impact: final report to the consumer product safety commission.* US Consumer Product Safety Commission, 1986.
13. Green ED, et al. 1980. Cardiac concussion following softball blow to the chest. Ann Emerg Med 9(3):155–157.
14. Karofsky PS. 1990. Death of a high school hockey player. Phys Sportsmed 18(2):99–103.
15. Edlich RF Jr, et al. 1987. Commotio cordis in a lacrosse goalie. J Emerg Med 5(0):181–184.
16. Van Camp SP. Sudden death. In *Clinics in sports medicine*, edited by JC Puffer, vol. 11, no. 2. Philadelphia: WB Saunders, 1992.
17. Van Camp SP, et al. 1995. Nontraumatic sports death in high school and college athletes. Med Sci Sports Exerc 27(5):641–647.
18. Ray R, and Lemire JE. 1995. Liver laceration in an intercollegiate football player. J Ath Train 30(4):324–326.
19. Klein S, Hons S, Fujitani R, and State D. 1988. Hematuria following blunt abdominal trauma: the utility of intravenous pyelography. Arch Surg 123(9):1173–1177.
20. York JP. 1990. Sports and the male genitourinary system: kidneys and bladder. Phys Sportsmed 18(9):116–129.
21. Bergman RT. 1996. Assessing acute abdominal pain: a team physician's challenge. Phys Sportsmed 24(4):72–82.

Special Conditions Related to Sports

Special Conditions Related to Sports

Chapter 17: **Conditions Related to the Reproductive System**

Chapter 18: **Other Health Conditions Related to Sports**

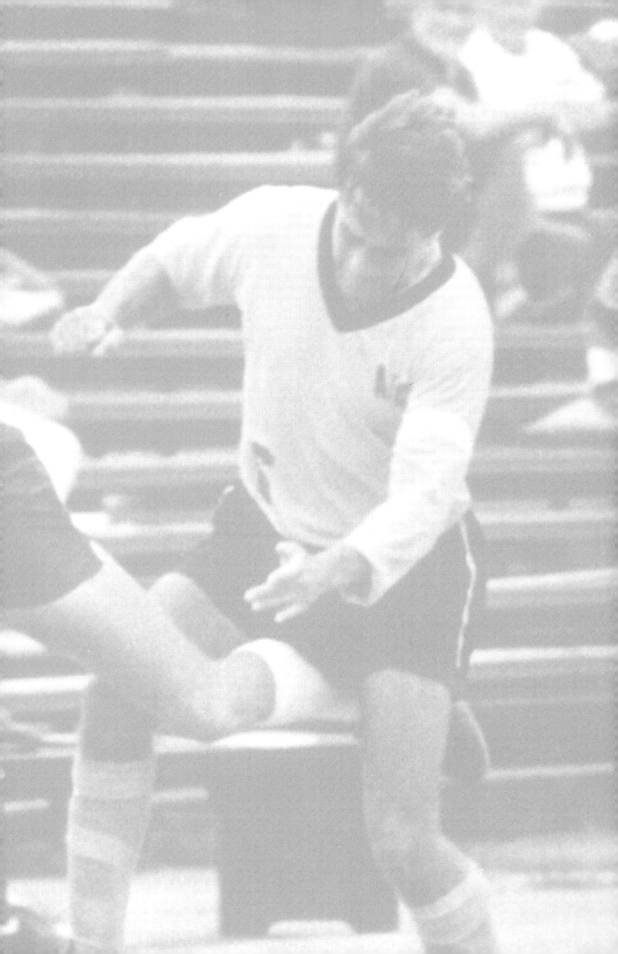

Marsha Grant, MEd, ATC

While playing field hockey at East Stroudsburg University, I got hurt twice within a 2-week period. As I visited the training room daily, I got to see the trainer, Lois Wagner, in action. What she did really sparked an interest in me. After talking with her about the field, I switched from wanting to be a health and physical education instructor to an athletic trainer. After completing my master's degree in education at the University of Virginia, I got my first taste of training and teaching at Western Illinois State University.

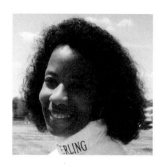

Marsha Grant was the first African-American Woman certified by the NATA. As a noted educator, she has served as an athletic trainer at the Division I, II, and III levels. She is currently the Head Athletic Trainer at Sterling High School in Somerdale, New Jersey.

Although I've worked at all three competitive levels of intercollegiate sports, I really enjoy my job at the high school level. I work full-time with a tremendous staff of administrators and coaches. Typically, I start my day at 1 o'clock in the afternoon and go until all the practices are over. I travel with the football team unless there is a home game, in which case I stay home to provide coverage there. It's a heavy workload in the fall, but because of the limited daylight I don't go quite as late. I make up for it in the winter season, however. We have a large variety of sports, and each sport may suit-up three different levels of teams, so the number of athletes I service daily is immense.

One great thing about this position is that we have a superb staff. Our school nurse always comes to the games and takes an active interest in the athletes. She also communicates with me daily about any player who may see her during the day. The athletic director also visits practice, often to see how things are going, and holds the coaches and athletes responsible for their actions. The athletes are aware of this sincere interest in their welfare, and are grateful for what I do for them. It is really fun to see these athletes enjoy participating in sports for the love of it. They have a good time, and I like being a part of that.

Although working on the college level was exciting because I got to travel all over the United States and interact with some outstanding colleagues, it just doesn't compare to working with this level. On the college level, I put in very long hours, seven days a week, for three seasons. Most people don't understand that you need a life outside of the training room and classroom. I honestly don't recall any coach ever asking me what time would be good for me to schedule a weekend practice. There is also a significant financial disparity in training on the college level. Some coaches with whom I worked were making $80,000 and up, and there I was, responsible for the entire health care of the scholarship athletes, making less than half of their salary.

It's different on the high school level. Salaries are more equitable, and there seems to be more respect from the coaches and administrators about the value you bring to their program. Parents, however, still do not necessarily see the importance of your daily presence. There are budget and equipment limitations, and it is sometimes difficult to convince parents to purchase needed protective braces for their daughters or sons. It may take two to three weeks to convince them to purchase the brace, whereas on the college level, I could walk into the storeroom and pull one out and fit the athlete right there.

Each level of competition has its pros and cons. As a woman in athletic training, you still have to fight the subtle notion that women aren't supposed to be trainers for men's intercollegiate teams. Had I not had the academic preparation and support at a school with an approved curriculum, I think my transition into the marketplace would have been more difficult. To succeed, you need to apply yourself in the classroom and in the clinical rotations. Utilize your resources and ask questions. Do clinical rotations at a variety of settings, including summer sports camps, to find out where you feel most comfortable. And most importantly, respect your skills and your profession. You are qualified to work with athletes, regardless of gender. Don't let anyone tell you that you can't. If you apply yourself, you will succeed and have fun doing it. It's a great profession.

Conditions Related to the Reproductive System

After completing this chapter, you should be able to:

- List the primary and accessory organs in the female and male reproductive systems

- Explain how hormones affect the human body

- Identify the signs and symptoms of common injuries to the female and male genitalia and explain their management

- Explain the risks associated with hepatitis and acquired immunodeficiency syndrome (AIDS) and indicate specific steps to prevent the spread of these diseases

- Describe menstrual irregularities and how contraceptive use and pregnancy may impact sport participation

Key Terms:

Accessory sex organs	Osteopenia
Amenorrhea	Osteoporosis
Androgens	Primary sex organs
Dysmenorrhea	Progesterone
Endometriosis	Retroviruses
Estrogens	Steroids
Menses	Tinea cruris

Injuries to the reproductive organs in sport participation are rare, particularly in the female. Diseases, however, such as hepatitis and AIDS, may be transmitted during sexual intercourse or via blood or blood products; these remain a concern for all health-care providers. Strictly following universal safety precautions can prevent the onset of many of these diseases. Sport participation can also be affected by menstrual disorders, contraceptive use, and pregnancy, although physicians believe a regular exercise program can be beneficial for the active woman.

This chapter begins with an anatomical review of the female and male reproductive systems and discusses the role of hormones in the overall development of the body. Common injuries or conditions associated with the various structures are then discussed. Next, hepatitis B and acquired immunodeficiency syndrome (AIDS) is presented, followed by information on sport participation during menstruation, ingestion of oral contraceptives, and pregnancy.

ANATOMY OF THE GENITALIA

? *Can the pelvic girdle totally protect the male and female reproductive systems from injury? Which structures may not be protected?*

The reproductive organs of the female and male include the primary and accessory sex organs. The **primary sex organs**, the ovaries and testes, produce gametes (specifically ovum and sperm, respectively) that, when joined together, develop into a fetus. Important sex hormones influence sexual differentiation, development of secondary sex characteristics, and, in the female, regulate the reproductive cycle. All sex hormones are predominantly produced by the primary sex organs and belong to the general family known as **steroids**. In the female, estrogen and progesterone are produced by the ovaries. In the male, the adrenal cortex and testes produce hormones known as **androgens**, the most active being testosterone. The **accessory sex organs** transport, protect, and nourish the gametes after they leave the ovaries and testes. In females, the accessory sex organs include the fallopian tubes, uterus, vagina, and vulva (**Fig. 17.1**). In males, the accessory sex

Primary sex organs
Reproductive organs responsible for producing gametes (ova and sperm)

Accessory sex organs
Organs that transport, protect, and nourish gametes

Steroids
A large family of chemical substances including endocrine secretions and hormones

Androgen
A class of hormones that promotes development of male genitals and secondary sex characteristics, and influences sexual motivation

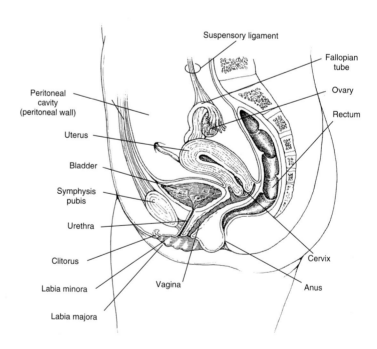

Figure 17.1. Median section of the female pelvis.

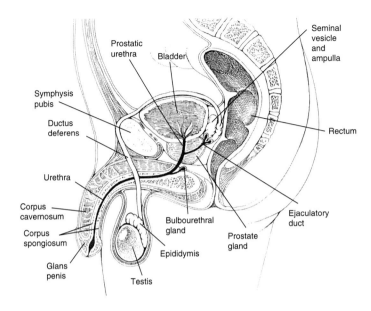

Figure 17.2. Median section of the male pelvis.

organs include the epididymis, ductus deferens, seminal vesicles, prostate gland, bulbourethral glands, scrotum, and penis **(Fig. 17.2)**.

Female Reproductive System

The female reproductive system includes: the ovaries, which produce ova (female eggs); the fallopian tubes, which transport, protect, and nourish the ova; the uterus, which provides an environment for the development of the fertilized embryo; and the vagina, which serves as the receptacle for the sperm **(Fig. 17.1)**. These structures are protected by the pelvic girdle and are seldom injured during sport participation.

The ovarian cycle begins at puberty, with a release of an ovum, or egg, from the ovary. The ovum, released at ovulation, travels through a fallopian tube to the uterus, where it embeds itself in the uterine wall. The menstrual cycle, lasting anywhere from 28 to 40 days, involves a repeated series of changes within the lining of the uterus, and is controlled by the ovarian cycle. **Menses**, or the menstrual flow, is a phase in the menstrual cycle lasting 3 to 6 days, when the thickened vascular walls of the uterus, the unfertilized ovum, and blood from the damaged vessels of the endometrium are lost.

The hormones estrogen and progesterone are produced by the ovaries. **Estrogens** help regulate the menstrual cycle and influence the development of female physical sex characteristics, such as the appearance of breasts, pubic and axillary hair, increased

Menses
Phase in the menstrual cycle when the thickened vascular walls of the uterus, the unfertilized ova, and blood from damaged vessels are lost during the menstrual flow

Estrogens
Hormones that produce female secondary sex characteristics and affect the menstrual cycle

Estrogens are responsible for the rapid growth spurt in girls between the ages of 12 and 13 years

Progesterone
Hormone responsible for thickening the uterine lining in preparation for the fertilized ovum

subcutaneous fat—especially in the hips and breasts—and widening and lightening of the pelvis. Estrogens are also responsible for the rapid growth spurt seen in girls between the ages of 12 and 13 years. This growth is short-lived, however, as increased levels of estrogen cause earlier closure of the epiphyses of long bones, leading to females reaching their full height between the ages of 15 to 17 years. In contrast, males may continue to grow until the age of 19 to 21 years. **Progesterones** are responsible for regulating the menstrual cycle and stimulating the development of the uterine lining in preparation for pregnancy.

The external genital organs of the female are known as the vulva, or pudendum. The outer rounded folds, the labia majora, protect the vestibule into which the vagina and urethra open.

Male Reproductive System

The male reproductive system includes: the testes, which produce spermatozoa; a number of ducts that store, transport, and nourish the spermatozoa; several accessory glands that contribute to the formation of semen; and the penis, through which urine and semen pass (**Fig. 17.2**). Testosterone, the primary androgen produced by the testes, stimulates the growth and maturation of the internal and external genitalia at puberty, and is responsible for sexual motivation. Secondary sex characteristics that are testosterone-dependent include the appearance of pubic, axillary, and facial hair, enhanced hair growth on the chest or back, and a deepening of the voice as the larynx enlarges. Androgens also increase bone growth, bone density, and skeletal muscle size and mass.

The pelvic girdle does provide strong protection for internal structures of the reproductive systems. Pelvic fractures, however, can seriously damage these structures. The external male genitalia are virtually unprotected from direct blows and can be injured with direct trauma.

INJURIES AND CONDITIONS OF THE GENITALIA

A soccer player was struck in the groin by an opponent's foot. He was not wearing a protective cup at the time. He immediately fell to the ground and drew the knees to the chest while grasping the genital region. How should this injury be managed? What signs or symptoms would indicate that immediate referral to a physician is warranted?

The male genitalia are more susceptible to injury than female genitalia because several structures are external to the body, thus exposed to direct trauma. Protective cups can protect the penis and scrotum from injury and are required for baseball catchers and hockey goalies (see **Fig. 6.14**). Direct trauma can damage the penis, urethra, and scrotum, which holds the testes. In addition, congenital variations in testicular suspension make certain individuals susceptible to torsion of the testicle.

Male Genital Injuries

Direct trauma to the groin from a knee, implement, or straddle-like injury, such as falling on a bar, can cause severe pain and dysfunction to the testes and penis (**Fig. 17.3**). Lacerations are rare; however, swelling and hemorrhage inside the scrotal sac can occur. To assist in assessment and follow-up management of an injury to the male genital organs, the individual should be instructed to do periodic self-assessment for pain and swelling and should be given guidelines on seeking further medical care, if necessary.

Penis Injuries

Superficial wounds to the penis or urethra may involve a contusion, abrasion, laceration, avulsion, or penetrating wound. Most injuries resolve without specific treatment. Superficial bleeding may be controlled with a sterile dressing and a cold compress with mild compression to control swelling. Referral to a physician is only necessary if hemorrhage persists or swelling impairs function of the urethra.

Scrotal Injuries

Blunt scrotal trauma can cause a contusion, hematoma, torsion, dislocation, or rupture of the testicle. Commonly, a knee, foot, or elbow to the groin compresses the testicle against the pelvis, leading to a nauseating, painful condition. Immediate internal hemorrhage, effusion, and muscle spasm occurs. Testicular spasm can be relieved by placing the individual on his back and flexing the knees toward the chest to relax the muscle spasm (**Fig. 17.4**).

> Blunt scrotal trauma can cause a contusion, hematoma, torsion, dislocation, or rupture of the testicle

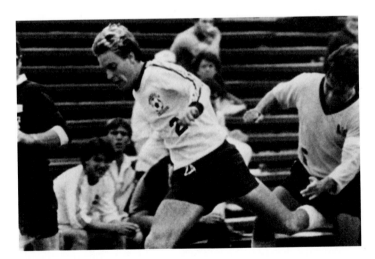

Figure 17.3. Direct trauma to the groin region can injure the penis or lead to swelling and hemorrhage in the scrotal sac.

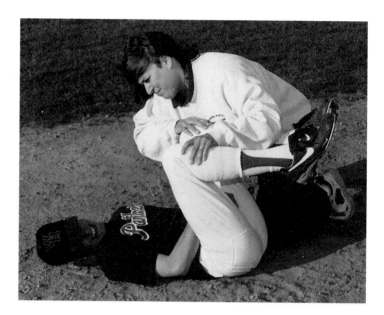

Figure 17.4. To relieve testicular spasm, place the individual on his back and flex the knees toward the chest. After pain has diminished, apply ice to control swelling and hemorrhage.

After pain subsides, a cold compress should be placed on the scrotum to reduce swelling and hemorrhage.

A scrotal mass may also be indicative of testicular cancer, the most common malignancy in 16- to 35-year-old males (1). Men who have an undescended or partially descended testicle are at a higher risk of developing testicular cancer than others. The first sign is a slightly enlarged testicle and a change in its consistency. Often a dull ache or sensation of dragging and heaviness is present in the lower abdomen or groin. Diagnosis is made with transillumination with a bright light or ultrasound. Early detection and surgical treatment yields an excellent survival rate.

> A scrotal mass may be indicative of testicular cancer, the most common malignancy in 16- to 35-year-old males

Female Genital Injuries

Injuries to the vulva usually involve straddling or penetration trauma or can be sustained by falls, resulting in tears from forced perineal stretching during sudden leg abduction. These injuries have occurred in gymnastics, water-skiing, snowmobiling, motorcycling, bicycling, sledding, cross-country skiing, and riding horses (2). Nearly all injuries are easily treated by ice application, mild compression, and bed rest. Occasionally, high-speed waterskiing injuries result in water being forced under high pressure into the vulva and vagina, leading to rupture of the vaginal walls. The water may also be forced through the fallopian tubes, leading to localized pelvic peritonitis. These injuries are easily preventable by wearing a neoprene wetsuit or nylon-reinforced suit.

Dermatologic Conditions

Tinea cruris (jock itch) is a common fungal infection involving the genitalia, seen more commonly in men than women. Perspiration can accumulate between the scrotum and skin of the thigh. This condition is augmented by wearing constrictive clothing, such as an athletic supporter, tight shorts, or spandex, which encourages fungal growth. In addition, tight garments cause chafing and irritation. The crual or perineal folds between the scrotum and inner thighs are usually the first areas to exhibit small patches of erythema and scaling. Other signs and symptoms include diffuse thick and dark lesions, weeping vesicles or pustules on the margins of inflammation, and severe itching. Topical anti-fungal medications may include Tinactin, Micatin, Lamisil, or Nizoral. These are typically applied twice daily for 2 to 6 weeks. During treatment, the groin area should be kept clean and dry, and loose, absorbent clothing should be worn. **Field Strategy 17.1** summarizes the signs, symptoms, and management of tinea cruris.

Intertrigo is a superficial dermatitis caused by moisture, warmth, sweat retention, or constant friction in the body's skinfolds. The condition may occur between the creases of the neck, in the axillary region, or beneath large breasts, but is primarily seen in the groin region in individuals with muscular thighs or in obese individuals, hence the nickname "chub rub." The condition is characterized by erythema, maceration, burning, and itching. In severe cases, the skin becomes eroded and weeping. The sweat pores become blocked, causing small sweat gland cysts. The condition can be prevented by wearing loose, soft, cotton underwear to keep the skin dry, clean, and friction free. The area should be cleansed daily with mild soap and water, followed by an application of hydrocortisone cream. Talcum powders should be avoided, as they can be abrasive and do not absorb moisture well.

Tinea cruris
Common fungal infection of the genitalia

Signs and symptoms of tinea cruris include thick, dark lesions, weeping vesicles, and severe itching

---

 ### Field Strategy 17.1. Management of Tinea Cruris

Signs and Symptoms

Erythema and scaling between the scrotum and inner thighs
Skin may appear thickened and dark
Weeping vesicles or pustules may appear at the margins of the
    inflammation
Severe itching

Management

Wash the region daily and after physical exertion. Rinse all soap residue
    from the region and completely dry the area. Apply powder liberally
Frequently change and wash the athletic supporter and undergarments.
    Wear loose, non-restrictive clothing
Apply ointments twice daily for at least a month. Use over-the-counter
    medications, such as Tinactin, Micatin, Lamisil, or Nizoral
If the condition does not clear up, seek medical assistance to rule out
    candidiasis, dermatitis, psoriasis, or other skin disorders

The position of the player will relieve testicular spasm. After the spasm has eased, remove the player from the field, apply cold compresses to reduce swelling and hemorrhage, and encourage the individual to do periodic self-assessment. If swelling of the testicle occurs, the individual should seek immediate medical attention.

BLOODBORNE VIRAL DISEASES

A basketball player is complaining of general muscle and joint pain, diarrhea, nausea, and dark urine. During the assessment you notice that the athlete's eyes appear yellowish and the skin is jaundiced. What condition may be present? What major abdominal organ may be damaged?

Viral diseases, particularly hepatitis B and AIDS, can be transmitted during sexual intercourse or via blood and blood products. Because of the very nature of managing sports injuries, any individual who supervises sport participants must be aware of these conditions and follow universal safety precautions to prevent their transmission.

Hepatitis B

Hepatitis B (HBV) is transmitted via blood or blood products, semen, vaginal secretions, and saliva and has an incubation period ranging from 45 to 160 days

There are five major types of hepatitis, with the hepatitis B virus (HBV) being the most common. HBV is transmitted via blood or blood products, semen, vaginal secretions, and saliva. The incubation period ranges from 45 to 160 days. Hepatitis primarily attacks the liver, severely impairing function. Early signs include mild, flu-like symptoms, such as malaise, fatigue, and loss of appetite. Progressive signs include severe fatigue, anorexia, nausea, vomiting, diarrhea, general muscle and joint pain, high fever, vomiting,

---

Table 17.1. Individuals at Risk for Hepatitis B and HIV Diseases

Individuals exposed to blood, including athletic trainers, student athletic trainers, nurses, and physicians
Staff and residents of institutions for the developmentally disabled
Staff and patients in kidney dialysis units
Intravenous drug users
Gay men
Sexually active heterosexuals with multiple partners
Recipients of blood transfusions or blood products on a regular basis
Anyone who has resided in Haiti or central Africa (HIV virus)
Heterosexual women and men who:
  Have anal intercourse
  Have multiple sexual partners
  Have multiple contacts with an infected partner
  Use oral contraceptives

---

severe abdominal pain, and dark urine. Among the most notable signs is a yellowing of the whites of the eyes and a yellowish, or jaundiced, skin appearance in light-complexioned individuals (3).

Currently there is no specific drug therapy to cure viral hepatitis B. Bed-rest and adequate fluid intake can prevent dehydration, but the disease must run its course. Immunoglobulin B (IGB) can prevent hepatitis B and should be administered to those individuals listed in **Table 17.1** who may be at risk for coming in contact with the virus. Although not specifically mentioned, coaches, referees, officials, and recreational sport supervisors should also be vaccinated, because they are often first on the scene of an acute injury involving hemorrhage. In 1992, this vaccine became a standard childhood immunization. Other preventative measures that can be followed in the athletic training room may be seen in **Field Strategy 17.2**.

> A noticeable sign of hepatitis is a yellowing of the whites of the eyes and a yellowish, or jaundiced, skin appearance in light-complected individuals

 ### Field Strategy 17.2. Preventing the Spread of Infectious Diseases in the Athletic Training Room

Immunization

Athletic training staff and student athletic trainers should receive the Hepatitis B inoculations and have up-to-date immunizations

Hygiene

Hands should be washed with an appropriate germicidal soap and warm water before treating each athlete and prior to wearing water-impervious latex gloves. Hands should be washed after glove removal

If bleeding occurs, the individual's participation should be interrupted until the bleeding has stopped and the wound is both cleansed and covered securely or occluded. Uniforms saturated with blood should be changed

Skin exposed to blood or other body fluids visibly contaminated with blood should be promptly cleansed with soap and water. Antiseptic hand cleansers or moist towelettes may be used if soap and water are unavailable; however, the individual must wash with soap and warm water as soon as possible

Eating, drinking, smoking, applying cosmetics or lip balm, and handling contact lenses are prohibited in all areas where blood or other infectious materials may be located

After sport participation, athletes should shower before receiving treatment

Protective Equipment

Water-impervious latex gloves should be readily available for staff when handling blood or other body fluids visibly contaminated with blood, and should be worn by individuals with nonintact skin

In situations of increased risk of exposure (i.e., heavy bleeding or use of Sharps) double gloving is recommended

At anytime when blood or other bodily fluids could be splashed, spurted, or sprayed, the use of a mask and/or protective eye guard with side shields, apron, and gown should be worn

CPR microshields, resuscitation bags, and oral airways should be used whenever possible during cardiopulmonary resuscitation

Field Strategy 17.2. Preventing the Spread of Infectious Diseases in the Athletic Training Room (continued)

Cleaning and Caring for Equipment

Disinfect all surfaces in the athletic training room with antiseptic/germicidal solutions following any exposure to blood or infectious materials

All tables, work space, and floors should be cleaned on a regular basis, particularly after patient use and immediately after any blood or infectious spills or soiling occurs

Commercial cleansers are available; however, a 1:10 (10%) bleach solution is adequate. Use caution when applying this solution near therapeutic modalities or skin, because of its corrosive properties

Athletic equipment (e.g., wrestling mats) visibly contaminated with blood should be wiped clean with a fresh bleach solution and allowed to dry before using

A Sharps container should be available at all times, including travel. It should be leakproof, puncture-resistant, red in color, and have a visible biohazard sign

Reusable Sharps, such as scissors and tweezers, should be sterilized after each use and stored in a container, such as an autoclave tray, that precludes the athletic trainer from retrieving the item with his/her hands

All disposable soiled products (i.e., gauze, paper towels, cotton) should be handled only with gloves and placed in leakproof bags with a visible biohazard sign

Soiled linens and towels should also be handled with gloves and placed in a leakproof bag with a visible biohazard sign. All items should be washed separately from the regular laundry, with detergent and hot water (71°C), for a minimum of 25 minutes. Additional disinfectant solution may be added to the water for heavily contaminated items

Soiled pullover scrubs, aprons, or gowns should be removed in such a way as to avoid contact with the outer surface and placed in an appropriately designated area or container

AIDS

Retroviruses
Any virus of the family *Retroviridae*, known to reverse the usual order of reproduction within the cells they infect

HIV can be transmitted in blood, semen, and vaginal secretions

AIDS results from the viral infection *human immunodeficiency virus* (HIV) and falls within a special category of viruses called **retroviruses**. In the United States, high risk groups include those individuals listed in **Table 17.1**. Currently, HIV has only been found to be transmitted in blood, semen, and vaginal secretions. In sports, the risk of AIDS is rare, although AIDS was recently reported in a body builder who injected anabolic-androgenic steroids into his body with a contaminated needle (4). In boxing, football, or wrestling, where participants may have a bloody nose or open cuts, close contact with the competitor may also pose a health risk. Individual's uniforms that become saturated with blood must be changed before returning to competition. Small amounts of bloodstain on a uniform, however, do not require removal of the participant from the game or uniform change. **Field Strategy 17.2** includes several measures to prevent the spread of infectious diseases in an athletic setting.

Signs and symptoms vary, depending on the degree to which the immune system is impaired. Common symptoms include those listed in **Table 17.2**. To date, there is no effective cure or vaccine

Table 17.2. Common Signs and Symptoms Indicating the HIV Virus

Persistent fever or night sweats
Unexplained weight loss and loss of appetite
Extreme fatigue not explained by physical activity or mental depression
White spots or unusual blemishes in the mouth, or a whitish coating on the tongue
A persistent, dry cough unrelated to smoking
Persistent unexplained diarrhea or bloody stools
Easy bruising or atypical bleeding from any body opening
Blotches or bumps on or under the skin
Persistent severe headaches

for AIDS. The best defense against the virus is education and prevention through behavioral changes and practicing universal precautions in dealing with blood and blood products.

For further information and publications on AIDS, contact:

National AIDS Hotline (CDC)
1-800-342-AIDS
1-800-344-7432 (Spanish)
1-800-243-7889 (Deaf Access, TTY)
National AIDS Information Clearing House (for AIDS publications/educational material)
1-800-458-5231

The basketball player complained of general muscle and joint pain, diarrhea, nausea, and dark urine. The eyes appeared yellowish and the skin was jaundiced. If you suspected possible hepatitis and liver damage, you are correct. This individual should be seen immediately by a physician.

MENSTRUAL IRREGULARITIES

A lean 16-year-old distance runner has reported she has not had a menstrual period in 3 months and is concerned she may be pregnant. What other menstrual irregularities could account for this absence of menses?

There continues to be a high participation rate of girls and women at all levels of sport. Many of these participants will, at one time or another, be affected by menstrual irregularities. Research is just beginning to explore the effects of conditioning and training on gynecologic function, yet much needs to be done. The two most common menstrual irregularities are dysmenorrhea and exercise-associated amenorrhea.

Dysmenorrhea

Dysmenorrhea, or menstrual cramps, is caused when the muscles of the uterus contract due to the overproduction of prostaglandins,

Dysmenorrhea
Difficult or painful menstruation; menstrual cramps

Regular exercise and a diet high in fluids and fiber and low in salt can alleviate the bloating and swelling caused by water retention

a group of chemicals produced in the body. Under most conditions, the contractions are minor and go unnoticed. With more severe contractions, abdominal aching or pain results during the first days of a woman's period. Other symptoms include bloating, nausea, vomiting, diarrhea, headache, breast tenderness, fatigue, irritability, or nervousness. The condition is very common in adolescent girls.

Regular exercise and a diet high in fluids and fiber and low in salt can alleviate bloating and swelling caused by water retention. Over-the-counter medications, such as Midol, Advil, Ibuprofen, aspirin, or Tylenol can relieve pain and cramping. Severe or persistent discomfort may necessitate physician referral to rule out pelvic inflammatory disease (PID), benign uterine tumors, obstruction of the cervical opening, and **endometriosis**, a condition whereby endometrial cells from the uterine lining implant themselves in the abdominal cavity.

Endometriosis
Condition whereby endometrial cells from the uterine lining implant themselves in the abdominal cavity, frequently forming cysts containing altered blood

Amenorrhea
Absence or abnormal cessation of menstruation

Secondary amenorrhea involves the disruption of an established menstrual cycle, resulting in the absence of menstruation for 3 to 6 consecutive menstrual periods

Osteopenia
Condition of reduced bone mineral density that predisposes the individual to fractures

Osteoporosis
Pathologic condition of reduced bone mass and strength

Amenorrhea and decreased estrogen predispose women to reduced bone density, leading to increased stress fractures and musculoskeletal injuries

Exercise-associated Amenorrhea

Amenorrhea is the absence of menstruation and is more prevalent among athletes, particularly runners, than the general population. Amenorrhea is a symptom, not a disease, and has been linked to prepubertal exercise, premature ovarian failure, central nervous system tumors, infections, pituitary or hypothalamic hormonal imbalances, chronic diseases, and malnutrition (5). Amenorrhea can lead to premature bone loss, lower peak bone mass, increased fractures in the vertebra and lower extremity, increased musculoskeletal injuries, and scoliosis (5–9). Delayed menarche results in prolonging the hypoestrogenic state of menses, which can lead to **osteopenia** at an age when bone density should be increasing (10). Osteopenia, or reduced bone mass, does not necessarily demonstrate fractures, but is considered a precursor to **osteoporosis**, which is the end-stage disease that does demonstrate deformations or fractures, particularly in the vertebrae.

There are two types of amenorrhea, primary and secondary. Primary amenorrhea is the failure to begin menstruation at puberty or by age 16. Secondary amenorrhea involves the disruption of an established menstrual cycle, resulting in the absence of menstruation for 3 to 6 consecutive menstrual months. This can result from pregnancy or dysfunction in the ovaries, endometrium, pituitary gland, or hypothalamus. A recent study reported that smoking one or more packs of cigarettes per day, multiple binge-eating behaviors combined with laxative use or self-induced vomiting, and weight fluctuation due to weight control in an adolescent population contributed to secondary amenorrhea (10).

Exercise-associated amenorrhea is a form of hypothalamic amenorrhea and has been reported in women participating in virtually every sport. Amenorrhea has been shown to affect up to 50% of competitive runners, 44% of ballet dancers, 25% of noncompetitive runners, and 12% of cyclists and swimmers (9).

Within the first 3 months of amenorrhea, a woman should be fully evaluated to rule out pregnancy and abnormalities in the thyroid gland, uterus, or vagina. The individual should be counseled to decrease her activity level to allow for a slight weight gain until normal menstrual cycles occur, and to consider a calcium and estrogen-progesterone supplement (11).

💡 *Secondary amenorrhea is common in adolescent distance runners. The woman, however, should be referred to a physician to rule out pregnancy and then counseled accordingly.*

BIRTH CONTROL AND SPORT PARTICIPATION

❓ *Many women use oral contraceptives for birth control. Think for a minute about what implications this may have on athletic performance. What adverse effects might occur?*

Intrauterine devices (IUDs) and oral contraceptives are two birth control methods used by women who participate in sport. Use of an IUD has been shown to increase the risk for PID, ectopic pregnancies, chlamydia, gonorrhea, endometriosis, anemia, uterine fibroids, and heart disease. In addition, IUDs have been associated with increased prevalence of heavy menstrual bleeding and dysmenorrhea, each of which can adversely affect sport performance (12).

Oral contraceptives (OCs) are used by fewer women athletes than the general population. Much of this is due to early studies that reported decreased maximal oxygen uptake and decreased isometric strength and endurance time with OC use (13). Most trained women have lower arterial blood pressures, lower body fat, higher lean body weight, and do not smoke—all factors that put sedentary women at risk for complications (13). Recent studies have reported that certain adverse effects are counteracted by exercise (14,15). The pills prohibit ovulation, reduce menstrual cramps, and decrease the amount and duration of the menstrual flow. Their use has been shown to decrease the frequency of skeletal injuries and loss of vertebral bone mineral density related to osteopenia (9). As such, it is not surprising that healthy active women, young amenorrheic women, and older postmenopausal women benefit from the use of oral contraceptives.

> IUDs have been associated with increased prevalence of heavy menstrual bleeding and dysmenorrhea, each of which can adversely affect athletic performance

> Oral contraceptives prohibit ovulation, reduce menstrual cramps, and decrease the amount and duration of the menstrual flow

💡 *Oral contraceptives can increase risk for certain conditions; however, low-dose oral contraceptives and regular exercise can offset many of the risks, providing a safe, effective birth control method for the active woman.*

PREGNANCY AND SPORT PARTICIPATION

❓ *A recreational tennis player is 3 months pregnant. She plays at least three times a week. Can her body's physiological needs during exercise harm the fetus? What steps can be taken to avoid any complications?*

The impact of exercise on an active pregnant women and her developing fetus is an area of concern, particularly when chemicals and nutrients pass freely in placental blood flow. Studies have shown that oxygen uptake by the uteroplacental tissues and fetus during exercise is maintained by a facilitated unloading of oxygen from the available maternal blood supply. For a previously active, healthy woman during an uncomplicated pregnancy, moderate aerobic exercise does not produce circulatory alterations that compromise fetal oxygen supply. In looking at fetal development, fetoplacental growth, prematurity, fetal stress/distress, and condition during labor and at birth, it was found that women who exercise regularly do not experience an increase in abortion, congenital abnormalities, abnormal placentation, premature rupture of the membranes, or preterm labor (16). Although increases were found in fetal heart rate after exercise, no adverse affects were seen.

Gains in body weight and fat accumulation are an obvious adaptation to pregnancy and can have some effect on weight-bearing exercise. In addition, postural adaptations to compensate for the weight of the uterus may lead to increased lordosis and upper spine extension. As the woman's center of gravity shifts upward and forward, lower back pain may ensue. Exercises to strengthen the abdominal and hip extensors (hamstrings, gluteus maximus), as well as relaxing and/or stretching the erector spinae and hip flexors (iliopsoas, rectus femoris), can relieve some of this pain. Proper lifting techniques to relieve stress on the low back area should be incorporated in daily activities. In addition to mechanical changes in the body during pregnancy, the hormones progesterone and relaxin increase joint laxity, making articulations widen and become more mobile during the later stages of pregnancy (17). Ballistic movements (bouncing) during daily activities and exercise should be avoided during the later stages of pregnancy.

Aerobic classes may be modified to decrease the amount of ballistic movements and time spent in exercising in the supine position. A 5- to 10-minute warm-up, low- or no-impact aerobics, and careful monitoring of heart rate, followed by a cool-down and stretching period, are recommended. Weight training with light weights and higher repetitions can be continued during pregnancy, when the goal is strength maintenance, not gain. In running programs, distance and intensity of the workout will need to be decreased as the pregnancy progresses. Many physicians believe that participation in moderate aerobic exercise during pregnancy at a level great enough to produce or maintain a training effect does not adversely affect birthweight or other maternal and infant outcomes, and may be associated with fewer perceived pregnancy-associated discomforts (18). All women should consult their physician about an exercise program.

The recreational tennis player should consult her physician about exercise during pregnancy. The physician will be able to identify any factors or health conditions that may compromise fetal blood supply during exercise as the pregnancy progresses.

Postural adaptations to compensate for the weight of uterus may lead to increased lordosis and upper spine extension, which can increase low back pain

Exercise programs for the pregnant woman need to be individualized

SUMMARY

Injuries to the reproductive organs in sport participation are rare, particularly in the female. Common diseases, such as hepatitis and AIDS, can be transmitted via blood or blood products and remain a major concern for all health-care providers. Individuals at risk for coming in contact with blood should be immunized against hepatitis B and use universal safety precautions in the training room to prevent the spread of contagious diseases.

Menstrual disorders, such as dysmenorrhea and amenorrhea, can also affect the sport participant. Amenorrhea, in particular, has been associated with reduced bone-mineral density, leading to an increased incidence of stress fractures and postural deviations. Evidence points to the fact that sport participation is not adversely affected by the use of oral contraceptives and can be beneficial to the pregnant woman.

REFERENCES

1. Melekos MD, Asbach HW, and Markou SA. 1988. Etiology of acute scrotum in 100 boys with regard to age distribution. J Urol 139(5):1023–1025.
2. Gianini GD, Method MW, and Christman JE. 1991. Traumatic vulvar hematomas: assessing and treating nonobstetric patients. Postgrad Med 89(4):115–118.
3. Buxton BP, Buxton BH, Okasaki EM, and Ho KW. 1994. Prevention of hepatitis B virus in athletic training. J Ath Train 29(2):107–112.
4. Sklarek HM, et al. 1984. AIDS in a bodybuilder using anabolic steroids, letter. N Engl J Med 311(26):1701.
5. Shangold M, Rebar RW, Wentz AC, and Schiff I. 1990. Evaluation and management of menstrual dysfunction in athletes. JAMA 263(12):1665–1669.
6. Ayers JWT, Gidwani GP, Schmidt IMV, and Gross M. 1984. Osteopenia in hyperestogenic young women with anorexia nervosa. Fertil Steril 41(2):224–228.
7. Fogelholm M, Lichtenbelt WV, Ottenheijm R, and Westerterp K. 1996. Amenorrhea in ballet dancers in the Netherlands. Med Sci Sports Exerc 28(5):545–550.
8. Lloyd T, et al. 1986. Women athletes with menstrual irregularity have increased musculoskeletal injuries. Med Sci Sports Exerc 18(4):374–379.
9. Fruth SJ, and Worrell RW. 1995. Factors associated with menstrual irregularities and decreased bone mineral density in female athletes. J Ortho Sports Phys Ther 22(1):26–38.
10. Johnson J, and Whitaker AH. 1992. Adolescent smoking, weight changes, and binge-purge behavior: associations with secondary amenorrhea. Am J Public Health 82(1):47–54.
11. Roberts WO. 1995. Primary amenorrhea and persistent stress fracture: a practical clinical approach. Phys Sportsmed 23(9):33–42.
12. Shangold MM. Gynecologic concerns in exercise and training. In *Women and exercise: physiology and sports medicine*, edited by MM Shangold and G Mirkin. Philadelphia: FA Davis, 1988.
13. Wells CL. *Women, sport, & performance: a physiological perspective*. Champaign, IL: Human Kinetics, 1991.
14. Gray DP, Harding E, and Dale E. 1983. Effects of oral contraceptive on serum lipid profiles of women runners. Fertil Steril 39(4):510–514.
15. Szoka P, and Edgren R. 1988. Drug interactions with oral contraceptives: compilation and analysis of an adverse experience report database. Fertil Steril 49(Suppl):31–37.

16. Clapp JF. 1991. Exercise and fetal health. J Dev Physiol 15(1):9–14.
17. Drinkwater BL, Nilson K, Ott S, and Chestnut CH III. 1986. Bone mineral density after resumption of menses in amenorrheic athletes. JAMA 256(3):380–382.
18. Sternfeld B, Quesenberry CP, Eskenazi B, and Newman LA. 1995. Exercise during pregnancy and pregnancy outcome. Med Sci Sports Exerc 27(5):634–640.

Chapter 18

Other Health Conditions Related to Sports

After completing this chapter, you should be able to:

- Describe the signs, symptoms, and management of common respiratory tract infections and disorders to the gastrointestinal tract

- Explain the physiological factors involved in diabetes and differentiate the management of diabetic coma from insulin shock

- Identify common contagious viral diseases

- Describe the signs and management of an individual experiencing an epileptic seizure

- Identify common substances abused by sport participants and the impact each will have on the individual's health and sport performance

- Describe the various eating disorders and explain guidelines for safe weight loss and weight gain

Key Terms:

Anemia	Hypertension
Anorexia nervosa	Hypoglycemia
Asthma	Infarcts
Bronchitis	Infectious mononucleosis
Bronchospasm	Influenza
Bulimia	Malaise
Clonic state	Pharyngitis
Constipation	Rhinitis
Diabetes	Rhinorrhea
Diarrhea	Sickle cell anemia
Epilepsy	Sinusitis
Gastroenteritis	Therapeutic drugs
Hay fever	Tonic state
Hyperglycemia	

There are several conditions unrelated to trauma that can influence the health of a sport participant. This chapter begins with a discussion of prevalent infections or conditions of the respiratory tract and gastrointestinal system, including their signs, symptoms, and management. Information on diabetes, epilepsy, hypertension, and anemia is then presented. Finally, an overview of substance abuse and eating disorders, relative to implications for the individual's health and sport performance, are discussed.

RESPIRATORY TRACT CONDITIONS

? *A 15-year-old asthmatic would like to improve his cardiovascular endurance. What activities might you recommend and what guidelines should be followed in developing the exercise program?*

Conditions of the respiratory tract are common in sport participants. Many factors, such as fatigue, chronic inflammation from a localized infection, environmental factors (allergens, dust, smog), and psychological stress brought on by stressful life events can suppress resistance to these conditions (1). The more common respiratory tract conditions will be presented here.

Common Cold

The common cold (coryza) is an acute infection that may result from aspirin sensitivity, use of oral contraceptives, topical decongestant abuse, cocaine abuse, presence of nasal polyps or deviated septum, or bacterial, viral, or allergic conditions. Symptoms include a rapid onset of a clear nasal discharge (**rhinorrhea**), nasal itching, sneezing, and associated itching and puffiness of the eyes. In the viral condition associated with the common cold, a low-grade fever, chills, and **malaise** (feeling lousy or tired) are often present.

Although there is no treatment or cure for the viral common cold, over-the-counter medications can alleviate or lessen symptoms. Vitamin C supplements have not been shown to decrease the incidence of colds; however, decreases in the duration and severity of symptoms have been found (2). **Field Strategy 18.1** provides several suggestions for preventing a cold.

Sinusitis

Sinusitis is an inflammation of the paranasal sinuses that may be secondary to an upper respiratory tract infection, allergy, or direct trauma **(Fig. 18.1)**. Signs and symptoms include nasal congestion and discharge (anterior or posterior), facial pain or pressure over the involved sinus, pain in the upper teeth or behind the eyes, coughing, and, in severe cases paranasal and eyelid swelling, fever, and chills (3). The individual will often pinch the bridge of the nose to demonstrate the area of discomfort or will report discomfort aggravated by eyeglasses.

Treatment involves controlling the infection, reducing mucosal edema, and allowing for nasal drainage. Oral antibiotics, such as amoxicillin, penicillin, or erythromycin, may be prescribed. Topical agents, such as phenylephrine hydrochloride (Neo-Synephrine)

The common cold is an acute infection that may result from aspirin sensitivity, use of oral contraceptives, topical decongestant abuse, cocaine abuse, presence of nasal polyps or deviated septum, or bacterial, viral, or allergic conditions

Rhinorrhea
Clear nasal discharge

Malaise
Lethargic feeling of general discomfort; out-of-sorts feeling

Vitamin C supplements do not decrease the incidence of colds, but can reduce the duration and severity of cold symptoms

Sinusitis
Inflammation of the paranasal sinuses

Field Strategy 18.1. Steps to Prevent a Cold

Avoid individuals with upper respiratory tract infections
Avoid touching or sharing objects touched by individuals with upper
respiratory tract infections
Wash the hands frequently in hot sudsy water
If exercising in cold weather, dress appropriately
Drink plenty of fluids
Although vitamin C supplements will not decrease the incidence of colds,
they have been found to decrease the duration and severity of
symptoms
Reduce environmental factors (dust, smog, allergens) that may preclude
you to rhinitis
Reduce stress
If using topical decongestant therapy, follow instructions carefully and do
not prolong its use, as rebound rhinitis may occur
Use decongestants during the day and antihistamines at night because of
their sedative effect
If cold symptoms include headache, fever, muscular aches, a hacking
productive cough, or loss of appetite, exercise should cease

or oxymetazoline hydrochloride (Afrin) can be used during the
first 3 to 4 days of treatment to facilitate drainage, but their value
is questionable (3,4). Longer use of decongestants can lead to a
rebound effect, whereby excessive mucus production and edema
are increased. In severe cases, surgical intervention may be necessary to drain the sinuses.

Pharyngitis (Sore Throat)

Pharyngitis results from a viral, bacterial, or fungal infection of
the pharynx, leading to a sore throat. If caused by a streptococcal
bacteria and inadequately treated, peritonsillar abscess, scarlet
fever, rheumatic fever, or rheumatic heart disease may result.

Pharyngitis
Viral, bacterial, or fungal
infection of the pharynx,
leading to a sore throat

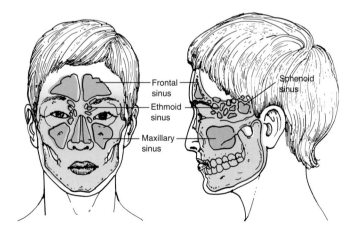

Figure 18.1. The frontal and ethmoid sinuses are more commonly involved in sinusitis.

Pharyngitis, if inadequately treated, can lead to peritonsillar abscess, scarlet fever, rheumatic fever, or rheumatic heart disease

Signs and symptoms include throat pain aggravated by swallowing that may radiate into the ears. The throat typically appears dark red and the tonsils appear red and swollen, and a pussy discharge may be visible. Other symptoms include rhinorrhea, swollen lymph glands, hoarseness, headache, cough, a low-grade fever, and malaise.

Treatment for streptococcal pharyngitis includes a 10-day administration of oral penicillin or erythromycin, or a single injection of benzathine penicillin (5). In cases not involving streptococcal pharyngitis, treatment involves bed rest, plenty of fluids, warm saline gargles, throat lozenges, and mild analgesics (aspirin, Advil, Ibuprofen).

Influenza

Influenza
Acute infectious respiratory tract condition characterized by malaise, headache, dry cough, and general muscle aches

Influenza, or "flu," is a specific viral bronchitis caused by *Haemophilus influenzae* type A, B, or C. It often occurs in epidemic proportions, particularly in school-age children. Immunization for the influenzae types A and B viruses is available for individuals at high risk, including pregnant women, individuals with chronic illness, such as diabetes mellitus and disorders of the pulmonary or cardiovascular system, children, and individuals with immunocompromised systems. Individuals with a fever should not be immunized until the fever has passed.

Influenza immunization should be administered to pregnant women, individuals with chronic illness, children, and individuals with immunocompromised systems

Signs and symptoms of influenza include a fever of 39 to 39.5°C (102 to 103°F), chills, malaise, headache, general muscle aches, a hacking cough, and inflamed mucosal membranes. Rapid onset of symptoms can occur within 24 to 48 hours after exposure to the virus. Sore throat, watery eyes, sensitivity to light (photophobia), and a nonproductive cough may linger up to 5 days. The cough may progress into bronchitis. Treatment consists of rest, plenty of fluids, saltwater gargles, cough medication, and analgesics (aspirin, Advil, Ibuprofen) to control fever, aches, and pains.

With influenza, a sore throat, watery eyes, photophobia, and a nonproductive cough may linger up to 5 days, with the cough progressing into bronchitis

Allergic Rhinitis (Hay Fever)

Rhinitis
Inflammation of the nasal membranes, with excessive mucus production resulting in nasal congestion and postnasal drip

Allergic **rhinitis** is a common upper respiratory tract condition affecting nearly 20% of all children and adults in the United States. It is often divided into seasonal allergic rhinitis, or "hay fever," and perennial allergic rhinitis. **Hay fever** usually involves a specific period of symptoms in successive years caused by airborne pollens and/or fungus spores associated with that season. In contrast, perennial allergic rhinitis occurs year-round if continually exposed to allergens, such as food allergens (e.g., shellfish, bread mold), dust, and animal emanations (e.g., cat hair, feathers).

Hay fever
Seasonal allergic rhinitis caused by airborne pollens and/or fungus spores

Postnasal drainage leads to a chronic sore throat and bronchial infection. In addition, the pharyngeal openings of the eustachian tubes can become blocked by swollen mucosa, enlarged lymphoid tissue, or exudate. Without normal air flow, increasing negative pressure in the middle ear results in fluid accumulation and chronic serous otitis, leading to a partial hearing loss and recurrent middle ear infections (6).

Management involves reducing exposure to the allergen or irritant, suppressive medication to alleviate symptom severity, and specific hypersensitization to reduce responsiveness to unavoidable allergens. Antihistamine drugs have been effective in reducing symptoms; however, in competitive athletes, drowsiness, lethargy, mucous membrane dryness, and occasional nausea and light-headedness may be unwanted side effects.

In children, the eustachian tubes can become blocked by swollen mucosa or exudate, leading to serous otitis, a partial hearing loss, or recurrent middle ear infections

Acute Bronchitis

Bronchitis is inflammation of the mucosal lining of the tracheobronchial tree resulting from infection or inhalants, and may be acute or chronic. Acute bronchitis, commonly seen in athletes, involves bronchial swelling, mucus secretion, and increased resistance to expiration. Coughing, wheezing, and large amounts of purulent mucus will be present (7). Once the stimulus is removed, the swelling decreases and airways return to normal.

Bronchitis
Inflammation of the mucosal lining of the tracheobronchial tree characterized by bronchial swelling, mucus secretions, and dysfunction of the cilia

With bronchitis, coughing, wheezing, and large amounts of purulent mucus are present

Infectious Mononucleosis

The Epstein-Barr virus (EBV) in the Herpes family is known to cause **infectious mononucleosis**, an acute viral disease manifested by a general feeling of malaise and fatigue. Infectious rates are found highest in individuals between 15 to 25 years of age, with 25 to 50% of these developing classic symptoms (8). The incubation period is 30 to 50 days, with peak incidence in females at age 16 and in males at age 18 (9). Signs and symptoms within the first 3 to 5 days include headache, fatigue, loss of appetite, malaise, and muscular aches and pains. Within 2 weeks, a sore throat, enlarged tonsils, fever, enlarged lymph nodes, swollen eyelids, spots on the palate, and, in 90% of patients, inflammation of the liver may be present. In addition, an enlarged spleen can be palpated and, in 10 to 15% of infections, jaundice and a rubella-like rash are present (9).

Individuals with mononucleosis should not participate in contact or collision sports in which trauma could rupture the enlarged vulnerable spleen. Splenic rupture usually occurs between 2 to 4 weeks of illness, when the splenic capsule is heavily infiltrated with lymphocytes (9). Most individuals with mononucleosis will recover uneventfully. Anti-inflammatory medication may be used to control headaches, fever, and general muscle aches and pain. Lozenges, saltwater gargles, and viscous lidocaine (Xylocaine) can ease throat pain. The decision to return to sport participation will rest with the supervising physician. Recent recommendations for return to contact sports range from 3 weeks to 3 months (9).

Infectious mononucleosis
Viral condition caused by the Epstein-Barr virus that attacks the respiratory system and leaves the spleen enlarged and weak

Advanced signs and symptoms of mononucleosis include severe sore throat, fever, swollen eyelids, abnormal liver chemistries, and enlarged lymph nodes, tonsils, and spleen

Asthma
Lung disease characterized by bronchospasm, increased bronchial secretions, and mucosa swelling, all leading to airway narrowing and inadequate airflow during respiration

Bronchial Asthma

Asthma is caused by a constriction of bronchial smooth muscles (**bronchospasm**), increased bronchial secretions, and mucosa swelling, all leading to an inadequate airflow during respiration

Bronchospasm
Contraction of the smooth muscles of the bronchial tubes, causing narrowing of the airway

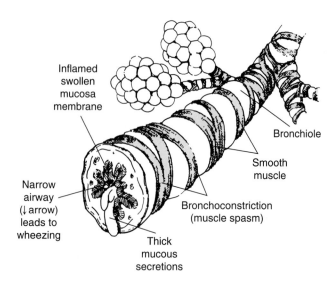

Figure 18.2. An asthma attack is due to bronchospasm that constricts the bronchiole tubes. This spasm, combined with increased bronchial secretions and mucosa swelling, results in a characteristic loud wheezing sound heard during expiration.

(especially expiration) **(Fig. 18.2)**. Wheezing is a common sign and results from air squeezing past the narrowed airways. Because the airways cannot fill or empty adequately, the diaphragm tends to flatten and the accessory muscles must work harder to enlarge the chest during inspiration. This increased workload leads to a rapid onset of fatigue when the individual can no longer hyperventilate enough to meet the increased oxygen need. Acute attacks may occur spontaneously, but are often provoked by a viral infection.

A large amount of thick yellow or green sputum is produced by the bronchial mucosa. As dyspnea (difficult breathing) continues, anxiety, panic, loud wheezing, sweating, rapid heart rate, and laboring to breathe are apparent. Individuals diagnosed with asthma typically carry medication delivered by a compressor-driven nebulizer or inhaler to alleviate the attack. The value of bronchodilators in children and young adults continues to be debated. Medications involve selective beta$_2$-agonists (albuterol, pirbuterol, terbutaline, and bitolterol); aerosol corticosteroids (budesonide, beclomethasne); or cromolyn sodium, an antiasthmatic drug that prevents the release of chemical mediators that cause bronchospasm and mucous membrane inflammatory changes (10,11). Once the attack has subsided, the lungs usually return to normal.

Exercise-induced Asthma

Exercise-induced asthma (EIA) affects up to 90% of asthmatics, developing shortly after 6 to 8 minutes of strenuous exercise between 65 and 85% of maximum workload (12). Factors contributing to the severity of EIA include ambient air conditions (cold air, low humidity, pollutants), duration, type, and intensity of exercise, exposure to allergen in sensitized individuals, overall control of asthma, poor physical conditioning, respiratory infections, time since the last episode of EIA, and any underlying bronchial hyperreactivity (13). Despite its prevalence, the precise mechanisms responsible for EIA are still unknown. It is thought that breathing dry, cold air through the mouth stimulates bronchospasm. Thus, breathing through the nose to warm and humidify air, or swimming in an indoor pool, may prevent the onset of symptoms. In addition, the use of a bronchodilator 15 minutes prior to activity can delay symptoms for 2 to 4 hours.

> EIA develops shortly after 6 to 8 minutes of strenuous exercise working between 65 and 85% of maximum workload

Signs and symptoms of EIA include chest pain, chest tightness, or a burning sensation with or without wheezing, a dry cough, lack of energy, and shortness of breath shortly after or during exercise. Medications include those used in regular asthma treatment, including beta$_2$-agonists, cromolyn sodium, and oral theophylline; however, athletes should check with the appropriate governing sport body to ensure the medication is legal for competition (13).

> Signs and symptoms of EIA include chest tightness or a burning sensation, wheezing, coughing, and shortness of breath shortly after or during exercise

Asthmatics who are physically fit and free of significant airway obstruction respond to exercise similar to nonasthmatic individuals. Activities such as tennis, running, and football are well-tolerated, provided exercise includes pre-exercise warm-up and postexercise warm-down, and repetitive bouts of exercise (less than 5 minutes) are performed no less than 40 minutes apart (12). **Field Strategy 18.2** summarizes exercise strategies for individuals with asthma.

The asthmatic individual should be seen by a physician before starting an exercise program. In general, the program can include a 5 to 10 minute warm-up of moderate stretching and 10

Field Strategy 8.2. Exercise Strategies for Exercise-induced Asthma

Before beginning an exercise program, consult a physician
Take medications for asthma as prescribed
Use a bronchodilator 15 minutes prior to exercise
Perform a 5 to 10 minute warm-up of moderate stretching before vigorous exercise
Work out slowly for the first 10 to 15 minutes, keeping the pulse rate below 140 beats per minute
Do continuous and rhythmic exercise for 20 to 30 minutes at least three times a week at 70 to 80% of maximum heart rate
Increase the time and intensity of the workout as tolerated
Breathe slowly through the nose to warm and humidify the air or exercise in a warm, humid environment
Avoid exposure to air pollutants and allergens whenever possible
Do a graduated 10 to 30 minute warm-down (or cool-down) after a vigorous workout to avoid rapid thermal changes in the airways

to 15 minutes of low-intensity exercise, keeping the pulse below 140 beats/minute. This can be followed by repetitive intensive exercise for less than 5 minutes performed 40 minutes apart, with a 10 to 30 minute cool-down. Use of a bronchodilator 15 minutes prior to exercise can also be used to delay symptoms for 2 to 4 hours.

THE GASTROINTESTINAL TRACT

? *A male distance runner has reported the consistent need to stop and have a bowel movement while training. Is this normal for runners? What can be done about it?*

The gastrointestinal tract extends from the mouth to the anus. Often nervous tension produces indigestion, diarrhea, or constipation that can adversely affect sport participation. Many seemingly minor disorders, however, can be the first sign of more serious underlying conditions. If symptoms persist with any disorder, referral to a physician is warranted.

Gastroenteritis

Gastroenteritis
Inflammation of the mucous membrane of the stomach and/or small intestine

Gastroenteritis is an inflammation of the mucous membrane of the stomach or small intestine. The condition may be caused by viruses, bacteria, allergic reactions, medications, ingested contaminated food (food poisoning), or emotional stress. In mild cases, increased secretion of hydrochloric acid in the stomach may lead to indigestion (dyspepsia), nausea, flatulence (gas), and a sour stomach. In moderate to severe cases, abdominal cramping, diarrhea, fever, and vomiting can lead to fluid and electrolyte imbalance. The condition usually clears up in 2 to 3 days. Treatment is symptomatic and includes eliminating irritating foods from the diet, avoiding factors that bring on anxiety and stress, and avoiding dehydration by drinking clear fluids or electrolyte-containing fluids.

Diarrhea

Diarrhea
Loose or watery stools resulting when food residue rushes through the large intestine before there is sufficient time to absorb the remaining water

Diarrhea is a common and troublesome disorder, particularly among runners, characterized by abnormally loose, watery stools. This is due to food residue rushing through the large intestine before that organ has had sufficient time to absorb the remaining water. Prolonged diarrhea can lead to dehydration and depletion of electrolytes, particularly sodium, bicarbonate, and potassium. Diarrhea may respond to Peptobismol, loperamide (Imodium), or diphenoxylate with atropine (Lomotil); however, these should not be used on a regular basis. Eliminating foods that trigger bowel irritation, including lactose intolerance, and improving hydration before and during exercise may increase plasma volume to decrease intestinal mucosal ischemia. Eating a low-fiber diet 24 to 36 hours prior to competition may also help. An attempt should be made to defecate at a regular daily time, taking advantage of the morning gastrocolic reflex. Peristalsis and defecation can be stimulated by drinking coffee or tea, or performing a light workout in the morning.

Constipation

Constipation is described as infrequent or incomplete bowel movements and is not a disease but rather a description of symptoms that may indicate more serious underlying conditions. Identifiable causes range from lack of fiber in the diet, improper bowel habits, lack of exercise, emotional distress, diabetes mellitus, pregnancy, or laxative abuse. It can also be drug-induced (diuretics, bile acid binders, drugs that lower serum cholesterol, and analgesics that slow bowel transit) (14).

Management of constipation depends on the origin. In most cases, eating high-fiber foods, such as cereals, vegetables, and grains, increasing daily exercise, particularly aerobic exercise, and adequate fluid intake can alleviate symptoms. Laxatives or suppositories are useful, but should be used sparingly.

The runner's condition is not unusual. Find out if there is a history of irregular bowel function, eating prior to running, or running before breakfast. A high-fiber diet, an increase in daily exercise and fluid intake, and over-the-counter medication may be recommended. If the condition continues, the individual should see a physician to rule out other conditions.

THE DIABETIC ATHLETE

A diabetic basketball player is halfway through a practice session when suddenly the player begins to feel weak and faint. The skin appears pale and moist and respirations are shallow. What may be occurring and how will you manage this athlete?

Diabetes mellitus is a chronic systemic disorder characterized by near or absolute lack of the hormone insulin, insulin resistance, or both. Insulin, secreted by the pancreas, is needed to transfer glucose from the blood, after carbohydrate ingestion, into the skeletal and cardiac muscles. In addition, insulin promotes glucose storage in muscles and the liver in the form of glycogen (see **Fig. 18.3**).

Diabetes mellitus is divided into two classes: Type I or insulin-dependent diabetes, and Type II or non-insulin-dependent diabetes **(Table 18.1)**. Type I has an onset prior to age 30 in people who are not typically obese and is associated with an absolute deficiency of insulin. Individuals generally have a more severe abnormal glucose homeostasis, the effects of exercise on the metabolic state are more pronounced, and the management of exercise-related problems are more difficult (15). Only 10% of these individuals have a family history of diabetes. Type II has an onset after age 30, with nearly 70 to 80% of affected people obese (16). This type is associated with significant resistance to insulin's actions, an abnormal but relatively well-maintained insulin secre-

Constipation
Infrequent or incomplete bowel movements

Diabetes
Metabolic disorder characterized by near or absolute lack of the hormone insulin, or insulin-resistance, or both

Insulin is needed to transfer glucose from the blood after carbohydrate ingestion into skeletal and cardiac muscles, and promotes glucose storage in muscles and the liver in the form of glycogen

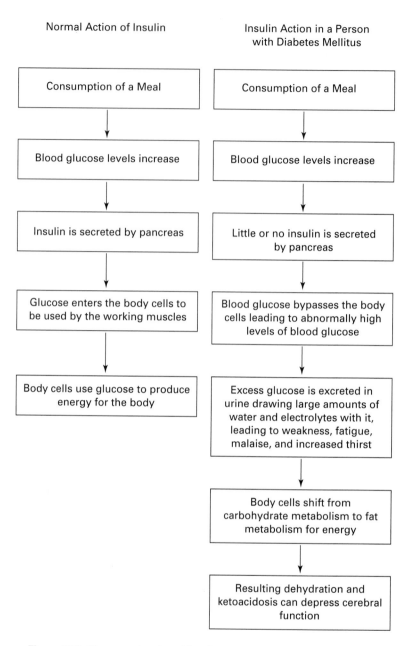

Figure 18.3. The normal action of insulin as compared to insulin action in a person with diabetes mellitus.

Type I diabetes has onset prior to age 30 in people who are not typically obese. Type II has onset after age 30, with nearly 70 to 80% of affected people obese

tion, and normal to elevated plasma insulin levels (15). Oral gliclazide used alone or in combination with insulin has had positive results in treating Type II diabetes (17). Several factors increase the frequency and severity of diabetes, including heredity, increasing age, obesity, being female, stress, infection, and a diet high in carbohydrates and fat.

Table 18.1. Comparison of Type I and Type II Diabetes

	Type I	Type II
Age of onset	Usually before 30	Usually after 30
Type of onset	Abrupt (days to weeks)	Usually gradual (weeks to months)
Nutritional status	Almost always lean	Usually obese
Insulin production	Negligible to absent	Present, but may be excessive and ineffective due to obesity
Insulin	Needed for all patients	Necessary in 20 to 30% of patients
Diet	Mandatory along with insulin for control of blood glucose	Diet alone is usually sufficient to control glucose
Family history	Minor	Common link

In diabetes, lack of insulin or insulin resistance leads to **hyperglycemia**. In essence, adequate amounts of glucose levels in the blood fail to enter the cells, causing blood glucose levels to increase to abnormally high levels. Increased osmotic blood pressure drives fluid from the cells into the vascular system, leading to cell dehydration. The excess glucose is passed into the kidneys and excreted in urine, drawing large amounts of water and electrolytes. An electrolyte imbalance leads to weakness, fatigue, malaise, and increased thirst. In response, the body shifts from carbohydrate metabolism to fat metabolism for energy. This produces an excess of ketoacids and results in acidosis. Acetone, formed as a by-product of fat metabolism, is volatile and blown off during expiration, giving the breath a sweet or fruity odor. If the condition is not rectified with insulin injection, further dehydration and ketoacidosis can depress brain function. The individual becomes confused, drowsy, and may lapse into a diabetic coma and die.

Controlled diabetes rests on a balance of glucose levels, insulin production, diet, and exercise. Alterations in this equilibrium can lead to two separate conditions: diabetic coma and insulin shock.

Hyperglycemia
Abnormally high levels of glucose in the circulating blood that can lead to diabetic coma

Acetone, formed as a by-product of fat metabolism, is volatile and blown off during expiration, giving the breath a sweet or fruity odor

Diabetic Coma

Without insulin, the body is unable to metabolize glucose, leading to hyperglycemia in the blood. The symptoms appear gradually and can occur over several days. The individual will often become increasingly restless, confused, and complain of dry mouth and intense thirst. Abdominal cramping and vomiting are common. As the individual slips into a coma, signs include dry, warm skin; eyes that appear sunken and deep; sighing respirations; a rapid, weak pulse; and a sweet acetone breath, similar to nail polish remover (18).

If in doubt, give sugar to the individual. The additional glucose will not worsen the condition, provided they are transported immediately

As the name implies, coma is a serious condition and is considered a medical emergency. If unsure of the condition and unable to determine if the individual is in insulin shock or a diabetic coma, give the individual glucose or glucose in orange juice. If recovery is not rapid, then a medical emergency exits and EMS should be summoned. The additional glucose will not worsen the condition, provided the individual is transported immediately.

Insulin Shock

Hypoglycemia
Abnormally low levels of glucose in the circulating blood that can lead to insulin shock

Exercise lowers blood sugar, hence, any exercise must be counterbalanced with increased food intake or decreased amounts of insulin. If blood glucose falls below normal levels, **hypoglycemia**, or insulin shock, results. Contrary to the slow onset of a diabetic coma, the signs and symptoms of hypoglycemia have a rapid onset and include dizziness; aggressive behavior; intense hunger; fainting; pale, cold, and clammy skin; and profuse perspiration, salivation, and drooling.

The signs and symptoms of insulin shock have a rapid onset and include dizziness; aggressive behavior; intense hunger; fainting; pale, cold, and clammy skin; and profuse perspiration, salivation, and drooling

Since glucose levels in the blood are low compared to high levels of insulin, treatment includes getting sugar into the system quickly. Use table sugar (sucrose), honey, sugared candy, orange juice or soda (only in a conscious person). Do not use a sugar substitute or diet soda, as artificial sweeteners will not help the individual (18). Place sugar or honey under the tongue in an unconscious person, as it will be absorbed through the mucosal membrane. Recovery is usually rapid; however, even when blood glucose has returned to normal, physical performance and judgement may still be impaired. **Field Strategy 18.3** compares the two conditions and provides additional information on the cause, signs and symptoms, and management of the condition.

Exercise and Diabetes

Aerobic low-resistance exercise can be a positive and rewarding experience for the diabetic athlete, provided certain precautions are followed

Prior to any exercise program, a physician should be consulted and normal blood glucose (BG) levels documented, as strenuous exercise is contraindicated for some diabetics. With the advent of blood glucose self-monitoring, however, exercise is encouraged if certain precautions are followed. Blood glucose levels should be taken before and after exercise. The diabetic athlete should eat a well-balanced diet of 55% to 65% complex carbohydrate, 20% fat, and less than 15% protein (19). A pregame meal should be ingested 1 to 3 hours prior to exercise and 15 to 30 grams of carbohydrates should be eaten every 30 minutes during intense exercise. A snack of carbohydrates should also follow the exercise period. To ensure adequate hydration during prolonged exercise, the athlete should drink an additional glass of fluid after he or she no longer feels thirsty. Emphasis should be placed on aerobic low-resistance activities, such as walking, jogging, cycling, or swimming. Gradual exercise over several weeks should precede any competitive sport participation. This allows better regulation of food intake and insulin dosage.

Field Strategy 18.3. Management of Diabetic Emergencies

Insulin Shock	Diabetic Coma
Causes	**Causes**
Too much insulin has been taken or not enough food was eaten to provide adequate sugar intake	Insulin was not taken or too much food was eaten, flooding the blood with glucose
The individual may have overexercised, reducing blood glucose levels, or vomited a meal	
Signs and Symptoms	**Signs and Symptoms**
Rapid onset of symptoms	Gradual onset of symptoms
Dizziness, headache, intense hunger	Dry mouth and intense thirst
Hostile or aggressive behavior	Abdominal pain and vomiting
Normal blood pressure and respirations	Confusion followed by stupor
Full, bounding pulse	Fever is common
Pale, cold, clammy skin with profuse sweating	Coma with these signs:
Fainting or convulsions	Deep, exaggerated respirations
Severe salivation and drooling	Rapid, weak pulse
	Dry, red, warm skin
	Eyes that appear sunken
	Slightly lower blood pressure
	Sweet, fruity acetone breath
Management	**Management**
Look for a medical alert tag	*Look for a medical alert tag*
In a conscious person:	Administer sugar. If no response, summon EMS and transport immediately to the nearest hospital
Administer sugar, honey, a lifesaver, or other sugared candy under the tongue, or have them drink orange juice or a soda	
In an unconscious person:	
Do not give liquids	
Place sugar under the tongue	
Transport to the nearest hospital	

The diabetic basketball player suddenly felt weak and faint. The skin was pale, moist, and respirations were shallow. If you determined possible insulin shock, you are correct. Get the player to the sideline and provide a source of sugar, such as a candy bar, orange juice, or sugared candy. If the condition does not rapidly improve, summon EMS.

EPILEPSY

During warm-up, a softball player suddenly gets a glassy stare on the face, begins to smack the lips, and walks aimlessly around the field as if intoxicated. What condition might this individual have? How will you manage the situation?

Epilepsy is a brain disorder characterized by recurrent episodes of sudden, excessive discharges of electrical activity in the

Epilepsy
Disorder of the brain characterized by recurrent episodes of sudden, excessive discharges of electrical activity

brain. The discharge may trigger altered sensation, perceptions, behavior, mood, level of consciousness, or convulsive movements. There are three recognizable types of epileptic seizures: absence attacks (petit mal), complex partial seizures (psychomotor), and tonic-clonic seizures (grand mal).

Absence attacks are characterized by blank staring into space for 5 to 10 seconds. Slight twitching of the facial muscles or fluttering of the eyelids may occur. Onset is usually about age 5, with attacks most prevalent in childhood. Complex partial seizures are characterized by disorientation; loss of contact with reality; uncontrolled motor activity in isolated muscle groups, such as hand clapping or lip smacking; or walking about aimlessly. The average seizure is 1 to 5 minutes, and may be followed by disorientation. Tonic-clonic seizures are the most severe form of epilepsy. Many individuals experience a sensory phenomenon, such as a particular taste, smell, or aura, prior to the seizure. The person loses consciousness and displays intense convulsions, either clonic or tonic. A **clonic state** is movement marked by repetitive muscle contractions and relaxation in rapid succession. A **tonic state** involves steady, rigid muscle contractions with no relaxation. Loss of bowel and bladder control is common and severe biting of the tongue may occur, although this is relatively uncommon. The average seizure lasts from 50 to 90 seconds, then muscles relax and the person awakens, but may not remember what happened (20).

Management of any seizure is directed toward protecting the individual from self-injury. Nearby objects should be removed so the individual does not strike them during uncontrollable muscle contractions. Protect the individual's head at all times, but do not stop or restrain the person, or place any object into the mouth. Wait until the seizure has come to an end and ensure an adequate airway. **Field Strategy 18.4** summarizes the management of a seizure.

In nearly all instances, epilepsy can be controlled with proper medication. Participation in sports, particularly those with a danger of falling, contact sports, and water sports, should be carefully evaluated with a neurologist prior to participation. Individuals who experience frequent seizures should choose activities accordingly.

The softball player is probably having a complex partial seizure. Do not stop or restrain the person, but help her lie down and place something soft under the head. Clear the other ball players away from the area. The person may be confused or disoriented after the seizure. If this is her first seizure, refer the individual to a physician.

Clonic state
Movement marked by repetitive muscle contractions and relaxations in rapid succession

Tonic state
Steady, rigid muscle contractions with no relaxation

Protect the individual's head at all times, but do not stop or restrain the person, or place any object into the mouth

HYPERTENSION

During the preparticipation exam, a gymnast learned that her blood pressure was very high. What implications will this have on her participation?

Field Strategy 18.4. Management of an Epileptic Seizure

During the Seizure

Remove harmful objects near the person
Do not stop or restrain the person
Help the individual lie down and place something soft under the head
Remove glasses and loosen tight clothing
Do not place your fingers or any other object into the mouth

After the Seizure

Ensure an adequate airway
Turn the individual to one side to allow saliva to drain from the mouth
Protect the person from curious bystanders
Do not leave the person until the individual is fully awake
If this is a first-time seizure, the individual should be seen by a physician
If seizure activity is continuous or if another attack occurs in rapid
  succession, the individual should be transported to the nearest medical
  facility by ambulance
If transported:
  A written description of the type of seizure activity should be sent with
  the individual. Include whether it was generalized or localized, how it
  started, the length of time from the moment of onset until the individual
  regained consciousness, and the number of seizures experienced by the
  individual

Hypertension is defined as sustained elevated blood pressure above the accepted norms of 140 mm Hg systolic or 90 mm Hg diastolic. The onset is generally between ages 20 and 50, with the frequency greater in African Americans. Certain prescribed medications, anabolic steroids, amphetamines, oral contraceptives, chronic alcohol or tobacco use, nasal decongestants containing sympathomimetic amines, and some non-steroidal anti-inflammatory drugs (NSAIDs) may elevate blood pressure (21). Longstanding hypertension often attacks the heart, brain, kidneys, and eyes. Any individual who has mild or moderate hypertension should not participate in competitive sports until cleared by a physician.

Aerobic-type exercises have been shown to modestly reduce high blood pressure. Twenty to thirty minutes of aerobic exercise at 60 to 85% of maximum heart rate, 3 to 4 times a week, is recommended. Daily walking at a moderate speed is excellent; however, isometric exercises and heavy-resistance training should be avoided. In more serious cases, sodium and alcohol restrictions, weight loss, reduction of other cardiovascular risk factors, and other medications are used to manage the condition.

The gymnast should see the physician to determine the degree of severity. A supervised exercise program may include sodium restrictions, weight control, and possible medications. The individual should not participate in activity until cleared by the physician.

Hypertension
Sustained elevated blood pressure above the norms of 140 mm Hg systolic or 90 mm Hg diastolic

Twenty to thirty minutes of aerobic exercise at 60 to 85% maximum heart rate, 3 to 4 times a week, has been shown to reduce high blood pressure

ANEMIA

❓ *A 15-year-old female volleyball player is complaining of chronic fatigue and malaise, particularly during practice. She appears somewhat pale and tired, but otherwise is fine. While taking her history, she reports that she tends to have a heavy menstrual flow. What condition might you suspect?*

A reduction in either the red blood cell volume (hematocrit) or hemoglobin concentration is called **anemia**. Although there are several classifications of anemia, all are caused by either impaired red blood cell (RBC) formation or excessive loss or destruction of RBCs. A family history of anemia, past history of anemia, inadequate iron intake, heavy menstrual loss or gastrointestinal bleeding, oral contraceptive use, impaired iron absorption, and iron losses in urine and sweat are all risk factors for developing the disorder (22). In sport participation, anemia reduces maximum aerobic capacity and anaerobic threshold, which decreases physical work capacity, increases lactic acidosis, and increases fatigue. Two common types of anemia occur in sport participants.

Iron-deficiency Anemia

The most common cause of anemia in the world is iron-deficiency, characterized by deficient hemoglobin synthesis. This condition is more common in female athletes than in male athletes, with as many as 90% of elite women athletes having an inadequate intake of dietary iron. In infancy and early childhood, inadequate diet may be an underlying factor; in older children and adults, blood loss or impaired absorption of iron should be suspected (22). Iron-deficiency anemia is prevalent in women of childbearing age, secondary to menstrual losses, and is seen in endurance athletes and in those who maintain a lower percent body fat.

Clinical manifestations of iron deficiency are rare unless anemia is severe. Signs and symptoms include exercise fatigue, muscle burning, nausea, dyspnea, blood mixed with feces, and pallor (22). Later symptoms include tachycardia, cardiac murmurs, congestive heart failure, loss of hair, and pearly sclera. Treatment may involve dietary iron supplementation and ascorbic acid (Vitamin C) on an empty stomach to enhance iron absorption. Foods high in iron content include red meat, turkey and chicken (dark meat), liver, lima beans, shellfish, and green vegetables. Avoid colas, coffee, or tea, as caffeine hampers iron absorption.

Sickle Cell Anemia

Sickle cell anemia, more commonly seen in African Americans, results from abnormalities in hemoglobin structure that produce a characteristic sickle- or crescent-shaped red blood cell that is fragile and unable to transport oxygen. Because of its rigidity and irregular shape, sickle cells clump together and block small blood

---

Anemia
Abnormal reduction in red blood cell volume or hemoglobin concentration

---

Individuals at risk for anemia include those who have a family history of anemia, a past history of anemia, intermittent jaundice early in life, and chronic blood loss through heavy menstruation or gastrointestinal bleeding

---

Iron-deficiency anemia is commonly seen in women of childbearing age secondary to menstrual losses, pregnant women, endurance athletes, and athletes maintaining a lower percent body fat

---

Sickle cell anemia
Abnormalities in hemoglobin structure resulting in a characteristic sickle- or cresent-shaped red blood cell that is fragile and unable to transport oxygen

vessels, leading to vascular occlusion, or **infarcts**, in organs such as the heart, lungs, kidneys, spleen, and central nervous system. Although an individual with the sickle cell trait may be asymptomatic for their entire life, exercising in excessively high heat, humidity, and/or altitude may lead to dehydration, predisposing an individual to increased protein in the circulating blood cells. This high concentration increases blood viscosity and impairs blood flow, which can lead to a stroke, congestive heart failure, acute renal failure, pulmonary embolism, or sudden death (23).

Signs and symptoms include swollen, painful, and inflamed hands and feet, irregular heart beats, severe fatigue, headache, skin pallor, and muscle weakness, or severe pain due to oxygen deprivation. Currently, there is no known treatment to reverse the condition. Since dehydration can complicate the condition, individuals should hydrate maximally before, during, and after exertion. Liquids with caffeine, such as colas, coffee, and tea, should be avoided because of their potential diuretic effect. Individuals with sickle cell trait should limit running to no more than one-half mile without rest, and should avoid activity in extremely hot, humid weather, and at altitudes greater than 2500 ft (23).

💡 *The volleyball player may have iron-deficiency anemia. Her age, activity level, and heavy menstrual flow are all factors that put her at risk for the condition. Refer her to a physician to rule out other underlying conditions.*

SUBSTANCE ABUSE

❓ *An 18-year-old football player returned from summer vacation 30 pounds heavier and able to bench press 50 additional pounds. He reported he was on an aggressive weight training program over the summer, but you question how these gains were made in such a short time. What implications might this have on his health and performance?*

Drugs are divided into three types: (1) therapeutic drugs—those taken to manage an injury or illness; (2) performance-enhancing drugs—those used to enhance one's athletic performance; and (3) recreational drugs—those taken to alter one's mood (for entertainment or to escape reality). These are not exclusive categories, as some therapeutic and performance enhancing drugs may be used recreationally to alter one's mood. Drugs sold over-the-counter, or nonprescription drugs, are designed to relieve pain and inflammation. Prescription drugs are designed to relieve symptoms and cure a disease or condition. In most cases, the coach or athletic trainer will only be concerned with nonprescription medication; however, extreme caution must be exercised with all medications.

Therapeutic Drugs

Therapeutic drugs are used to treat an injury or illness and, depending on the dosage, may be prescribed or over-the-counter

Infarcts
Clumping together of cells that block small blood vessels, leading to vascular occlusion, ischemia, and necrosis in organs

Drugs are divided into three types: therapeutic, performance-enhancing, and recreational

Therapeutic drugs
Prescription or over-the-counter medications used to treat an injury or illness

medications. Prescribed medications include NSAIDs, major pain relievers, diuretics, beta-agonists, corticosteroids, barbiturates or tranquilizers, amphetamines, and oral contraceptives. Over-the-counter medications include analgesics, decongestants and antihistamines, laxatives and antidiarrheal agents, and weight-loss medications (24). The use and side effects of the more common therapeutic drugs are listed in **Table 18.2**.

Performance-enhancing Drugs

Performance-enhancing drugs include anabolic-androgen steroids (AAS); growth hormones; stimulants, including some amphetamines, caffeine, nicotine, and beta-sympathomimetics; erythropoietin (EPO); and beta-blockers (24). The use and side effects of the more common performance-enhancing drugs are listed in **Table 18.3**. There is little to no research proving food supplements, such as amino acids, protein or carbohydrate powders, herbs, vitamins, and minerals, enhance performance; therefore, they will not be discussed. Reported side effects of food supplements include stomach pain, nausea, dizziness, vomiting, diarrhea, and cardiovascular problems (25).

> Research has not proven that food supplements enhance performance

Recreational Drugs

Recreational drugs are nonprescription drugs used for mood-altering purposes. Alcohol is the major drug abused in the United States and falls within this category. Tobacco, nicotine, and illegal drugs, such as marijuana/hashish, heroin, barbiturates, amphetamines, cocaine/crack, hallucinogens (LSD), and PCP (phencyclidine hydrochloride), also fall within this category (24). The use and side effects of the more common recreational drugs are listed in **Table 18.4**.

Signs of Substance Abuse

The coach, athletic trainer, and sport supervisor must be alert to the signs of possible drug abuse. It is imperative to intervene and get prompt professional help for the individual. Signs that indicate possible drug abuse are included in **Table 18.5**. Be prepared for the denial of use by the individual. This barrier, however, must be overcome if the individual is to seek help. It is best to document any suspicions by noting behavioral or physical changes in the individual prior to counseling them. If confronting the individual is uncomfortable, it may be best to discuss the situation first in confidentiality with a professional counselor. The counselor may then intervene to help the suspected user.

Drug Testing

Drug testing began at the 1968 Olympic Games and was adopted by the National Collegiate Athletic Association (NCAA) in 1986. The major goals of drug testing are to make competition fair and

Table 18.2. Therapeutic Drugs

Drug	Intended Use	Side/Adverse Effects
NSAIDs	Reduce inflammation, pain, & fever	Gastrointestinal bleeding, drowsiness, prolonged clotting time, dizziness, tinnitus, headaches
Diuretics	Control hypertension, reduce edema	Hyperglycemia, decreased sport performance, reduced blood volume, dehydration, electrolyte imbalance, muscle cramps
Beta-agonists	Asthma and bronchospasm	Dizziness; swelling of the face, lips, or eyelids; headache; tremors; tachycardia
Corticosteroids	Chronic inflammation and pain reduction	Gastrointestinal bleeding, nausea, retention, insomnia, hyperglycemia, depression
Barbiturates	Seizures, tremors, depression, and insomnia	Decreased attention span, slurred speech, blurred vision, drowsiness, dependence, addiction
Amphetamines	Narcolepsy and short-term appetite suppression	Insomnia, hyperactivity, headache, tremors, nausea, palpitations, constipation, and drug dependence
Oral contraceptives	Prevent unwanted pregnancies and osteopenia in amenorrheic athletes	Dizziness, migraine headaches, lethargy, hypertension, urinary tract infections, and dysmenorrhea
Analgesics	Reduce pain, inflammation, fever	Nausea, GI bleeding, prolonged clotting, tinnitus, diarrhea, renal failure, convulsions, death
Decongestants & antihistamines	Control upper respiratory tract infections, colds, allergies	Nervousness, dizziness, headaches, tachycardia, confusion, cerebral hemorrhage, stroke
Laxatives & antidiarrheal	Relieve or control constipation and diarrhea	Gas pains, pain with bowel movement, fluid and electrolyte imbalance, dry mouth, constipation
Weight-loss drugs	Control and lose weight	Hyperactivity, tremors, headache, nausea, constipation

equitable and safeguard the health of participants. Drug testing involves analyzing a urine sample with thin-layer chromatography (TLC) or gas-liquid chromatography (GLC) for the presence of performance-enhancing and illegal drugs. The athletic trainer should not be involved in the testing process, as it compromises their role as an impartial, unbiased health provider.

Institutions may have mandatory testing for all athletes—announced or random—or test only those athletes for whom reasonable suspicion is present. Drug-testing policies should be clearly documented and made available to all student athletes. Student athletes may be totally unaware of what drugs may be on the banned substance list until they have tested positive for their

Table 18.3. Performance-enhancing Drugs

Drug	Intended Use	Side/Adverse Effects
Anabolic/androgen steroids (AAS)	Increase lean body mass & strength	Acne, psychologic changes (increased aggression, mood swings, depression, delusions), changes in serum cholesterol and clotting factors, hypertension, risk of cardiovascular disease
Amphetamines	Treat narcolepsy, delay onset of fatigue, appetite suppression	Insomnia, headache, tremors, twitches, tachycardia, nausea, addiction
Erythropoietin (EPO)	Anemia and AIDS	Hypertension, tachycardia, headache, dehydration, pelvic and limb pain, death
Beta-blockers	Reduce tremors, hypertension, angina	Hypotension, nausea, impotence, diarrhea, constipation, insomnia

use. A positive test can result in ineligibility for an extended period of time. Further information on drugs and the athlete, and drug-testing, can be obtained from the NCAA, P.O. Box 1906, Mission, Kansas, 66201.

You suspect the football player used anabolic steroids over the summer to increase his size and strength. Did you determine you should talk to him about it? There is no set process. You

Table 18.4. Recreational Drugs

Drugs	Intended Use	Side/Adverse Effects
Alcohol	CNS depressant; mood altering to aid in socializing and escape from reality	Decreases alertness, reaction time, hand-eye coordination, accuracy, balance, judgement
Tobacco	No role in clinical medicine	Oral and lung cancer, cerebrovascular disease, chronic pulmonary disease; neoplasms in the respiratory and GI systems
Stimulants	Attention-deficit disorders, certain CNS diseases to overcome drowsiness	Increases pulse, respirations, and blood pressure; blurred vision, insomnia, headache, dry mouth
Sedatives	Seizure disorders	Sedation, slurred speech, impaired gait/balance, confusion, impaired memory, drug dependence
Marijuana	Bronchodilator, decrease intraocular pressure and muscle spasms, reduce side effects of chemotherapy	Tachycardia, impaired motor coordination, chest pains, short-term memory loss, immune system compromised, asthma, bronchitis, emphysema
Cocaine/crack	Used with epinephrine as topical anesthetic for nasal surgery	Myocardial infarction, cerebral infarction, addiction, seizures, blindness, liver toxicity, sudden death

Table 18.5. Signs of Possible Substance Abuse

Abrupt changes in attendance at school, practice, or place of
   employment
Deterioration in work performance and mood swings
Deterioration of physical condition, i.e., less stamina, dressing poorly,
   unclean or unkept
Overt protection of personal possessions
Wearing sunglasses in inappropriate weather or indoors
Wearing long-sleeved garments in inappropriate weather
Borrowing money often or stealing items that can be pawned or sold
   for money to pay for a drug habit
Social withdrawal from the usual circle of friends, or association with
   known drug users
Frequent trips to the bathroom, basement, bedroom
Blood-shot eyes, slurred speech, excessive acne, red raw nostrils, hair
   loss, visible needle marks
Dilated pupils (alcohol, marijuana, barbiturates). Constricted pupils
   (heroin and other narcotics)
Rapid weight gain or frequent complaints of "feeling sick"
Appears intoxicated or tends to fall asleep easily

*might want to show your concern about his health, discuss the
short- and long-term health consequences of using performance-
enhancing drugs, and let him know you are there to help.*

DISORDERED EATING

? *There are rumors that a swimmer was seen eating a large
amount of food, then disappeared to the restroom to vomit.
There is noticeable bilateral soft tissue swelling over the angle of
her mandible and calluses over the metacarpophalangeal (MCP)
joint of the middle finger. Her weight appears normal. Do these
rumors need to be addressed? Why or why not?*

Disordered eating habits have become more prevalent in both
competitive and recreational sport participants, particularly in the
young female athlete driven to excel. Although disordered eating
is often linked to sports that stress leanness, such as gymnastics,
distance running, swimming, diving, ballet, and wrestling, no sport
is exempt. The term *disordered eating* is preferred to the term
eating disorder, because of its emphasis on the spectrum of pathologic patterns of eating. Classification is defined by the strict *Diagnostic and Statistical Manual (DSM-IV)* criteria, of which there are
four specific categories: disordered eating not otherwise specified
(NOS), bulimia nervosa, anorexia nervosa, and combined disorders
of anorexia plus bulimia (26). Disordered eating patterns are typically associated with single, white, college-educated females from
middle- to upper-class families; however, more recent findings
indicate gender, race, and social class are becoming less of a
factor (27).

> Atypical eating patterns
> may be categorized as
> disordered eating not
> otherwise specified (NOS),
> bulimia nervosa, anorexia
> nervosa, or combined
> disorders of anorexia plus
> bulimia

Disordered Eating Not Otherwise Specified (NOS)

Many athletes have signs of disordered eating habits, but do not meet the criteria established for bulimia nervosa or anorexia nervosa. This person may have an average weight, does not have binge-eating episodes, but frequently engages in self-induced vomiting. In addition, the individual exhibits all of the features of anorexia nervosa in a female except the absence of menses, and all of the features of bulimia nervosa except the frequency of binge-eating episodes (26). Studies by the American College of Sports Medicine (ACSM) have shown the prevalence of atypical disordered eating among female athletes ranges from 15 to 62% of sport participants (27). Many of these individuals exhibit symptoms that indicate a disorder eating pattern, which can be seen in **Table 18.6**.

Bulimia Nervosa

People with bulimia tend to have a high need of approval, low self-esteem, emotional expressiveness, frustration tolerance, affective instability (depression, anger, anxiety), and tend to come from families with conflict resolution problems (26,28). They strive for thinness; however, this fear manifests itself in either a restrictive eating pattern or purging behavior. Weight fluctuations are common.

Table 18.6. Signs and Symptoms of Disordered Eating

Physical Features

Weight that is too low for athletic performance
Extreme fluctuations in weight
Swollen salivary glands or puffy cheeks
Amenorrhea
High incidence of stress fractures
Sores or callouses on the knuckles from inducing vomiting
Increased cavities with dental or gum disease
Gastrointestinal complaints (abdominal cramps, constipation, diarrhea)
Dehydration and electrolyte loss (headaches, dizziness, muscle weakness, or fatigue)
Loss or thinning of the hair, or downy hair appearing on the face, back or extremities

Psychological and Behavioral Symptoms

High need for approval
Low self-esteem and low frustration tolerance
Excessive dieting, weighing, guilt about eating, or excessive eating without weight gain
Obsessive about exercise and pursuit of thinness
Claiming to "feel fat" even though their weight may be normal
Evidence of self-induced vomiting
Use of drugs to attempt to control weight (abuse of laxatives, diet pills, diuretics, emetics)

Bulimia nervosa is defined as recurrent episodes of binge eating, with a minimum average of two binge-eating episodes a week for at least 3 months (26). The person with bulemia maintains a cyclical pattern of ingesting large quantities of food, usually greater than 5000 calories during a single eating episode, then fasting. Purging may or may not occur. Other symptoms include strict dieting, vigorous exercise to prevent weight gain, and obsession with body shape and weight (27). People with bulemia often lose their gag reflex and can purge without mechanical stimulation, or Ipecac may be used. Irregular menses is common, rather than amenorrhea, as seen in people with anorexia. Gastrointestinal complications from this behavior may include swollen parotid glands, abdominal cramps, bloating, esophagitis, possible esophageal perforation, pancreatitis, and constipation secondary to chronic laxative abuse (28,29).

The three most common physical signs associated with people with bulemia include:

1. Russell's sign, which is an elongated hyperpigmented lesion on the dorsum of the MCP joint of the hand caused by repetitive trauma to the area during self-induced vomiting
2. Hypertrophy of the salivary glands, particularly the parotid glands. The individual often has a "chipmunk"-like face
3. Dental erosion and increased cavities caused by acidic gastric secretions that decalcify the teeth during recurrent vomiting episodes

Anorexia Nervosa

Anorexia nervosa is defined as a refusal to maintain body weight over a minimal normal weight for age and height, with body weight being 15% below what is expected (26). The disorder is typically seen in females during adolescence. People with anorexia have a distorted body image and maintain a great fear of gaining weight, even though they are underweight. They view themselves as "fat," and equate body appearance with self-worth. An obsessive-compulsive nature for perfection and achievement leads many individuals to develop a highly ritualized exercise program for continuation over an entire day.

Amenorrhea often occurs prior to significant weight loss and continues for at least 3 consecutive months. Amenorrhea is related to bone mineral density loss and can lead to an increased incidence of stress fractures and osteoporosis. There is a desire to control the body and eating, and remain in a prepuberty state, resulting in a near-starvation behavior. Many complain of being cold even on hot days (hypothermia). Others suffer from severe constipation because of poor food intake.

Detection of anorexia is easier than bulimia nervosa because of the deteriorated physical state of the individual. Treatment for both conditions is dependent on the presence of a personality disorder. The multidisciplinary team of primary care physician,

Bulimia
Personality disorder manifested by episodic bouts of binging large amounts of food, followed by purging and feelings of guilt, self-disgust, and depression

Anorexia nervosa
Personality disorder manifested by extreme aversion toward food, resulting in extreme weight loss, amenorrhea, and other physical disorders

psychologist, and nutritionist must work closely together in treating these athletes. When recognized early, intervention counseling can help. Bulimia nervosa and anorexia nervosa may not be curable, but can be managed with a well-structured and supervised rehabilitation program. **Table 18.7** compares bulimia nervosa with anorexia nervosa and lists medical complications that can result from these eating disorders. In extreme cases of eating disorders, the mortality rate is 10 to 18% (27).

Exercise and Weight Management

Weight management is best achieved with a supervised program of exercise and food intake. Sport performance can be adversely affected by improper weight reduction. Rapid weight loss can dehydrate the body and deplete muscle glycogen stores. This can reduce blood volume, which in turn can adversely affect renal function, electrolyte balance, thermal regulation, and decrease strength, endurance, speed, and coordination (28). To lose weight,

Table 18.7. Comparison of Bulimia Nervosa and Anorexia Nervosa

Bulimia Nervosa	Anorexia Nervosa
Normal weight for age and height	Body weight 15% below what is normal
Irregular menses is common	Amenorrhea is common
Distorted body image	Intense fear of becoming "fat" even when emaciated
Low self-esteem, depression, and compulsive behavior is common	Low self-esteem is common; obsessed with perfection and achievement
Recurrent binge eating, followed by fasting	Near-starvation is commonly seen
Weight fluctuations are common	Weight diminishes steadily
Purging may or may not occur; laxatives, diuretics, and self-induced vomiting may be used	Purging is not common
	Depression, fear, anger, anxiety, and irritability

Complications of Eating Disorders

Related to Purging	Related to Weight Loss
Electrolyte disturbances due to decreased blood volume, metabolic alkalosis, and magnesium deficiency	Loss of fat and muscle mass, including heart muscle
Inflammation of the salivary glands and pancreas	Bloating, constipation, abdominal pain, nausea
Erosion of the esophagus and stomach, which can lead to severe GI bleeding	Amenorrhea
Erosion and decay of dental enamel and discoloration due to gastric juices	Osteopenia, osteonecrosis, and femoral head collapse
	Peripheral neuropathy
	Loss of scalp and pubic hair

one must increase activity or decrease food intake. The average American consumes 3300 calories a day, much more than is necessary for normal activity.

Weight loss should not exceed three pounds per week. Eating foods low in fat can significantly decrease caloric intake. In addition, fresh fruits, vegetables, water, and foods high in complex carbohydrates (potatoes, rice, and pasta) should provide the bulk of food intake. Competitive athletes should start weight reduction prior to the beginning of the competitive season so as not to affect sport performance.

Individuals who want to gain weight should consume extra servings at mealtime, preferably primarily carbohydrate with some protein, and eat frequent snacks that are low in fat. Good food choices include bagels, muffins, English muffins, pretzels, a turkey or lean beef sandwich, fresh fruit, chopped vegetables, soup (tomato, bean, or vegetable), yogurt, low-fat crackers, and popcorn (with little or no butter) (27). Weight gain of lean body mass may only increase one to two pounds per week. In addition to increasing dietary intake, the sport participant should continue to exercise and weight train. **Field Strategy 18.5** lists guidelines for safe weight loss and weight gain.

 Field Strategy 18.5. Guidelines for Safe Weight Loss and Weight Gain

One pound of body fat contains approximately 3500 calories

Moderate exercise for one-half hour, three times a week, burns over 1050 calories. Consequently, one need only reduce weekly caloric intake by 2450 calories to lose one pound per week. Exercise 5 days a week, coupled with reduced caloric intake (1200 to 1500 calories/day), would result in more weight loss. Weight reduction should not exceed 3 to 4 lbs/week in the off-season; 2 to 3 lbs/week during the season

Aerobic exercise, such as walking, running, rope-skipping, cycling, and swimming is excellent. Weight reduction without exercise causes a significant loss in muscle mass

Drink plenty of water and avoid caffeine

A well-balanced diet should include fresh fruits, vegetables, cereal, grains, milk and milk products, and high-protein foods. Avoid fried foods

Rapid weight loss to "make weight," is often achieved through water losses which can be harmful. Dehydration can lead to muscle cramping, fatigue, weakness, and impaired heat regulation

Laxatives or diuretics should never be used in weight loss, as chronic abuse can lead to serious complications

To gain weight, eat three meals a day and consume extra servings at mealtime. Eat frequent snacks that are low in fat and primarily carbohydrate, along with some protein, such as granola, GrapeNuts, and bananas. Drink whole milk, cranberry and grape juice, or calorie-containing fluids. Weight gain should not exceed 1 to 2 pounds per week, and should be combined with continued exercise and weight training

There was noticeable bilateral soft tissue swelling on the cheeks of the swimmer, and a callus over the MCP joint of the middle finger. This individual is showing definite physical and behavioral signs of an eating disorder. Intervene and talk with her, letting her know you are there to help. Express concern for her health and recommend professional counseling.

SUMMARY

As a health-care provider you will be confronted with numerous daily health problems unrelated to trauma. Upper respiratory tract infections can be contagious and affect other team members. Gastrointestinal tract problems can lead to indigestion, diarrhea, or constipation. Sport participants may also have systemic conditions, such as diabetes mellitus, epilepsy, hypertension, or anemia, that may require special adaptations to their exercise program or require immediate care, should their health status rapidly deteriorate.

There is no place in sport for substance abuse. Being under the influence of drugs can lead to self-injury or injury to other players through unintentional actions. In addition, current drug-testing can lead to expulsion from sport participation. Likewise, individuals who may have an eating disorder should be identified and counseled accordingly.

REFERENCES

1. Cohen S, Tyrrell DAJ, and Smith AP. 1991. Psychological stress and susceptibility to the common cold. N Engl J Med 325(9):606–611.
2. Hemila H. 1992. Vitamin C and the common cold. Br J Nutr 67(1):3–16.
3. Oppenheimer RW. 1991. Sinusitis: how to recognize and treat it. Postgrad Med 91(5):281–286, 289–292.
4. Herr RD. 1991. Acute sinusitis: diagnosis and treatment update. Am Fam Physician 44(6):2055–2062.
5. Lang SDR, and Singh K. 1990. The sore throat: when to investigate and when to prescribe. Drugs 40(6):854–862.
6. Solomon W. Familiar allergic disorders: anaphylaxis and the atopic diseases. In *Pathophysiology: clinical concepts of disease processes*, edited by SA Price and LM Wilson. St. Louis: Mosby-Year Book, 1992.
7. Renfroe DH. Obstructive alterations in pulmonary function. In *Pathophysiology: adaptations and alterations in function*, edited by BL Bullock and PP Rosendahl. Philadelphia: JB Lippincott, 1992.
8. Peterslund NA. 1991. Herpes virus infection: an overview of the clinical manifestations. Scan J Infect 80(Suppl):15–20.
9. Eichner ER. 1996. Infectious mononucleosis: recognizing the condition, 'reactivating' the patient. Phys Sportsmed 24(4):49–58.
10. Weinberger M. 1991. Day-to-day management of asthma. Pediatr 18(4):301–311.
11. Murphy S, and Kelly HW. 1991. Management of acute asthma. Pediatr 18(4):287–300.
12. Gong H Jr. 1992. Breathing easy: exercise despite asthma. Phys Sportsmed 20(3):159–167.
13. Rupp NT. 1996. Diagnosis and management of exercise-induced asthma. Phys Sportsmed 24(1):77–87.

14. Tremaine WJ. 1990. Chronic constipation: causes and management. Hosp Prac Off Ed 25(4A):89–100.

15. McArdle WD, Katch FI, and Katch VL. *Exercise physiology: energy, nutrition, and human performance*. Philadelphia: Lea & Febiger, 1995.

16. Heaman D. Normal and altered functions of the pancreas. In *Pathophysiology: adaptations and alterations in function*, edited by BL Bullock and PP Rosendahl. Philadelphia: JB Lippincott, 1992.

17. Rifkin H. 1991. Current status of non-insulin-dependent diabetes mellitus (type II): management with gliclazide. Am J Med 90(Suppl 6A):3–7.

18. Grant HD, Murray RH, and Bergeron JD. *Brady emergency care*. Englewood Cliffs, NJ: Prentice Hall, 1995.

19. Small E, and Bar-Or O. The young athlete with chronic disease. In *Clinics in sports medicine*, edited by LJ Micheli, vol. 14, no. 3. Philadelphia: WB Saunders, 1995.

20. Gates JR. 1991. Epilepsy and sports participation. Phys Sportsmed 19(3):98–104.

21. Daniels SR, and Loggie JMH. 1992. Hypertension in children and adolescents. Part II: pharmacologic control—what works and why. Phys Sportsmed 20(4):97–110.

22. Harris SS. Helping active women avoid anemia. Phys Sportsmed 23(5):35–48.

23. Browne RJ, and Gillespie CA. 1993. Sickle cell trait: a risk factor for life-threatening rhabdomyolysis? Phys Sportsmed 21(6):80–88.

24. Jones AP, Sickles T, and Lombardo JA. Substance abuse. In *Clinics in sports medicine*, edited by JC Puffer, vol. 11, no. 2. Philadelphia: WB Saunders, 1992.

25. Cowart VS. 1992. Dietary supplements: alternative to anabolic steroids? Phys Sportsmed 20(3):189–198.

26. American Psychiatric Association. *Diagnostic and statistical manual of mental disorders*. Washington DC, 1987.

27. Wichmann S, and Martin DR. 1993. Eating disorder in athletes: weighing the risks. Phys Sportsmed 21(5):126–135.

28. Thompson RA, and Sherman RT. *Helping athletes with eating disorders*. Champaign: Human Kinetics, 1993.

29. Yen JL. 1992. General overview and treatment considerations of anorexia and bulimia. Comp Ther 18(1):26–29.

30. Steen SN, Oppliger RA, and Brownell KD. 1988. Metabolic effects of repeated weight loss and regain in adolescent wrestlers. JAMA 260(1):47–50.

Credits

Chapter 1. From American Academy of Pediatrics Committee on Sports Medicine, Pediatrics, 81:737–739, 1988, Table 1.5.

Chapter 2. Courtesy of Hall SJ, Figs. 2.12B & C; Adapted from Salter RB, Textbook of Disorders and Injuries of the Musculoskeletal System, Baltimore: Williams & Wilkins, 1983, Fig. 2.14.

Chapter 3. From McArdle MD, Katch FI, and Katch VL, Exercise Physiology: Energy, Nutrition, and Human Performance, Philadelphia: Lea & Febiger, 1991, Tables 3.3 and 3.5 (modified); From Grant HD, Murray RH, and Bergeron JD, Brady Emergency Care, Englewood Cliffs, NJ: Prentice-Hall, 1990, Table 3.4 (adapted).

Chapter 4. Courtesy of Springfield College Sports Medicine Department, Springfield, MA, Figs. 4.1 and 4.9; From Clarkson HM and Gillewich GB, Musculoskeletal Assessment: Joint Range of Motion and Manual Muscle Strength, Baltimore: Williams & Wilkins, 1989, Tables 4.4 and 4.5 (adapted).

Chapter 5. Courtesy of Biodex Medical Systems, Shirley, NY, Fig. 5.4C; Courtesy of Aircast, Inc., Summit, NJ, Fig. 5.8; From Knight KL, Guidelines for rehabilitation of sports injuries, in Clinics in Sports Medicine, edited by J.S. Harvey, Vol. 4, No. 3, 1985, Table 5.3 (adapted).

Chapter 6. Courtesy of Polonchek JP, Bridgewater, MA, Figs. 6.6 and 6.15A; Courtesy of Brace International, Scottsdale, AZ, Fig. 6.8; Courtesy of Mueller Sports Medicine, Inc., Prairie du Sac, WI, Figs. 6.9A and 6.18A; Courtesy of Pro Orthopedic

Devices, Inc., Tucson, AZ, Figs. 6.13B, 6.15A, 6.16A, and 6.18B; Courtesy of Jbi, Williston, VT, Fig. 6.12; Courtesy of Adams, U.S.A., Cookeville, TN, Figs. 6.14A & B; Courtesy of Innovation Sports, Irvine, CA, Fig. 6.15B; Courtesy of Aircast, Inc., Summit, NJ, Fig. 6.18C; Courtesy of Foot Management, Pittsville, MD, Fig. 6.19A.

Chapter 7. No credits.

Chapter 8. Courtesy of Dr. D. Adelberg, Hawthorn Physical Therapy and Sports Medicine, N. Dartmouth, MA, Fig. 8.20.

Chapter 9. Courtesy of Dr. B. Saperia, Morton Hospital and Medical Center, Taunton, MA, Fig. 9.16; From Norkin CC and Levangie PK, Joint Structure and Function: A Comprehensive Analysis, Philadelphia: F.A. Davis, 1992, Table 8.1 (adapted); From American Academy of Orthopaedic Surgeons, Athletic Training and Sports Medicine, Philadelphia: American Academy of Orthopaedic Surgeons, 1991, Table 8.3.

Chapter 10. Courtesy of Dr. D. Adelberg, Hawthorn Physical Therapy and Sports Medicine, N. Dartmouth, MA, Figs. 10.9 and 10.12; Courtesy of Dr. M. Ehrlich, Rhode Island Hospital, Providence, RI, Fig. 10.14.

Chapter 11. Courtesy of Hinshaw W, Salisbury Evening Post, Salisbury, NC, Fig. 11.12A; Courtesy of Dr. D. Adelberg, Hawthorn Physical Therapy and Sports Medicine, N. Dartmouth, MA, Figs. 11.17, 11.19, and 11.20.

Chapter 12. Courtesy of Dr. B. Saperia, Morton Hospital and Medical Center, Taunton, MA, Fig. 12.11.

Chapter 13. Courtesy of Dr. D. Adelberg, Hawthorn Physical Therapy and Sports Medicine, N. Dartmouth, MA, Fig. 13.19.

Chapter 14. Courtesy of Dr. D. Titelbaum, Shields Health Care, Brockton, MA, Figs. 14.8A & B. From Cantu RC, Criteria for return to competition after a closed head injury, in Athletic Injuries to the Head, Neck, and Face, edited by J.S. Torg, St. Louis: Mosby Yearbook, 1991, Table 14.6.

Chapter 15. Courtesy of Dr. D. Adelberg, Hawthorn Physical Therapy and Sports Medicine, N. Dartmouth, MA, Fig. 15.9; Courtesy of Dr. B. Saperia, Morton Hospital and Medical Center, Taunton, MA, Fig. 15.13.

Chapter 16. No credits.

Chapter 17. Courtesy of Springfield College Sports Medicine Department, Springfield, MA, Fig. 17.3.

Chapter 18. From Alfaro-Levre R, Blicharz ME, Flynn NM, and Boyer MJ, Drug Handbook: A Nursing Process Approach, Redwood City, CA: Addison-Wesley Nursing, 1992, Tables 18.2 and 18.3 (adapted); From Wadler G and Hainline B, Drugs and the Athlete, Philadelphia: F.A. Davis, 1989, Table 18.4 (adapted); From National Collegiate Athletic Association, Drugs and the Athlete . . . A Losing Combination, Mission, KS, 1988, Table 18.5 (adapted); From Garner DM and Rosen LW, Eating disorders among athletes: research and recommendations, J Appl Sport Sci Res, 5(2):100, 1991, Table 18.6.

Glossary

Abrasion
Skin wound in which the external layers have been rubbed or scraped off

Abscess
Localized accumulation of pus and necrotic tissue

Accessory sex organs
Organs that transport, protect, and nourish gametes

Acclimatization
Physiologic adaptations of an individual to a different environment, especially one of climate or altitude

Active inhibition
Technique whereby an individual consciously relaxes a muscle prior to stretching

Active movement
Joint motion performed voluntarily by the individual through muscular contraction

Acute injury
Injury from a specific event, leading to a sudden onset of symptoms

Adhesions
Tissues that bind the healing tissue to adjacent structures, such as other ligaments or bone

Afferent nerves
Nerves carrying sensory input from receptors in the skin, muscles, tendons, and ligaments to the central nervous system

Alveoli
Air sacs at the terminal ends of the bronchial tree, where oxygen and carbon dioxide are exchanged between the lungs and surrounding capillaries

Amenorrhea
Absence or abnormal cessation of menstruation

Analgesia
Conscious state in which normal pain is not perceived, such as a numbing or sedative effect

Analgesic
Agent that produces analgesia

Analgesic effect
Condition whereby pain is not perceived; a numbing or sedative effect

Anatomical position
Standardized position with the body erect, facing forward, with the arms at the sides, palms facing forward

Anatomical snuff box
Region directly over the scaphoid bone bounded by the extensor pollicis brevis medially and the extensor pollicis longus laterally

Androgen
A class of hormones that promotes development of male genitals and secondary sex characteristics, and influences sexual motivation

Anemia
Abnormal reduction in red blood cell volume or hemoglobin concentration

Anesthesia
Partial or total loss of sensation

Anisotropic
Having different strengths in response to loads from different directions

Annulus fibrosis
Tough outer covering of the intervertebral disc, composed of fibrocartilage

Anorexia nervosa
Personality disorder manifested by extreme aversion toward food, resulting in extensive weight loss, amenorrhea, and other physical disorders

Anoxia
Deficiency or absence of oxygen

Antalgic gait
Walking with a limp to avoid pain

Antihistamine
Medication used to counteract the effects of histamine; it relieves the symptoms of an allergic reaction

Antipyresis
Action whereby body temperature associated with a fever is reduced

Antipyretic
Medication used to relieve or reduce a fever

Appendicitis
Inflammation of the appendix

Appendicular segment
Relates to the extremities of the body, including the arms and legs

Aseptic necrosis
The death or decay of tissue due to a poor blood supply in the area

Asthma
Lung disease characterized by bronchospasm, increased bronchial secretions, and mucosal swelling, all leading to airway narrowing and inadequate airflow during respiration

Atria
Two superior chambers of the heart that pump blood into the ventricles

Atrophy
A wasting away or deterioration of tissue due to disease, disuse, or malnutrition

Avascular
Devoid of blood vessels

Avascular necrosis
Death of tissues due to insufficient blood supply

Avulsion
A tearing away or forceful separation of a body part or structure

Axial force
Force acting along the long axis of a structure

Axial loading
Loading directed along the long axis of a body

Axial segment
Central part of the body, including the head and trunk

Ballistic stretch
Increasing flexibility by utilizing repetitive bouncing motions at the end of the available range of motion

Bandage
Material used to cover a wound

Bankart lesion
Avulsion or damage to the anterior lip of the glenoid as the humerus slides forward in an anterior dislocation

Battle's sign
Delayed discoloration behind the ear due to basilar skull fracture

Bending
Loading that produces tension on one side of an object and compression on the other side

Bennett's fracture
Fracture-dislocation to the proximal end of the first metacarpal at the carpal-metacarpal joint

Bilateral
Pertaining to both sides

Bipartite
Having two parts

Blister
Fluid accumulation under the skin caused by friction of the skin over a hard or rough surface, causing the epidermis to separate from the dermis

Boutonnière deformity
Rupture of the central slip of the extensor tendon at the middle phalanx, resulting in no active extensor mechanism at the proximal interphalangeal joint

Brachial plexus
Large mass of interwoven spinal nerves (C_5–T_1) that innervate the upper extremity

Bronchitis
Inflammation of the mucosal lining of the tracheobronchial tree characterized by bronchial swelling, mucus secretions, and dysfunction of the cilia

Bronchospasm
Contraction of the smooth muscles of the bronchial tubes, causing narrowing of the airway

Bucket-handle tear
Longitudinal meniscal tear of the central segment that can displace into the joint, leading to 'locking' of the knee

Bulimia
Personality disorder manifested by episodic bouts of binging large amounts of food, followed by purging and feelings of guilt, self-disgust, and depression

Bunion
Swelling and prominence of the 1st metatarsal head associated with lateral shift of the great toe (hallus valgus)

Burner
Burning or stinging sensation characteristic of a brachial plexus injury

Bursa
A fibrous sac membrane containing synovial fluid, typically found between tendons and bones; acts to decrease friction during motion

Bursitis
Inflammation of one or more bursae

Calcific tendinitis
Accumulation of mineral deposits in a tendon

Callus
Localized thickening of skin epidermis due to physical trauma; fibrous tissue containing immature bone tissue that forms at fracture sites during repair and regeneration

Cancellous
Bone tissue of relatively low density

Cardiac tamponade
Acute compression of the heart caused by effusion of fluid or blood into the pericardium from rupture of the heart or penetrating trauma

Cardiovascular endurance
The body's ability to sustain submaximal exercise over an extended period of time

Carpal tunnel syndrome
Compression of the median nerve as it passes through the carpal tunnel, leading to pain and tingling in the hand

Cauda equina
Lower spinal nerves, resembling a horse's tail, that course through the lumbar spinal canal

Cauliflower ear
Hematoma between the perichondrium and cartilage of the outer ear; auricular hematoma

Chemosensitive
Sensitive to chemical stimulation

Chondral fracture
Fracture involving the articular cartilage at a joint

Chondromalacia patellae
Degenerative condition in the articular cartilage of the patella caused by abnormal compression or shearing forces

Chronic injury
Injury characterized by a slow, sustained development of symptoms that culminates in a painful inflammatory condition

Chyme
Paste-like substance that food is churned into in the stomach

Circumduction
Circular motion of a body segment resulting from sequential flexion, abduction, extension, and adduction, or vice versa

Cirrhosis
Progressive inflammation of the liver, usually caused by alcoholism

Claw toes
A toe deformity characterized by hyperextension of the metatarsophalangeal (MTP) joint and hyperflexion of the interphalangeal (IP) joints

Clonic state
Movement marked by repetitive muscle contractions and relaxations in rapid succession

Closed-chain exercises
Weight-bearing exercises in which movement at one joint will produce predictable motion at another joint

Cold allergies
Hypersensitivity to cold, leading to superficial vascular reaction manifested by transient itching, erythema, hives, or whitish swellings (wheals)

Collateral ligaments
Major ligaments that cross the medial and lateral aspects of the knee

Colles' fracture
Fracture of the radius and ulna, just proximal to the wrist, that results in the distal segment displacing in a dorsal and radial direction

Compartment syndrome
Condition in which increased intramuscular pressure impedes blood flow and function of tissues within that compartment

Compressive force
Axial loading that produces a squeezing or crushing effect on a structure

Concussion
Violent shaking or jarring action of the brain, resulting in immediate or transient impairment of neurologic function

Congenital
Existing since birth

Conjunctivitis
Bacterial infection leading to itching, burning, watering, and inflamed eye; pinkeye

Constipation
Infrequent or incomplete bowel movements

Contracture
Adhesions occurring in an immobilized muscle, leading to a shortened contractile state

Contraindication
A condition adversely affected by a specific action

Contralateral
Pertaining to the opposite side

Contrecoup injuries
Injuries away from the actual injury site due to axial rotation and acceleration

Contusion
Compression injury involving accumulation of blood and lymph within a muscle; a bruise

Coordination
The body's ability to execute smooth, fluid, accurate, and controlled movements

Core temperature
Internal body temperature regulated by the hypothalamus

Cortical
Bone tissue of relatively high density

Corticosteroid
Any of the steroid hormones secreted by the adrenal cortex

Cramp
Painful involuntary muscle contraction, either clonic or tonic

Crepitus/Crepitation
Cracking or grating sound heard during palpation that indicates a possible fracture

Cruciate ligaments
Major ligaments that criss-cross the knee in the anteroposterior direction

Cryokinetics
Use of cold treatments prior to an exercise session

Cryotherapy
Cold or ice application

Cyanosis
A dark blue or purple tinge to the skin due to insufficient oxygen in the blood

Cyclist's nipples
Nipple irritation caused by the combined effects of perspiration and windchill, producing cold, painful nipples

Cyclist's palsy
Seen when bikers lean on the handlebars for an extended period of time, resulting in paresthesia in the ulnar nerve distribution

Dead arm syndrome
Common sensation felt with a recurrent anterior shoulder dislocation

Debridement
Removal of foreign matter and dead tissue from a wound

Decompression
Surgical release of pressure caused by fluid or blood accumulation

Deformation
Change in the original shape of a structure due to mechanical strain

de Quervain's tenosynovitis
An inflammatory stenosing tenosynovitis of the abductor pollicis longus and extensor pollicis brevis tendons

Dermatome
A region of skin supplied by a single afferent neuron

Detached retina
Neurosensory retina is separated from the retinal epithelium by swelling

Diabetes
Metabolic disorder characterized by near or absolute lack of the hormone insulin, or insulin resistance, or both

Diagnosis
Definitive determination of the nature of the injury or illness made only by physicians

Diarrhea
Loose or watery stools resulting when food residue rushes through the large intestine before there is sufficient time to absorb the remaining water

Diastole
Residual pressure in aorta between heart beats

Diathermy
Local elevation of temperature in the tissues produced by therapeutic application of high-frequency electric current, ultrasound, or microwave radiation

Diffuse injury
Injury over a large body area, usually due to low-velocity–high-mass forces

Diplopia
Double vision

Dislocation
Separation of a joint so that the bone ends are no longer in contact; third degree sprain

Diuretics
Chemicals that promote the excretion of urine

Dorsal
Relating to the back or posterior surface of a body part

Dressing
Covering over a wound used to hold a bandage in place

Drug
A therapeutic agent used in the prevention, diagnosis, cure, treatment, or rehabilitation of a disease, condition, or injury

Dural sinuses
Formed by tubular separations in the inner and outer layers of the dura mater, these sinuses function as small veins for the brain

Dysmenorrhea
Difficult or painful menstruation; menstrual cramps

Dyspnea
Labored or difficult breathing

Ecchymosis
Superficial tissue discoloration

Ectopic bone
Proliferation of bone ossification in an abnormal place

Edema
Swelling resulting from collection of exuded lymph fluid in the interstitial tissues

Efferent nerves
Nerves carrying stimuli from the central nervous system to the muscles

Effusion
The escape of fluid from the blood vessels into a cavity or joint

Elastic limit
The maximum load that a material can sustain without permanent deformation

Emergency plan
A process that activates emergency health care services of the facility and community

Endometriosis
Condition whereby endometrial cells from the uterine lining implant themselves in the abdominal cavity, frequently forming cysts containing altered blood

Epicondylitis
Inflammation and microrupturing of the soft tissues on the epicondyles of the distal humerus

Epilepsy
Disorder of the brain characterized by recurrent episodes of sudden, excessive discharges of electrical activity

Epiphyseal fracture
Injury to the growth plate of a long bone in children and adolescents; may lead to arrested bone growth

Epistaxis
Profuse bleeding from the nose; nosebleed

Estrogens
Hormones that produce female secondary sex characteristics and affect the menstrual cycle

Exostosis
A cartilage-capped bony projection arising from any bone that develops from cartilage

Expressed warranty
Written guarantee that states the product is safe for consumer use

Extensor mechanism
Complex interaction of muscles, ligaments, and tendons that stabilize and provide motion at the patellofemoral joint

Extrasynovial
Structures found outside of the synovial cavity and synovial fluid

Extrinsic
Originating outside of the part where it is found or upon which it acts; particularly denoting a muscle

Extruded disc
Condition in which the nuclear material moves into the spinal canal and runs the risk of impinging adjacent nerve roots

Exudate
Material composed of fluid, pus, or cells that has escaped from blood vessels into surrounding tissues following injury or inflammation

Failure
Loss of continuity; rupturing of soft tissue or fracture of bone

Fasciitis
Inflammation of the fascia surrounding portions of a muscle

Flexibility
Total range of motion at a joint dependent on normal joint mechanics, mobility of soft tissues, and muscle extensibility

Focal injury
Injury in a small, concentrated area, usually due to high-velocity–low-mass forces

Force
A push or pull that causes or tends to cause motion, or a change in motion

Foreseeability of harm
Condition whereby danger is apparent, or should have been apparent, resulting in an unreasonably unsafe condition

Fracture
A disruption in the continuity of a bone

Gamekeeper's thumb
Rupture of the volar ligament at the metacarpophalangeal joint, due to forceful abduction of the thumb while the thumb is extended

Ganglion cyst
Benign tumor mass commonly seen on the dorsal aspect of the wrist

Gastroenteritis
Inflammation of the mucous membrane of the stomach and/or small intestine

Glenoid labrum
Soft tissue lip around the periphery of the glenoid fossa that widens and deepens the socket to add stability to the joint

Goniometer
Protractor used to measure joint position and available joint motion (range of motion)

Hallux
The first, or great, toe

Hammer toes
A flexion deformity of the distal interphalangeal (DIP) joint of the toes

Hay fever
Seasonal allergic rhinitis caused by airborne pollens and/or fungus spores

Heat cramps
Painful, involuntary muscle spasms caused by excessive water and electrolyte loss

Heel bruise
Contusion to the subcutaneous fat pad located over the inferior aspect of the calcaneus

Hemarthrosis
Collection of blood within a joint or cavity

Hematoma
Localized mass of blood and lymph confined within a space or tissue

Hematuria
Blood or red blood cells in the urine

Hemothorax
Condition involving the loss of blood into the pleural cavity, but outside the lung

Hepatitis
Inflammation of the liver

Hernia
Protrusion of abdominal viscera through a weakened portion of the abdominal wall

High-density material
Materials that absorb more energy from higher impact intensity levels through deformation, thus transferring less stress to a body part

Hip pointer
Contusions caused by direct compression to an unprotected iliac crest that crushes soft tissue and, sometimes, the bone itself

Hyperesthesia
Excessive tactile sensation

Hyperglycemia
Abnormally high levels of glucose in the circulating blood that can lead to diabetic coma

Hypermobility
Increased motion at a joint; joint laxity

Hypertension
Sustained elevated blood pressure above the norms of 140 mm Hg systolic or 90 mm Hg diastolic

Hyperthermia
Elevated body temperature

Hypertrophic cardiomyopathy
Excessive hypertrophy of the heart, often of obscure or unknown origin

Hypertrophy
Increase in general bulk or size of an individual tissue, such as a muscle, not due to tumor formation

Hyperventilation
Respiratory condition in which too much carbon dioxide is exhaled, leading to an inability to catch one's breath

Hyphema
Hemorrhage into the anterior chamber of the eye

Hypoesthesia
Decreased tactile sensation

Hypoglycemia
Abnormally low levels of glucose in the circulating blood that can lead to insulin shock

Hypomobility
Decreased motion at a joint

Hypothermia
Decreased body temperature

Hypothenar
Mass of intrinsic muscles of the little finger, including the abductor digiti minimi, flexor digiti minimi brevis, and opponens digiti minimi

Hypovolemic shock
Shock caused by excessive loss of whole blood or plasma

Hypoxia
Having a reduced concentration of oxygen in air, blood, or tissue; less severe than anoxia

Idiopathic
Of unknown origin

Impingement syndrome
Chronic condition caused by repetitive overhead activity that damages the glenoid labrum, long head of the biceps brachii, and subacromial bursa

Implied warranty
Unwritten guarantee that the product is reasonably safe when used for its intended purpose

Incision
A wound with smooth edges; a surgical wound

Indication
A condition that could benefit from a specific action

Infarcts
Clumping together of cells that block small blood vessels, leading to vascular occlusion, ischemia, and necrosis in organs

Infection
Invasion of a host or host tissue by organisms such as bacteria, fungi, viruses, or parasites

Infectious mononucleosis
Viral condition caused by the Epstein-Barr virus that attacks the respiratory system and leaves the spleen enlarged and weak

Inflammation
Pain, swelling, redness, heat, and loss of function that accompany musculoskeletal injuries

Influenza
Acute infectious respiratory tract condition characterized by malaise, headache, dry cough, and general muscle aches

Informed consent
Consent whereby an injured adult, or parents of minor children, are reasonably informed of needed treatment, possible alternative treatments, and advantages and disadvantages of each course of action, and give written consent to receive treatment

Innervation
Nerve supply to a body part

Innominate bones
Without a name; used to describe anatomic structures

Inspection
Refers to factors seen at the actual injury site, such as redness, swelling, bruising, cuts, or scars

Interstitial tissues
Relating to spaces within a tissue or organ

Intracapsular
Structures found within the articular capsule; intra-articular

Intrinsic
Inherent; belonging entirely to a part; muscles with proximal and distal attachments located within the body part

Iontophoresis
Technique whereby direct current is used to drive charged molecules from certain medications into damaged tissue

Ipsilateral
Situated on, pertaining to, or affecting the same side, as opposed to contralateral

Ischemia
Local anemia due to decreased blood supply

Jaundice
A yellowish discoloration of the skin, sclera, and deeper tissues, often due to liver damage

Jersey finger
Rupture of the flexor digitorum profundus tendon from the distal phalanx, due to rapid extension of the finger while actively flexed

Jones fracture
A transverse stress fracture of the proximal shaft of the fifth metatarsal

Kehr's sign
Referred pain down the left shoulder indicative of a ruptured spleen

Kinematics
Study of the spatial and temporal aspects of movement

Kinetics
Study of the forces causing and resulting from motion

Kyphosis
Excessive curve in the thoracic region of the spine

Laceration
Wound that may leave a smooth or jagged edge through the skin, subcutaneous tissues, muscles, and associated nerves and blood vessels

Larsen-Johansson disease
Inflammation or partial avulsion of the apex of the patella due to traction forces

Legg-Calvé-Perthes disease
Avascular necrosis of the proximal femoral epiphysis, seen especially in young males ages 3 to 8

Little league elbow
Tension stress injury of the medial epicondyle, seen in adolescents

Little league shoulder
Fracture of the proximal humeral growth plate in adolescents caused by repetitive rotational stresses during the act of pitching

Lordosis
Excessive convex curve in the lumbar region of the spine

Low-density material
Materials that absorb energy from low-impact intensity levels

Lumbar plexus
Interconnected roots of the first four lumbar spinal nerves

Maceration
Softening of tissues that may result in breaking, tearing, or wasting away

Magnetic resonance imaging (MRI)
Diagnostic technique using magnetism to produce high-quality, cross-sectional images of organs or structures within the body without x-rays or other radiation

Malaise
Lethargic feeling of general discomfort; out-of-sorts feeling

Mallet finger
Rupture of the extensor tendon from the distal phalanx, due to forceful flexion of the phalanx

Malocclusion
Inability to bring the teeth together in a normal bite

Malpractice
Committing a negligent act while providing care

Marfan's syndrome
Inherited connective tissue disorder affecting many organs, but commonly resulting in the dilation and weakening of the thoracic aorta

McBurney's point
A site one-third the distance between the anterior superior iliac spine (ASIS) and umbilicus that, with deep palpation, produces rebound tenderness, indicating appendicitis

Mechanosensitive
Sensitive to mechanical stimulation

Meninges
Three protective membranes that surround the brain and spinal cord

Meningitis
Inflammation of the meninges of the brain and spinal column

Menisci
Fibrocartilagenous discs within the knee that reduce joint stress

Menses
Phase in the menstrual cycle when the thickened vascular walls of the uterus, the unfertilized ova, and blood from damaged vessels are lost during the menstrual flow

Metatarsalgia
A condition involving general discomfort around the metatarsal's heads

Microtrauma
Injury to a small number of cells due to accumulative effects of repetitive forces

Modalities
Therapeutic physical agents that promote optimal healing, such as thermotherapy, cryotherapy, electrotherapy, or manual therapy, while reducing pain and disability

Motion segment
Two adjacent vertebrae and the intervening soft tissues; the functional unit of the spine

Muscle spindle
Encapsulated receptor found in muscle tissue sensitive to stretch

Muscle strength
The ability of a muscle to produce resulting force in one maximal effort, either statically or dynamically

Muscular endurance
The ability of muscles to exert tension over an extended period

Muscular power
The ability of muscles to produce force at a given time

Myopia
Nearsightedness

Myositis
Inflammation of connective tissues within a muscle

Myositis ossificans
Accumulation of mineral deposits in muscle tissue

Myotome
A group of muscles primarily innervated by a single nerve root

Necrosis
Death of a tissue due to deprivation of a blood supply

Negligence
Breach of one's duty of care that causes harm to another individual

Neoplasm
Mass of tissue that grows more rapidly than normal and may be benign or malignant

Nerve root
The portion of a nerve associated with its origin in the spinal cord, such as C_6 or L_5

Neuritis
Inflammation or irritation of a nerve; commonly found between the third and fourth metatarsal heads

Neuroma
A nerve tumor

Nociceptors
Specialized nerve endings that transduce pain

Nonunion fracture
A fracture in which healing is delayed or fails to unite at all

NSAID
Nonsteroidal anti-inflammatory drug

Nucleus pulposus
Gelatinous-like material comprising the inner portion of the intervertebral disc

Nystagmus
Abnormal jerking or involuntary eye movement

Observation
Visual analysis of overall appearance, symmetry, general motor function, posture, and gait

Oligomenorrhea
Menstruation involving scant blood loss

Open-chain exercises
Nonweight-bearing exercises in which the distal joints function independently of the other joints

Orthosis
Devices or appliances used to correct or straighten a deformity

Orthotics
The science concerned with the making and fitting of orthopedic appliances

Osgood-Schlatter disease
Inflammation or partial avulsion of the tibial apophysis due to traction forces

Osteitis pubis
Stress fracture to the pubic symphysis caused by repeated overload of the adductor muscles or repetitive stress activities

Osteochondral fracture
Fracture involving the articular cartilage and underlying bone

Osteochondritis dissecans
Localized area of avascular necrosis resulting from complete or incomplete separation of joint cartilage and subchondral bone

Osteochondrosis
Any condition characterized by degeneration or aseptic necrosis of the articular cartilage due to limited blood supply

Osteopenia
Condition of reduced bone mineral density that predisposes the individual to fractures

Osteoporosis
Pathologic condition of reduced bone mass and strength

Overload principle
Physiologic improvements occur only when an individual physically demands more of the muscle than is normally required

Overuse injury
Any injury caused by excessive, repetitive movement of the body part

Painful arc
Pain located within a limited number of degrees in the range of motion

Pallor
Ashen or pale skin

Palpation
Act of feeling a region with the fingers to detect temperature, swelling, point tenderness, deformity, crepitus, and cutaneous sensation

Paralysis
Partial or complete loss of the ability to move a body part

Paresthesia
Abnormal sensations, such as numbness, tingling, itching, or burning

Paronychia
A fungal/bacterial infection in the folds of skin surrounding a fingernail or toenail

Parrot-beak tear
Horizontal meniscal tear typically in the middle segment of the lateral meniscus

Partial airway obstruction
Choking in which the individual has some air exchange in the lungs and is able to cough

Passive movement
A limb or body part is moved through the range of motion with no assistance from the individual

Passive stretching
Stretching of muscles, tendons, and ligaments produced by a stretching force other than tension in the antagonist muscles; stretching of body part done by a clinician without the help of the patient

Patellofemoral joint
Gliding joint between the patella and the patellar groove of the femur

Patellofemoral stress syndrome
Condition whereby the lateral retinaculum is tight or the vastus medialis oblique is weak, leading to lateral excursion and pressure on the lateral facet of the patella, causing a painful condition

Percussion
Used to assess abdominal injuries; performed by tapping the nondominant hand with the dominant hand to determine presence and location of hollow versus solid organs, or masses in the abdomen

Periorbital ecchymosis
Swelling and hemorrhage into the surrounding eyelids; black eye

Peristalsis
Periodic waves of smooth muscle contraction that propel food through the digestive system

Peritonitis
Inflammation of the peritoneum that lines the abdomen

Pes cavus
High arch

Pes planus
Flat feet

Pharyngitis
Viral, bacterial, or fungal infection of the pharynx, leading to a sore throat

Phonophoresis
The introduction of medication through the skin with the use of ultrasound

Photophobia
Abnormal sensitivity to light

Plantar fascia
Specialized band of fascia that covers the plantar surface of the foot and helps support the longitudinal arch

Plyometric training
Exercises that employ explosive movements to develop muscular power

Pneumothorax
Condition whereby air is trapped in the pleural space, causing a portion of a lung to collapse

Point tenderness
Specific painful area at an injury site that can be palpated

Postconcussion syndrome
Delayed condition characterized by persistent headaches, blurred vision, irritability, and inability to concentrate

Posttraumatic memory loss
Forgetting events after an injury

Primary sex organs
Reproductive organs responsible for producing gametes (ova and sperm)

Primary survey
Immediate assessment to determine unresponsiveness and status of the ABCs (Airway, Breathing, Circulation, and severe arterial bleeding)

Progesterone
Hormone responsible for thickening the uterine lining in preparation for the fertilized ovum

Prognosis
Probable course or progress of an injury or disease

Prolapsed disc
Condition when the eccentric nucleus produces a definite deformity as it works its way through the fibers of the annulus fibrosus

Pronation
Inward rotation of the forearm; palms face posteriorly. At the foot, combined motions of calcaneal eversion, foot abduction, and dorsiflexion

Prophylactic
Preventative or protective

Proprioceptive neuromuscular facilitation (PNF)
Exercises that stimulate proprioceptors in muscles, tendons, and joints to improve flexibility and strength

Proprioceptors
Specialized deep sensory nerve cells in joints, ligaments, muscles, and tendons sensitive to stretch, tension, and pressure, which are responsible for position and movement

Pulmonary circuit
Blood vessels that transport unoxygenated blood to the lungs from the right heart ventricle and oxygenated blood from the lungs to the left heart atrium

Pulmonary contusion
Contusion to the lungs due to compressive force

Pulmonary embolism
A blood clot that travels through the circulatory system and lodges in the lungs

Pupillary light reflex
Rapid constriction of pupils when exposed to intense light

Q-angle
Angle between the line of quadriceps force and the patellar tendon

Raccoon eyes
Delayed discoloration around the eyes from anterior cranial fossa fracture

Raynaud's phenomenon
Intermittent bilateral attacks of ischemia in the digits marked by severe pallor, burning, and pain brought on by cold

Referred pain
Pain felt in a region of the body other than where the source or actual cause of the pain is located

Reflex
Action involving stimulation of a motor neuron by a sensory neuron in the spinal cord without involvement of the brain

Resilience
The ability to bounce or spring back into shape or position after being stretched, bent, or impacted

Resisted movement
Any form of active motion in which a dynamic or static muscular contraction is resisted by an outside force applied manually or mechanically

Resting position
Slightly flexed position of a joint that allows for maximal volume to accommodate any intra-articular swelling

Retrograde amnesia
Forgetting events that happened before an injury

Retroviruses
Any virus of the family *Retroviridae*, known to reverse the usual order of reproduction within the cells they infect

Rhinitis
Inflammation of the nasal membranes, with excessive mucus production resulting in nasal congestion and postnasal drip

Rhinorrhea
Clear nasal discharge

Rotator cuff
The SITS (supraspinatus, infraspinatus, teres minor, and subscapularis) muscles that hold the head of the humerus in the glenoid fossa and produce humeral rotation

Rubor
Reddish skin

Runner's nipples
Nipple irritation due to friction when the shirt rubs over the nipples

Sacral plexus
Interconnected roots of the L_4–S_4 spinal nerves

Saddle joint
Joint at which one bone surface has a convex, saddle-like shape, and the articulating bone surface is reciprocally shaped

Scapulohumeral rhythm
Coordinated rotational movement of the scapula that accompanies abduction and adduction of the humerus

Sciatica
Compression of a spinal nerve due to a herniated disc, a muscle-related or facet joint disease, or compression between the two parts of the piriformis muscle

Scoliosis
Lateral rotational spinal curvature

Screwing-home mechanism
Rotation of the tibia on the femur during extension that produces an anatomic 'locking' of the knee

Secondary survey
Detailed head-to-toe assessment to detect medical and injury-related problems that, if unrecognized and untreated, could become life-threatening

Sesamoid bones
Short bones embedded in tendons; largest is the patella (knee cap)

Sesamoiditis
Inflammation of the sesamoid bones of the 1st metatarsal

Sever's disease
A traction-type injury, or osteochondrosis, of the calcaneal apophysis, seen in young adolescents

Shear force
A force that acts parallel or tangent to a plane passing through an object

Shin bruise
A contusion to the tibia, sometimes referred to as tibial periostitis

Shock
Collapse of the cardiovascular system when insufficient blood cannot provide circulation for the entire body

Sickle-cell anemia
Abnormalities in hemoglobin structure resulting in a characteristic sickle- or crescent-shaped red blood cell that is fragile and unable to transport oxygen

Sign
Objective measurable physical findings that you can hear, feel, see, or smell during the assessment

Sinusitis
Inflammation of the paranasal sinuses

Smith's fracture
Fracture of the radius and ulna, just proximal to the wrist that results in the distal segment displacing in a volar direction; opposite of Colles' fracture

Snapping hip syndrome
A snapping sensation either heard or felt during motion at the hip

Snowball crepitation
Sound similar to that heard when crunching snow into a snowball; indicative of tenosynovitis

Solar plexus punch
A blow to the abdomen that results in an immediate inability to breathe freely

Somatic pain
Pain originating in the skin, ligaments, muscles, bones, or joints

Spasm
Transitory muscle contractions

Spica
Figure-eight pattern to limit motion around two body parts of differing sizes

Spondylolisthesis
Anterior slippage of a vertebra, resulting from complete bilateral fracture of the pars interarticularis

Spondylolysis
A stress fracture of the pars interarticularis

Sports medicine
Area of health and special services that applies medical and scientific knowledge to prevent, recognize, manage, and rehabilitate injuries related to sport, exercise, or recreational activity

Sprain
Injury to ligamentous tissue

Standard of care
What another minimally competent professional educated and practicing in the same profession would have done in the same or similar circumstances to protect an individual from harm

Static position
Stationary position in which no motion occurs

Static stretch
Slow, sustained muscle stretching used to increase flexibility

Stenosing
Narrowing of an opening or stricture of a canal

Steroids
A large family of chemical substances, including endocrine secretions and hormones

Sticking point
Insufficient strength to move a body segment through a particular angle

Stitch in the side
A sharp pain or spasm in the chest wall, usually on the lower right side, that occurs during exertion

Strain
Amount of deformation with respect to the original dimensions of the structure

Stress
The distribution of force within a body; quantified as force divided by the area over which the force acts

Stress (fatigue) fracture
Fracture resulting from repeated loading with relatively lower magnitude forces

Subconjunctival hemorrhage
Minor capillary ruptures in the eye globe

Subcutaneous emphysema
Presence of air or gas in subcutaneous tissue, characterized by a crackling sensation on palpation

Subungual hematoma
Collection of blood under the fingernail, caused by direct trauma

Sudden death
Nontraumatic, unexpected death occurring instantaneously or within a few minutes of an abrupt change in an individual's previous clinical state

Supination
Outward rotation of the forearm; palms facing forward. At the foot, combined motions of calcaneal inversion, foot adduction, and plantar flexion

Symptom
Subjective information provided by an individual regarding their perception of the problem

Syncope
Fainting or lightheadedness

Syndesmosis
A joint where the opposing surfaces are joined together by fibrous connective tissue

Syndrome
An accumulation of common signs and symptoms characteristic of a particular injury or disease

Synovitis
Inflammation of a synovial membrane, particularly at a joint

Systemic circuit
Blood vessels that transport unoxygenated blood to the right heart atrium and oxygenated blood from the left heart ventricle

Systole
Pressure in aorta when left ventricle contracts

Tendinitis
Inflammation of a tendon

Tenosynovitis
Inflammation of a tendon sheath

Tensile force
Axial loading that is the opposite of compressive force; a pulling force that tends to stretch the object to which it is applied

Tension pneumothorax
Condition in which air continuously leaks into the pleural space, causing the mediastinum to displace to the opposite side, compressing the uninjured lung and thoracic aorta

Thenar
Mass of intrinsic muscles of the thumb, including the flexor pollicis brevis, abductor pollicis brevis, and opponens pollicis

Therapeutic drugs
Prescription or over-the-counter medications used to treat an injury or illness

Thermotherapy
Heat application

Thrombophlebitis
Acute inflammation of a vein

Tibiofemoral joint
Dual condyloid joints between the tibial and femoral condyles that function primarily as a modified hinge joint

Tinea
Ringworm; a fungal infection of the hair, skin, or nails, characterized by small vesicles, itching, and scaling; tinea pedis—athlete's foot; tinea cruris—jock itch; tinea capitis—ringworm of the scalp

Tinnitus
Ringing or other noises in the ear due to trauma or disease

Tonic state
Steady, rigid muscle contractions with no relaxation

Torsion
Twisting of a structure around its longitudinal axis

Tort
A wrong done to an individual whereby the injured party seeks a remedy for damages suffered

Total airway obstruction
Choking in which the individual has no air passing through vocal cords and is unable to speak or cough

Traumatic asphyxia
Condition involving extravasation of blood into the skin and conjunctivae due to a sudden increase in venous pressure

Triage
Assessing all injured individuals to determine priority of care

Unconsciousness
Impairment of brain function wherein the individual lacks conscious awareness and is unable to respond to superficial sensory stimuli

Valgus laxity
An opening on the medial side of a joint caused by the distal segment moving laterally

Varus laxity
An opening on the lateral side of a joint caused by the distal segment moving medially

Vasoconstriction
Narrowing of blood vessels

Vasodilation
Increased diameter of the blood vessels

Ventricles
Two inferior chambers of the heart that pump blood out of the heart, one to the pulmonary circuit and one to the systemic circuit

Visceral pain
Pain resulting from injury or disease to an organ in the thoracic or abdominal cavity

Viscoelastic
Responding to loading over time with changing rates of deformation

Vital signs
Objective measurements of pulse, respirations, blood pressure, and skin temperature, indicating normal body functions

Volar
Referring to the palm of the hand or the sole of the foot

Volkmann's contracture
Ischemic necrosis of the forearm muscles and tissues, caused by damage to the blood flow

Wedge fracture
A crushing compression fracture that leaves a vertebra narrowed anteriorly

Wheal
A smooth, slightly elevated area on the body that appears red or white and is accompanied by severe itching; commonly seen in allergies to mechanical or chemical irritants

Zone of primary injury
Initial region of injured tissue composed of blood and necrotic tissue

Zone of secondary injury
Region of damaged tissue following vasodilation

Index

Italic page numbers indicate figures; page numbers with *t* indicate tables.

ABCs (Airway, Breathing, Circulation), 64
Abdominal thrusts, *90, 91*
Abdominal wall injuries
  appendicitis, *589,* 604
  bladder injuries, 604
  hernias, *601,* 601–602
  kidney injuries, 604
  liver contusion and rupture, 603–604
  muscle strains, 600
  skin wound and contusions, 600
  solar plexus contusion, 601
  splenic rupture, 603
Abduction
  glenohumeral, *384,* 393
  of hip, 345–346
Abrasions, 41–42
  of cornea, 533
  of wrist and hand, 473
Acceleration, 507
Accessory sex organs, 618
Accident reports, 21, 23
  information needed on, *26t*
Acclimatization, 78–79
Acetabulum, 340–341
Acetaminophen, 178
Achilles tendinitis, 262, 279–280
Achilles tendon, 253
  rupture of, 277–278, *278*
    Thompson's test for, 290–291, *291*
  taping of, 225–226, *228*
Acquired immunodeficiency syndrome (AIDS), 618, 626–627, *627t*
Acromioclavicular (AC) joint, 382, *382, 383*
  distraction/compression, 416, *418, 418*
  sprain of, 398, 400, 401, *401*
  taping of injury to, 236, *238*
Active inhibition, 154, *156*
Active movement, 132–133
Activities
  protected, 150
  restricted, 150
Activities of daily living (ADLs), 124–125
Acute injury, 124
Adam's apple, 582, *583*

Adduction
  glenohumeral, *385,* 393
  of hip, 346, *346*
  of knee, 304
Adductor brevis, 346
Adductor longus, 346
Adductor magnus, 346
Adductor strains, 357–358
Adhesions, 45–46
Adrenocorticosteroids, 178
Afferent nerves, 54
Airway, obstructed, 65–66
  opening, 88–91
Allergic rhinitis, 636–637
Alveoli, 584, 585
Amenorrhea, 51, 282, 655
  exercise-associated, 628–629
American Society for Testing and Materials (ASTM), 184
Amnesia, 519
  retrograde, 515
Analgesic effect, 150
Analgesics, 178
Anatomical position, 115
Anatomical snuff box, 485, *485*
Anconeus, 435
Ando, Yoshitaka, 380
Androgens, 618
Anemia
  iron-deficiency, 648
  sickle cell, 648–649
Anesthesia, 135
  local, 178
Anisotropic, 33
Ankle. (*See* Foot, ankle, and lower leg)
Annulus fibrosus, 541
Anorexia nervosa, 655–656
  comparison of bulimia nervosa and, *656t*
Anterior cruciate ligament (ACL), 311–312
Anterior cruciate ligament (ACL) braces, 199
Anterior drawer test
  for ankle, 291
  for knee, 331, *332*
Anterior impingement test for shoulder, 420, *420*
Anterior superior iliac spine (ASIS), 341
Antipyresis, 178

Aorta, 590
Apley's Scratch test, 413–414, *414*
Aponeuroses, 40
Apophyses, 52
Apophysitis, thoracic spinal, 560–561, *561*
Appendicitis, *589,* 604, 609
Appendicular segment, 115, *115*
Apprehension test for anterior shoulder dislocation, *418,* 418–419
Arachnoid mater, 503
Arches
  plantar, 252–253, *254*
  support of ankle, 218, 220, *220*
  zygomatic, 524
Arterial bleeding, 68
Aseptic necrosis, 484
Aspirin, 178
Asthma
  bronchial, 637–638
  exercise-induced, 638–639
Athlete's foot, 272
Athletic shoes, factors in selection and fit of, 205
Athletic trainer, 8–9, *9, 10t*
  career opportunities for, 27–29
  duties of, *10t*
  NATA certification for, 13–14
  respiration of, in sports-related injuries, 113, *114*
Atrophy, 127
Avulsion fractures, 323
Avulsions, 50–51
Axial force, 33
Axial segment, 115, *115*
Axillary artery, 388
Axillary nerve, 388

Ballistic stretches, 40, 153
Ballotable patella test, 327
Bankart lesion, 402
Batting helmets, 186
Battle's sign, 509
Bending, 36–37
Bennett's fracture, 485, *486*
Biceps brachii, 384, 434
Biceps femoris, 303, 345
Bicipital tendinitis, Speed's test for, 420, *420*

Bicipital tendon injuries, 406
Bicycle helmets, *186*, 186–187
Bilateral palpation, 129–130
Bipartite, 282
Birth control and sport
    participation, 629
Black eye, *531*, 531–532
Bleached tape, 211
Bleeding
  arterial, 68
  external, 68
  venous, 68
Blisters, 42, 267, 269
Blood pressure in secondary injury
    assessment, 105–106
Blood supply
  for elbow, 431–432, 432*t*, *433*
  for foot, ankle, and lower leg,
    255, 257, *259*, *260*
  for head and face, 505*t*,
    505–506, *506*
  for knee, 301, *303*, 303–304
  for shoulder, 387*t*, *388*, *388*, *389*
  for thigh, hip, and pelvis, 342,
    342, *344*
  for wrist and hand, 465, 467,
    469
Bloodborne viral disease, 624–625
Blowout fracture, 534
Body cooling, systemic, 84–85
Bones. (*See also specific*)
  anatomical properties of, 46–47,
    47, *48*, *49*
  cancellous, 47
  concha, 503
  cortical, 47
  ectopic, 437
  ethmoid, 502
  of foot, ankle, and lower leg,
    250, *251*, *252*
  frontal, 502
  injuries to, 46–53
    classifications, 49–51, *50*
  innominate, 341
  occipital, 502
  parietal, 502
  skull, *502*, 502–503
  sphenoid, 502
  of wrist and hand, 464–465, *465*
Bony palpations
  for elbow, 451, 453
  for foot, ankle, and lower leg,
    287
  for knee, 327
  in secondary injury assessment,
    102, *103*, *104*
  for shoulder, 413
  for thigh, hip, and pelvis, 367
  for wrist and hand, 489
Bony tissue, healing, 52–53
Boutonniere deformity, 478, *478*
Brachial artery, 432
Brachial plexus, 388, 431, 465, 467,
    469
  injuries to, 558–559, *559*
Brachioradialis, 435

Brain, 503–504
Breast injuries, 594
Breathing, 91–93, *93*
Bronchial asthma, 637–638
Bronchitis, acute, 637
Bronchospasm, 637
Bulimia nervosa, 654–655
  comparison of anorexia nervosa
    and, 656*t*
Bunions, 270, *271*
Burner, 559
Bursa
  infrapatellar, 310
  olecranon, 440
  pes anserinus, 310
  prepatellar, 310, *310*
  shoulder, *385*, 386–387
  subacromial, 386–387, *388*
  trochanteric, 341, 354
Bursitis, 44
  in foot, 270–271, *271*
  in knee, 306, 310, *310*
  olecranon, *440*, 440–441
  in shoulder, 406
  in thigh, hip, and pelvis, *354*,
    354–355

Calcaneofibular ligament, 251
Calcaneus, 253
Calcific tendinitis, 43
Calcium, 58
Calluses, 267, 269
Cancellous bone, 47
Carbohydrates, 57
Cardiac tamponade, 599
Cardiopulmonary emergencies, 66
Cardiovascular endurance, 165, 166
Career opportunities in athletic
    training, 27–29
Carotid artery, 505, 592
Carpal tunnel compression test of
    wrist and hand, 493
Carpal tunnel syndrome, 480,
    481–482, *482*
Carpometacarpal (CM) joint, 465
  motion of, 471
Cauda equina, 544
Cauliflower ear, 529, *530*
Centinela test, 420
Cerebral hematomas, 510–511,
    512, 513*t*
Cervical compression test for
    spine, 574, *575*
Cervical distraction test for spine,
    574, *575*
Cervical neck rolls, 191, *191*
Cervical spine
  fractures and dislocations,
    557–558, 558*t*
  injuries to, 555–558, *556*, *557*
  strains and sprains, 556–557
Chemical packs, 171
Chemosensitive nociceptors, 56
Chondral fracture, 323
Chondromalacia patellae, *318*,
    318–319

Choroid, 505
Chronic injury, 124
Chyme, 587, 589
Circulation, establishing, 93–94, *94*
Circumduction, 470
Cirrhosis, 589
Clavicular fractures, 407, *407*, *408*
Claw toe, 267, *267*
Clonic state, 646
Closed basketweave, 223–224, *224*
Closed-chain exercises, 162, *162*
  in rehabilitation of elbow, 458
  in rehabilitation of hand and
    wrist, 495
  in rehabilitation of shoulder,
    421, 424
Cloth ankle wrap, 225, *227*
Coach, 9, 11
Cold allergies, 167
Cold whirlpools, 169
Cold-gel packs, 171
Cold-related injuries, preventing,
    82–83
Collagen, 46
Collagenous scar formation,
    149–150
Collateral ligaments, 301
  support for knee, 230, *231*
Collegiate settings, opportunities in
    athletic training in, 27–28
Colles fracture, 483, *484*
Commercial ear plugs, 530
Commission on Accreditation of
    Allied Health Educational
    Programs (CAAHEP),
    13–14
Common cold, 634
Compartment syndrome
  acute, 273
  exercise-induced, 280–281
Compressive force, 33–34
Concha bones, 503
Concussions, 513–516, 514*t*
Condyloid joint, 464
Confidentiality, 18–19
Congenital problems, 127
Conjunctiva, 504
Conjunctivitis, 533
Consciousness, loss of, 519
Constipation, 641
Continuing education
    requirements, 14
Continuous passive motion (CPM),
    167, 177, *177*
Contoured cryo cuffs, 168–169,
    169
Contractility of muscle, 41
Contracture, 153
Contraindication, 128–129, 165
Contrast baths, 174
Contrecoup injuries, 508, *508*
Contusions
  of elbow, 436–437, 440
  facial, 524
  of foot, ankle, and lower leg,
    272–274

lumbar, 563–564
of thigh, hip, and pelvis,
351–354, *352, 353*
thoracic, 560
of wrist and hand, 473
Coordination, 163–164
Coracoacromial ligament, 383, 387,
388
Coracobrachialis, 384
Coracoclavicular joint, 382, *382,*
383
Coracoclavicular ligament, 383
Coracohumeral ligament, 383–384
Cornea, 505
abrasions of, 533
Cortical bone, 47
Cortisone, 178
Costal cartilages, 584
Costochondral injury, 594–595,
595
Cramps, 43
heat, 79–80
Cranial injury mechanisms, *507,*
507–508, *508*
Cranial nerve, 505, 505*t*
Cranium, 502
Crepitus, 71
Cruciate ligaments, 300–301
Cryokinetics, 165, 168
Cryotherapy, 165, *167,* 167–169,
168*t, 170,* 171, *172,* 172*t,*
173, 174, 175
Cutaneous sensation, *136*
in secondary injury assessment,
105
Cyanosis, 65
Cyclist's nipples, 594
Cyclist's palsy, 483

Daily treatment logs, 27
de Quervain's tenosynovitis, 479
Dead arm syndrome, 404
Decompression, 511
Deformation, 507
Deltoid ligament, 250, 384
Dental injuries, 527–528, *528, 529*
Dermatologic conditions, 623
Dermatomes, 57, 135, *136*
Dermis, 39
Derotation, 199
Detached retina, 533–534
Diabetes mellitus, 641
comparison of Type I and Type
II, 643*t*
Diabetic athlete, 641–643, *642,*
643*t*
coma, 643–644
exercise and diabetes, 644
insulin shock, 644
Diabetic coma, 643–644
Diagnosis, 139
Diagnostic and Statistical Manual
(DSM-IV), 653
Diaphragm, 585
Diaphysis, 46
Diarrhea, 640–641

Diastole, 585
Diastolic blood pressure, 105
Diathermy, 174
Diffuse injuries, 182, 508
Diplopia, 101, 534
Directional terms, 116, 116*t,* 117*t*
Disability resulting from injury,
124–125
Disc injuries, lumbar, 565, *576*
Dislocations
cervical, 557–558, 558*t*
of elbows, 441–442, *442*
of hand and wrist, *475,* 475–477,
476
lumbar, 565
Disordered eating, 653–658, 654*t*
Displaced contact lens, 534
Disqualifying conditions for sport
participation, 25*t*
Distal interphalangeal (DIP) joint,
250, 465
Distal radioulnar joint, 464
Dorsal radiocarpal ligament, 465
Dorsal scapular nerve, 388
Dorsiflexion and plantar flexion,
260, *261*
Drug testing, 650–652
Dual high school/clinic athletic
trainer, opportunities in
athletic training in, 28–29
Dura mater, 503
Dural sinuses, 503
Durrant, Earlene, 4
Duty of care, 15–16, 19
Dysmenorrhea, 627–628
Dyspnea, 638

Ear injuries, 529–530, *530*
Ear wear, 190, *191*
Ecchymosis, 42, 129
Ectopic bone, 437
Efferent nerves, 54
Effusion, 129
Elastic limit, 33
Elastic tape, 211
Elastic wrap, 213
Elbow, 430, *430*
assessment of, 449
bony structure of, 430, *431*
fractures of, 448–449, 452, 453
history in assessing, 449–450
hyperextension of, 238, *240*
ligaments of, 430
major muscle actions of,
433–434
flexion and extension, *434,*
434–435
pronation and supination,
435–436
muscles of, 431, 432*t*
nerves and blood vessels of,
431–432, 432*t, 433*
observation and inspection,
450–451
olecranon bursitis in, *440,*
440–441

overuse conditions, 444
impingement of ulnar nerve,
448
lateral epicondylitis, 445–446,
447
medial epicondylitis, 444–445,
445
palpations
bony, 451
soft tissue, 453
prevention of injuries
contusions, 436–437, 440
exercises for, 437–439
protection of, 192–193, *195, 196*
rehabilitation of, *458,* 458–459
special tests for, 453–454
joint range of motion, 454
neurologic testing, 454
resisted manual muscle
testing, 454
stress and functional tests,
454–457
sprains and dislocations,
441–442, *442*
management of, 442
strains, 443–444
Emergency medical services
(EMS), 63–64
Emergency plan, 85–86
Emergency procedures, 63–65
Emphysema, subcutaneous, 597
Empty can test, 420
Endometriosis, 628
Endurance, muscular, 160
Epicondylitis, 429, 444
lateral, 445–446, *447*
management of, 446
medial, 444–445, *445*
Epidermis, 39
Epidural hematoma, 511, *512*
Epilepsy, 645–646
Epiphyseal centers, 407–408, *408*
Epiphyseal fracture, 361
Epiphyseal injury, classifications of,
51, 52
Epiphyseal plates, 46
Epiphyses, 46
Epistaxis, 526
Estrogens, 619–620
Ethmoid bones, 502
Exercise
and diabetes, 644
and weight management, 656,
657
Exercise-associated amenorrhea,
628–629
Exercise-induced asthma, 638–639
Exercise-induced compartment
syndrome, 280–281
Expressed warranty, 18
Extension
of elbow, *434,* 434–435
glenohumeral, *384, 385,* 393
of hand and wrist, *468,* 470
of knee, 304, *305*
spinal, 546

Extension *continued*
of thigh, hip, and pelvis, 345, *346*
toe, 259
Extensor carpi radialis, 471
Extensor carpi radialis brevis, 470
Extensor carpi radialis longus, 470
Extensor carpi ulnaris, 470
Extensor digiti minimi, 470
Extensor digitorum, 470
Extensor digitorum brevis, 259
Extensor digitorum longus, 255, 259
Extensor hallucis longus, 255, 259
Extensor indicis, 470
Extensor mechanism, 317
Extensor pollicis longus, 470
Extensor tendon rupture, 321
External bleeding, 68
External ear injury, 529
External hemorrhage, management of, 71
Extrinsic muscles, 465
Extruded disc, 565
Eye wear, 189–190, *190*
Eyes, *504*, 504–505
evaluation of, 535
injuries to
conjunctivitis, 533
corneal abrasion, 533
detached retina, 533–534
displaced contact lens, 534
foreign bodies in, 532
hemorrhage into anterior chamber, 533
orbital fracture, 534
periorbital ecchymosis, *531*, 531–532
subconjunctival hemorrhage, 533

Face. (*See* Head and face)
Face guards, *186*, 187, *187*
Failure, mechanical, 33
Failure to warn, 16
Fasciitis, 43
Femoral artery, 257
Femoral nerve, 304
Femur, 297, 340
Fibrocartilaginous disc, 541
Fibula, 250, 251, 303
Finger sweep, 91, *91*
Finger taping technique, *242*, 242–243, *243*
Finger to nose test, 521, *521*
Fingertip injuries, 480
Flexibility, 153–154
Flexion
of elbow, *434*, 434–435
of knee, 304, *305*
spinal, 546
toe, 259
of toe, 259
in wrist and hand, *467*, 470
Flexor carpi radialis, 471
Flexor carpi ulnaris, 467

Flexor digitorum brevis, 259
Flexor digitorum longus, 255, 259
Flexor digitorum profundus, 431, 467, 470
Flexor digitorum superficialis, 470
Flexor hallucis longus, 255
Fluid hydration, 79
Focal injuries, 182, 508
Food guide pyramid, 58, *58*
Foot, ankle, and lower leg, 249–250
acute strains of, 276–277
Achilles tendon rupture, 277–278, *278*
muscle cramps, 277
tendon strains, 277
ankle strapping
closed basketweave, 223–224, *224*
game strapping, 225, *226*
open basketweave, 221–223, *222*
assessment of, 284
bones of foot, 250, *251*, *252*
bunions (hallux valgus), 270, *271*
bursitis (pump bump, runner's bump), 270–271, *271*
athlete's foot, 272
cloth ankle wrap, 225, *227*
contusions, 272
acute compartment syndrome, 273
foot, 273
lower leg, 273
contusions of, 273
and foot protection, 202–205, *203*, *204*, *206*
fractures, 281–284, *283*
history, 284–285
ligaments in, 250–251, *253*
lower leg protection, 201–202, *202*
major muscle actions of, 257, 259
dorsiflexion and plantar flexion, 260, *261*
inversion and eversion, 261, *261*
pronation and supination, 261–262
toe flexion and extension, 259
Morton's neuroma, 270, *270*
muscles of, 255, *255*, *256*, 257, 258*t*
nerves and blood supply of, 255, 257, 259, *260*
observation and inspection, 285–286
overuse conditions, 278
Achilles tendinitis, 279–280
exercise-induced compartment syndrome, 280–281
medial tibial stress syndrome (MTSS), 280, 281
plantar fasciitis, 278–279
palpations, 286

bony, 287
soft tissue, 287
plantar arches, 252–253, *254*
prevention of injuries, 262–265
rehabilitation, 292–294
special tests
joint range of motion, 288
neurologic assessment, 288, 290, *290*
resisted manual muscle testing, 288
stress and functional, 290–292, *292*
sprains
lateral, 274–275, *275*, 276
medial, 275
toe and foot sprains/ dislocations, 274
toe and foot conditions, 266, *267*, 268
blisters and calluses, 267, 269
claw toes, 267, *267*
hammer, 267, *267*
ingrown toenail, 267, 268
turf, 266–267
Foot contusions, 273
Football helmets, 184–185
proper fitting of padded, 185
Force and its effects, 32–36, *34*, *35*
Forearm protection, 192–193, *195*, *196*
Foreign bodies
in ear, 529
in eye, 532
Foreseeability of harm, 17–18, *18*
Fox, Kathy, 62
Fractures, 49–51, *50*, 70–73
cervical, 557–558, 558*t*
of elbow, 448–449
of foot, ankle, and lower leg, 281–284, *283*
greenstick, 50
lumbar, 565
of shoulder, *407*, 407–409, *408*, *409*
stress, 51
thoracic spinal, 560–561, *561*
of wrist and hand, 483–486
Frontal bones, 502
Frostbite injuries, 83–84
Functional tests, 138
for elbow, 457
for foot, ankle, and lower leg, 291–292
for shoulder, 420–421
for spine, 576
for thigh, hip, and pelvis, 373
for wrist and hand, 493–494

Gallbladder, 589
Game strapping, 225, *226*
Gamekeeper's thumb, 474, *474*
Ganglion cysts, 479
Gas-liquid chromatography (GLC) in drug testing, 651
Gastroenteritis, 640

Gastrointestinal (GI) tract
  constipation, 641
  diarrhea, 640–641
  gastroenteritis, 640
Gemellus inferior, 346
Gemellus superior, 346
Genicular, 304
Gerdy's tubercle, 321
Glasgow Coma Scale, 67, 67t, 518, 518t
Glenohumeral joint, 382, 383, 383–384, 390, 391, 393, 394
  dislocations of, 402–404, 403
  range-of-motion exercises for, 422
  sprain of, 401–402, 402
Glenoid fossa, 383, 384
Glenoid labrum, 383, 383–384
Gluteal muscles, 358
Gluteus maximus, 341, 345
Goniometer, 133
Grant, Marsha, 616
Gravity drawer test for knee, 331, 332
Great toe, 250
  taping of, 218, 219
Greenstick fractures, 50
Grind test for knee, 332, 333
Groin wrap, 234, 236, 237
Guards
  face, 186, 187, 187
  mouth, 188, 188–189, 189

Hallux, 250
Hallux valgus, 270, 271
Hammer toe, 267, 267
Hamstrings, strain of, 356–357
Hamstrings contracture test, 372, 373
Hand. (See Wrist and hand)
Harm, foreseeability of, 17–18, 18
Hay fever, 636–637
Head and face, 501–502
  assessment of cranial injuries, 517–518, 518t
    determination of findings, 510t, 521–524
    history, 519–520
    observation, 520
    palpation, 520
    special tests, 520–521
    vital signs, 518–519
  bones of skull, 502, 502–503
  brain, 503–504
  cerebral hematomas, 510–511, 512, 513t
  concussions, 513–516, 514t
  cranial injury mechanisms, 507, 507–508, 508
  ear injuries, 529–530, 530
  eye injuries, 531–535
    conjunctivitis, 533
    corneal abrasion, 533
    detached retina, 533–534
    displaced contact lens, 534

foreign bodies, 532
hemorrhage into anterior chamber, 533
orbital "blowout" fracture, 534
periorbital ecchymosis, 531, 531–532
subconjunctival hemorrhage, 533
eyes, 504, 504–505
facial injuries
  fractures, 524–525
  soft tissue, 524
nasal injuries, 525–526
  epistaxis, 526
  fractures, 526, 526–527
nerves and blood vessels of, 505t, 505–506, 506
oral and dental injuries
  dental injuries, 528, 529
  lacerations of mouth, 527–528
prevention of injuries, 506
protective equipment for, 184–192, 186, 187, 188, 190, 191
scalp, 503
  injuries to, 516–517
skull fractures, 508–510, 509, 510t
Head tilt/chin lift method, 88–89, 89
Heart, 584
  injuries of, 599
Heat cramps, 79–80
Heat emergencies, preventing, 78–79
Heat exhaustion, 80
Heat stress, emergency care for, 81
Heat stress index, measuring, 78, 78t
Heat stroke, 80–81
Heel bruise, 273
Heel/toe walking, 521
Heimlich maneuver, 90, 90
Helmets, 550
  batting, 186
  bicycle, 186, 186–187
  football, 184–185
    proper fitting of padded, 185
  ice hockey, 186, 186
  lacrosse, 186
Hemarthrosis, 313
Hematomas, 42
  cerebral, 510–511, 512, 513t
  epidural, 511, 512
  subdural, 511, 512, 513t
Hematuria, 604
Hemorrhage, 68
  control of, 68
  external, 68
    management of, 71
  in eye
    into anterior chamber, 533
    subconjunctival, 533
  internal, 70
    management of, 72
Hemothorax, 598–599

Hepatitis, 589
Hepatitis B, 618, 624–625, 627t
Hernias, 601, 601–602
High school settings, opportunities in athletic training in, 27–28
High velocity, 182
Higher-density material, 182–183, 183
Hip. (See Thigh, hip, and pelvis)
Hip abductors, 345–346
Hockey Equipment Certification Council (HECC) of the Canadian Standards Association (CSA), 184
HOPS format, 114, 120
Humeral fractures, 408–409
Humeroradial joint, 430
Humeroulnar joint, 430
Hutsick, Maria, 500
Hydrocollator packs, 172, 173
Hydrocolloids, 70
Hydrocortisone, 178
Hyperesthesia, 135
Hyperextension
  of elbow, 238, 240
  of knee, 230, 232–233, 233
  spinal, 546
  of wrist and hand, 468, 470
Hyperglycemia, 643
Hypermobility, 153
Hypertension, 646–647
Hyperthermia, 74–85
Hypertrophic cardiomyopathy, 599
Hypertrophy, 127
Hyperventilation, 596–597
Hypesthesia, 135
Hyphema, 533
Hypoglycemia, 644
Hypomotility, 153
Hypothenar mass, 482–483
Hypothermia, 81–85, 82
Hypovolemic shock, 362
Hypoxia, 44

Ibuprofen, 178
Ice hockey helmets, 186, 186
Ice immersion, 169
Ice massage, 168
Ice packs, 168
Idiopathic injuries, 547
Iliotibial band friction syndrome, 321, 321–322
Iliotibial tract, 341
  contracture, 333–334
Impingement
  rotator cuff, 404–406, 405
  of ulnar nerve, 448
Impingement syndrome in shoulder, 405
Implied warranty, 18
Incisions, 42
Indication, 165
Industrial health care programs, opportunities in athletic training in, 29

Infarcts, 649
Infectious mononucleosis, 603, 637
Inflammation, controlling, 148–151
Influenza, 636
Informed consent, 17
Infrapatellar bursa, 310
Infraspinatus, 384, 391, 393
Ingrown toenail, 267, 268
Injured participant
    moving, 107, *108,* 109, *109*
    and psychology, 146–147
Injuries
    diffuse, 182
    focal, 182
    mechanisms, 32
        force and its effects, 32–36,
            34, 35
        torque and its effects, *36,*
            36–38, *37*
        rehabilitation of, and progress
            charts, 24, *25t*
Innominate bones, 341
Inspection, 125
    of injury site, 129, *129*
Insulin shock, 644
Intermittent compression, 167
Intermittent compression units,
    176, 177
Internal bleeding, management of,
    72
Internal ear injuries, 530
Internal heat regulation, 75, 77–78
Internal hemorrhage, 70
Interossei, 259
Interphalangeal collateral ligament
    sprains, 474–475, *475*
Interphalangeal (IP) joint, 465
    motion of, 472
Interstitial tissues, 44, *45*
Intertrigo, 623
Intra-abdominal injuries, 602, *603t*
Intracranial pressure, 519
Intrauterine devices (IUDs), 629
Intrinsic muscles, 465
Iontophoresis, 176
Ipsilateral straight-leg raising test,
    564, *576*
Iris, 505
Iron-deficiency anemia, 648
Irritability of muscle, 41
Ischiofemoral ligament, 341–342
Isokinetic training, 159
Isometric exercises in rehabilitation
    of shoulder, 421
Isometric training, 157, 159
Isotonic training, 159

Jaw thrust method, *89,* 90
Jersey finger (profundus tendon
    rupture), 477
Joint movement terms, *118–119,*
    119
Joint range of motion, 132–133,
    153, *154*
    for assessing elbow, 454

for foot, ankle, and lower leg,
    288
for knee, 328
for shoulder, 413–414
for spine, 572
for thigh, hip, and pelvis, 368
for wrist and hand, 491
Jones fracture, 283
Jugular vein, 592
Jumper's knee, 319–320

Kehr's sign, 603
Kendall test for rectus femoris
    contracture, 371–372,
    372
Kidney, 590
    and bladder injuries, 604
Kinematics, 259
Knee, 297–298
    assessment of, 325
    contusions and bursitis, 306,
        310, *310*
    fractures of, 322–325, *324*
    history, 325
    hyperextension of, 230, 232–233,
        233
    iliotibial band friction syndrome,
        321, 321–322
    joint capsule and bursae, 300
    ligaments of, 300–301
        injuries to, 311
            management of, 314–315
            unidirectional, 311–313,
                312, 313, 314t
    major muscle actions of
        flexion and extension, 304, *305*
        patellofemoral joint motion,
            305–306
        rotation and passive abduction
            and adduction, 304
    meniscal injuries, 316, *316*
    menisci, 300
    muscles crossing, 301, *302t*
    nerves and blood supply of, 301,
        303, 303–304
    observation and inspection,
        325–326
    palpations, 327
        bony, 327
        soft tissue, 327
        for swelling, 327, *328*
    patella and related injuries
        acute patellar subluxation and
            dislocation, 319
        chondromalacia patellae, *318,*
            318–319
        extensor tendon rupture, 321
        Osgood-Schlatter disease, 320
        patellar tendinitis, 319–320
        patellofemoral stress
            syndrome, 317–318
    and patella protection, 198–201,
        200, 201
    patellofemoral joint, 301, *302*
    prevention of injuries, 306,
        307–309

rehabilitation, 334–337, *335, 336*
    special tests, 328,
        joint range of motion, 328
        neurologic assessment, 330
        resisted manual muscle
            testing, 328, *329–330*
        stress and functional,
            330–334, *331, 332, 333,*
            334
    taping and wrapping techniques
        for, 230–233, *231, 232,*
        233
    tibiofemoral joint, 298, *298–299*
Kyphosis, 547

Lacrimal ducts, 504
Lacrimal glands, 504
Lacrosse helmets, 186
°Larsen-Johansson disease, 320
°Larsen-Johansson syndrome, 52
Lasègue's test, 373, *374*
Lateral ankle sprains, 262
Lateral epicondylitis, 445–446, *447*
    tennis elbow test for, 455–456
Latissimus dorsi, 391, 393
Leg length measurement, 371, *371*
Legal liability, 15–16
    confidentiality, 18–19
    failure to warn, 16
    foreseeability of harm, 17–18, *18*
    informed consent, 17
    negligence, 16, *17t*
    preventing litigation, 19, *20t*
    product, 18
Legg-Calvé-Perthes' disease, 52,
    359, 359–360
Levator scapula, 384
Lifting techniques, proper,
    550–551
Ligamentous instability tests
    for assessing elbow, 455, *456*
    for wrist and hand, 493
Ligaments, 40. (*See also specific*)
    of elbow, 430
    of foot, ankle, and lower leg,
        250–251, *253*
    of knee, 300–301
    spinal, *541,* 542
Little league elbow, 52, 429, 445
Little league shoulder, 408, *408*
Liver, 589
    contusion and rupture, 603–604
Local anesthetics, 178
Longitudinal bone growth, 46
Lordosis, 547–548
Low back pain, 562
Low velocity, 182
Low-density material, 182, *183*
Lower body, protective equipment
    for, 198–205, *199, 200,*
    201, 202, 203, 204, 206
Lower leg. (*See* Foot, ankle, and
    lower leg)
Lumbar disc injuries, 565, *576*
Lumbar plexus, 342
Lumbar spine

injuries to, 561–566
protection for, 195, *196*
Lumbricals, 259
Lunate, 464
Lungs, 584

Maceration, 223
Malaise, 440, 634
Mallet finger, 477, *478*
Malocclusion, 524
Mandibular fractures, 524
Massage, 167, 177
  ice, 168
McBurney's point, 604, 609
Mechanosensitive nociceptors,
  55–56
Medial epicondylitis, 52, 444–445,
  445
Medial epicondylitis test, 457
Medial tibial stress syndrome
  (MTSS), 280, 281
Median nerve, 431
Medical data information cards, 21,
  26
Medical records and record
  keeping, 19
Medications, 167
Meningeal artery, 505
Meninges, 503
Meningitis, septic, 509
Meniscal injuries, 316, *316*
Meniscal test for knee, 332
Menisci, 300
Menses, 619
Menstrual cycle, 619
  irregularities in, 627–629
Metacarpal fractures, 485–486, *486*
Metacarpophalangeal (MP) joint,
  465
  motion of, 471, *471*
Metatarsalgia, 270
Metatarsals, 250
Metatarsophalangeal (MTP) joint,
  250
Midfoot sprains, 274
Modalities, 141
Morton's neuroma, 270, *270*
Motion, restoration of, 151–158
Motion segment, 541, *541*
Motor function, 127–129
Motor testing, 135
Mouth guards, *188*, 188–189
  fitting mouth-formed, 189
Muscle, 40–41, *41*
Muscle contusions, 42
Muscle spindles, 138
Muscular endurance, 160
Muscular movement in secondary
  injury assessment, 105
Muscular power, 160–161
Muscular strength, 157, *158*, 159*t*
Musculocutaneous nerve, 388, 431
Myopia, 534
Myositis, 43
Myositis ossificans, 43, 351, 353, *353*
Myotome, 135

Nasal fractures, *526*, 526–527
Nasal injuries, 525–526
National Athletic Trainers'
  Association (NATA), 6–7,
  14
Board of Certification
  (NATABOC), 14
certification
  for athletic trainer, 8–9,
    13–14
  continuing education
    requirements, 14
  registration and licensure,
    14–15
legal liability, 15–16
  confidentiality, 18–19
  failure to warn, 16
  foreseeability of harm,
    17–18, *18*
  informed consent, 17
  negligence, 16, 17*t*
  preventing litigation, 19, 20*t*
  product, 18
medical records and record
  keeping, 19
  accident reports, 21, 23
  data information cards, 21
  injury management,
    rehabilitation, and
    progress charts, 24, 25*t*
  preparticipation exams,
    20–21, 22
certified athletic trainer, 13
National Collegiate Athletic
  Association (NCAA),
  650–652
National Operating Committee on
  Standards for Athletic
  Equipment (NOCSAE),
  184
Neck protectors, 190–191, *191*
Necrosis, 44
Negligence, 16, 17*t*
Nerve entrapment syndromes, 480
Nerve root, 135
Nerves. (*See also specific*)
  afferent, 54
  anatomical properties of, 54
  efferent, 54
  of elbow, 431–432, 432*t*, *433*
  in foot, ankle, and lower leg,
    255, 257, *259, 260*
  in head and face, 505*t*, 505–506,
    506
  healing, 55
  injuries, 53–55
    classifications, 54–55
  in knee, 301, *303*, 303–304
  sensory, 54
  for shoulder, 387*t*, 388, *388, 389*
  for thigh, hip, and pelvis, 342,
    342, 344
  for wrist and hand, 465, 467,
    469
Neuritis, 270
Neurologic assessment, 135–136

for elbow, 454
for foot, ankle, and lower leg,
  288, 290, *290*
for knee, 330
for shoulder, 415, *417*
for spine, 573
for thigh, hip, and pelvis,
  369–370
for wrist and hand, 491–492
Neurological basis of pain, 55–56
Neuroma, 55
Neuromuscular electrical
  stimulation, 167, 175, *176*
Nonelastic tape, 211
Nonelastic wrap, 213
Nonsteroidal anti-inflammatory
  drugs (NSAIDS), 178
  for bicipital tendon injuries, 406
  for contusions, 437, 440
  for glenohumeral joint sprain,
    402
  for impingement syndrome, 405
  for sprains and dislocations, 441
Nonunion fracture, 283
Nucleus pulposus, 541
Nutrition, 57–58
Nystagmus, 515

Ober's test for iliotibial tract
  contracture, for knee,
    333–334
Observation, 125, 127–129
  in secondary injury assessment,
    99
Obstructed airway, 65–66
Obturator externus, 346
Obturator internus, 346
Occipital bones, 502
Off-the-field assessment, 120–121
Olecranon bursa, 440
Olecranon bursitis, *440*, 440–441
Olecranon process, 435
Oligomenorrhea, 282
100 minus 7 test, 521
O'Neil, Ron, 248
On-the-field assessment, 120–121·
Open basketweave ankle strapping,
  221–223, *222*
Open-chain exercises, 161–162,
  162
Oral contraceptives (OCs), 629
Oral injuries, 527–528
Orbital fracture, 534
Osgood-Schlatter disease, 52, 320
Osteitis pubis, 362
Osteoblasts, 47
Osteochondral fracture, 323
Osteochondritis dissecans, 323, *324*
Osteochondrosis, 52
Osteoclasts, 47
Osteopenia, 51, 560, 628
Osteoporosis, 628, 655
Ovarian cycle, 619
Overload principle, 157
Overuse injuries
  for elbow, 436, 444–448

Overuse injuries continued
  for foot, ankle and lower leg,
    278–281
  for shoulder, 404–406, *405*

Pain, 55
  factors that mediate, 56
  neurological basis of, 55–56
  radiating, 56–57
  referred, 56–57, 123
  somatic, 123
  visceral, 123
Painful arc, 135
Pallor, 100
Palpations, 129–132
  of elbow, 451
    bony, 451, 453
    soft tissue, 453
  of foot, ankle, and lower leg
    bony, 287
    soft tissue, 287
  of knee, 327
    bony, 327
    soft tissue, 327
    for swelling, 327, *328*
  in secondary injury assessment,
    102
  of shoulder, 411–412
    bony, 413
    soft tissue, 413
  spinal, 570–571
  of thigh, hip, and pelvis, 366
    bony, 367
    soft tissue, 367
  of wrist and hand, 488–489
    bony, 489
    soft tissue, 489
Pancreas, 590
Paraffin baths, 172–174, *174*
Paresthesia, 135
Parietal bones, 502
Paronychia, 267, 480
Pars interarticularis fractures,
    548–549
Partial airway obstruction, 65–66
Passive range of motion (PROM),
    133
Patella apprehension test for knee,
    332, *333*
Patella compression test for knee,
    332, *333*
Patellar subluxation and
    dislocation, acute, 319
Patellar tendinitis, 319–320
Patellofemoral joint, 301, *302*
  motion of, 305–306
Patellofemoral joint motion,
    305–306
Patellofemoral stress syndrome,
    317–318
Pectoral nerve, 388
Pectoralis major muscle, strain of,
    594
Pectoralis minor, 384
Pelvic girdle, 341
  muscles of, 590, 591*t*

Pelvic inflammatory disease (PID),
    628
Penis injuries, 621
Performance-enhancing drugs, 650,
    652*t*
Pericranium, 503
Periorbital ecchymosis, *531,*
    531–532
Periosteum, 47
Peristalsis, 589
Peritonitis, 602
Peroneal nerve, 303
Peroneus brevis, 261
Peroneus longus, 261
Peroneus tertius, 255
Pes anserinus bursa, 310
Pes planus, 262
Petroleum jelly, 213
Phalanges, 250
  fractures of, 486
Phalen's (wrist flexion) test of wrist
    and hand, 493
Pharyngitis, 635–636
Phonophoresis, 175
Photophobia, 514–515
Physical therapist, 11–12
Pia mater, 504
Pinkeye, 533
Piriformis, 346
Plantar arches, 252–253, *254*
Plantar fascia, 253, *254*
Plantar fasciitis, 262, 278–279
Plantar flexion and dorsiflexion,
    260, *261*
Pleura, 584
Plyometric exercises in shoulder
    rehabilitation, 425
Plyometric jumping, 336
Plyometric training, 161
Pneumothorax, 597, *598*
Popliteal artery, 257, 304
Popliteal fossa, 303
Postconcussion syndrome, 515
Posterior cruciate ligament (PCL),
    312–313
Posterior deltoid, 391
Posterior drawer test for knee, 331,
    332
Posterior superior iliac spine
    (PSIS), 341
Posttraumatic memory loss, 515
Power, muscular, 160–161
Prednisone, 178
Pregnancy and sport participation,
    629–630
Preparticipation exams, 20–21, *22*
Prepatellar bursa, 310, *310*
Primary care physician, 8
Primary injury assessment, 87–96
Primary sex organs, 618
Primary survey, 64, *95*
  flow chart for, 96
Product liability, 18
Professional practice, standards of,
    12–15
Professional sport teams,

opportunities in athletic
    training in, 29
Profundus tendon rupture, 477
Progesterones, 620
Prognosis, 141
Prolapsed disc, 565
Pronation, 262
  of forearm, 435–436
Pronator quadratus, 435
Pronator teres, 435, *435*
Prophylactic, 209
Prophylactic devices, 182
Prophylactic knee braces (PKBs),
    198
Proprioception, 335
Proprioceptive feedback, 210–211
Proprioceptive neuromuscular
    facilitation (PNF), 154
  exercises in shoulder
    rehabilitation, 425
  stretching techniques, 394
Proprioceptors, 138
Protective cups, 620
Protective equipment, 181
  for head and face, 184–192, *186,*
    187, 188, 190, 191
  for lower body, 198–205, *199,*
    200, 201, 202, 203, 204,
    206
  principles of, 182*t*, 182–183, *183*
  for upper body, 192–195, *194,*
    195, 196, 197
Proteins, 57
Proximal interphalangeal (PIP)
    joint, 250, 465
Proximal radioulnar joint, 430
Psychology and injured participant,
    146–147
Pulmonary circuit, 584, *586*
Pulmonary contusion, 597
Pulmonary embolism, 360
Pulse in secondary injury
    assessment, 102
Pump bump, 271
Pupillary light reflex, 101
Pupils, 505
  abnormalities of, 519
  in secondary injury assessment,
    101

Q-angle, 301, *302*
Quadratus femoris, 346
Quadratus plantae, 259
Quadriceps
  contusion of, 351, 352, *352*
  and hamstrings wrap, 233–234,
    234, 235
  strain of, 356

Raccoon eyes, 509
Radial arteries, 432
Radial collateral ligament, 465
Radial nerve, 431
Radiating pain, 56–57
Radius, 464
  stress fractures to, 448

Range-of-motion exercises
  for elbow, 458, *458*
  for glenohumeral joint, 422
  in rehabilitation of hand and
      wrist, 495
Raynaud's phenomenon, 167
Recreational drugs, 650, 652*t*
Rectus femoris contracture,
      Kendall test for,
      371–372, *372*
Referred pain, 56–57, 123, 609,
      610*t*
Reflex actions, 544–545
Reflex testing, 135–136, 136*t*, *137*
Regional terms, *118*, 119
Registration and licensure, 14–15
Rehabilitation
  of elbow, *458*, 458–459
  focus of, 210
  of knee, 334–337, *335*, *336*
  of shoulder injury, 421–426
  of spinal injury, 577–578
  of thigh, hip, and pelvis,
      374–375
  of wrist and hand, 494–495
Rehabilitative braces, *200*, 200–201
Reproductive system, 617–618
  anatomy of genitalia, *618*,
      618–619, *619*
  female, *618*, 619–620
  male, 620
  birth control and sport
      participation, 629
  bloodborne viral disease,
      624–625
  injuries and conditions of, 620
  dermatologic, 623
  female genital injuries, 622
  male genital injuries, *621*,
      621–622
  menstrual irregularities, 627–629
  pregnancy and sport
      participation, 629–630
Resilience, 183
Resisted manual muscle testing,
      133–135
  for elbow, 454
  for foot, ankle, and lower leg,
      288
  for knee, 328, *329–330*
  for shoulder, 414–415, *415*, *416*
  for spine, 572–573, *573*, *574*
  for thigh, hip, and pelvis, 368,
      368
  for wrist and hand, 491, *492*
Resisted movement, 133
Respiration in secondary injury
      assessment, 99
Respiratory tract conditions, 634
  acute bronchitis, 637
  allergic rhinitis, 636–637
  bronchial asthma, 637–638
  common cold, 634
  exercise-induced asthma,
      638–639
  infectious mononucleosis, 637

influenza, 636
pharyngitis, 635–636
sinusitis, 634–635, *635*
Resting position, 450–451
Restoration of motion, 151–158
Restricted activity, 150
Retina, 505
  detached, 533–534
Retinacula of wrist, 467–468
Retrograde amnesia, 515
Retroviruses, 626
Rhinorrhea, 634
Rhomboids, 384, 386, 390
Rib fractures, 595–596, *608*
Romberg test, 521, *522*
Rotary knee instability taping, 230,
      232
Rotator cuff muscles, 384
Rotator cuff/impingement injuries,
      404–406, *405*
Rounded back, 547
Rubor, 100
Runner's bump, 271
Runner's nipples, 594
Russell's sign, 655

Sacral plexus, 342
Sacral protection, 195, *196*
Sacrum and coccyx injuries,
      566
Saddle joint, 465
Scalp, 503
  injuries of, 516–517
Scan exam, 569
Scaphoid, 464
  fractures of, *484*, 484–485
Scapular fractures, 407
Scapular muscles, 384–385
Scapulohumeral rhythm, 391, *392*
Scapulothoracic joint, 382, 384,
      384, *385*, *386*, *386*
Scar formation, healing through, 45
Sciatic nerve, 257, 303, 358
Sciatica, 564–565
Sclera, 505
Scoliosis, 547
Screwing-home mechanism, 298
Scrotal injuries, 621–622, *622*
Second impact syndrome, 516
Secondary injury assessment,
      96–97, 98*t*
  determination of findings,
      106–107
  history of, 97
  observation, 99
    pupils, 101, *101*
    respiration, 99
    skin color, 100–101
  palpation, 102
    bony, 102, *103*, 104
    cutaneous sensation, 105
    pulse, 102
    temperature, 102, *103*
  special tests
    blood pressure, 105–106
    muscular movement, 105

Secondary survey, 64
Semimembranosus, 345
Semitendinosus, 345
Sensory nerves, 54
Sensory testing, 135
Septic meningitis, 509
Serratus anterior, 384
  weakness of, 416, *417*
Sever's disease, 52, 282
Shear force, 34, *34*
Shin bruise, 273
Shin guards, 201, 202, *202*
Shin splints taping, 227–228, *229*,
      230
Shock, 73–74
  hypovolemic, 362
  management of, 76
Shoulder, 381–382
  acromioclavicular joint, 382, *383*
  assessment of, 410
  bursae, 385, 386–387
  coracoclavicular joint, 382, *383*
  fractures, *407*, 407–409, *408*,
      409
  glenohumeral joint, *383*,
      383–384
  history, 410, *411*
  major muscle actions of, 389,
      390
    coordination of movements,
      391–392, *392*
    glenohumeral abduction, 384,
      393
    glenohumeral adduction, 385,
      393
    glenohumeral extension, 384,
      385, 393
    glenohumeral flexion, 385,
      386, 392–393
    lateral and medial rotation of
      humerus, *384*, 393
    throwing, 389–391, *391*, 392*t*
  muscles of, 386, 387*t*
  nerves and blood vessels of,
      387*t*, 388, *388*, *389*
  observation and inspection,
      410–411, *412*
  overuse injuries
    bicipital tendon, 406
    bursitis, 406
    rotator cuff/impingement,
      404–406
  palpations, 411–412
    bony, 413
    soft tissue, 413
  prevention of injuries, 394–397
    flexibility exercises for
      shoulder region, 395
    strengthening exercises for
      complex, 396–397
  rehabilitation, 421–426
  scapulothoracic joint, 384, *384*,
      385, 386, *386*
  special tests
    joint range of motion,
      413–414

Shoulder continued
neurologic assessment, 415, 417
resisted manual muscle testing, 414–415, *415, 416*
stress and functional tests, 415–416, 417
sprains to, 398, *399*
acromioclavicular joint, 398, 400, 401, *401*
glenohumeral dislocations, 402–404, *403*
glenohumeral joint, 401–402, *402*
recurrent subluxations and dislocations, 404
sternoclavicular joint, 398, 400
sternoclavicular joint, 382, *382*
taping and wrapping techniques for, 236, *237, 238, 239*
Shoulder pads, 192, *194*
fitting football, 193
Shoulder pointer, 398
Shoulder protection, 192, *194*
Shoulder spica wrap, 236, 238, 239
Sickle cell anemia, 648–649
Sign, 64
Sinusitis, 634–635, *635*
Skin, 39, *39*
bruises of, 42
classification of injuries, 41–42
color in secondary injury assessment, 100–101
Skull
bones of, *502,* 502–503
fractures of, 508–510, *509, 510t*
Small intestine, 587, 589
Smith fracture, 483, *484*
Snapping hip syndrome, 354–355
Snowball crepitation, 277
SOAP notes
assessment, 141
objective evaluation, 140–141
plan, 141
subjective evaluation, 140
Soft tissue
anatomical properties of, *38, 38–41, 39, 40, 41*
healing, 44–46, *45*
injuries, 38–46
palpation of
for elbow, 453
for foot, ankle, and lower leg, 287
for knee, 327
for shoulder, 413
for thigh, hip, and pelvis, 367
for wrist and hand, 489
Solar plexus contusion, 601
Somatic pain, 123
Sore throat, 635–636
Spasms, 43
Special tests in secondary injury assessment, 105

Speed's test for bicipital tendinitis, 420, *420*
Sphenoid bones, 502
Spica, 210
Spinal loading, 550–551
Spine, 539–540, *540*
anatomical variations predisposing individuals to injuries, 547
curvatures, 547–548
pars interarticularis fractures, 548–549
assessment of, 566–567
brachial plexus injuries, 558–559, *559*
cervical injuries, 555–558, *556, 557*
history, 567–568
ligaments of, *541,* 542
lumbar injuries, 561–566
major muscle actions of, 545, *546*
flexion, extension, and hyperextension, 546
lateral flexion and rotation, 546
muscles of, 542, 543–544t, *544*
observation and inspection, 568
gross neuromuscular assessment, 570
of injury site, 569
posture, 568–569, *569*
scan exam, 569
palpations, 570–571
prevention of injuries, 549–555
rehabilitation, 577–578
sacrum and coccyx injuries, 566
special tests
joint range of motion, 572
neurologic assessment, 573
resisted manual muscle, 572–573, *573, 574*
stress and functional, 573–576
spinal cord and spinal nerves, 542, 544–545, *545*
thoracic injuries, 560–561
vertebrae and intervertebral discs, *547,* 547–548, *548, 549*
Spleen, 589–590
rupture of, 603
Splints, 72–73
Spondylolisthesis, 548, *549,* 569
Spondylolysis, 548, *548*
Sport bras, 194, *197*
Sport participation, 11
disqualifying conditions for, *25t*
Sport supervisor, 9, 11
Sports injury assessment, 113–114, *114*
anatomical foundations, 114–115
body segments and position, 115, *115, 116*

directional terms, 116, *116t, 117t*
joint movement terms, *118–119,* 119
regional terms, *118,* 119
functional testing, 138
history of, 121–122, *122*
characteristics of symptoms, 123–124
disability resulting from, 124–125
mechanism of, 123
primary complaint, 123
related medical history, 125
injury recognition, 138–140
joint range of motion, 132–133
neurologic testing, 135–136
observation and inspection, 125–129
on-the-field vs. off-the-field, 120–121
palpation, 129–132
resisted manual muscle testing, 133–135
SOAP notes, 140
assessment, 141
objective evaluation, 140–141
plan, 141
subjective evaluation, 140
stress tests, 136–137
Sports medicine, definition of, 6–7
Sports medicine clinics, opportunities in athletic training in, 28, *28*
Sports medicine specialists, 5
Sports medicine team, responsibilities of primary, *7t,* 7–8
athletic trainer, 8–9, *9, 10t*
coach, 9, 11
participants, 11
physical therapist, 11–12
physician, 8
primary care physician, 8
student athletic trainer, 11, *12*
supervisor, 9, 11
Sport-specific skill conditioning, 164
Sprains, 42–43
cervical, 556–557
and dislocations of thigh, hip, and pelvis, 355, 355–356
of elbows, 441–442
foot and ankle, 274–276, *275*
lumbar, 563–564
to shoulder complex, 398
thoracic, 560
of wrist and hand, 473–477
Standard of care, 15
Static position, 133
Static stretch, 40, 153
Stenosing, 479
Sternal fractures, 595–596, *608*
Sternoclavicular joint, 382, *382*
sprains of, 398, 400
Sternocostal pectoralis, 393

Steroids, 618
Sticking point, 159
Stitch in side, 593
Stomach, 587, 589
Stork stand, 521
Straight-leg raising test, 373, *374*
  for spine, 574, 576, *576*
Strains, 35, 42–43
  cervical, 556–557
  of elbow, 443–444
  of hand and wrist, 477–479
  lumbar, 563–564
  of pectoralis major muscle, 594
  of thigh, hip, and pelvis,
    356–357, *357t*
  thoracic, 560
Strength, 157
  muscular, 157, *158*, 159, *159t*
Strengthening exercises, 397
  for cervical region, 550
Stress, 34–35, *35*
  valgus, 457
Stress and functional tests,
    135–136, 138
  for elbow, 454–457
  for foot, ankle, and lower leg,
    290–292, *292*
  for knee, 330–334, *331, 332,
    333, 334*
  for shoulder, 415–416, 417
  for spine, 573–576
  for thigh, hip, and pelvis,
    370–373
  for wrist, 492–494
Stress fractures, 51
Student athletic trainer, 11, *12*
Subacromial bursa, 386–387, *388*
Subclavian artery, *388*
Subclavius, 384
Subconjunctival hemorrhage, 533
Subcutaneous emphysema, 597
Subdural hematoma, 511, *512,
    513t*
Subscapular nerve, *388*
Subscapularis, 384, *393*
Substance abuse, 649
  performance-enhancing drugs,
    650, *652t*
  recreational drugs, 650, *652t*
  signs of, 650, *653t*
  therapeutic drugs, 649–650, *651t*
Subtalar joint, 251
Subungual hematoma, 480, *481*
Sudden death in athletes, 599–600
Supination, 262, 435–436
Supinator, *435*, 435–436
Supracondylar fractures, 448–449
Suprascapular nerve, *388*
Supraspinatus, 384, *391*
Supraspinatus tendon, *388*
Supraspinatus testing, *419*,
    419–420
Sustentaculum tali, 251
Sutures, 502
Swimmer's back, 547
Swimmer's ear, 530

Symptom, 64
Systemic body cooling, 84–85
Systemic circuit, 584, *586*
Systole, 585
Systolic blood pressure, 105

Talar tilt, 291
Talocrural joint, 250
Talofibular ligament, 251
Taping and wrapping
  common techniques, 217
    for lower extremity, 218, *219,
      220*, 220–228, *221, 222,
      224, 226, 227, 228, 229,
      230, 231*, 232–234, *234,
      235, 236, 237*
  principles of, 209–217, *210*
    application of tape, 213–316,
      214, 215, 216
    application of wraps, 216–217
    types of tape and wraps, 211,
      213, *213*
    uses of, 211, *212*
  for upper extremity, 236, *237,
    238*, 238–240, *239, 240,
    241, 242*, 242–243, *243*
T-bar exercises in rehabilitation of
    shoulder, 421
Team physician, 8
Temperature in secondary injury
    assessment, 102, *103*
Tendinitis, 43
  calcific, 43
  and stenosing tenosynovitis,
    478–479, *479*
Tendons, 39–40
Tennis elbow, 429
Tennis elbow test for lateral
    epicondylitis, 455–456
Tenosynovitis, 43, 276
Tensile force, 34, *34*
Tension, 34, *34*
Tension pneumothorax, 598
Teres major, 384, *391, 393*
Teres minor, 384, *391, 393*
Testosterone, 620
Therapeutic drugs, 178–179,
    649–650, *651t*
Therapeutic exercise
  developing program, 147–148,
    148, 149t
  phase one, controlling
    inflammation, 148–151
  phase two, restoration of motion,
    151–158
  phase three, developing
    muscular strength,
    endurance, and power,
    156–157, *158, 159t*,
    159–162, *160, 162*
  phase four, return to sport
    activity, 163–165
  ultimate goal of, 146
Therapeutic modalities and
    medications, 165
  cryotherapy, *167*, 167–169, *168t*,

    170, 171, *172, 172t, 173,
    174, 175*
Thermomoldable plastics, 183
Thermotherapy, 167, 171–175,
    172, 172t, 173, 174, 175
Thigh, hip, and pelvis, 339–340,
    341
  assessment of, 364
  bony structure of, *340*, 340–341
  bursitis, *354*, 354–355
  and buttock protection, 198,
    199
  contusions
    hip pointers, 353
    myositis ossificans, 351, 353,
      353
    quadriceps, 351, 352, *352*
  hip fractures, 360, *360, 361*, 362,
    363t
  hip joint, 340, *341*, 341–342,
    343t
    sprains of, 355–356
  hip pointers, 353
  history, 364
  major muscle actions of, 344,
    346
    abduction, 345–346
    adduction, 346, *346*
    extension, 345, *346*
    flexion, 344, *346*
    medial and lateral rotation of
      femur, 346, 351
  nerves and blood vessels of, 342,
    342, 344
  observation and inspection,
    364–365
  palpations, 366
    bony, 367
    soft tissue, 367
  rehabilitation, 374–375
  special tests, 367
    joint range of motion, 368
    neurologic assessment,
      369–370
    resisted manual muscle
      testing, 368, *368*
    stress and functional tests,
      370–373
  sprains and dislocations, *355*,
    355–356
  strains, 356–358, *357t*
  Thomas test for hip flexion
    contractures, 371, *372*
  vascular disorders of, 359–360
Thigh protection, 198, *199*
Thin-layer chromatography (TLC)
    in drug testing, 651
Thomas test for hip flexion
    contractures, 371, *372*
Thompson's test for Achilles
    tendon rupture, 290–291,
    291
Thoracic spine injuries, 560–561
Thoracodorsal artery, *388*
Thorax. (*See* Throat, thorax, and
    visceral injuries)

Throat, thorax, and visceral
        injuries, 581–582
    abdominal wall
        hernias, *601,* 601–602
        muscle strains, 600
        skin wound and contusions,
            600
        solar plexus contusion, 601
    anatomy of, 582–583, 583–585,
            584, 585, 586, 587*t, 590,*
            591
        of thorax, 583–585, *584, 585,*
            586, 587*t*
        of throat, 582–583, *590, 591*
        of visceral region, 585, 587,
            589, 589–590
    assessment of, 605
    history, 605–606
    internal complications, 596–597
        heart injuries, 599
        hemothorax, 598–599
        hyperventilation, 596–597
        pneumothorax, 597, *598*
        pulmonary contusion, 597
        sudden death in athletes,
            599–600
        tension pneumothorax, 598
        traumatic asphyxia, 598
    intra-abdominal, 602, 603*t*
        appendicitis, *589,* 604
        kidney and bladder, 604
        liver contusion and rupture,
            603–604
        splenic rupture, 603
    observation and inspection, 607
    palpations, 607–609
    prevention of injuries, 591–592
    rib and abdominal protection,
        193, *196*
    special tests, 609–611
        thoracic injuries, 593
        breast, 594
        costochondral, 594–595,
            595
        sternal and rib fractures,
            595–596, *608*
        stitch in side, 593
        throat injuries, 592–593
Throat protectors, 190–191, *191*
Thrombophlebitis, 360
Throwing, 389–391, *391,* 392*t*
Thumb, wrapping of, 239–240, *242*
Tibia, 250, 251, 297
Tibial tuberosity, 323
Tibialis anterior, 255, 261
Tibialis posterior, 255, 261
Tibiofemoral joint, 298, *298–299*
Tibiofibular articulations, 251
Tibiofibular ligament, 251
Tinea cruris, 623
Tinea pedis, 272
Tinel's sign for ulnar neuritis, 457,
        457
Tinnitus, 513
Tissues, interstitial, 44, *45*
Toenail, ingrown, 267

Toes
    claw, 267, *267*
    flexion and extension, 259
    hammer, 267, *267*
    taping and wrapping technique
        for, 218, *219*
    turf, 266–267
Tonic state, 646
Torque and its effects, *36,* 36–38,
        37
Torsion, 37
Torso injuries, 581–582
Tort, 15
Total airway obstruction, 66
Transcutaneous electrical nerve
        stimulation (TENS),
        176–177
Trapezius, 384
Traumatic asphyxia, 598
Triage, 87
Triceps, 435
Triceps brachii, 384
Triquetrum, 464
Trochanteric bursa, 341, 354
Turf toe, 266–267

Ulna, stress fractures to, 448
Ulnar entrapment, 480
Ulnar nerve, 431
    impingement of, 448
Ulnar neuritis, Tinel's sign for,
        457, *457*
Ulnar neuropathy, 482–483
Ultrasound, 174–175, *175*
Unconscious athlete, 66–67
Unconsciousness, 67
Upper body, protective equipment
        for, 192–195, *194, 195,*
        196, 197

Valgus laxity, 311
Valgus stress, 457
Valgus stress test for knee, 330,
        331, *331*
Vapocoolant sprays, 171
Varus laxity, 311
Vascular disorders of thigh, hip,
        and pelvis, 359–360
Vastus medialis oblique (VMO),
        305
Venous bleeding, 68
Ventricles, 585
Vermiform appendix, 589
Vertebrae and intervertebral disc,
        547, *547–548, 548, 549*
Vertebral arteries, 505
Visceral injuries. (*See* Throat,
        thorax, and visceral
        injuries)
Visceral pain, 123
Visceral region, anatomy of, 585,
        587, *589,* 589–590
Viscoelastic fashion, 40
Vital signs, 518–519

Vitamins, 57–58
Volar radiocarpal ligament, 465
Volkmann's contracture, 449

Warranty
    expressed, 18
    implied, 18
Wedge fracture, 560, *561*
Whirlpools, 171, *172*
Wounds
    cleansing, 68–69
    dressing, 70
    universal safety precautions in
        treating, 69
Wrap. (*See* Taping and wrapping)
Wrist and hand, 463–464, *464*
    abrasions, 473
    assessment of, 486–487
    bones and articulations of,
        464–465, *465*
    contusions, 473
    fingertip injuries, 480
    fractures
        carpal, 483–485, *484*
        distal radial and ulnar, 483,
            484
        metacarpal, 485–486, *486*
        phalangeal, 486
    history in assessing, 487–488
    major muscle actions of, 470,
        470
        carpometacarpal joint motion,
            471
        extension and hyperextension,
            468, 470
        flexion, *467,* 470
        interphalangeal joint motion,
            472
        metacarpophalangeal joint
            motion, 471, *471*
        radial and ulnar deviation,
            467, 468, 471
    muscles of, 465, 466*t, 467, 468*
    nerve entrapment syndromes,
        480
        carpal tunnel, 481–482, *482*
        ulnar neuropathy, 482–483
    nerves and blood vessels of, 465,
        467, *469*
    observation and inspection, 488
    palpations, 488–489
        bony, 489
        soft tissue, 489
    prevention of injuries, 472
    protection for, 192–193, *195,*
        196
    rehabilitation, 494–495
    retinacula of, *467–468*
    special tests
        joint range of motion, 491
        neurologic, 491–492
        resisted manual muscle, 491,
            492
        stress and functional, 492–494
    sprains, 473–477

dislocations, *475*, 475–477, *476*
Gamekeeper's thumb, 474, *474*
interphalangeal collateral ligament, 474–475, *475*
wrist, 473–474
strains
boutonniere deformity, 478, *478*

ganglion cysts, 479
jersey finger (profundus tendon rupture), 477
mallet finger, 477, *478*
tendinitis and stenosing tenosynovitis, 478–479, *479*
wrapping techniques for, 238–239, *241*

Wrist flexion test of wrist and hand, 493

Zones
of primary injury, 44
of secondary injury, 44
Zygomatic arch, 524